CEREBROVASCULAR INSUFFICIENCY

GRUNE & STRATTON
RAPID MANUSCRIPT REPRODUCTION

CEREBROVASCULAR INSUFFICIENCY

Edited by

John J. Bergan, M.D.

Magerstadt Professor of Surgery
Chief, Division of Vascular Surgery
Northwestern University Medical School
Chicago, Illinois

James S. T. Yao, M.D., Ph.D

Professor of Surgery
Director, Blood Flow Laboratory
Northwestern University Medical School
Chicago, Illinois

G&S

Grune & Stratton
A Subsidiary of Harcourt Brace Jovanovich, Publishers
New York London
Paris San Diego San Francisco São Paulo
Sydney Tokyo Toronto

Grune & Stratton, Inc.
111 Fifth Avenue
New York, New York 10003

Distributed in the United Kingdom by
Grune & Stratton, Inc. (London) Ltd.
24/28 Oval Road, London NW 1

Library of Congress Catalog Number 82-83967
International Standard Book Number 0-8089-1540-1
Printed in the United States of America

Contents

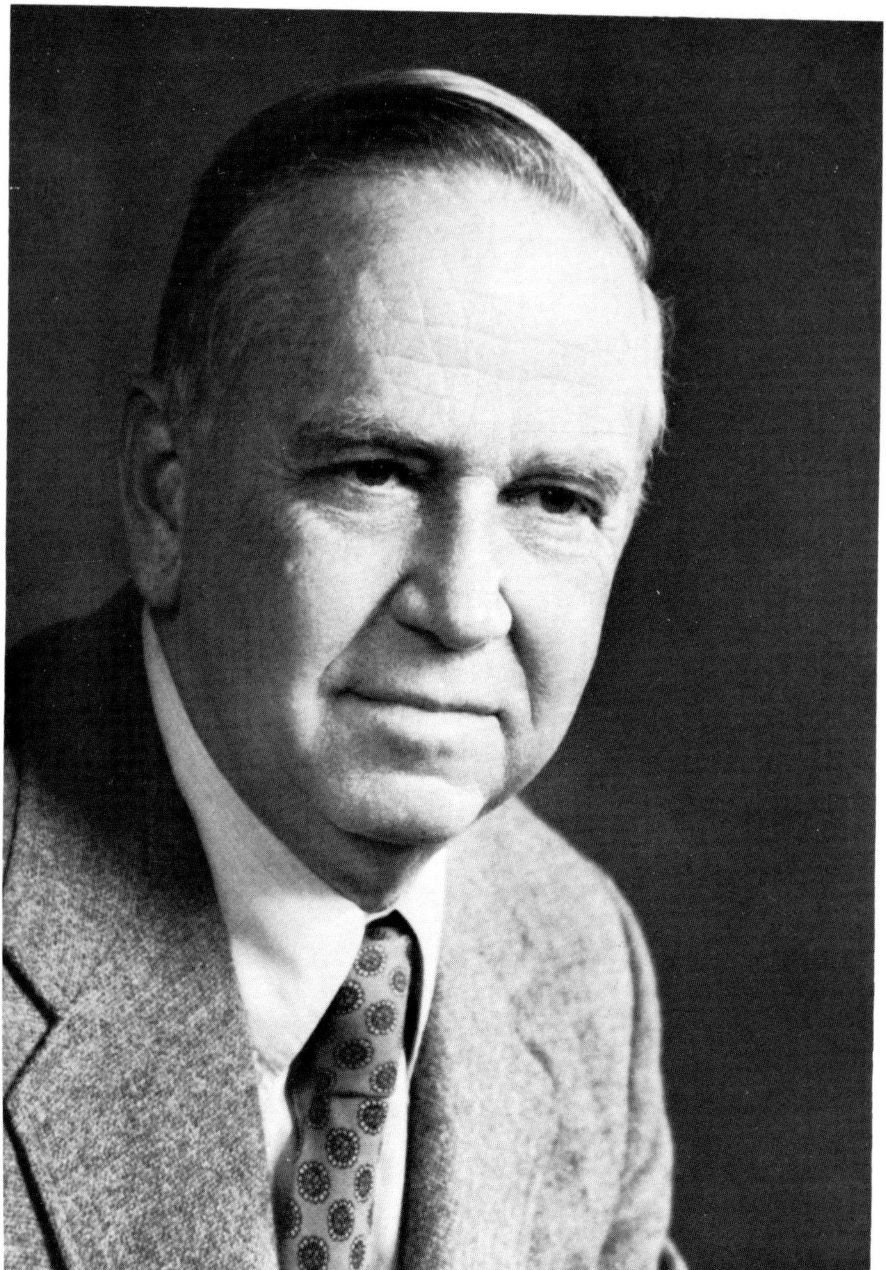

Edwin J. Wylie, M.D., 1918–1982

Dedication

To Jack Wylie,
surgeon, pioneer in vascular surgery, scholar, yachtsman,
a man of many parts, and a good friend.

Jack Wylie died on September 2, 1982. He had been performing surgery that morning, appropriately enough, correcting cerebrovascular insufficiency. His death was unexpected, a shock to his wife, his colleagues at the University of California in San Francisco, and his many friends in vascular surgery throughout the world. For more than 30 years, he had been at the frontier of vascular surgery. His influence was strongly positive as the field emerged as an important subspecialty in surgery. It is hard to imagine vascular surgery without Jack.

John Cid dos Santos wrote about Jack Wylie in 1975. Because his words, so beautifully eloquent, have not received wide publication, they are reprinted here in edited form:

My dear Jack,

You are a pioneer in vascular surgery and you have dedicated the best of your life to it. This means that, for almost 30 years, you have lived in a peculiar world—a world that you were obliged to build by yourself, step by step, independent of other vascular surgeons of the time. Peculiar worlds demand peculiar natures. This is no truism though it is a commonplace. But commonplaces often are most difficult to realize. I was born of general surgery and I still consider myself today a general surgeon. You also come from general surgery. Consequently, we both know well that the peculiarity of vascular surgery and of the vascular surgeon is a fundamental truth, independent of any tendency to overestimate one's field of activity.

Let us both remember, dear Jack, why vascular surgery is peculiar. We are already old in this business and quite well aware of these truths. But, in order to discover the strict laws of our job, we had to endure a long suffering. Forty years ago, there was still no experience, no knowledge, and thence, no rules. Modern vascular surgery was but darkness in the 1940s. Then it was revealed to each one of us under its true form: a sacred monster. And we either took it as it was or abandoned it.

The peculiarity of vascular surgery lies, above all, in its being mainly a surgery of ruins. *One has to work and build with deeply lesioned vascular walls. One has to suture those walls, or the crumbling remnants of them after endarterectomy, as if they were sound stuff. Meanwhile the inner surface of the artery may remain like a garden full of rich vegetation. Then these fragile sutures are immediately submitted to blood pressure and, consequently, they have to be resistant and hemostatic. Healing must take place under unfavorable and delicate conditions. As soon as the operation is over, one must be prepared for the possibility of secondary thrombosis developing at once, or of an embolism that could block the distal blood flow. When this happens the operation must be continued at once, sometimes with a different technique, and usually at the cost of much extra time. All these accidents are liable to happen, notwithstanding angiography, because the true macroscopic pathology of atherosclerosis is full of mystery, and when the real truth becomes apparent, it is sometimes impossible to retrocede; this surgery being contrary to many corrections. Then it may already be too late, the operation may have gone too far. On account of all these existing possibilities, the patient's condition may be worse at the end of the operation than prior to it. Or, the "best side" in bilateral operations may become worse than the "bad side," and amputation may finally be necessary. In addition, once the patient has left the operating theater, one must be prepared for the occurrence of secondary thrombosis, hemorrhage from different causes and of various types, dilatation of the vascular wall, and even the unmanageable infection. All these accidents may happen within minutes or several years later. In fact, vascular surgery is a surgery of repetition. Even so, and notwithstanding all these drawbacks, the final result is often a positive one. As unbelievable as this may seem, it is the miracle of this specialty. What I have described and have experienced, and most probably has been experienced by others, is a matter that I have repeatedly considered and that has led me to think that we are performing, on occasions, an impossible surgery that, under certain of its aspects, compels the vascular surgeon to face a dilemma: when to attempt surgery and when to refrain from it.*

Vascular surgery is a world apart under every point of view: examination, medical and surgical treatment, postoperative period, and follow-up. This accounts for the necessity of having a single independent unit for this particular surgery, as the dispersion of the necessary means seems to me unacceptable. And a separate department of angiography is just as in-

admissible, although this is the case in many places in the world. A vascular service without its own angiographic unit is like a body without a limb. We vascular surgeons must have our angiograms always at our close disposal, before, during, and after their performance; and our patients' records and angiograms must be around us at all times; otherwise, it will mean the loss of important and ready information. Angiograms are the eyes of the vascular surgeon; without them, he at once becomes a mole.

Modern times yielded several new surgical specialties, vascular surgery being one of them. We who have intensively lived its beginnings are aware of its bewildering character and complexity. Then, in the midst of all the storms and hard victories of vascular surgery, what a quiescence of the soul to think of general surgery! There sutures are made with sound tissues and diseased areas are either removed or bypassed. There one has the possibility of putting a zone at rest by drainage or temporary diversion. Only those who have performed both surgeries are able to appraise this sound world so completely apart. General surgery thus appears as the image of a liner cruising the peaceful Mediterranean Sea under infinitely blue skies.

Given what I say about vascular surgery, it is obvious that I expect a vascular surgeon should possess some singularities of his own. Just as we all know that not just anyone can become a surgeon, it is my belief that not every surgeon is gifted to become a vascular surgeon. It demands of the man an appropriate mentality, rather than a marked skillfulness, because vascular surgery is a mental affair—"e cosa mentale," *as Leonardo da Vinci so accurately said about painting. Perhaps one of the main qualities pertaining to the vascular surgeon should be his endurance to defy constant mental stress; although this is not sometimes apparent, it is always part of an unconscious background. Furthermore, he should possess some other attributes: an intense shrewdness, a strong and broad mind for decision, the art of controlling insecurity, and a powerful moral courage. He must also be of an amiable nature and have an unabashed frame of temper, as he may easily be called upon to perform a reoperation, at any time of the day or night, which may ask of him long hours of work over the estimated time. All this he must endure without becoming nervous, impatient, or angry. Furthermore, he must have total control of his team and inspire in all his aides not only complete understanding of what goes on but also the necessary good will and patience, only surpassed by that of the surgeon himself. Once loaded with such attributes, which must be cultivated (although they have to exist partly innately), he may attempt to navigate these thunderous seas. But as the practice of vascular surgery involves tremendous difficulties and hazards, this specialty stands sharply in contrast with the world of general surgery and, for this reason, there is still another factor that may put great strain upon the mentality and sensitivity of the vascular surgeon: environment. The patient for vascular surgery and his relatives often do not realize they are treading very delicate ground, as they tend to compare it with general surgery. A primary amputation may be accepted quite easily, but a secondary one will probably be considered as failure on the surgeon's part, instead of as a consequence of the disease itself. The patient is not the only hindrance, however. General surgeons themselves often misunderstand the problems within the vascular scope, being used to the routine of their operations, and they may cripple the poor vascular surgeon with their disdainful disapprobation.*

All these reasons indicate that in order to proceed with his work according to the ethics of vascular surgery, the surgeon should possess a steel armor under his skin and have one constant preoccupation: to look far beyond his scope and never at the passing moment—except for many useful "examens de conscience." *He may then advance with his Sisyphean task.*

My dear Jack, these are my feelings about the life we both partake. Certainly this is how I have seen it and how I have lived it. Your own life cannot have differed very much from my own. As a pioneer, you entered on the practice of vascular surgery solidly based upon sympathetic ganglionectomy and guided by the hand of Reynaldo (as we called Dos Santos, senior), Howell, and Murray, who told us that there probably was a new field for research lying before us. Our minds worked in unison and our dreams went far materializing the unknown. So you tried your first steps with arteriography and heparinization. Where arteriography is concerned, you studied the method thoroughly and you soon established the notion, still little spread in 1958, of the importance of seriography and of complete arteriography of the lower part of the body—aortoarteriography, as I wrongly named it, but the term remained. Since then, your interest in this particular field, without which we are so helpless, has never diminished. As to heparinization, you have studied and compared general and regional heparinization, experimentally and clinically, clearly demonstrating the advantages of the regional use of heparin. Already in 1949, you published an excellent result of a long thrombectomy of the lower limb, still an uncommon feature at the time.

Then you took your major step in vascular surgery: the introduction of endarterectomy in this country. This practice was still in its very early beginnings, and every surgeon of consequence considered its attempt an act of pure madness or lack of consciousness. After an experimental study to demonstrate the regeneration of the intima, you performed your first endarterectomy in January of 1951. At that very moment, you saw the door that opened the way and you got through it. Based upon your first few cases, you were able to demonstrate the regeneration of the intima after endarterectomy in man. This occurred approximately at the same time as I succeeded in demonstrating it in Lisbon. This early work of yours already contains some new ideas for that time. First, the notion that heparinization was not an absolute necessity during the postoperative period after endarterectomy. Second, the utmost importance of blood flow "free from eddies," a most fundamental notion that took a long time to be understood. And finally, I found in your drawings (just as I did in Wiley Barker's some time later, and still later semiconsciously expressed by Otto Trippel in 1963) that which I described, in 1964, under the name of "overpass." All this serves to prove that young brains may at once see very far even if they are not aware of the real value of their statements or of their drawings at the time of their conception. You were also sagacious in the choice of the main vessels of the pelvis for most of your first attempts, as this enabled you at once to obtain considerably better results; therefore you grew steadily more confident in your work, as opposed to myself, who experienced successive failures with the abominable femoral arteries, about which you have always remained apprehensive, contrary to some surgeons who would refer to femoral disobliteration as if that was a settled matter.

During this period of your life, you also showed us the importance of direct vascular surgery in early cases of obstructive disease, thus improving the average results as compared to the surgery of widely obstructed cases. This indication for early operations was already a sign of the great confidence you had in your work. Then came your main contribution to endarterectomy, besides the fact that you introduced it in the United States: the appraisal of the method, in 1955, four years after you first attempted it. *This appraisal is a pure product of the mind, and your capacity as a thinker and as a critic was already clearly apparent. In this work of yours, one can find many concepts and principles about the macroscopic pathology of atherosclerosis, methods of examination, heparinization, and operative judgment and technique that still stand today. Every word translates your perspicacity and common sense. You should be proud today of that "appraisal," which certainly demanded of you a powerful effort.*

Later, in 1965, you had the idea of using arterial autografts with the main arteries of the pelvis. This idea involved a certain risk, as the artery that was to be removed as graft had to be replaced by a Dacron tube, and thus the sound side of the patient became exposed to some disastrous occurrence. Still, you went ahead with your Hunterian "try" and you succeeded in demonstrating, most brilliantly, the usefulness of your idea.

You investigated many other aspects of obliterative and aneurysmal diseases of the abdomen, thorax, and limbs. In fact, all I have related until now may be considered as the backbone of your work.

Then, you shot out in several directions and also became a pioneer in other vascular fields, of which I stress your work on the renal and carotid arteries, and on the renal and cerebral circulation. You were the first to attempt an operation of a fibromuscular hyperplasia localized in a carotid artery, and in addition, you accomplished a very remarkable work, which has become a classic, on the development of this disease.

I have probably failed to value some other aspects of your scientific work in this short appraisal, for you certainly touched upon every surgical chapter of vascular disease. Furthermore, with regard to the venous system, you performed a long thrombectomy of the iliac veins, and you probably remained with the same feeling of incredulity, like myself, as to its real usefulness.

Throughout your scientific work I have found simplicity—never sophistication—clearness, inventiveness, demonstrativeness, and a powerful background of material and spiritual effort.

Your long experience and the development of your meditations over many years had to lead you, some day, to expose your ideas about the education of the vascular surgeon, his training and environment. In your Presidential Address of 1970 to the International Cardiovascular Society in Chicago, you developed your thoughts about the education of the vascular surgeon and the possible solutions to obtain a better standard of training for the younger surgeons in this country. Reading between the lines, I had the feeling that perhaps what I have said myself about vascular surgery and the vascular surgeon meets with your agreement. Your own center was one of the first foci of formation of vascular surgeons in the United States. Your students and collaborators have dispersed throughout the country, but they continue to honor you.

Thus, yours has been a fruitful life. As a pioneer in vascular surgery, you have contributed powerfully to the development of this branch of science through your own personal work. In addition, you have trained a new generation of vascular surgeons.

Jack Wylie continued his leadership after 1975, becoming President of the Society for Vascular Surgery, producing two volumes of a magnificent atlas of vascular surgery, and leading the struggle to achieve certification in vascular surgery by the American Board of Surgery.

As this volume was being completed, the news came of Jack's passing away. It seemed appropriate to dedicate this book to his memory, his pioneering work in carotid surgery, and his secure place in the history of this very special surgical art. Those of us who were privileged to know Jack will carry his memory, our many memories of him, with a smile.

John J. Bergan, M.D.
James S. T. Yao, M.D., Ph.D.
Chicago, September, 1982

Preface

Medicine is dependent upon changing concepts for progress in treatment of patient problems. Perhaps nowhere in medicine is conceptual change so obvious as in study of the cerebral vasculature and its effects upon brain physiology.

The ancients were particularly confused about the brain, and although the Egyptians described pulsations of the brain during life, they were ignorant of brain circulation. This was because they did not differentiate between tendons, nerves, and blood vessels. Similarly, though Pythagoras characterized the brain as an organ of reasoning, this concept was denied by no less a figure than Aristotle 200 years later.

Even the anatomical distribution of the cerebral blood vessels has been subject to changing concepts. For example, Galen felt that the *rete mirable*, seen in lower animals such as the dog and cat, was present in man. This concept stood for a thousand years, until Vesalius described the course of the internal carotid artery and changed forever Galen's erroneous concept. Even Vesalius himself was in error. The most cursory study of his drawings will show a large communication between the internal carotid artery and the tranverse sinus, a concept that demanded change.

Changing concepts and ideas are a part of our time, and many of these are the focus of the chapters in this volume. Eastcott, who was present at the birth of carotid surgery, begins a discussion of these changing concepts in his contribution on the beginning of this surgical art. Further examples of changing ideas with regard to the genesis of carotid artery plaques and the mechanisms of production of transient ischemic attacks are detailed in the contributions of Zarins, Giddens, and Glagov on atherosclerotic plaque distribution, and of Salzman on the role of platelet-vessel interaction in cerebrovascular disease. The increasing importance of intraplaque hemorrhage in the genesis of neurologic deficit is emphasized by Lusby, Ferrell, and Wylie in their chapter on this subject, and a neurologist's explanation of methods of evaluation of cerebral ischemia is given by Dyken, long a student of clinical syndromes of cerebrovascular insufficiency. Antiplatelet therapy has been explored thoroughly in treatment of transient cerebrovascular insufficiency, and no one knows more about this subject than the author of the chapter in this volume on medical treatment of patients with transient ischemic attacks. Fields, a professor of neurology at the University of Texas, Houston, details this subject and points out how concepts have changed in this field of treatment, as they have in surgical practices.

Investigations of the cerebral vasculature are becoming dependent upon imaging techniques. The differing roles of Doppler imaging and angiographic techniques, including digital subtraction angiography, are the subject of chapters by Turnipseed and by Hertzer and Modic on the former subject, and by Sumner, Russell, and Miles, by Zierler, Roederer, and Strandness, and Hobson, Berry, and Lynch on the latter. A comparison of direct and indirect tests for carotid artery lesions is summarized by a chapter from Yao's laboratory at Northwestern.

Although there has been very little change in the operation of carotid endarterectomy, there has been a great deal of controversy about elements of that surgical procedure. This ranges from controversy over the treatment of asymptomatic lesions, which is discussed by Thompson, to treatment of ulcerated plaque, described by Moore, and to surgery for crescendo TIAs and stroke in evolution, as described by McIntyre and Goldstone.

There are many elements of specialized management during carotid surgery that have been the subject of controversy and change. Among these is the thinking about tandem lesions affecting the cervical and intracranial carotid arteries, which is discussed by Schuler, Flanigan, and Williams, and cerebral protection during carotid surgery, as described by Sundt, by Javid, and by Callow and O'Donnell.

At one time, the external carotid artery was ignored in discussion of methods of revascularizing the ischemic brain, but it has assumed a proper place and the surgeon's armamentarium now includes endarterectomy of the external carotid in specialized circumstances. This is discussed by O'Mara. A special technique for carotid artery reconstruction comes to this volume from Paris, from the very busy service of Cormier.

In the past, intraoperative arteriography, discussed in this volume by Gaspar's group, was used to assure the totality of the carotid endarterectomy. In the future, intraoperative ultrasonic carotid artery imaging, discussed by Flanigan, Sigel, and Schuler, may very well have a place in the surgeon's laboratory, the operating room.

Cerebrovascular insufficiency is not always due to carotid artery atherosclerosis. Sometimes fibromuscular dysplasia can produce transient ischemic attacks and stroke. An enormous experience with this condition is described by Krupski, Effeney, and Ehrenfeld, and from Paris comes the contribution on supraaortic trunk lesions producing Takayasu's disease and cerebrovascular insufficiency, written for this volume by Kieffer and Natali. Another special problem affecting surgery on the carotid artery is the simultaneous occurrence of severely symptomatic coronary artery disease and carotid artery lesions. This is discussed from the huge background of experience given by the Cleveland Clinic to Hertzer, Beven, and their colleagues.

Occasionally, high exposure of the carotid artery is necessary in performing surgery, especially for internal carotid aneurysms. An intriguing technique to achieve this is described for this volume by Welsh of Buenos Aires.

During and after carotid artery surgery, special problems occur that have received attention and about which there is some controversy. The avoidance of cranial nerve injury is described by Bergan, Flinn, and Yao, and the controversy about changing speech and mentation patterns before and after carotid reconstruction is discussed in evenhanded fashion by Evans and his group. Blood pressure changes occurring in the perioperative period may be due to neurologic deficit at the time of surgery, incomplete control of preoperative hypertension, and other causes. This is discussed by Eskind and Dean from Vanderbilt, and management of frank stroke occurring during and after carotid surgery is detailed by Baker. Fortunately, carotid endarterectomy can be performed with an acceptable mortality and morbidity. This is emphasized by Swenson and Gundlach's chapter describing experience with this operation in a community hospital.

The long-term results of carotid artery surgery have been studied in detail by DeWeese, who summarizes his findings in his contribution on the subject.

A variety of techniques have emerged to improve cerebral blood flow. Among these are the extra-anatomic bypasses, described in a chapter by Rich's group from Walter Reed Army Medical Center, the revascularization of vertebral and subclavian artery occlusions, described by Imparato and Riles, and the technique of vertebrocarotid reimplantation, described by Bergan and Yao. Extracranial–intracranial bypass, performed brilliantly and described lucidly by Reichman, is a most important procedure, and a vascular surgeon's view of this operation by Greenhalgh is a valuable addition to this volume.

Thus change in concept, change in diagnostic approach, change in therapy, and even change in expectations of therapy become the thread that binds these contributions together. They are collected here for use by physicians as they attempt to decrease the enormous physical and economic drain caused by stroke.

Contributors

William H. Baker, M.D.
Professor of Surgery and Chief
Section of Peripheral Vascular Surgery
Loyola University Medical Center
Maywood, Illinois

Donald D. Bell, M.D.
Assistant Clinical Professor of Surgery
University of Southern California School of Medicine
Los Angeles, California

John J. Bergan, M.D.
Magerstadt Professor of Surgery and Chief
Division of Vascular Surgery
Northwestern University Medical School
Chicago, Illinois

Silvia M. Berry, M.Sc.
Associate, Division of Vascular Surgery
University of Medicine and Dentistry of New Jersey
New Jersey Medical School
Newark, New Jersey

Edwin G. Beven, M.D.
Department of Vascular Surgery
The Cleveland Clinic Foundation
Cleveland, Ohio

Donna Blackburn, R.N.
Assistant Director, Blood Flow Laboratory
Northwestern Memorial Hospital
Chicago, Illinois

Allan D. Callow, M.D.
Vice Chairman, Department of Surgery
Tufts University School of Medicine
Chief of Vascular Surgery
New England Medical Center Hospital
Boston, Massachusetts

G. Patrick Clagett, M.D.
Associate Professor of Surgery
Uniformed Services University of the Health Sciences
Chief, Peripheral Vascular Surgery Service
Co-Director, Vascular Fellowship Training Program
Walter Reed Army Medical Center
Washington, D.C.

Richard G. Considine, B.S.
Blood Flow Laboratory
Division of Vascular Surgery
Northwestern University Medical School
Chicago, Illinois

Prof. Agr. J. M. Cormier
Vascular Surgery Service
Hôpital Saint-Joseph
Paris, France

Peter Dawson
Department of Surgery
Charing Cross Hospital Medical School
London, England

Richard H. Dean, M.D.
Professor of Surgery and Head
Division of Vascular Surgery
Vanderbilt University School of Medicine
Nashville, Tennessee

James A. DeWeese, M.D.
Professor and Chairman
Division of Cardiothoracic Surgery
University of Rochester Medical Center
Rochester, New York

Mark L. Dyken, M.D.
Professor and Chairman
Department of Neurology
Indiana University School of Medicine
Indianapolis, Indiana

H.H.G. Eastcott, M.S., F.R.C.S., F.R.C.O.G., F.A.C.S. (Hon.), F.R.A.C.S. (Hon.)
Consultant Surgeon
St. Mary's Hospital
London, England

David J. Effeney, M.B., B.S., F.R.A.C.S.
Assistant Professor in Residence
Department of Surgery
University of California School of Medicine
San Francisco, California

William K. Ehrenfeld, M.D.
Professor of Surgery
University of California School of Medicine
San Francisco, California

Steven J. Eskind, M.D.
Chief Resident Surgeon
Vanderbilt University School of Medicine
Nashville, Tennessee

William E. Evans, M.D.
Clinical Professor of Surgery
Ohio State University
Chief of Vascular Surgery and Director
Vascular Laboratory
St. Anthony Hospital
Columbus, Ohio

Linda D. Ferrell, M.D.
Assistant Professor of Pathology
University of California School of Medicine
San Francisco, California

William S. Fields, M.D.
Professor of Neurology
Director
Neuro-oncology Center
MD Anderson Hospital
Houston, Texas

D. Preston Flanigan, M.D.
Associate Professor of Surgery
Chief, Division of Vascular Surgery
Abraham Lincoln School of Medicine
University of Illinois at the Medical Center
Chicago, Illinois

William R. Flinn, M.D.
Assistant Professor of Surgery
Northwestern University Medical School
Chicago, Illinois

Wilson V. Garrett, M.D.
Clinical Instructor in Surgery
University of Texas Southwestern Medical School
Associate Attending Surgeon
Baylor University Medical Center
Dallas, Texas

Max R. Gaspar, M.D.
Clinical Professor of Surgery
University of Southern California School of Medicine
Los Angeles, California

Don P. Giddens, Ph.D.
Regents Professor of Aerospace Engineering
School of Aerospace Engineering
Georgia Institute of Technology
Atlanta, Georgia

Seymour Glagov, M.D.
Professor of Pathology
University of Chicago
Chicago, Illinois

Jerry Goldstone, M.D.
Professor of Surgery and Chief
Section of Vascular Surgery
University of Arizona Health Sciences Center
Staff Surgeon
Veterans Administration Medical Center
Tucson, Arizona

R. M. Greenhalgh, M.A., M. Chir., F.R.C.S.
Director of the Department of Surgery
Charing Cross Hospital Medical School
London, England

William J. Gundlach, M.D.
Assistant Clinical Professor of Medicine
University of North Dakota School of Medicine
Division of Hematology
Quain and Ramstad Clinic
Bismarck, North Dakota

James Hayes, B.S., M.S.
Vascular Surgery Service,
St. Anthony Hospital
Columbus, Ohio

Norman R. Hertzer, M.D.
Department of Vascular Surgery
The Cleveland Clinic Foundation
Cleveland, Ohio

Robert W. Hobson, II, M.D.
Professor and Vice Chairman, Department of Surgery
Director, Division of Vascular Surgery
University of Medicine and Dentistry of New Jersey
New Jersey Medical School
Newark, New Jersey

John E. Hutton, Jr., M.D.
Vice Chairman and Associate Professor of Surgery
Uniformed Services University of the Health Sciences
Chief, Department of Surgery
Walter Reed Army Medical Center
Washington, D.C.

Anthony M. Imparato, M.D.
Professor of Surgery and Director
Division of Vascular Surgery
New York University Medical Center
New York, New York

Hushang Javid, M.D., Ph.D.
Professor of Surgery
Rush Medical College
Senior Attending Surgeon
Department of Cardiovascular-Thoracic Surgery
Rush-Presbyterian-St. Luke's Medical Center
Chicago, Illinois

Terry Jones
MRC Cyclotron Unit
Hammersmith Hospital
London, England

Dr. Edouard Kieffer
Professeur Agrége a la Faculté et Chirurgien des Hôpitaux de Paris
Service de Chirurgie Vasculaire
Groupe Hospitaliér Pitié-Salpetrière
Paris, France

William C. Krupski, M.D.
Assistant Professor of Surgery
University of California School of Medicine
San Francisco, California

Steven R. Larson, M.D.
Clinical Research Fellow
University of Southern California School of Medicine
Los Angeles, California

Guy G. Lemire, M.D.
Attending Surgeon
St. Mary Medical Center
Long Beach, California

Floyd D. Loop, M.D.
Department of Thoracic and Cardiovascular Surgery
The Cleveland Clinic Foundation
Cleveland, Ohio

Robert J. Lusby, F.R.C.S.
Fogarty International Research Fellow in Vascular Surgery
University of California School of Medicine
San Francisco, California

Thomas G. Lynch, M.D.
Assistant Professor of Surgery
Division of Vascular Surgery
University of Medicine and Dentistry of New Jersey
New Jersey Medical School
Newark, New Jersey

Charles Mate-Kole
Departments of Psychiatry and Surgery
Charing Cross Hospital Medical School
London, England

Kenneth E. McIntyre, Jr., M.D.
Assistant Professor of Surgery
University of Arizona Health Sciences Center
Staff Surgeon
Veterans Administration Medical Center
Tucson, Arizona

Richard D. Miles, Ph.D.
Assistant Professor and Biomedical Engineer
Department of Surgery
Southern Illinois University School of Medicine
Springfield, Illinois

Michael T. Modic, M.D.
Department of Radiology
The Cleveland Clinic Foundation
Cleveland, Ohio

Wesley S. Moore, M.D.
Professor of Surgery and Chief
Section of Vascular Surgery
University of California School of Medicine,
Los Angeles, California

Herbert J. Movius, M.D.
Clinical Professor of Surgery
University of Southern California School of Medicine
Los Angeles, California

Dr. Jean Natali
Professeur et Chirurgien des Hôpitaux de Paris
Vascular Surgery Service
Groupe Hospitaliér Pitié-Salpetrière
Paris, France

Thomas F. O'Donnell, Jr., M.D.
Associate Professor of Surgery
Director, Noninvasive Vascular Laboratory
Tufts-New England Medical Center
Boston, Massachusetts

David W. Olson, M.D.
Instructor of Surgery
Uniformed Services University of the Health Sciences
Fellow, Peripheral Vascular Surgery Service
Walter Reed Army Medical Center
Washington, D.C.

Charles S. O'Mara, M.D.
Assistant Professor of Surgery
Director, Vascular Laboratory
The Johns Hopkins Medical Institutions
Baltimore, Maryland

William H. Pearce, M.D.
Assistant Professor of Surgery
University of Cincinnati Medical Center
Cincinnati, Ohio

David G. Piepgras, M.D.
Professor of Neurosurgery
Cerebral Vascular Research Center
Mayo Clinic and Mayo Foundation
Rochester, Minnesota

Roberto Pradier, M.D.
Assistant Professor of Surgery
University of Buenos Aires
Chief, Head and Neck Surgery
Institute of Oncology
Buenos Aires, Argentina

O. Howard Reichman, M.D.
Professor and Chief
Division of Neurological Surgery
Loyola University Medical Center
Maywood, Illinois

Roberto Repetto, M.D.
Assistant Professor of Surgery
University of Buenos Aires
Vascular Surgeon
Instituto Pombo and CEMIC
Buenos Aires, Argentina

Jean-Baptiste Ricco, M.D.
Fellow in Peripheral Vascular Surgery
Northwestern University Medical School
Chicago, Illinois

Norman M. Rich, M.D.
Professor and Chairman
Department of Surgery
Chief, Division of Vascular Surgery
Uniformed Services University of the Health Sciences
Bethesda, Maryland
Co-Director, Vascular Fellowship Training Program
Walter Reed Army Medical Center
Washington, D.C.

Thomas S. Riles, M.D.
Assistant Professor of Surgery
New York University
Director of Vascular Surgery
Bellevue Hospital
New York, New York

Ghislaine O. Roederer, M.D.
Research Fellow, Department of Surgery
University of Washington School of Medicine
Seattle, Washington

John J. Rosental, M.D.
Associate Clinical Professor of Surgery
University of Southern California School of Medicine
Los Angeles, California

James B. Russell, B.S.
Researcher, Department of Surgery
Southern Illinois University School of Medicine
Springfield, Illinois

James M. Salander, M.D.
Assistant Professor of Surgery
Uniformed Services University of the Health Sciences
Assistant Chief
Peripheral Vascular Surgery Service
Walter Reed Army Medical Center
Washington, D.C.

Edwin W. Salzman, M.D.
Professor of Surgery
Harvard Medical School
Associate Director of Surgery
Beth Israel Hospital
Boston, Massachusetts

James J. Schuler, M.D.
Assistant Professor of Surgery
Division of Vascular Surgery
Abraham Lincoln School of Medicine
University of Illinois at the Medical Center
Chicago, Illinois

Frank W. Sharbrough, M.D.
Associate Professor of Neurology
Cerebral Vascular Research Center
Mayo Clinic and Mayo Foundation
Rochester, Minnesota

Bernard Sigel, M.D.
Professor of Surgery
Abraham Lincoln School of Medicine
University of Illinois at the Medical Center
Chicago, Illinois

D. Eugene Strandness, Jr., M.D.
Professor of Surgery
University of Washington School of Medicine
Seattle, Washington

David S. Sumner, M.D.
Professor of Surgery and Chief
Section of Peripheral Vascular Surgery
Southern Illinois University School of Medicine
Springfield, Illinois

Thoralf M. Sundt, Jr., M.D.
Professor of Neurological Surgery
Cerebral Vascular Research Center
Mayo Clinic and Mayo Foundation
Rochester, Minnesota

Wayne M. Swenson, M.D.
Associate Professor of Surgery
University of North Dakota School of Medicine
Chairman, Department of Surgery
Quain and Ramstad Clinic
Bismarck, North Dakota

C. M. Talkington, M.D.
Clinical Assistant Professor of Surgery
University of Texas Southwestern Medical School
Associate Attending Surgeon
Baylor University Medical Center
Dallas, Texas

Paul C. Taylor, M.D.
Department of Thoracic and Cardiovascular Surgery
The Cleveland Clinic Foundation
Cleveland, Ohio

Jesse E. Thompson, M.D.
Clinical Professor of Surgery
University of Texas Southwestern Medical School
Chief of Surgery and Director of Graduate Education in Vascular Surgery
Baylor University Medical Center
Dallas, Texas

William D. Turnipseed, M.D.
Associate Professor of Surgery
University of Wisconsin
Chief of Vascular Surgery
University and Veterans Administration Hospitals
Madison, Wisconsin

Blair D. Vermilion, M.D.
Vascular Surgery Service
St. Anthony Hospital
Columbus, Ohio

Patricio A. Welsh, M.D.
Assistant Professor of Surgery
University of Buenos Aires
Chief, Vascular Surgery
Instituto Pombo and CEMIC
Buenos Aires, Argentina

Larry R. Williams, M.D.
Resident in Surgery
Abraham Lincoln School of Medicine
University of Illinois at the Medical Center
Chicago, Illinois

Richard Wise
MRC Cyclotron Unit
Hammersmith Hospital
London, England

Edwin J. Wylie, M.D.
Professor of Surgery
University of California School of Medicine
Center for the Health Sciences
San Francisco, California

James S. T. Yao, M.D., Ph.D.
Professor of Surgery
Northwestern University Medical School
Director, Blood Flow Laboratory
Northwestern Memorial Hospital
Chicago, Illinois

Jerry R. Youkey, M.D.
Instructor of Surgery
Uniformed Services University of the Health Sciences
Fellow, Peripheral Vascular Surgery Service
Walter Reed Army Medical Center
Washington, D.C.

Christopher K. Zarins, M.D.
Professor of Surgery
Chief of Vascular Surgery
University of Chicago
Chicago, Illinois

R. Eugene Zierler, M.D.
Instructor in Surgery
University of Washington School of Medicine
Seattle, Washington

PART I

History

H.H.G. Eastcott

1

The Beginning of Carotid Surgery

The Concise Oxford Dictionary, defining the carotid as "of or near the two great arteries carrying blood to the brain," tells us also that they are so named from the Greek *karotides, karoo* meaning stupefy, compression of these arteries being thought to do this. Some association between these vessels and the function of the brain itself, therefore, seems to have existed in the minds of men since classical times, but their scientific elucidation did not come until a millenium and a half brought the world into the month of January, 1621. In a charming country cottage in the village of Great Bedwyn, Wiltshire (Fig. 1-1), was born Thomas Willis, into troubled times, for the Civil War was soon to come, yet it did not prevent him from studying hard and graduating Bachelor of Arts at Oxford and later as Bachelor of Medicine also.[1] At some time he became a friend of Christopher Wren, and to him he turned when his greatest work, *Cerebri Anatome,* was in preparation for the illustration that shows so clearly the free communication beneath the brain of the four arteries that supply it. From a later work[2] comes this important quotation: "if the Carotid of one side should be obstructed, then the vessels of the other side might provide for either Province . . . further, if both the Carotids should be stopt, the offices of each might be supplied through the Vertebrals."

That the large branches over the hemispheres could also serve this function was clear to Willis, for he described the case of a man, dead of abdominal cancer, at whose post-mortem examination the right carotid was found to be occluded, yet he had suffered no stroke or mental impairment but had been troubled with a left-sided headache, and, Willis suggested, "the blood excluded from the right carotid . . . rushed more impetuously in the left and had distended the membrane."

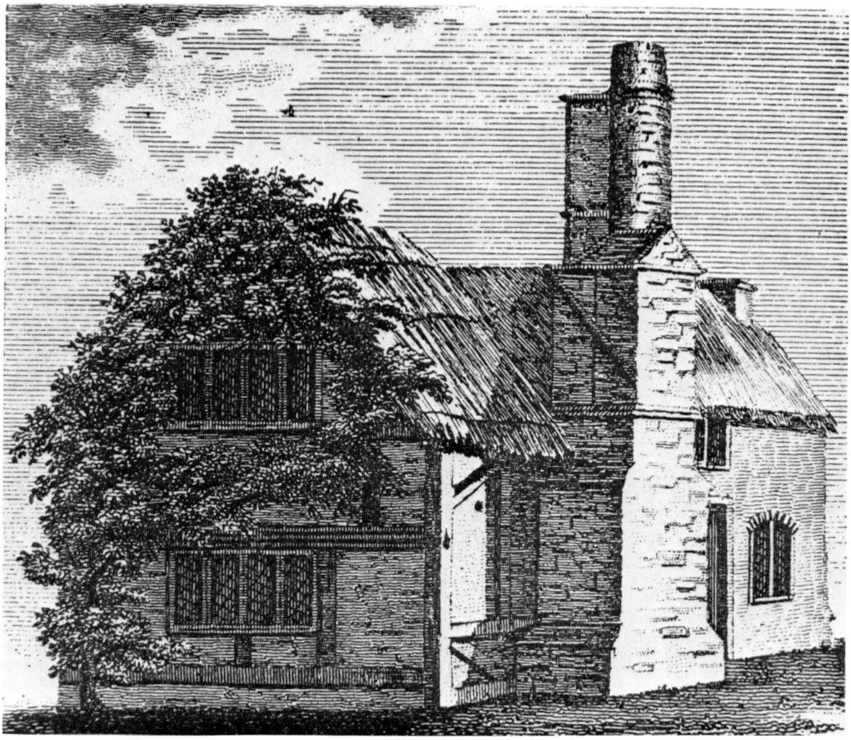

Figure 1–1. The birthplace of Thomas Willis. From a drawing made in 1798, and first published by Sir Charles Symonds and Dr. W. Feindal in 1969.[1] By kind permission of the British Medical Journal.

THE CONTRIBUTIONS OF GUY'S HOSPITAL

The opening articles in the first volume of the Guy's Hospital Reports in 1838 are by Dr. Richard Bright, on the effects of cerebrovascular disease, with particular reference to diagnosis during life[3] and the pathological findings after death; and a thirteen-year follow-up, also with autopsy confirmation, on the world's first successful carotid operation by Sir Astley Cooper.[4]

Bright, a rich man's son, well-travelled and highly intelligent, joined the staff as Assistant Physician in 1820. At Guy's Hospital, he worked in the company of 2 colleagues who were also to become famous, Thomas Addison and Thomas Hodgkin. In cases of threatened apoplexy, he realized, headache is a common warning symptom. In two such instances that involved women who had each suffered a fatal stroke in later life, Bright saw that the vessels beneath the brain were hard and brittle, particularly the carotids as they left the neck and entered the skull. He knew also that a sudden onset, with loss of conciousness, is prognostically grave. Although blood pressure measurement was still in the future, he saw the effects of chronic renal disease on cardiac hypertrophy and that the patient who suffered those effects often succumbed to stroke. Today, we know that of all the preventive and also surgically supportive measures against stroke, control of hypertension is the most important.

Astley Cooper, in 1808, undertook the treatment of a man of 50 who had a painful, pulsating swelling beneath the left mandibular angle. There was increasing hoarseness and a drooping of the left eyelid. Carefully sparing the vagus, Cooper ligated the common carotid doubly, with transfixion, and divided the artery. The patient's pain left him at once and never returned, though the pulsation did not wholly cease, it steadily diminished, until 3 months after the operation neither it, nor the swelling itself, could be recognised beneath the scar. Meanwhile, the hoarseness abated and the eye improved. When, in 1821, the patient succumbed to a painful apoplexy, Cooper obtained the pathological examination that proved the correctness of Thomas Willis's views on the purpose of the cerebral anastomoses that he had discovered (Fig. 1-2). The left posterior communicating artery was very large in comparison with the right; indeed, the "left side of the Circle of Willis was much more developed . . . and the left side of the brain received its full share of arterial blood."

LESSONS FROM CAROTID LIGATION FOR INTRACRANIAL ANEURYSM

Later in the nineteenth century, the indications for ligation extended to the treatment of trigeminal neuralgia and epilepsy and in these circumstances, apparently, the complication rate was low. With more serious structural disease, such as aneurysm or hemorrhage, however, contemporary reports on a total of several hundred patients agree on a mortality figure of between 30 and 40 percent, and 20 and 30 percent of severe cerebral symptoms.[5] Modern experience has been more favorable. Sir Geoffrey Jefferson of Manchester[6] found that of 142 patients undergoing carotid ligation for intracranial saccular aneurysm, there were no deaths that could be attributed to the ligation, though there were 11 instances of hemiplegia, 7 of which were severe. By now, it was possible to measure the effect of clamping on the distal carotid pressure, and an early finding in this case series showed a reduction of from 40 to 60 percent, which was a suitable objective for the control or prevention of intracranial bleeding.

By 1976, the clinical problem had still not been resolved, though Professor Bryan Jennett and his colleagues at the University of Glasgow had measured the effects of carotid ligation, common or internal, upon distal carotid arterial pressure and cerebral blood flow, and a set of guidelines was

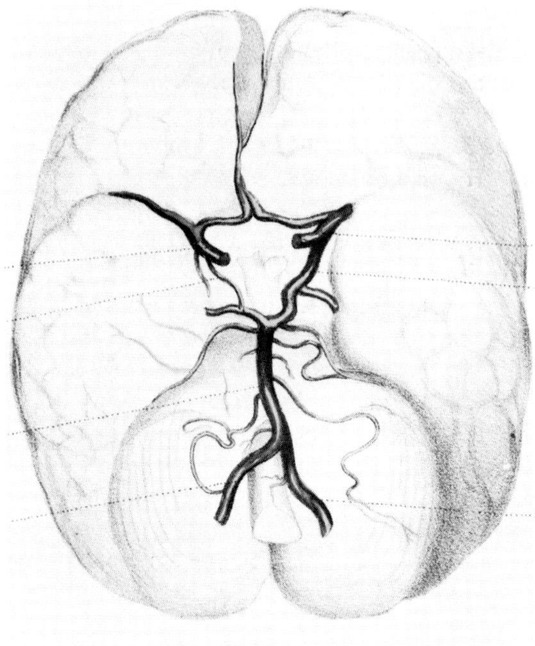

ACCOUNT

OF THE

FIRST SUCCESSFUL OPERATION,

PERFORMED ON THE COMMON CAROTID ARTERY,

FOR

ANEURISM,

IN THE YEAR 1808:

WITH THE POST-MORTEM EXAMINATION, IN 1821.

FROM THE NOTES OF

SIR ASTLEY COOPER, BART.

H. HUMPHREYS, aged 50, who had been used to carry heavy burdens in the streets of London, perceived, about six months ago, a tumor, about the size of a walnut, possessing a pulsatory motion, on the left side of the neck, just below the angle of the jaw, and extending down as low as the thyroid cartilage. It was productive of great pain on the

Figure 1-2. Title heading and plate from Astley Cooper's report. The left posterior communicating artery is much larger than the right.

established: the carotid could be ligated if flow was maintained at 40 ml/100g/min, but not if less than 20 ml; between 20 and 40 ml, if the flow reduction was less than 25 percent, or 11 ml; and in cases where flow reduction lay between 25 and 35 percent, provided that the carotid stump pressure was more than 60 mm Hg, in a normotensive patient.[5]

THE THIRD KILLER: ISCHEMIC THROMBOEMBOLIC STROKE

It is surprising that with all the concern and study of the nineteenth-century neurologists, stroke disease of the common kind remained an enigma, there being almost no concept that the carotid could be playing a major part. Not until 1913, when Ramsay Hunt of Columbia University, New York was addressing the American Neurological Association[7] (Fig. 1-3) did it begin to dawn upon the medical profession that the cerebral lesion in most stroke victims could be the effect and not the cause. Perhaps to convey his meaning better, he reminded his audience of the work with which they were already familiar, on the consequences of carotid artery ligation. In one large group, he said, though there might be some minor early symptoms, there are no permanent effects, though "it would be interesting to know the subsequent neurological histories in such patients." From four case series available at that time, he had found permanent symptoms to have developed in from 9.6 to 27 percent. Regarding the circle of Willis, Hunt agreed that it could be sufficient

704 HUNT: THE ROLE OF THE CAROTID ARTERIES

THE ROLE OF THE CAROTID ARTERIES, IN THE CAUSATION OF VASCULAR LESIONS OF THE BRAIN, WITH REMARKS ON CERTAIN SPECIAL FEATURES OF THE SYMPTOMATOLOGY.[1]

By J. Ramsay Hunt, M.D.,

ASSOCIATE PROFESSOR OF NERVOUS DISEASES, COLLEGE OF PHYSICIANS AND SURGEONS, COLUMBIA UNIVERSITY, NEW YORK.

Introduction. In recent years, special attention has been given to the more exact localization of vascular lesions of the brain, and as a result a number of new syndromes have been added to the literature of this subject. The object of the present study is to emphasize the importance of obstructive lesions of the main arteries of the neck (the innominate, common carotid, and internal carotids), in the causation of softening of the brain, and

Figure 1-3. Title heading of Ramsay Hunt's paper.

to compensate for obstruction more proximally in the young, but that in "individuals with diseased or weakened hearts and sclerotic vessels, compensatory changes may not develop." Even so, the young could be at serious risk also, for he cited the cases of two youthful patients with traumatic carotid artery thrombosis, both of whom succumbed—something that is familiar to all accident surgeons today.

The great message of Ramsay Hunt's paper was to bring emphasis to the importance of obstructive lesions of the main arteries of the neck in cases of cerebrovascular disease with softening of the brain, and to urge the routine examination of these vessels, both clinically and pathologically, whenever possible. Palpation of the carotids, especially in the area between the upper border of the thyroid cartilage and the angle of the jaw, would generally be found to show equal pulsation, except in hemiplegics, where a distinct weakness was noted on the side corresponding to the cerebral lesion. Four out of 20 such patients examined in a home for old people in New York showed such diminution of the relevant carotid pulsation. The clinical examination should include palpation of the temporal pulse, advised Hunt, if involvement of the external carotid is suspected. Here again, he was years ahead of his time when he reminded his audience of the importance of main artery disease in lower limb ischemia, with intermittent claudication or gangrene, and urged the same attitude of mind in the search for clinical evidence in cerebrovascular cases: "and never omit a detailed examination of the main arterial stem." We shall later consider one of these details, the carotid bruit, but first the scene must be set for that which came sooner, the clinical and radiological elucidation of carotid insuffiency in stroke of various degrees of severity.

EARLY CAROTID ARTERIOGRAPHY: A FALSE DAWN

Recognition of cervical internal carotid atheroma remained mainly retrospective long after Ramsay Hunt's lecture. Reduced pulsation in the neck, as he knew, was an insensitive test, with many false negatives. Positive findings, when they could be elicited, all too often meant that the carotid was already occluded.

The Portuguese school of angiography was founded by Egaz Moniz during the early 1920's. By 1937, he and his colleagues using thorotrast injection into the carotid were able to report the following[8] (Fig. 1-4):

> Thrombosis of the internal carotid, though rare, is nevertheless commoner than is thought. We have seen at least 4 cases in a total of 537 patients on whom we have performed cerebral angiography. The diagnosis is otherwise impossible. Excluding the first 37 cases in our early experience the incidence was 0.8 percent. If we had studied a series of hemiplegics this figure would certainly have been higher. For a while the cerebral circulation was our first concern, but before long

HÉMIPLÉGIES PAR THROMBOSE DE LA CAROTIDE INTERNE

PAR MM.

Egas MONIZ, Almeida LIMA
et Rui de LACERDA
(Lisbonne)

La thrombose de la carotide interne, bien que rare, est, cependant, plus fréquente qu'on ne l'avait pensé. En effet, nous l'avons rencontrée, au moins dans 4 cas, depuis que nous faisons l'épreuve de l'angiographie cérébrale, c'est-à-dire sur un total de 537 malades.

Figure 1-4. The first report of arteriography for stroke. By kind permission of Presse Medicale.

> we began to suspect the possibility of seeing lesions in the internal carotid, so we decided to take neck pictures as well.

This loose translation is my own.

Fig. 1-5a shows their findings in a man aged 46, who had a complex previous neurological history that included neurosyphilis and an attempted suicide by shooting himself into his right ear, the bullet lodging behind the right mandible where it could have damaged the carotid. The right internal carotid was seen to be occluded in this case. Another patient, a man aged 43, suffered left hemiplegia following prodromal symptoms during the three preceding days. His arteriogram (Fig. 1-5b) showed an apparent stenosis of the right internal carotid in its mid-cervical portion, while the left was occluded from its origin.

THE CLINICAL AWAKENING AFTER WORLD WAR II

Vascular surgery continued its long sleep, begun it seems when the first World War interrupted the stream of creative thought that flowed from the work of Alexis Carrel. With the second return of peace in 1945, and the vastly

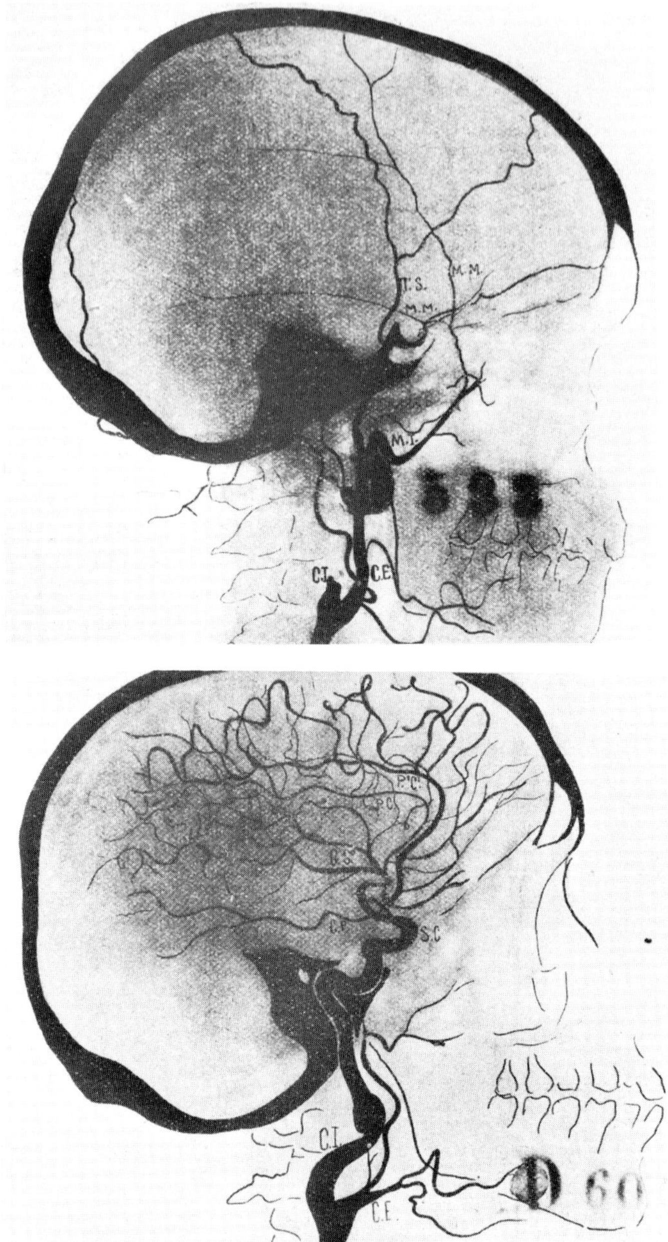

Figure 1-5. a) Complete occlusion of the right internal carotid from an old bullet wound. b) Stenosis or looping of the right internal carotid in a previously fit man with right hemiplegia and aphasia. The left internal carotid was shown to be completely occluded. By kind permission of Presse Medicale.

improved communications that were one of the better legacies of the recent war, medicine was poised for great developments; a different attitude of mind at last prevailed. Always at the forefront of intellectual excellence, Boston and the Harvard Medical School at that time shone a great searchlight upon the areas of greatest promise. C. Miller Fisher, a Canadian neurologist, working with Dr. Raymond D. Adams at the Massachusetts General Hospital, on the afternoon of Sunday, June 11th, 1950, was addressing the American Association of Neuropathologists' Annual Meeting at Atlantic City. They had examined the brains of 373 patients who had succumbed after having been diagnosed as suffering from cerebrovascular occlusion and had found hemorrhagic infarcts in 66. Their conclusion was that nearly all such cases were of embolic origin, and that some of the transient clinical phenomena were related to the temporary proximal arrest of such emboli. The essential importance of Ramsay Hunt's teaching was recalled in their statement that "No case of vascular disease of the brain is completely investigated if the carotid arteries have not been examined."[9]

The following year, Miller Fisher wrote again:

> My interest in this subject was aroused while working in the Mallory Institute under the direction of Dr. R.D. Adams . . . in case after case neuropathological examination failed to confirm the clinical impression of disease of the middle cerebral artery . . . not a single case in 200 examined over nine months . . . it was logical to look more proximally, namely in the internal carotid artery for unrecognised disease.

He went on to describe eight such cases.[10]

THE BOSTON-LONDON LINK: AND THE RETURN OF THE MESSAGE

The Shattuck Lecture of the Massachusetts Medical Society on May 21, 1951, was delivered by an Englishman, D. Denny-Brown, whose professional career was in Boston though he had returned to serve throughout the 1939-45 War with the British Royal Army Medical Corps. The subject of his address was "The Changing Pattern of Neurologic Medicine"[11]; in it he considered the role of insufficiency of the circle of Willis in the causation of intermittent cerebral attacks, with particular reference to more widespread cardiovascular disturbances, a theme which he developed in a later article[12], including the significance of external-internal carotid collateral pathways, the fact that patients may be quite young (these perhaps may have been examples of fibromuscular carotid dysplasia), and a note of caution on the risks of direct carotid arteriography in elderly patients, in whose extensively atheromatous vessels thrombosis might thus be induced. He also showed that when the opposite carotid is supplying an ophthalmic artery, the branches of which are under fundoscopic examination, compression of that carotid can produce visible narrowing of the retinal vessels. Noninvasive carotid artery testing had arrived.

Denny-Brown's close friend and colleague was another distinguished neurologist, on the staff of the National Hospital for Nervous Diseases, Queen Square, London, and also at St. Mary's Hospital, where he was dean of the Medical School. His name was Dr. Denis Brinton, and he now lives in happy retirement in the New Forest, in Hampshire in the south of England. The two Dennys, as they were known when on the Resident Staff of the National Hospital before the War, kept in touch over the eventful years that followed, and it is certain that Brinton had his friend's ideas much in mind when Sir George Pickering called him in consultation over the case of a woman aged 66, who in March 1954, presented having had 33 attacks in which heaviness or tightness of the chest was immediately followed by blindness of the left eye, loss of her speech, and loss of the use of the right arm and leg—the episodes lasting between 10 and 30 minutes. There were no abnormal neurological signs, but the left carotid, superficial temporal, and facial arterial pulses were diminished. Aware of the new possibilities for the elucidation of the syndrome, Denis Brinton advised that arteriography should be done. Only a year or so before, a new radiologist had joined the St. Mary's Hospital staff; his name was Dr. David Sutton, and his skill in angiography has since played an important part in the development of vascular surgery at our hospital. Sutton performed a left carotid arteriogram, first with intracranial views, noting delay in the filling that made him decide to obtain special neck views, which showed atheromatous obstruction of the origin of the left internal carotid. Consultation with Professor Charles Rob followed, and the decision was made to attempt the surgical cure of the condition.

THE OPERATION OF MAY 19TH, 1954

The events of that day afford another example of the links between Boston and London that have proved so fruitful in the years that have since passed. During late 1949 and early 1950, I was fortunate enough to have the opportunity of working under Dr. Francis D. Moore and Dr. Charles A. Hufnagel at the Peter Bent Brigham Hospital and in the Surgical Laboratory of Harvard Medical School where I learned the techniques of arterial reconstructive surgery. My first carotid operation was in September, 1949, under the instruction of the late David Hume and consisted in the excision and replacement by suture anastomosis of the left carotid artery of one of our laboratory dogs. Returning to St. Mary's a year later, I joined the Professorial Surgical Unit under its new Director, Charles Rob, who, after much experience with the vascular surgery of war wounds, could see the future that lay ahead for reconstructive operations, and together we did several of the first cases of various kinds to be done in Britain. There had in fact been a previous carotid resection in 1952, in a man aged 82, for adherent metastatic lymph nodes whose favorable course showed us that the 20 minutes required to clamp, resect, and anastomose the common carotid could be well tolerated.

This, however did little to reassure me, and I must confess to having had misgivings about the risks of such a procedure in a patient who was already having hemiplegic attacks. Rob and Pickering, however, could see that since the probable outcome without operation was likely to be a permanent stroke, the venture was fully justified, and so it proved to be.

May in England can be a cold month, and with all the operating theater windows open, ice bags and fans and cold sheets over the patient to reduce her body temperature, the same effect was soon noticed by the nursing staff and by the several visitors who were with us that day. One of these was Dr. George Dunlop, of Worcester, Massachusetts, later to become President of the American College of Surgeons and a close personal friend. Dr. Dunlop had his camera with him and quite unknown to us took several fine photographs on that memorable occasion.

The operative details are reported in our article.[13] Under hypothermia at 28° C, the 28 minutes of carotid clamping required to resect the carotid bifurcation and anastomose the common and internal carotids end-to-end proved acceptable, and the patient made a smooth recovery, and lived comfortably, free from any neurological symptoms, for another 20 years, during which time her condition was regularly reviewed for mild continuing cardiovascular symptoms, mainly from her hypertension. Her eventual death was unaccompanied by cerebrovascular features.

OTHER EARLY OPERATIONS

Endarterectomy for complete carotid occlusion was reported in 1953, by Strully and his colleagues from New York[14] though in this case the wise decision was made to ligate the internal carotid when it was clear that thrombus remained in its upper reaches, rather than to complete the repair with risk of cerebral embolism. In the same year, Dr. DeBakey and his colleagues in Houston succeeded in establishing back flow in a similar case, and in 1959 reported a satisfactory outcome, together with a much larger subsequent experience, including the aortic arch branches.[15]

The first published report of carotid endarterectomy for stenosis came out in 1956 and was by Dr. Denton Cooley and his colleagues.[16] The patient was a man aged 71 years who suffered dizziness on standing and a pulsatile tinnitus. The bruit was clinically confirmed, and a thorotrast angiogram of the kind practiced by Moniz showed tight narrowing of the left common carotid just below its bifurcation. Notable features of this report include the bruit, mention of the use of the Matas test (left carotid compression produced dizziness and partial aphasia), and also the use of a temporary arterial shunt at operation.

THE END OF THE BEGINNING

By the early 1960s, two further basic concepts had been defined that were to help define the scope of carotid endarterectomy and to identify more patients for its possible benefits.

First came the recognition *that recent, major completed stroke is an important contraindication,* particularly when the level of consciousness is impaired. The 1959 Houston paper[15] mentioned that a fatal outcome had followed operation in 3 patients who were comatose and extensively paralysed before it. The reason for such catastrophes was examined by Wylie et al.,[17] who by 1964, had learned from 5 cases who died within a few hours or days of endarterectomy. Three had suffered a recent major stroke; the other 2 had not, though one was known to have a complete occlusion of his right internal carotid and a stenosis on the left, the repair of which led to severe right-sided headaches on the third postoperative day, with the development of a left hemiplegia and death within 12 hours. A large right hemisphere infarct of hemorrhagic type was confirmed at autopsy. This combination of occlusion and contralateral stenosis is now known to carry a higher operative risk, which to some extent can be assessed by computer scanning and reduced by intraoperative shunting if no recent infarct is identified.

The second great leap forward in simple clinical terms was the realization that *in most patients with transient hemisphere or ocular ischemia, a systolic arterial bruit can be detected* with the stethoscope placed a little below and behind the angle of the jaw. This, too, was realized in the early Houston experience[15] where it was found to be present "in all patients with partial occlusions" though not with a complete occlusion unless there was stenosis of the opposite carotid. In our experience at St. Mary's Hospital, of 40 patients reviewed in 1960,[18] no neck bruits were recorded though there were two with murmurs over the eye, something that had been observed by Miller Fisher in 1957.[19] The second series of 57 St. Mary's patients reviewed in 1962[20] contained 18 with neck bruits mentioned in their clinical records. In my own case notes, the first mention of a carotid bruit was in 1960.

SOME EARLY PROBLEMS THAT REMAIN

The ultimate disaster in a preventive operation is the precipitation by it of the very complication that it was designed to avoid. *Perioperative stroke* is with us still, and various methods of avoiding it will be familiar to every reader. The common factor seems to be the technical skill and experience of the operator more than the particular method that he chooses to use. *Control of hypertension* is now realized to be one of the most important needs after operation, just as it has been shown to be in the wider world of preventive epidemiology.[21] *Associated ischemic heart disease,* as we knew in our patient of 1954, must bring an extra operative danger; in fact, the coronary mortality today, in the major centers, should exceed that from stroke. The planning of combined treatment methods is still a matter of concern.

CONCLUSION

The fact that a whole symposium can now be devoted to aspects of the surgery of the bifurcation of one artery is evidence that many questions remain to be answered. Twenty-eight years ago, much was uncertain in our minds. Today, some of those doubts have been resolved, though others have succeeded them. I am made very glad by this opportunity to present the past in the light of the future.

REFERENCES

1. Symonds C, Feindal W: Birthplace of Thomas Willis. Br Med J 2:648, 1969
2. Symonds C: The circle of Willis. Br Med J 1:119, 1955
3. Bright R: Cases illustrative of the effects produced when the arteries and brain are diseased: Selected chiefly with a view to the diagnosis in such affections. Guy's Hosp Rep 1:9, 1836
4. Cooper A: Account of the first successful operation, performed on the common carotid artery, for aneurism, in the year 1808: With the post mortem examination, in 1821. Guy's Hosp Rep 1:53, 1836
5. Jennett B, Miller JD, Harper AM (eds): Effect of Carotid Artery Surgery on Cerebral Blood Flow. Amsterdam, Excerpta Medica 1976, p6
6. Jefferson G: The pathology, diagnosis and treatment of intracranial saccular aneurysms. Proc Roy Soc Med 45:300, 1952
7. Hunt JR: The role of the carotid arteries, in the causation of vascular lesions of the brain, with remarks on certain features of the symptomatology. Amer J Med Sci 147:704, 1913
8. Moniz E, Lima A, de Lacerda R: Hémiplégies par thrombose de la carotide interne. Presse Medicale 45:977, 1937
9. Fisher M, Adams RD: Observations on brain embolism with special reference to the mechanism of hemorrhagic infarction. J Neuropath Exp Neurol 10:92, 1951
10. Fisher CM: Occlusion of the internal carotid artery. Arch Neurol Psychiat 65:346, 1951
11. Denny-Brown D: The changing pattern of neurologic medicine. New Eng J Med 246:839, 1952
12. Denny-Brown D: Symposium on specific methods of treatment; treatment of recurrent cerebrovascular symptoms, and the question of vasospasm. Med Clin N Amer 35:1457, 1951
13. Eastcott HHG, Pickering GW, Rob CG: Reconstruction of internal carotid artery in a patient with intermittent attacks of hemiplegia. Lancet 2:994, 1954
14. Strully KJ, Hurwitt ES, Blankenberg HW: Thromboendarterectomy for thrombosis of the internal carotid artery in the neck. J Neurosurg 10:474, 1953

15. Crawford ES, DeBakey ME, Fields WS, et al: Surgical treatment of arterial occlusive lesions in patients with cerebral artery insufficiency. Circulation 20:168, 1959
16. Cooley DA, Al-Naaman YD, Carton CA: Surgical treatment of arteriosclerotic occlusion of common carotid artery. J Neurosurg 13:500, 1956
17. Wylie EJ, Hein MF, Adams JE: Intracranial hemorrhage following surgical revascularisation for treatment of acute strokes. J Neurosurg 21:212, 1964
18. Edwards CH, Gordon NS, Rob CG: The surgical treatment of internal carotid artery occlusion. Quart J Med 29:67, 1960
19. Fisher CM: Observations of the fundus oculi in transient monocular blindness. Neurol 9:333, 1959.
20. Edwards CH, Gordon NS: Surgical treatment of narrowing of the internal carotid artery. Brit Med J 1:1289, 1962
21. Rose G: Strategy of prevention: lessons from cardiovascular disease. Brit Med J 282:1847, 1981

PART II

Basic Considerations

Christopher K. Zarins
Don P. Giddens
Seymour Glagov

2

Atherosclerotic Plaque Distribution and Flow Velocity Profiles in the Carotid Bifurcation

The carotid bifurcation is particularly prone to the development of atherosclerotic plaques.[1] Lesions are found in the carotid sinus early in life[2] and are a very common finding in adults.[3] Extensive and complex plaques may be present in the carotid bifurcation with little or no plaque formation in the proximal common carotid artery or distal internal carotid artery.[4] The particular susceptibility of this site to plaque deposition has been attributed to local hemodynamic conditions which exist at the carotid bifurcation. While flow studies in model bifurcations demonstrate regions of high flow velocity, low flow velocity, flow separation and disordered or turbulent flow,[5,6,7,8] there is as yet no consensus as to which specific hemodynamic condition potentiates plaque formation. Both high shear stress and fluctuation in shear stress[9] as well as low shear stress with boundary layer separation[10] have been implicated. We have studied the distribution of intimal thickening and early plaque formation in the human carotid bifurcation in individuals without symptoms of carotid artery disease and correlated the findings with hemodynamic observations in a model of the human carotid bifurcation under steady flow conditions. Our findings support the concept that carotid lesions localize in regions of low flow velocity and flow separation and not in regions of high velocity and elevated shear stress.

CAROTID BIFURCATION ATHEROSCLEROSIS

The extent, severity, and distribution of intimal thickening was studied in 14 human carotid bifurcations removed at autopsy. The age of the subjects ranged from 17 to 78 years. Each bifurcation was excised, cannulated, and rewarmed by perfusing the artery with buffered saline solution at body temperature (37°C). Normal vessel configuration was restored by increasing intraluminal pressure to 100 mmHg and maintaining that pressure during fixation with formalin.[11] The redistended and fixed carotid bifurcation was filled with a liquid radiopaque barium-gelatin mixture at 37°C which solidified at room temperature and formed a cast of the lumen. Multiple projection angiograms were then obtained to provide information on bifurcation angle, lumen contour, and vessel dimensions. In order to characterize early intimal lesion localization, this study was limited to carotid bifurcations without significant lumen stenosis on postmortem angiography.

Transverse sections for light microscopy were removed at standard locations in the common carotid, proximal internal, and distal internal carotid arteries (Fig. 2-1). Histologic sections were cut at 7 μm and stained with hematoxylin and eosin, as well as with the Gomori trichrome-aldehyde-fucshin and Verhoff VanGieson stains for connective tissue. Mounted tissue sections were projected onto a digitizing plate coupled to a micro-computer.

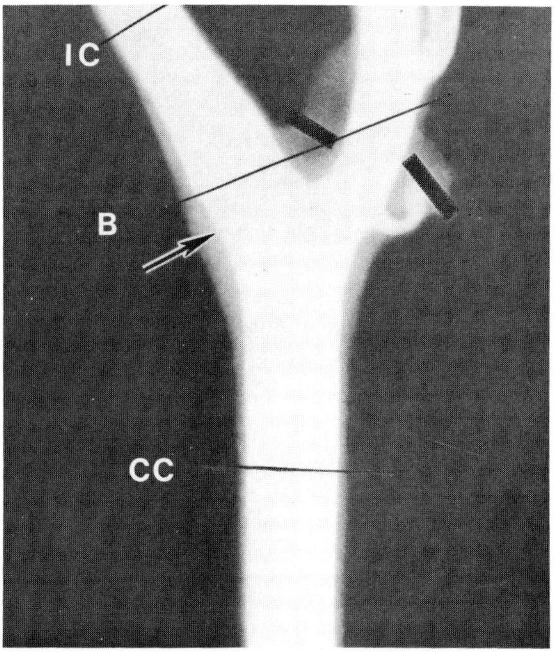

Figure 2-1. Postmortem angiogram of a pressure-perfusion fixed human carotid artery bifurcation. Note lumen contour irregularity (arrow) due to early plaque formation in the internal carotid artery sinus opposite the bifurcation flow divider. Lines denote standard tissue section sites in the common carotid (CC), proximal carotid bifurcation (B) and distal internal carotid (IC).

Contour tracings of the lumen, internal elastic lamina, and outer media were made and quantitative information was obtained using a program designed to compute lumen radius, plaque thickness, and wall thickness at selected positions around the vessel circumference.[12] Measurements were made on transverse sections of the common carotid artery and the distal internal carotid, and on sections at the level of the bifurcation which included both the internal and external carotid arteries. The *inner wall* of the internal carotid artery sinus at the level of the bifurcation was defined as that sector closest to the bifurcation (flow divider of the carotid artery), while the *outer wall* was defined as the sector lying at 180° opposite the bifurcation.

Intimal Plaque Thickness

In the *common carotid* artery, intimal thickness was uniform about the circumference of the vessel, and there was no eccentric atherosclerotic plaque deposition. In the *proximal internal carotid* artery, within the carotid sinus, intimal thickness along the inner wall was no different from that noted in the common carotid artery. Along the outer wall of the carotid sinus, however, there was a fourfold increase in intimal thickness compared to the inner wall at the same level ($p<.01$) (Table 2-1). This intimal thickening was often associated with the appearance of lipid containing atherosclerotic plaques (Fig. 2-2). Selective increase in intimal thickness and/or plaque formation in the carotid sinus opposite the flow divider was evident in 13 of the 14 specimens (93 percent), and was already present in the carotid artery of the 27-year-old-subject. Furthermore, the extent of intimal thickening along the outer wall appeared to be independent of age or gender. In the *distal internal carotid* artery, beyond the carotid sinus, intimal thickness was once again uniform about the circumference with little evidence of atheromatous plaque deposition.

Table 2-1
Carotid Bifurcation Intimal Thickness (mm)

Common Carotid	
Inner Wall	0.10 ± 0.02
Outer Wall	0.12 ± 0.03
Carotid Sinus	
Inner Wall	0.14 ± 0.06
Outer Wall	0.62 ± 0.14*
Internal Carotid	
Inner Wall	0.07 ± 0.02
Outer Wall	0.08 ± 0.04

± SEM
*$p<.01$

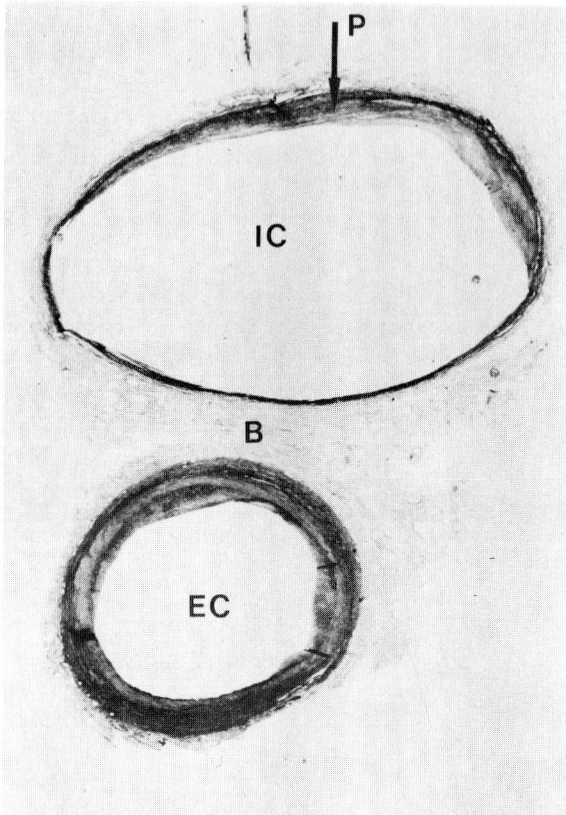

Figure 2-2. Transverse section though carotid bifurcation. Note the localized areas of intimal plaque (P) along the outer wall of the internal carotid artery (IC) opposite the bifurcation. There is no intimal thickening along the inner wall of the carotid sinus. The wall of the external carotid artery (EC) is thicker than the wall of the carotid sinus.

CAROTID BIFURCATION FLOW DYNAMICS

Using measurements obtained from 57 biplanar carotid angiograms in adults, two models of the human carotid bifurcation were constructed: a blown glass model for flow visualization and a machined plexiglass model for laser Doppler anemometry determinations of fluid velocity profiles.[5] Model dimensions were scaled from the angiograms, and the average bifurcation angle was computed from measurements of the biplanar views. A bifurcation angle of 50° was used in the models. The mean angle measured on the postmortem specimens was 45 ± 6°. Studies were conducted under steady flow conditions at varying Reynolds numbers (Re). The Reynolds number relates velocity, diameter, and viscosity and varies with pulsatile flow at differing points in the cardiac cycle. Studies were performed at Re 400 to reflect conditions likely to exist during diastolic flow, and studies were performed at Re 1200 to reflect conditions which might prevail during peak systolic flow. A flow division ratio between the internal and external carotid arteries of 70:30 was used in these studies.

Carotid Flow Visualization

Flow visualization was carried out using a hydrogen bubble technique.[13] Hydrogen bubbles were generated at a cathode wire stretched across the common carotid artery proximal to the bifurcation. The pattern of hydrogen

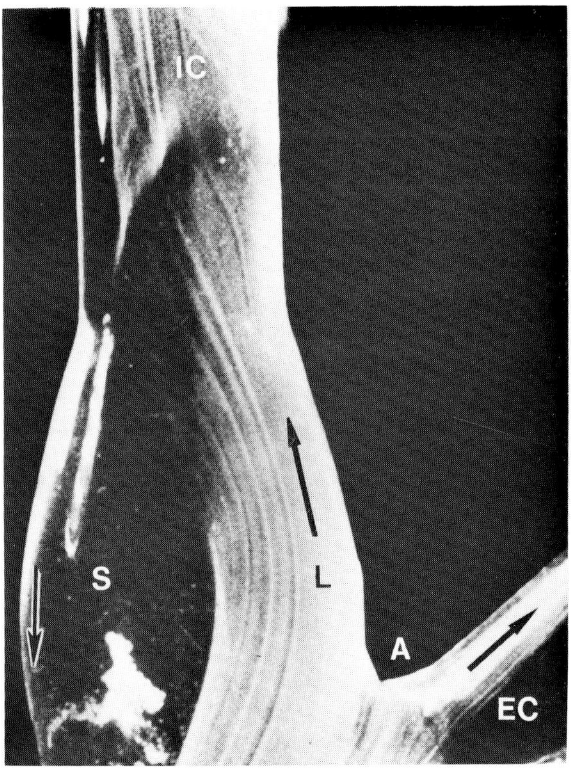

Figure 2-3. Hydrogen bubble flow visualization in a glass model carotid bifurcation. Note skewing of the velocity profile towards the apex (A) of the bifurcation and laminar flow along the inner wall of the carotid sinus. There is a large area of flow separation (S) along the outer wall of the carotid sinus. Arrow denotes direction of flow. Internal carotid (IC):external carotid (EC) flow division ratio is 70:30.

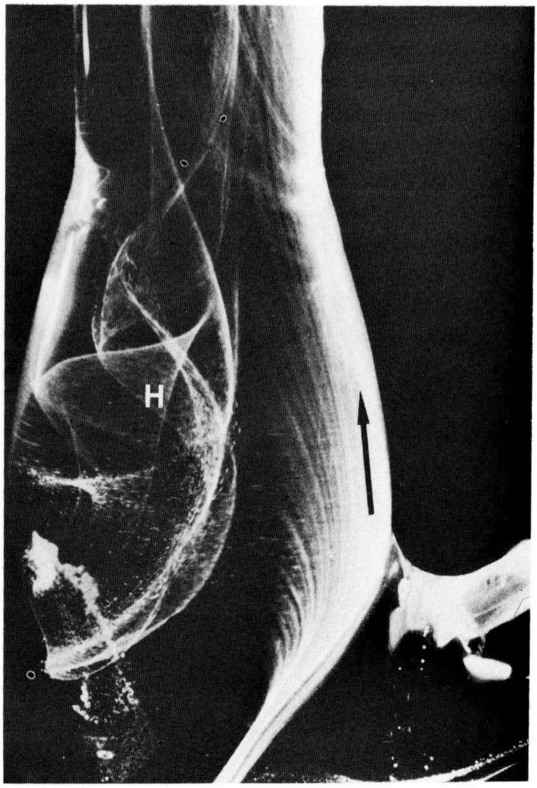

Figure 2-4. Hydrogen bubble flow visualization of the carotid bifurcation under conditions similar to that shown in Figure 2-3. The area of flow separation in the carotid sinus contains low flow velocities and complex flow patterns including counter-rotating helical (H) trajectories which carry the bubbles downstream. Arrow indicates direction of laminar flow along the inner wall of the carotid sinus.

bubble distribution downstream corresponded to alterations in the flow field induced by the bifurcation and carotid sinus. Rotation of the wire permitted flow visualization in any desired plane. Visualization studies revealed that the central lines of rapid flow were compressed toward the apex of the carotid bifurcation and inner wall of the internal carotid artery. Rapid, laminar flow was present along the *inner wall* of the carotid sinus (Fig. 2-3). Along the *outer wall* of the carotid sinus, a large area of flow separation developed which was characterized by a reversal of axial flow and fluid movement upstream along the outer wall. This, however, was not a zone of stasis and recirculation since there was no entrapment of bubbles. Rather, this was a zone of complex secondary and tertiary flow patterns, including counter-rotating helical trajectories, which carried the bubbles downstream (Fig. 2-4). In the *internal*

Table 2-2
Carotid Bifurcation Flow Velocity (cm/sec)

	Mean Flow (Re 400)	Peak Flow (Re 1200)
Common Carotid	43 ± 2	128 ± 4
Carotid Sinus		
Inner Wall	39 ± 2	115 ± 4
Outer Wall	-2 ± 1	-6 ± 2
Internal Carotid		
Inner Wall	47 ± 2	143 ± 4
Outer Wall	28 ± 2	82 ± 3

± est. exp. error

carotid artery distal to the sinus, circumferential flow reattachment occurred and a laminar flow profile redeveloped.

Flow Velocity Measurements

Flow velocity measurements were performed using a laser Doppler anemometer under flow conditions similar to those used in the flow visualization studies.[14] Velocity profiles were measured at cross-sections in the model which corresponded to the location of tissue sections in the cadaver carotid bifurcations.

In the *common carotid* artery there was a fully developed laminar flow velocity profile. At the carotid bifurcation, the axial flow velocity profile became skewed towards the apex of the bifurcation with the development of negative flow velocity along the outer wall of the carotid sinus. In the *internal carotid artery,* flow velocity along the *inner wall* of the sinus was similar to that observed in the common carotid artery at both Re 400 and Re 1200 (Table 2-2). Along the *outer wall* of the carotid sinus, however, flow velocity was greatly reduced and even reversed at both Re 400 and 1200. The tendency to reversal of flow was greater at Re 1200. *Distal* to the carotid sinus, where flow reattachment occurred, flow velocity along the inner wall of the carotid artery was similar to that observed in the common carotid artery. Along the outer wall, the velocity vector was once again directed cephalad both at Re 400 and Re 1200 and approached common carotid velocity values.

Wall Shear Stress

Fluid moving near a vessel wall creates a drag or shear stress upon the surface of the lumen which is proportional to the velocity gradient at the wall. From the laser Doppler velocity profiles, the velocity gradient at the wall was extrapolated and using appropriate viscosity and scaling factors, wall shear stresses were calculated.[14] In the *common carotid* artery, wall shear stresses at both diastolic (Re 400) and peak systolic (Re 1200) flow rates were relatively

Table 2-3
Carotid Bifurcation Shear Stress (dynes/cm²)

	Mean Flow (Re 400)	Peak Flow (Re 1200)
Common Carotid	10 ± 1	29 ± 3
Carotid Sinus		
Inner Wall	23 ± 5	203 ± 61
Outer Wall	0 ± 2	-2 ± 2
Internal Carotid		
Inner Wall	50 ± 10	565 ± 170
Outer Wall	39 ± 8	50 ± 10

± est. exp. error.

low (Table 2-3). At the apex of the flow divider and along the *inner wall* of the carotid sinus, however, shear stress was high and was accentuated at peak systolic flow rates, due to the very high velocity gradient at the vessel wall. Along the *outer wall* of the carotid sinus, shear stress was very low, principally due to the low flow velocities at this location. In the internal carotid artery beyond the carotid sinus, outer wall shear stress was again restored to common carotid levels. Along the inner wall of the distal internal carotid artery, calculated wall shear stress at Re 1200 was 565 dynes/cm^2 which exceeded the value for shear stress reported by Fry to cause endothelial damage.[9]

RELATION BETWEEN FLUID DYNAMICS AND PLAQUE LOCALIZATION

The model carotid bifurcation contained well-defined regions in which there were marked differences in flow patterns, velocities, and shear stresses (Fig. 2-5). The apex of the bifurcation, inner wall of the carotid sinus, and distal internal carotid artery were exposed to high velocity laminar flow and high wall shear stress. These regions in the cadaver carotid bifurcations had little or no intimal thickening and were free of plaque formation. The outer wall of the carotid sinus, on the other hand, was a region of flow separation, low flow velocity, low shear stress, and disordered flow patterns. Early, localized intimal thickening and plaque formation was noted in this region of the carotid bifurcation.

Similar patterns of plaque localization along the outer wall of the carotid sinus with little plaque formation at the bifurcation flow divider have been noted by others studying more extensive carotid atherosclerosis[4,15] and can be seen on cerebral angiography in patients with severe carotid stenosis.[16] Examination of severe lesions removed by carotid endarterectomy confirms the selective deposition of plaque in the outer wall of the sinus with relative sparing of the inner wall (Fig. 2-6).

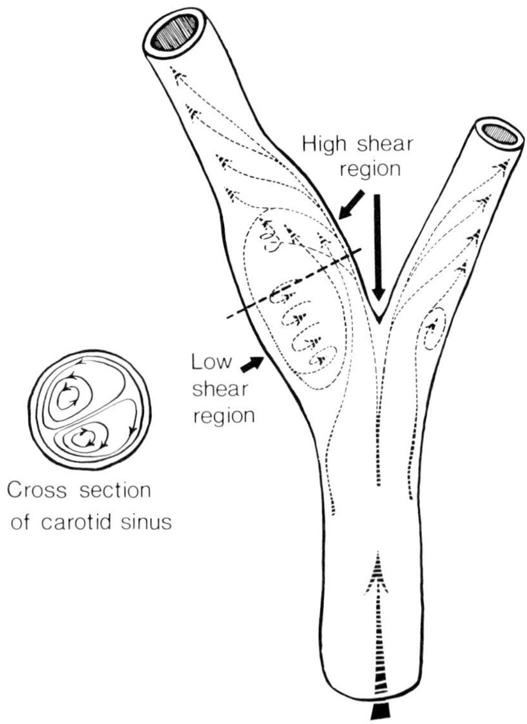

Figure 2-5. Diagrammatic representation of flow patterns in the carotid bifurcation. The inner wall of the carotid sinus is a region of high shear stress, while the outer wall is a low shear region.

These findings suggest a close relation between intimal plaque formation and regions of flow separation and low shear stress.[17] Caro et al. have suggested that low shear rates may adversely affect transport mechanisms away from the wall and result in the accummulation of metabolic products and lipids at the vessel wall.[10] Flow separation has also been shown to be a site for the accummulation of platelet aggregates in vitro.[18] Static zones and boundary layer separation have been demonstrated radiographically at the outer wall of the carotid sinus in patients with intracranial disease, and Fox and Hugh have suggested that atheromatous disease develops in these areas of stasis.[7] LoGerfo et al. using a plexiglass model carotid bifurcation and dye injection techniques also have demonstrated boundary layer separation in the outer wall of the sinus and related this finding to plaque formation.[8]

These findings are in contrast to the suggestion by Fry[9] and others[19,20] that high wall shear stresses may produce endothelial damage and may, thus, predispose to plaque formation. While it may be possible under certain experimental circumstances to elevate shear stress in vivo and cause endothelial injury,[9,19] there is no convincing evidence that endothelial injury

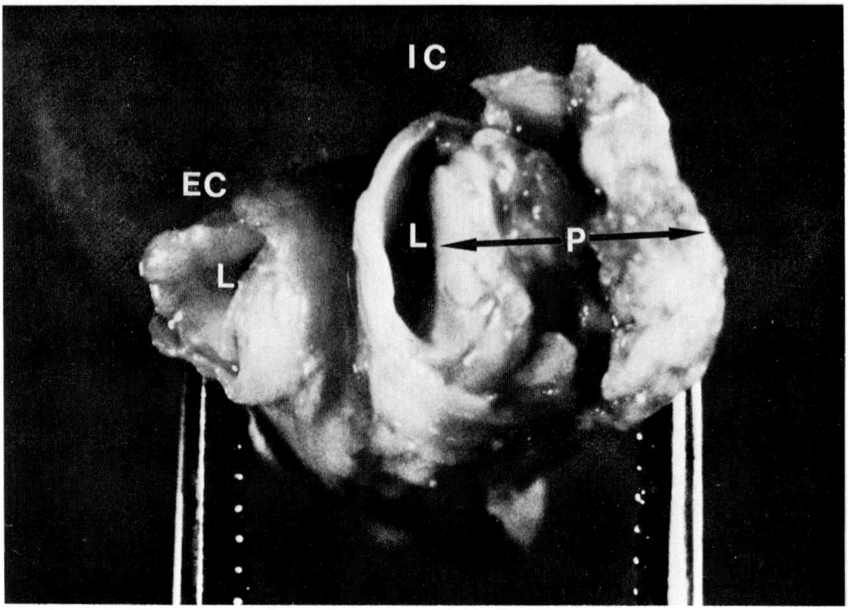

Figure 2-6. Carotid plaque removed during carotid endarterectomy. The plaque is viewed on end with external carotid (EC) and internal carotid (IC) branches visible. Note extensive plaque (P) on outer wall of carotid sinus and thin intima along the inner wall. The lumen is indicated by (L).

results in plaque formation. Although shear stresses as high as those shown to produce endothelial damage in vivo appear to exist in the carotid bifurcation, these areas were spared from plaque formation. The observation that high shear areas are less likely to develop plaques is further supported by experimental evidence from monkeys with aortic coarctations fed an atherogenic diet. Flow velocity and shear stress were greatly increased within the coarct channel, but the channel was found to be free of plaque formation despite extensive plaque development elsewhere in the same aorta.[21]

DISCUSSION

Precise description of blood flow through the human carotid artery is difficult due to the complex geometry of the bifurcation, the pulsatile nature of flow, distensibility of the arterial wall, and non-Newtonian characteristics of blood. Of these factors, bifurcation geometry has the most dominant influence on the flow field, while the non-Newtonian characteristics have the least effect. We modeled the specific geometry of the human carotid bifurcation but utilized a rigid model, a Newtonian fluid, and a steady flow system. Although vessel distensibility is an important factor in pulse wave propagation, its effect on local velocity profiles is small and should not greatly alter our observations. Similarly, use of a Newtonian fluid should have little effect. The assumption of steady flow, however, may lead to inaccuracies. To address this problem, we used a range of Reynolds numbers and flow conditions to simulate conditions as they may exist at varying points in the cardiac cycle. At each Reynolds number studied, there was a region of flow separation in the carotid sinus, and this region increased in size with increasing Reynolds numbers and decreasing flow through the internal carotid. Our own preliminary experiments utilizing pulsatile flow reveal an area of flow separation in the carotid sinus in the same location as seen with steady flow. Despite variation in the point of flow reattachment and accentuation of flow field fluctuations, the qualitative changes and relative velocity profiles were similar under both steady flow and pulsatile flow conditions. LoGerfo has also found little difference in the qualitative findings in the carotid bifurcation flow field between steady and pulsatile flow.[8] Thus, it is unlikely that further refinement of studies using pulsatile flow will alter the general conclusion that plaques tend to develop in areas of flow separation and low shear and not in areas of laminar flow and high shear.

CLINICAL IMPLICATIONS

If flow separation, low shear stress, and flow instabilities are indeed predisposing factors to plaque deposition, intimal thickening and plaque formation may themselves promote further flow disorder and accelerate the rate of plaque formation. Slow flow and turbulence in the carotid bifurcation may, in addition, influence surface characteristics on existing carotid plaques and may contribute to the tendency for such lesions to ulcerate, embolize, or thrombose and lead to symptomatic cerebrovascular disease.

Several implications with regard to operative therapy for carotid artery disease are suggested by our findings. Removal of a large carotid plaque by endarterectomy may result in an increase in carotid sinus lumen diameter. A large carotid sinus would result in a large region of flow separation which may favor recurrent plaque deposition. Indeed, we have seen recurrent carotid stenosis several years after endarterectomy due to atherosclerotic plaque formation in the same carotid sinus location as the initial intimal lesion. In addition, if carotid artery closure is performed using a vein or Dacron patch angioplasty, a large sinus diameter may result and create a low velocity region which may promote the development of flow separation. Whether this will have a bearing on lesion reappearance in the future is unclear but merits further study and attention.

REFERENCES

1. Schwartz CJ, Mitchell JRA: Observations on localization of arterial plaques. Circulation Research 11:63, 1962
2. Peterson RE, Livingston KE, Escobar A: Development and distribution of gross atherosclerotic lesions at cervical carotid bifurcation. Neurology 10:955, 1960
3. McGill HC, et al: General findings of the International Atherosclerosis Project. Laboratory Investigation 18:498, 1968
4. Heath D, Smith P, Harris P, et al: The atherosclerotic human carotid sinus. Journal of Pathology 110:49, 1973
5. Balasubramanian K, Giddens, DP, Mabon RF: Steady flow at the carotid bifurcation, in Schneck DJ, (ed): Bio-Fluid Mech, vol. 6, New York, Plenum Press, 1980, p 475
6. Ferguson GG, Roach MR: Flow conditions at bifurcations as determined in glass models with reference to the focal distribution of vascular lesions, in Bergel DH, (ed): Cardiovascular Fluid Dynamics, vol. 2, New York, Academic Press, 1972
7. Fox JA, Hugh AE: Static zones in the internal carotid artery: correlation with boundary layer separation and stasis in model flows. British Journal Radiology 43:370, 1976
8. LoGerfo FW, Nowak MD, Quist WC, et al: Flow studies in a model carotid bifurcation. Arteriosclerosis 1:235, 1981
9. Fry DL: Acute vascular endothelial changes associated with increased blood velocity gradients. Circ Res 22:165, 1968
10. Caro CG, Fitzgerald JM, Schroter RC: Atheroma and arterial wall shear: Observation, correlation and proposal of a shear dependent mass transfer mechanism for atherogenesis. Proc R Soc Lond (Biol) 117:109, 1971
11. Wolinsky H, Glagov S: Structural basis for the static mechanical properties of the aortic media. Circ Res 14:400, 1964
12. Glagov S, Grande J, Vesselinovitch D, et al: Quantitation of cells and fibers in histologic sections of arterial walls: Advantages of contour tracing on a digitizing plate, in McDonald TF, Chandler AB, (eds): Connective Tissues in Arterial Pulmonary Disease, New York, Springer-Verlag, 1981, p 57
13. Bharadvaj BK, Mabon RF, Giddens DP: Steady flow in a model of the human carotid bifurcation, Part I-flow visualization. J Biomechanics, 1982 (in press)
14. Bharadvaj BK, Mabon RF, Giddens DP: Steady flow in a model of the human carotid bifurcation, Part II-laser Doppler anemometer measurements. J Biomechanics, 1982 (in press)
15. Solbert LA, Eggen DA: Localization and sequence of development of atherosclerotic lesions in the carotid and vertebral arteries. Circulation 43:711, 1971
16. Bauer RB, et al: Arteriographic study of sites, incidence and treatment of atherosclerotic cerebro-vascular lesions. Neurology 12:698, 1962
17. Zarins CK, Giddens DP, Balasubramanian K, et al: Carotid plaques localize in regions of low flow velocity and shear stress. Circ 64(suppl. IV):44, 1981
18. Parmentier EM, Morton WA, Petschek HE: Platelet aggregate formation in a region of separated blood flow. Phys Fluids 20:2012, 1977
19. Joris E, Zand T, Majno G: Hydrodynamic injury of the endothelium in acute aortic stenosis. Am J Path 106:394, 1982
20. Reidy MA, Bowyer DE: Scanning electron microscopy of arteries. The morphology of aortic endothelium in haemodynamically stressed areas associated with branches. Atherosclerosis 26:181, 1977
21. Zarins CK, Bomberger RA, Glagov S: Local effects of stenoses: Increased flow velocity inhibits atherogenesis. Circulation 64(suppl. II):221, 1981

Edwin W. Salzman

3

Platelet-Vessel Interaction in Cerebrovascular Disease: the Role of Prostaglandins

It is now established that platelets play a major role in the genesis and progression of arteriosclerosis. Although the contribution of blood elements to arteriosclerosis was suggested by German pathologists in the 19th century and the contribution of plasma coagulation to this process was emphasized by Duguid[1] more than 30 years ago, the significant involvement of platelets and the mechanism of their participation have been appreciated only more recently.

The contribution of platelets to arteriosclerosis may take several forms:

1. Platelets may adhere to one another and to damaged or diseased vessel walls to produce a partially or totally occluding thrombus, which is often the terminal event for progressive arterial obliterative disease in that vessel.
2. Dislodgement of a thrombus from the site of its formation or aggregation of platelets suspended in the blood may give rise to remote embolization.
3. Through secretion of vasoactive amines stored in specialized granules within platelets or by synthesis of vasoconstrictive metabolic products, platelets may contribute to arterial spasm, which aggravates the narrowing of the vessel lumen produced by arteriosclerosis.
4. A growth factor for smooth muscle cells may be secreted by platelets in response to their interaction with collagenous components of damaged vessel walls, leading to intimal thickening, which is the first visible manifestation of the arteriosclerotic lesion.

Platelets normally circulate as discrete cytoplasmic fragments that adhere neither to each other nor to the healthy endothelial lining of the vessel wall. Exposed to underlying layers of the vessel from which endothelial cells have been removed, however, as a result of abrasion by mechanical trauma or by poorly understood chemical injury (for example, in homocystinemia or hypercholesterolemia), platelets adhere to subendothelial connective tissue, chiefly to microfibrils and other components containing collagen [2] (Fig. 3-1). The initial adhesion of platelets to collagenous tissue is facilitated by a macromolecule, von Willebrand's factor,[3] a large protein complex deficient or, less often, functionally defective in the plasma of patients with an inherited autosomal bleeding disorder, von Willebrand's disease. The von Willebrand's factor contains a subunit with coagulant activity that is abnormal in patients with hemophilia. It may be noted parenthetically that a strain of pigs with a hereditary bleeding disorder that is apparently identical to von Willebrand's disease is resistant to the experimental production of arteriosclerosis by vascular injury and feeding of an atherogenic diet.[4]

Contact with collagen at the surface of a damaged vessel is enhanced by spreading and flattening of the platelet, which increase the area of contiguity and allow cooperative interactions of multiple platelet-collagen contact points.[5] Through mechanisms that are not entirely understood but that probably involve rearrangement of receptors in the plasma membrane, these events lead to reordering of the platelet cytoskeleton.[6] It is thought that there is a rise in the cytoplasmic ionized calcium concentration, which activates contractile proteins whose actions then result in central migration of storage granules to sites in intimate contact with an intracellular canalicular system

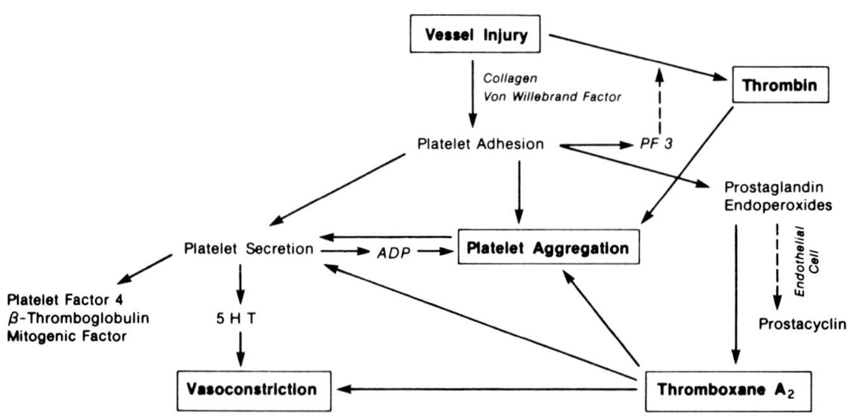

Figure 3-1. Mechanism of platelet interaction with the vessel wall. For details, see text. (From Lewis JL and Salzman EW: Antithrombotic therapy, in Rutherford R: Vascular Surgery. Philadelphia, PA, W.B. Saunders Co., 1982. In press. By permission.)

into which the contents of the granules are secreted and from which they enter the surrounding plasma.[7,8]

Many of the secreted substances have important biological activity. They include serotonin (5-hydroxy-tryptamine or 5-HT, a vasoconstrictor), adenosine diphosphate (ADP, which itself activates platelets and causes their aggregation), catecholamines, fibrinogen, calcium and potassium ions, an antiheparin (termed platelet factor 4), β-thromboglobulin (a platelet-specific protein of uncertain function), a mitogenic factor for smooth muscle cells (platelet-derived growth factor or PDGF), ATP, fibronectin, coagulation factor V, and probably other substances as well.[9] Accompanying these secretory phenomena is the acquisition by the platelet of the ability to accelerate blood coagulation, a property termed "platelet factor 3" (PF 3), which appears to be due to adsorption and local concentration of activated plasma protein clotting factors on the platelet surface.[10] There is increasing evidence that some of the clotting proteins are actually stored and secreted by the platelet itself.

In the course of this reaction, probably as a result of a local or generalized cytoplasmic elevation of the concentration of ionized calcium, phospholipase enzymes in the platelet are activated [11,12] (Fig. 3-2). Their hydrolytic action releases arachidonic acid from storage sites in their substrate membrane phospholipids, chiefly phosphatidylcholine and phosphatidylinositol. The free arachidonic acid then sets off down a metabolic pathway involving first its

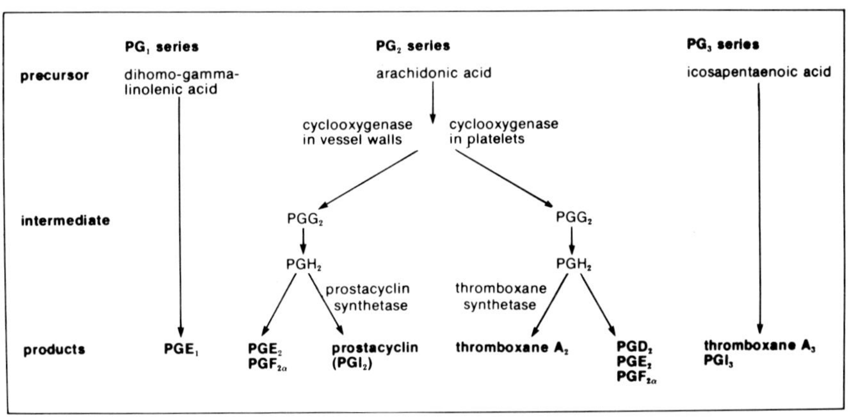

Figure 3-2. Prostaglandin precursors and products. In man, arachidonic acid (4 double bonds) is the major precursor and gives rise to prostaglandins of the PG_2 series as well as prostacyclin and thromboxane A_2.

Dihomogamma-linolenic acid (3 double bonds) and icosapentaenoic acid (5 double bonds) have products of the PG_1 or PG_3 series, which are platelet-inhibiting. (From Lewis JL, MacIntyre DE, Salzman EW: The role of prostaglandins in atherosclerosis and thrombosis. J Cardiovasc Med 6:601–614, 1981. By permission.)

reaction with molecular oxygen through the activity of the enzyme cyclo-oxygenase to form prostaglandin endoperoxides (PGG_2 and PGH_2) and then conversion of these labile compounds to a variety of lipid products of great diversity. These include the "stable prostaglandins," namely prostaglandin E_2, $F_{2\alpha}$, and D_2, the last of which is a potent inhibitor of platelet function, and, more important, thromboxane A_2, a powerful stimulant of platelet aggregation and secretion and a vasoconstrictor of impressive potency. There is evidence[13] that the generation of thromboxane A_2 is a final common path in the platelet response to a large number of agonists. For example, platelet stimuli as disparate as ADP, thrombin, collagen, and epinephrine all lead to production of thromboxane A_2. Certain of these agonists appear to owe most of their platelet aggregating ability to this action. Recruitment of additional mechanisms peculiar to specific stimuli also occurs, but the contribution of thromboxane formation is important.

Among the products secreted by platelets is adenosine diphosphate (ADP), which has for over twenty years been recognized as a powerful stimulant to platelet aggregation.[14] The action of ADP results in an alteration in platelet shape from disc to spiculated sphere and in exposure on the platelet surface of receptor sites for fibrinogen.[15] Platelets normally peacefully coexist in native blood indifferent to this dumb-bell-shaped protein molecule which surrounds them in high concentration. However, the platelet surface altered by the action of ADP acquires binding sites of high affinity for fibrinogen, and these sites, which apparently contain critical glycoproteins,[16] form a close attachment with fibrinogen that appears to be essential to platelet aggregation. Other stimulants to platelet aggregation, such as epinephrine and thrombin, also induce binding sites for fibrinogen, probably at least in part through the action of ADP secreted by the platelet. The mechanism of action of fibrinogen in promoting platelet aggregation is not established. The asymmetric molecule is probably long enough to bridge between adjacent platelets, but it is not certain that this is its role. It is, however, known that conversion to fibrin is not necessary.

Platelet participation in arteriosclerosis is also influenced by the biochemistry of the vessel wall. Pathways for oxidation of arachidonic acid also exist in endothelial cells, but, in contrast to the case in the platelet, the chief product of prostaglandin endoperoxide conversion is not the platelet stimulant thromboxane A_2 but rather a powerful inhibitor of platelet function and a vasodilator, prostacyclin (PGI_2).[17] Increasing evidence suggests the existence of a physiologic balance between the platelet stimulant and pressor, thromboxane A_2, and the platelet antagonist and depressor, prostaglandin I_2, the one derived from platelets and the other from vessel walls. In addition, it has been shown[18] that prostaglandin endoperoxides of platelet origin can be metabolized by the vessel wall and can contribute to the production of prostacyclin, a potentially effective negative feedback control on the platelet's aggressive tendencies. Other possibilities for feed-back control are suggested by the modulating effects of substances secreted by platelets, which may alter prostacyclin production by blood vessels. Two proteins contained in specific storage organelles ("alpha granules") in platelets have opposite effects: platelet-derived growth factor is reported to stimulate PGI_2 formation [19] and β-thromboglobulin to inhibit it.[20] Serotonin, secreted from other storage sites in platelets ("dense granules"), is also reputed to increase prostaglandin production by endothelial cells.

Many influences that operate as risk factors for arteriosclerosis can be explained by their ability to alter arachidonic acid metabolism in a direction consistent with their effect on thrombotic processes. It should be noted that Duncan et al. [21] have determined that risk factors previously identified with coronary arteriosclerosis (e.g., smoking, diabetes, hypertension, etc.) apply as well to carotid artery stenosis. For example, in diabetes mellitus, platelet stimulation leads to exaggerated formation of thromboxane A_2,[22] but prostacyclin production by blood vessels is reduced, compared to non-diabetics.[23] In uremia, in which platelet function is typically depressed, endothelial prostacyclin formation is enhanced [24]; presumably an explanation for the propensity of patients on dialysis to develop accelerated arteriosclerosis lies elsewhere. The ratio of thromboxane/prostacyclin production is tilted in favor of the former in patients with hypercholesterolemia.[25] Inhaled products of cigarette smoking enhance platelet thromboxane production by platelets and reduce vascular PGI_2 synthesis [26]; the latter is also a feature of advancing age [27]; the mechanisms are not understood.

In contrast, dietary manipulation which leads to substitution of ω:3 or ω:5 fatty acids for arachidonic acid (ω:4) may have an antithrombotic (and arteriosclerosis-suppressive) effect. For example, ingestion of large quantities of cold water fish results in replacement of arachidonic acid by icosapentaenoic acid in cell membranes [28]: the oxidation products of this ω:5 fatty acid do not stimulate platelet aggregation.[29] This phenomenon may account for the striking freedom from arteriosclerosis enjoyed by Greenland Eskimos.

Decreased levels of urinary prostacyclin metabolites (e.g., prostaglandin 6-keto-$F_{1\alpha}$), indicative of reduced PGI_2 synthesis, but normal urinary thromboxane B_2 (the stable metabolite of thromboxane A_2) are reported in patients with essential hypertension.[30] Such findings would be consistent with the recognized acceleration of arteriosclerosis in hypertensives. The well-known unfavorable effects of administration of estrogen on vascular disease may be an additional illustration of altered prostacyclin output.[31]

The complex plaque characteristic of arteriosclerosis may also contribute to its own progression. There is evidence [32] that arterial segments afflicted with such lesions are below par in their ability to synthesize prostacyclin and thus might have a relatively feeble capacity to prevent the local deposition of thrombus on an ulcerated plaque.

There are many reports that platelets are more reactive, on the average, in patients with vascular disease than in the normal population: i.e., that they respond to lower concentrations of stimulating substances such as ADP and that their response to a standard dose of an agonist is enhanced, both biochemically through the production of increased amounts of thromboxane A_2 [33] and functionally through more profound platelet aggregation and through secretion of increased amounts of platelet constituents.[34,35] There is also evidence of increased plasma levels of platelet-derived substances (e.g., β-thromboglobulin and platelet factor 4) in patients with various forms of arteriosclerosis, particularly in association with its more acute manifestations such as myocardial infarction[36] and unstable angina pectoris.[37] Increased plasma levels of these substances indicate platelet activation somewhere in the patient's circulation. Such observations often apply, of course, only to the average behavior of a population, and assessment of these traits may find them entirely normal in any particular patient. Their value is therefore not necessarily in diagnosis but more likely in providing clues to pathogenesis. Even here the situation is clouded, for there is a major cart vs. horse problem, and demonstration of platelet activation may not distinguish cause from effect.

It is also claimed that survival of platelets in the circulation is shorter than normal in patients with arteriosclerotic vascular disease,[38] presumably because of accelerated consumption of platelets interacting with deendothelialized plaques. There are also reports [39,40] that thrombotic disorders are sometimes associated with circulating aggregates of platelets (microembolism); this contention has given rise to considerable controversy. In many such instances, the demonstrated clumps of aggregated platelets may actually have formed in the collection apparatus during blood sampling; it is doubtful that aggregates of more than a few platelets could successfully traverse a capillary bed.

In cerebrovascular disease, the platelet's repertoire of prothrombotic actions is fully displayed. Arteriosclerotic plaques in the extracranial carotid artery or in the middle cerebral or other arteries within the skull are an obvious cause of transient cerebral ischemia and stroke by impeding flow in the narrowed vessels. They may owe their existence to earlier platelet interaction with a subtly injured vessel wall. If they ulcerate, they may serve as a nidus for platelet thrombus and embolism, which leads to transient cerebral ischemic attacks, retinal emboli with amaurosis fugax, and stroke.[41] By scintillation scanning, Davis et al. [42] demonstrated localization of ^{111}Indium-labelled platelets in the region of ulcerated atherosclerotic carotid plaques. There is also reason to believe that spasm of intracranial arteries may in some circumstances be induced by substances of platelet origin.[43]

Preston et al. [44] described transient neurological dysfunction in 12 patients with thrombocytosis and no other apparent explanation for their symptoms. They attributed their findings to "spontaneous" platelet aggregation and microembolism. The symptoms abated when the patients received drugs that inhibit platelet aggregation (see below). Al-Mefty and associates[45] reported a series of 22 patients with TIAs in whom there were no angiographically-detectable cerebrovascular disease, no discernable intracranial lesions, and no other apparent source of emboli, and in whom the only abnormality detected was platelet hyperreactivity. Treatment with antiplatelet drugs led to subsidence of symptoms. These observations are of interest in view of the report of deBono and Warlow[46] that, among 117 patients studied because of symptoms of transient cerebral or retinal ischemia, 25 percent had no angiographic, echocardiographic, or other evidence of cardiovascular disease.

On the other hand, Baconnet et al.[47] found no consistent pattern of unusually aggressive platelet activity in 101 patients with a history of TIA or stroke, including 19 in whom a stroke occurred less than 12 days before study. There was a modest increase in sensitivity to epinephrine of platelets from patients with recent stroke; the authors attributed this to a secondary platelet response to ischemic tissue. Platelet thrombosis can, of course, lead to arterial occlusion and distal ischemia or infarction, but it is also known[48] that platelet thrombosis may occur secondarily as a result of ischemic tissue necrosis, presumably in response to platelet-activating substances that originate in the damaged tissue. Gaudet and Levine[49] have demonstrated the production of prostaglandins by ischemic brain tissue in gerbils when blood flow was restored after bilateral carotid occlusion. It appeared necessary to have sufficient residual circulation to furnish molecular oxygen for oxygenation of arachidonic acid by cyclo-oxygenase. Both vasodilatory (e.g., PGI_2) and vasoconstrictive (e.g., thromboxane A_2) products were formed; a possible explanation is thus available no matter what net effect on the circulation is observed.

Pharmacological intervention through the administration of drugs that suppress platelet activity is a popular approach to the control of arteriosclerosis and its complications.[50] Several such drugs have been evaluated in cerebrovascular disease and will be discussed in more detail later in this conference. Of the agents available, aspirin and sulfinpyrazone have been most extensively evaluated. Both are thought to owe their principal antithrombotic activity to their capacity to inhibit platelet function. This resides in their ability to block conversion of arachidonic acid to endoperoxides and subsequently to thromboxane A_2 by inhibition of the enzyme cyclo-oxygenase. Among the other drugs available are inhibitors of cyclic AMP phosphodiesterase, such as dipyridamole, which block the breakdown of cyclic AMP within the platelet and thus raise the intracellular level of this nucleotide. In so doing, they stimulate and reinforce the biochemical effect of the platelet-inhibitory prostaglandins, including prostacyclin, which block platelet activity by stimulating adenylate cyclase, the enzyme that converts ATP to cyclic AMP. Elevation of platelet cyclic AMP, whether by stimulation of its formation or suppression of its destruction, is a general mechanism for inhibition of platelet activity, probably at multiple biochemical sites where it opposes the action or lowers the concentration of ionized calcium.[51]

Prostaglandins themselves are also promising as antithrombotic drugs. Prostacyclin prevents platelet adhesion and thrombus formation on exposed vascular subendothelium.[52,53] By inhibition of platelet aggregation, infusion of prostacyclin has been shown to prevent thrombotic occlusion of narrowed coronary arteries.[54] Vasodilation may also contribute to prostacyclin's antithrombotic effects, but unfortunately this action also may limit the clinical usefulness of PGI_2, since facial flushing and hypertension are unpleasant side effects of its administration. Stable analogs of PGE_2 have been developed; however, efforts to develop prostacyclin-like compounds with a greater therapeutic margin have so far been unsuccessful, as it has not been possible to separate the vasodilating and anti-platelet activities.

In addition to their acute effect on thrombus formation, prostaglandins and agents that alter prostaglandin production may be useful for their long-term effects on progression of arteriosclerosis. Aspirin and dipyridamole have been shown to reduce the intimal thickening that characteristically develops in aorto-coronary saphenous vein bypass grafts.[55] This lesion is thought to be analogous to the early smooth muscle hyperplastic stage in the genesis of the arteriosclerotic plaque. Evidence that the latter lesion can be suppressed in primates by aspirin has been provided by Pick.[56]

REFERENCES

1. Duguid JB: Thrombosis as a factor in the pathogenesis of coronary atherosclerosis. J Path Bact 58:207, 1946
2. Baumgartner HR, Muggli R, Tschopp TB, et al: Platelet adhesion, release and aggregation in flowing blood: Effect of surface properties and platelet function. Throm Hemos 35:124, 1976
3. Weiss HJ, Turitto VT, Baumgartner HR: Effect of shear rate on platelet interaction with subendothelium in citrated and native blood. I. Shear-dependent decrease of adhesion in von Willebrand's disease and the Bernard-Soulier syndrome. J Lab Clin Med 92:750, 1978
4. Santoro SA, Cunningham LW: Fibronectin and the multiple interaction model for platelet-collagen-adhesion. Proc Nat Acad Sci USA 76:2644, 1979
5. Fuster V, Bowie EJC, Lewis JC, et al: Resistance to arteriosclerosis in pigs with von Willebrand's disease. J Clin Invest 61:722, 1978
6. White JG: Fine structural alterations induced in platelets by adenosine diphosphate. Blood 31:604, 1968
7. Detwiler TC, Charo IF, Feinman RD: Evidence that calcium regulates platelet function. Throm Hemos 40:207, 1978
8. White JG: Indentification of platelet secretion in the electron microscope. Series Haemat 6:429, 1973

9. Fukami MH, Salganikoff L: Human platelet storage organelles: A review. Throm Haemo 38:963, 1977
10. Niewiarowski S. Proteins secreted by the platelets. Thromb Haemo 38:924, 1977
11. Feinstein MB: The role of calcium in blood platelet function, in Weiss GB (ed): Calcium in Drug Action, New York, Plenum Publishing Corp, 1978, p. 197
12. Walenga RW, Opas EE, Feinstein MB: Differential effects of calmodulin antagonists on phospholipases A_2 and C in thrombin-stimulated platelets. J Bio Chem 256:12523, 1981
13. Myers KM, Seachord CL, Holmsen H, et al: The dominant role of thromboxane formation in secondary aggregation of platelets. Nature 282:331, 1980
14. Gaarder A, Jonsen J, Laland S: Adenosine diphosphate in red cells as a factor in the adhesiveness of human blood platelets. Nature 192:531, 1961
15. Bennett JS, Vilaire G: Exposure of platelet fibrinogen receptors by ADP and epinephrine. J Clin Invest 64:1393, 1979
16. Nurden AT, Caen JP: Specific role for platelet glycoproteins in platelet function. Nature 255:720, 1975
17. Moncada S, Vane JR: Arachidonic acid metabolites and the interactions between platelets and blood vessel walls. NEJM 300:1142, 1979
18. Marcus AJ, Weksler BB, Jaffe EA, et al: Synthesis of prostacyclin from platelet-derived endoperoxides by cultured human endothelial cells. J Clin Invest 66:979, 1980
19. Coughlin SR, Moskowitz MA, Zetter BR, et al: Platelet-dependent stimulation of prostacyclin synthesis by platelet-derived growth factor. Nature, 288:600, 1980
20. Hope W, Martin TJ, Chesterman CN, et al: Human β-thromboglobulin inhibits PGI_2 production and binds to a specific site in bovine aortic endothelial cells. Nature 282:210, 1979
21. Duncan GW, Lees RS, Ojemann RG, et al: Concomitants of atherosclerotic carotid artery stenosis. Stroke 8:665, 1977
22. Ziboh VA, Maruta H, Lord J, et al: Increased biosynthesis of thromboxane A_2 by diabetic platelets. Euro J Clin Invest 9:223, 1979
23. Silberbauer K, Schernthaner G, Sinzinger H, et al: Decreased vascular prostacyclin in juvenile-onset diabetes. NEJM 300:366, 1979
24. De Gaetano G, Livio M, Donati MB, et al: Platelet and vascular prostaglandins in uraemia, thrombotic microangiopathy and pre-eclampsia. Phil Trans R Soc Lond B 294:339, 1981
25. Stuart MJ, Gerrard JM, White JG: Effect of cholesterol on production of thromboxane B_2 by platelets in vitro. NEJM 302:6, 1980
26. Hirsch PD, Campbell WB, Willerson JT, et al: Prostaglandins and ischemic heart disease. Am J Med 71:1009, 1981
27. Kent RS, Kitchell BB, Shand DG, et al: The ability of vascular tissue to produce prostacyclin decreases with age. Prostaglandins, 21:483, 1981
28. Seiss W, Scherer B, Bohlig B, et al: Platelet-membrane fatty acids, platelet aggregation, and thromboxane formation during a mackerel diet. Lancet 1:441, 1980
29. Needleman P, Raz A, Minkes MS, et al: Triene prostaglandins: Prostacyclin and thromboxane biosynthesis and unique biological properties. Proc Natl Acad Sci USA 76:944, 1979
30. Grose JH, Lebel M, Gbeassor FM: Variations in urinary metabolites of prostacyclin and thromboxane A_2 in essential hypertension (abst). Clin Res 28:685A, 1980
31. Elam MB, Lipscomb GE, Chesney CM, et al: Effect of synthetic estrogen on platelet aggregation and vascular release of PGI_2-like material in the rabbit. Prostaglandins 20:1039, 1980
32. D'Angelo V, Villa S, et al: Defective fibrinolytic and prostacyclin-like activity in human atheromatous plaques. Throm Haemo (Stuggart) 39:535, 1978
33. Szczeklik A, Gryglewski RJ, Musial J, et al: Thromboxane generation and platelet aggregation in survivors of myocardial infarction. Throm Haemos 40:66, 1979

34. Green LH, Seroppian E, Handin RI: Platelet activation during exercise-induced myocardial ischemia. NEJM 302:193, 1980
35. Kalendovsky Z, Austin J, Steele P: Increased platelet aggregability in young patients with stroke. Arch Neurol 32:12, 1975
36. Handin RI, McDonough M, Lesch M: Elevation of platelet factor four in acute myocardial infarction: measurement by radioimmunoassay. J Lab Clin Med 91:340, 1978
37. Sobel M, Salzman EW, Davies GC, et al: Circulating platelet products in unstable angina pectoris. Circ 63:300, 1981
38. Ritchie JL, Harker LA: Platelet and fibrinogen survival in coronary atherosclerosis: Response to medical and surgical therapy. Am J Cardiol 39:595, 1977
39. Wu KK, Hoak JC: Increased platelet aggregates in patients with transient ischemic attacks. Stroke 6:521, 1975
40. Gjesdal K: Platelet function and plasma free fatty acids during acute myocardial infarction and severe angina pectoris. Scand J Haemotol 17:205, 1976
41. McBrien DJ, Bradley RD, Ashton N: The nature of retinal emboli in stenosis of the internal carotid artery. Lancet 1:697, 1963
42. Davis HH, Siegel BA, Sherman LA, et al: Scintigraphic detection of carotid atherosclerosis with Indium-111-labeled autologous platelets. Circ 61:982, 1980
43. Boullin DJ, Buntin S, Blaso WP, et al: Responses of human and baboon arteries to prostaglandin endoperoxides and biologically generated and synthetic prostacyclin: Their relevance to cerebral arterial spasm in man. Br J Clin Pharmac 7:139, 1979
44. Preston FE, Martin JF, Stewart RM, et al: Thrombocytosis, circulating platelet aggregates, and neurological dysfunction. Brit J Med 2:1561, 1979
45. Al-Mefty O, Marano G, Rajaraman S, et al: Transient ischemic attacks due to increased platelet aggregation and adhesiveness. J Neurosurg 50:449, 1979
46. De Bono DP, Warlow CP: Potential sources of emboli in patients with presumed transient cerebral or retinal ischaemia. Lancet 1:343, 1981
47. Baconnet C, Bousser M-G, Conrad J, et al: Platelet aggregability in 101 patients with atherothrombotic ischemic cerebral disease. JAMWA 35:117, 1980
48. Petito CK: Platelet thrombi in experimental cerebral infarction. Stroke 10:192, 1979
49. Gaudet RJ, Levine L: Transient cerebral ischemia and brain prostaglandins. Biochem Biophys Res Comm 86:893, 1979
50. Fuster V, Cheseboro JH: Antithrombotic therapy: Role of platelet-induced drugs. Mayo Clin Proc 56:102, 1981
51. Steer ML, Salzman EW: Cyclic nucleotides in hemostasis and thrombosis, in Hamet P, Sands H (eds): Advances in Cyclic Nucleotide Research, vol. 12, New York, Raven Press, 1980, p 71
52. Weiss HJ, Turitto VT: Prostacyclin (prostaglandin I_2, PGI_2) inhibits platelet adhesion and thrombus formation on subendothelium. Blood 53:244, 1979
53. Tschopp TB, Baumgartner HR: Platelet adhesion and mural platelet thrombus formation on aortic subendothelium of rats, rabbits, and guinea pigs correlate negatively with the vascular PGI_2 production. J Lab Clin Med 98:402, 1981
54. Romson JL, Haack DW, Abrams GD, et al: Prevention of occlusive coronary artery thrombosis by prostacyclin infusion in the dog. Circ 64:906, 1981
55. Metke M, Lie JT, Fuster V, et al: Reduction of intimal thickening in canine coronary bypass vein grafts with dipyridamole and aspirin. Am J Cardiol 43:1144, 1979
56. Pick R, Chediak J, Glick G: Aspirin inhibits development of coronary atherosclerosis in cynomolgus monkeys (macaca fascicularis) fed an atherogenic diet. J Clin Invest 63:158, 1979

Robert J. Lusby
Linda D. Ferrell
Edwin J. Wylie

4

The Significance of Intraplaque Hemorrhage in the Pathogenesis of Carotid Atherosclerosis

Little attention has been directed to the atherosclerotic plaque changes at the carotid bifurcation with respect to their role in the acute onset of cerebral ischemic symptoms. Following the initial onset of symptoms, approximately 40 percent of patients progress then or at a later date to stroke while one third will die of other causes, and in the remainder, the disease remains quiescent.[1] The often rapid and unpredictable progression of disease has led us to suggest that factors such as mechanical stress and altered plaque structure, or a combination of the two, may be important precursors to the development of intraplaque hemorrhage,[2] a common finding in patients with transient cerebral ischemia.[3] It seems possible that the sudden change in luminal configuration secondary to an intraplaque hemorrhage may induce a thromboembolic event by one or more of three events: (1) protrusion of the plaque into the lumen causing local reduction in flow with luminal thrombus formation or occlusion; (2) through the production of luminal thrombus with distal embolization; or (3) through the breakdown of the luminal surface over a hemorrhage with ulceration and subsequent embolization of the degenerating hemorrhage.

BACKGROUND

Only recently has the role of intraplaque hemorrhage been appreciated. The emphasis of earlier investigators was directed toward documenting the more general relationship between carotid atheroma and cerebral symptoms.

Support for this work was in part given by the Fogarty International Center, National Institutes of Health, USA, Dr. R.J. Lusby. Grant No. 1F05TW 3103-01

In 1905, Chiari[4] demonstrated carotid artery thrombus as the only possible source of embolus in a patient with an ipsilateral middle cerebral artery embolus and contralateral hemiplegia. Ramsey Hunt,[5] in 1914, subsequently suggested a clinical relationship between transient ocular symptoms, with contralateral limb weakness and carotid artery occlusive disease. These reports, however, made little impact. In the early 1950s, Fisher[6,7,8] observed the occurrence of middle cerebral artery stroke without thrombosis of that vessel and confirmed an association between monocular visual loss and contralateral hemiplegia. He subsequently observed retinal artery emboli during episodes of amaurosis fugax and noted that the episodes of blindness abruptly ceased with the onset of hemiparesis. He stressed the importance of emboli in the generation of transient ischemia in the regions supplied by the internal carotid artery. The vascular nature of the atheromatous plaque was pointed out by Fisher in the first case report of monocular blindness associated with contralateral hemiplegia where he described an atheromatous mass with "abundant small endothelial lined capillaries scattered throughout." In 1955, Millikan and Siekart[9] suggested that cerebral ischemia may be transient as a result of an embolus lodging in an artery with subsequent fragmentation limiting the course of the ischemia. In 1961, Russell[10] reported a case of retinal artery embolus which, at autopsy, was associated with an internal carotid artery thrombus, the tail of which extended to the takeoff of the ophthalmic artery. Gunning et al.[11] suggested that friable micro-emboli, which arise from mural thrombi, were the commonest cause of symptoms. They noted fresh mural thrombus adherent to the wall in patients with recent symptoms that was not present in those vessels of patients with a longer interval prior to operation. They pointed out that unlike firm, fibrotic emboli of cardiac origin, carotid mural thrombi have a large platelet content that could dislodge, embolize, and with subsequent disaggregation, produce transient symptoms. Two types of retinal emboli appeared possible: (1) the platelet-rich embolus which McBrien et al.[12] suggested were the white bodies Fisher and others had seen in the retina and that Denny-Brown[13] had produced experimentally following trauma to the middle cerebral artery, and (2) atheromatous emboli. Witmer and Schmid[14] observed small refractile bodies lodged at retinal vessel bifurcations and suggested they were cholesterol crystals. Hollenhorst[15] concluded that these were flakes of cholesterol that had been washed into the retinal vascular bed from ulcerating atheromatous lesions in the neck.

In 1966, Ehrenfeld et al.[16] removed the carotid lesions from 32 patients with transient monocular blindness and demonstrated irregular intimal surfaces with ulceration in 18 patients. Aggregates of thrombus, fibrin, platelets, and cholesterol crystals were common findings in the specimens. They pointed out that symptoms may be present with or without a hemodynamically significant lesion. That the visual and cerebral ischemic attacks ceased following endarterectomy in 94 percent of the patients, provided convincing evidence that emboli were a major source of transient ischemia. Of interest is the presence of marked intraplaque hemorrhage in two of the illustrations in their report.

Cerebral hypoperfusion was shown to produce both global and focal ischemia by Denny-Brown, who induced symptoms in diseased patients with carotid compression and tilt table induced hypotension.[17] He also reported the development of symptoms in patients with cardiac arrhythmias. The presence of advanced disease and high-grade stenosis seem important contributing factors to the production of stroke. The precise relationship is uncertain, however, particularly in the presence of an adequate collateral flow. Schwartz and Mitchell[18] demonstrated that the incidence of carotid atheroma increased with age and that stenosis did not necessarily produce cerebral symptoms. These findings have been confirmed by several subsequent studies.[19,20,21] More recently, Busuttil et al.[22] have demonstrated a 16 percent risk of stroke in asymptomatic patients with a hemodynamically significant lesion of greater than 60 percent diameter reduction as detected by oculopneumoplethysmography compared to a 2 percent risk with lesser lesions. Batacharji, Hutchinson, and McCall[23] showed that atheromatous ulceration is significantly more frequent and severe in patients with cerebral infarction than in a control group without evidence of infarction. This suggests the intraplaque pathology associated with the stenosis is more important than the stenosis itself, and the embolism theory affords a more satisfactory explanation for most transient attacks than does repeated hemodynamic crises, although both mechanisms may cause symptoms.

MECHANICAL FACTORS

The carotid bifurcation is a site of predilection for the development of atheroma. Factors such as the asymmetrical nature of the bifurcation, the hemodynamic stress caused by the bulbous structure of the internal carotid artery origin, and differences in flow characteristics in the two major branches may all play some role in the unique changes that occur. Mechanical stress and intimal injury seem to be important initiating factors in the development of plaque along with platelet deposition, smooth muscle cell proliferation, and the slow accumulation of lipoproteins.

Carotid artery bruits commonly heard in the presence of atheroma are a result of vessel wall movements at high frequencies in the audible range.[24] There is evidence that particular frequencies cause changes in structural components of the vessel walls, particularly in elastin and collagen integrity.[25,26] These changes can lead to dilation and ulceration of the vessel wall. Heath et al.[27] showed that in atheromatous carotid arteries, the medial thickness of the carotid bulb is much less than that of the artery on either side, while the wall thickness, due to atheroma in the bulb, is much greater than in the common and distal internal carotid arteries. They pointed out that the medial thickness in the bulb is only some 5 percent of the external diameter of the artery, a figure more appropriate to the pulmonary than the systemic circulation, and felt that the microanatomical characteristic of localized thinning of the medial elements suggests that the bulb has an increased distensibility in the presence of atheromatous disease.

Recent studies using dynamic angiography and ultrasonic M mode distensibility[28] have shown variations in carotid artery diameter associated with pulsation to be much greater than previously appreciated. In particular, there appears to be much greater distensibility in the carotid bulb than in the adjacent common carotid artery even in the presence of disease. The segmental variations in distensibility probably indicate sudden differences in compliance at the origin of the internal carotid artery. Such abrupt changes in vessel compliance have been associated with disruptive stresses in the walls which may lead to dilation.[29] The tension in the wall of an artery, according to the law of La Place, depends on its diameter as well as the transmural

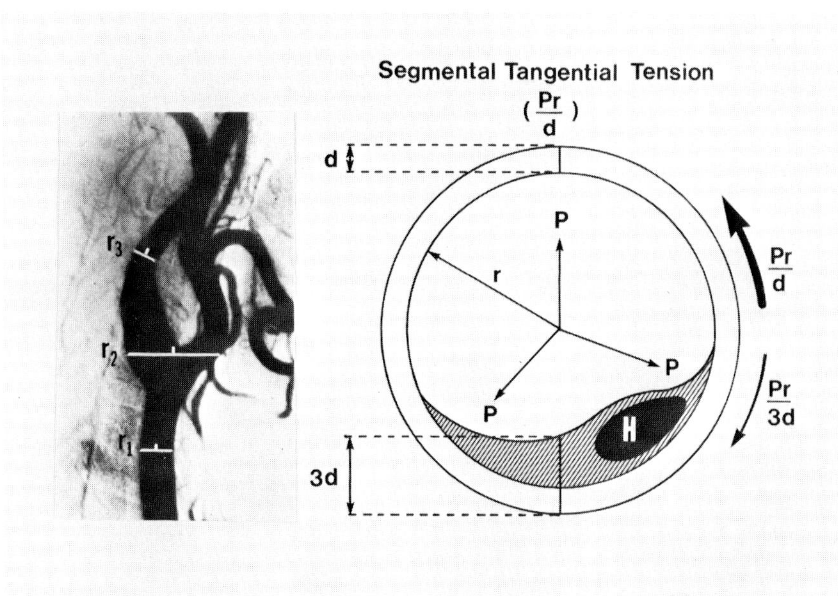

Figure 4-1. Angiogram of carotid bifurcation showing the increased radius (r) at the site of division of the artery along with a diagram showing the disparity in segmental tangential tension associated with posterior wall plaque. P=Pressure, d=Wall thickness, and r=Radius. The black area (H) represents the site where hemorrhages are often seen on sectioning carotid plaques.

pressure.[30] With pulsatile flow, this stress is greater in the bulbous origin of the internal carotid artery (Fig. 4-1). Furthermore, the composition and thickness of the vessel wall influence the tangential tension or force per unit area, tending to tear open the distended vessel wall. Changes in wall structure with the development of nondistensible atheroma, along with the asymmetric deposition of plaque, produce imbalances in wall tensions. Alterations in these forces, possibly associated with exacerbations in systemic blood pressure, may contribute not only to the gradual development of atheromatous plaque, but also to the sudden development of plaque fracture and intraplaque hemorrhage.[31]

HISTOPATHOLOGY

In defining the composition and structure of carotid atheromatous lesions, we have used an elastochrome stain, a combination of Verhoeff's Elastin, and the Gomori one-step trichrome, as well as routine hematoxylin and eosin staining.[2] The elastochrome stain shows elastin as black, collagen as blue, and hemorrhage as red-purple.

In an attempt to estimate the age of the hemorrhage, we have used the color changes seen with elastochrome and standard histological criteria based on the stage of the acute inflammatory response and healing characteristics.[2] Confirmation of the acute inflammatory response to intramural hemorrhage was sought in a series of canine vessel walls injected with fresh blood. Carotid and femoral arteries from 8 dogs were harvested at 24 and 48 hours, 7 and 14 days following injection of blood, and were examined microscopically for evidence of the inflammatory response.

Four pathological categories of hemorrhage have been defined, which although not totally precise, provide a framework for estimating the age of the hemorrhage:

1. Operative. Characterized by loose, intact red blood cells which stain yellow to red with elastochrome and have no associated inflammatory response.
2. Acute. (up to one week) Intact red blood cells staining light red with elastochrome, located within a plaque, and associated with a polymorphonuclear infiltrate and focal macrophage activity.
3. Recent. (one to six weeks) Hemorrhagic debris staining light to dark red with elastochrome and containing a mixture of intact and degenerating red blood cells. In addition, there is macrophage engulfment of hemosiderin, giant cell development, cholesterol crystal formation, and the appearance of angioneogenesis at the periphery of such recent hemorrhages (Fig. 4-2).

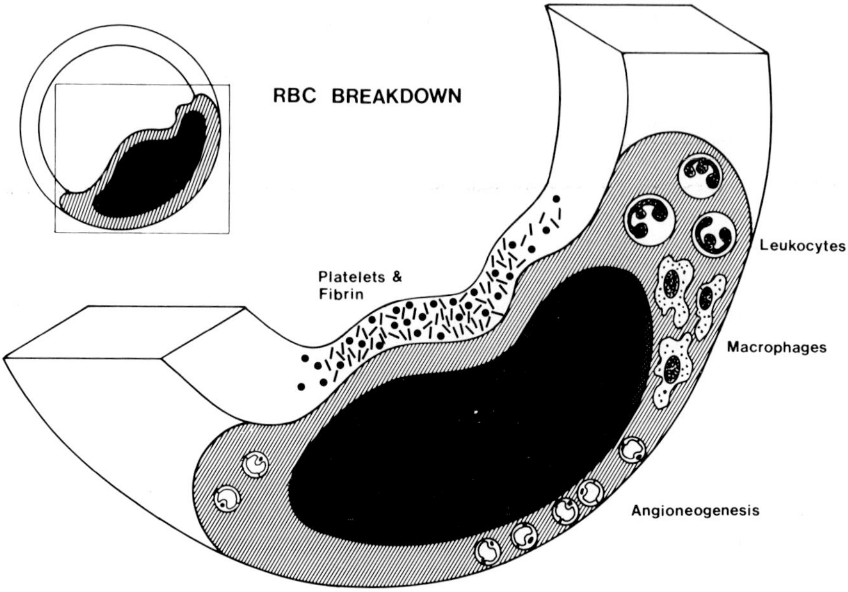

Figure 4-2. Diagram illustrating inflammatory response to an intraplaque hemorrhage with leukocyte cell and macrophage migration occurring as well as angioneogenesis. Platelets and fibrin are shown depositing on the luminal surface over the hemorrhage.

4. Remote. (greater than six weeks) Amorphous material staining purple, blue, or dark red with elastochrome, usually sharply demarcated and often surrounded by dense fibrous or calcified tissue. No evidence of inflammatory reaction is seen, but there may be dense cholesterol crystal formation with or without adjacent well-developed angioneogenesis.

RESULTS

A prospective evaluation of 79 atheromatous plaques removed from 69 consecutive patients undergoing carotid endarterectomy was recently reported.[2] Fifty-three plaques were associated with ipsilateral hemisphere or retinal symptoms with a median interval between onset of symptoms and operation of 2.9 weeks. Twenty-six plaques were obtained from asymptomatic patients or from the asymptomatic contralateral side of patients undergoing bilateral operations.

The presence of an acute or recent intramural hemorrhage (Fig. 4-3) was noted in 49/53 (92.5 percent) patients with symptoms of cerebral ischemia, in contrast to a low incidence 7/26 (27 percent) in asymptomatic patients

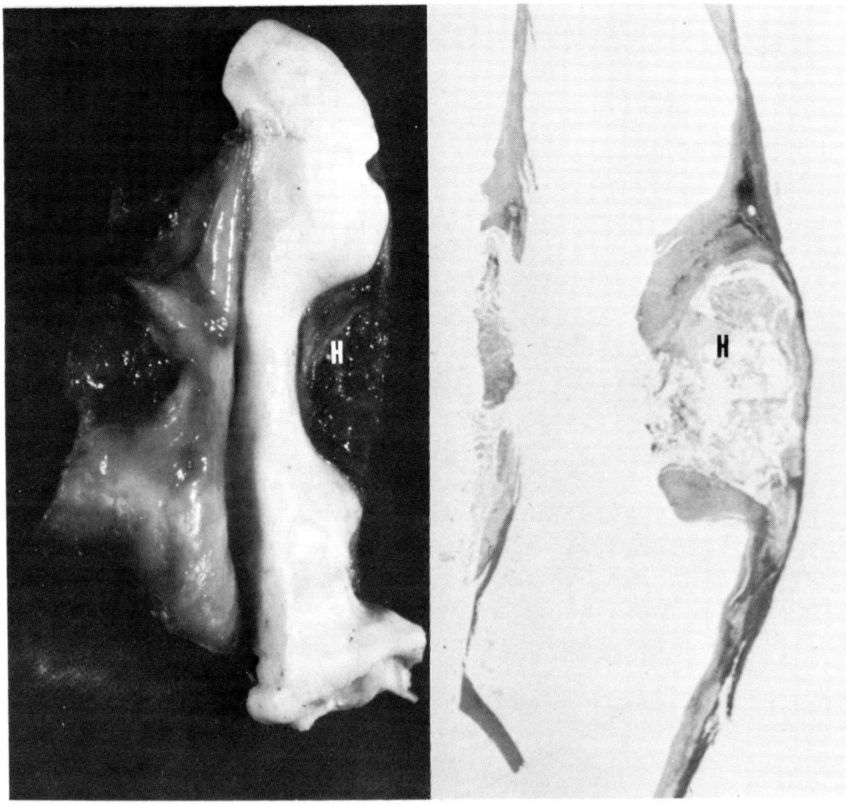

Figure 4-3. Opened carotid plaque with epoxy resin mold demonstrating luminal encroachment caused by intramural hemorrhage (H). A longitudinal histopathological section of the specimen is seen alongside with the hemorrhage lying in an atheromatous plaque.

($P < 0.005$ χ^2 test). Twelve of the 16 patients (75 percent) with symptoms occurring within a week of operation had evidence of an acute hemorrhage, while 27/36 (75 percent) of patients with symptoms occurring between 1 and 6 weeks had a recent intraplaque hemorrhage. Evidence of multiple hemorrhages based on pathological criteria was seen in 43/53 (81 percent) of symptomatic patients, many of whom had experienced several attacks of cerebral ischemia. Forty-six (86 percent) of the symptomatic patients had a lesion of greater than 50 percent diameter reduction. Hemorrhage of multiple ages was seen in 39 (84.7 percent) of these specimens. Analysis of the distribution of neurological symptoms showed no discernible difference in the neurological deficits sustained in 28/53 patients with luminal diameter reduction of 50-74 percent compared to the 18 patients with 75-99 percent diameter reduction.

Luminal thrombus formation, with or without ulceration, was seen on the intimal surface overlying subintimal hemorrhage in 11 symptomatic patients (20.7 percent) and on the luminal surface of one asymptomatic patient. Six of these symptomatic patients were on aspirin up to the time of operation. Histological evidence of early organization of such thrombus indicated its formation prior to operation. In the canine model, early thrombus formation was noted at 4 hours following sudden mural distension with saline, although there was no apparent intimal ulceration on light microscopy. In 2 patients, high grade stenosis secondary to recent hemorrhage was associated with thrombotic occlusion at operation, the thrombus being limited to the region of the stenosis and just beyond. Another patient with 3 areas of cerebral infarction demonstrated by computerized tomography had an initial angiogram suggesting total occlusion of the ipsilateral carotid artery. Doppler testing suggested a patent internal carotid artery which was confirmed at repeat angiography. Subsequent examination of the operative specimen revealed a recent intraplaque hemorrhage on the basis of the angiographic morphology (Fig. 4-4). A penetrating niche with a radiologic diagnosis of an ulcer in the vessel wall usually represented normal vessel wall between projecting mounds caused by subintimal hemorrhage. Histological

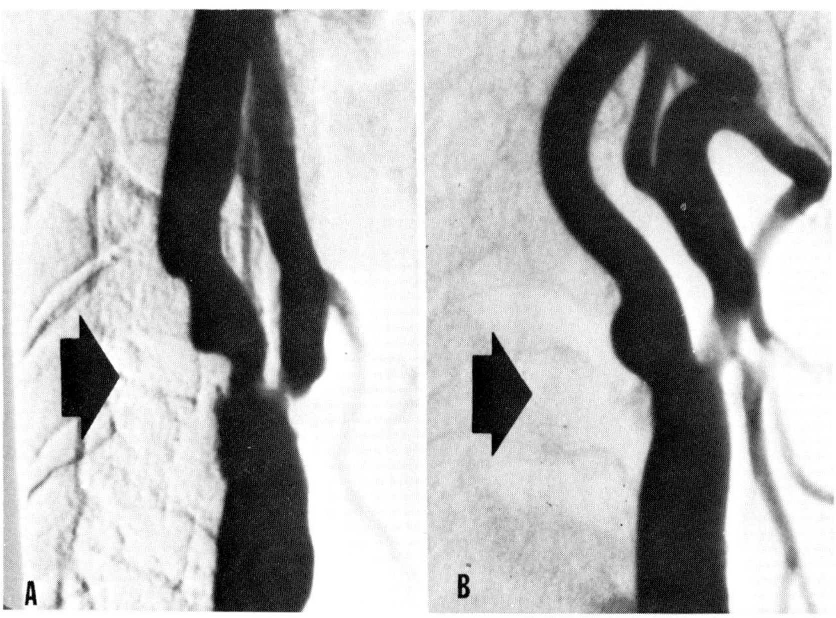

Figure 4-4. Angiograms of two carotid bifurcations showing similar morphological appearances. Angiogram A was taken from an asymptomatic patient and histologically the lesion showed remote hemorrhage, while Angiogram B from a symptomatic patient had evidence of recent hemorrhage.

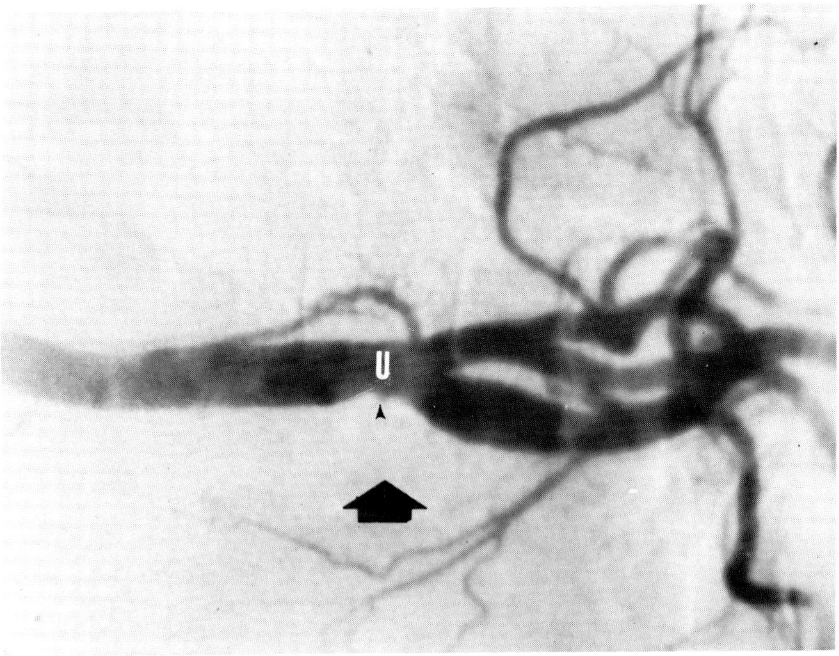

Figure 4-5. Carotid angiogram showing a protruding mound with a small ulcer (U) at the apex of the mound. The protrusion was caused by an intraplaque hemorrhage. Breakdown of the intimal surface over the hemorrhage produced the ulcer.

evidence of ulceration of the intimal surface was seen in 14/53 (26.4 percent) of symptomatic patients. Ulceration occurred over areas of subintimal hemorrhage with the intimal defect generally located at the apex or to 1 side of the protruding mound generated by the hemorrhage (Fig. 4-5). In only 1 patient was the ulcer located in the pit seen angiographically. Two patients with ulcerating lesions presented with attacks of monocular blindness associated with retinal artery cholesterol emboli. Five patients with a history of stroke had similar ulcerating lesions. Histologically, these ulcers lay over hemorrhages undergoing breakdown with cholesterol crystal formation (Fig. 4-6). Reendothelization was seen in five of the ulcerating plaques from patients with an interval of over 3 weeks between symptom onset and operation. Experimentally, intimal ulceration occurred in association with the acute production of a 50 percent flow-reducing lesion. While an early white cell response was noted, there was no evidence of blood dissecting into the vessel wall.

In lesions obtained from asymptomatic patients, a variety of atheromatous pathology was evident ranging from soft gruel to thick fibrous and calcified lesions with occasional bone formation. New vessel formation

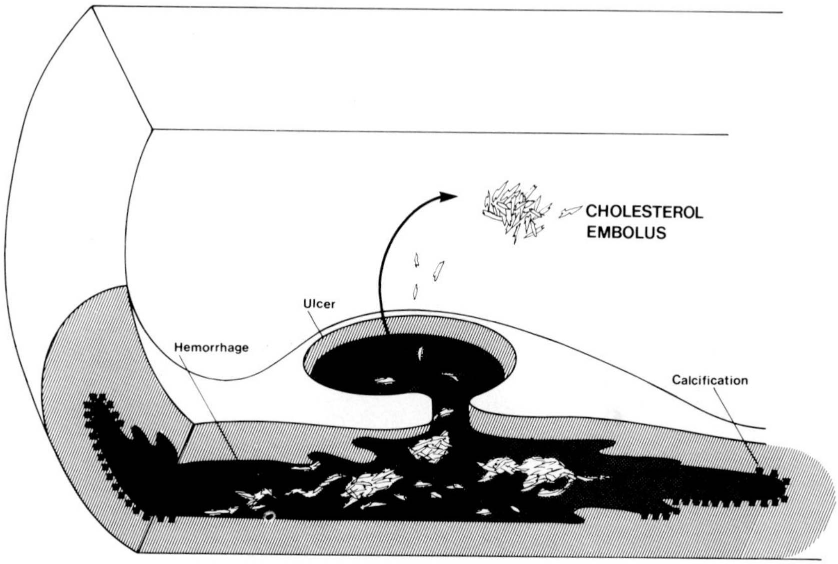

Figure 4-6. Diagram demonstrating the common appearance of an intimal ulcer over a mound produced by intraplaque hemorrhage. The breakdown products of the hemorrhage include cholesterol crystals which may be washed into the blood stream and embolize distally. Speckled calcification is often noted at the edge of such hemorrhages.

similar to that occurring in recent hemorrhages and in response to intramural injections of blood in the canine model was present in 17/26 specimens, often in areas adjacent to calcified and bony lesions. Evidence of remote hemorrhage was noted in 18/20 (90 percent) of the asymptomatic patients with greater than 50 percent diameter reduction. Seven of these patients had, in addition, evidence of recent hemorrhage.

Eighteen symptomatic patients continued to have ischemic attacks prior to operation while on antiplatelet therapy. Histological examination of the plaque revealed a recent hemorrhage in 16 of these patients, and 13 plaques had evidence of more than one hemorrhage (72 percent).

DISCUSSION

Many surgeons have noted the presence of hemorrhage in plaques removed at carotid endarterectomy. The use of the elastochrome stain in this study, however, has helped to identify the extent of involvement of such hemorrhages in symptomatic patients. In addition, this study has established a significant relationship between the development of a recent plaque

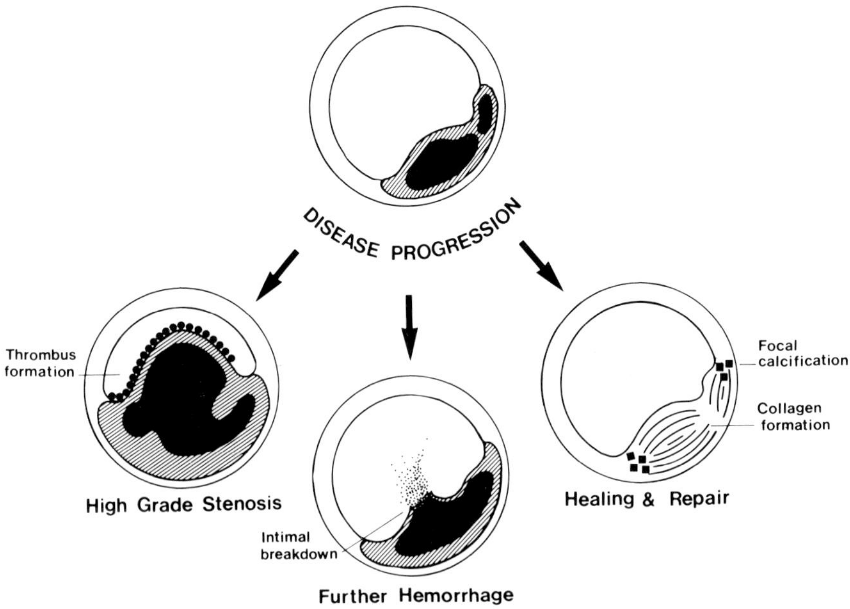

Figure 4-7. Diagram illustrating the possible sequence following an initial intraplaque hemorrhage.

hemorrhage and the onset of symptoms, suggesting a unique and major role for such hemorrhages in the development of symptoms.

Following the onset of intraplaque hemorrhage, an inflammatory response occurs which is characterized in part by the development of new capillary-like vessels. Experimentally, we have found these vessels to develop within 2 weeks of an intramural injection of blood. The presence of multiple hemorrhages seen in many symptomatic patients could be a consequence of subsequent tearing of these fragile new vessels, a possible mechanism for repeated transient ischemic attacks (TIAs). Such injury could result in part from increased mechanical stress associated with the development of turbulent blood flow or vessel wall vibration, as noted by the presence of a bruit. Again, the high risk of stroke in the first months following the onset of TIAs may be related to further hemorrhages (Fig. 4-7) leading to high-grade stenosis or thrombotic occlusion, the commonest cause of atherosclerotic induced stroke.[32] Two patients had progressed to thrombotic occlusion at the time of operation, and a third had the angiographic appearance of total occlusion. All 3 plaques had evidence of recent hemorrhage precipitating development of high-grade stenosis. In the third patient, this was associated with documented cerebral infarction, highlighting the relationship between plaque hemorrhage and the production of stroke.

Healing at the site of plaque hemorrhage resulted in a spectrum of end points ranging from remote hemorrhage surrounded by fibrous or calcified tissue to friable, compound, highly vascular atheromatous tissue. The lower incidence of stroke occurring 1 year or beyond following the onset of TIAs may be related to the development of a well-healed lesion. When progression to stroke does occur, it could be a result of further hemorrhage in the more friable vascular lesions. The difficulty for the clinician is to identify the type of lesion a patient may have.

The majority of asymptomatic lesions in this study had evidence of remote hemorrhage at the site of the stenosis. Many lesions were densely calcified with little evidence of recent intraplaque trauma. Two-thirds of these lesions had new vessel formation, however, and over a quarter had evidence of a recent intraplaque hemorrhage. The presence of fragile new vessels in a pathologically friable atheromatous mound and increased mechanical stress may explain the increased risk of stroke (up to 17 percent) and TIA (up to 30 percent) in high-grade asymptomatic lesions detected by oculoplethysmography.[22,33,34] The progression from a moderate asymptomatic lesion to a high-grade stenosis is often rapid and unpredictable,[35] suggesting an acute hemorrhage has occurred. Mechanical stresses operating at the carotid bulb may contribute to a loss of functional wall elements and structural integrity, leading to increased vulnerability in those lesions of greater than 50 percent diameter reduction. The increased mechanical stress might well lead to further intraplaque hemorrhages with subsequent stretching of the intima over the hemorrhage and further protrusion of the lesion into the lumen. These changes may result in reduction of blood flow, precipitate luminal thrombus formation, or lead to ulceration of the intima lying over the hemorrhage, all being possible causes of cerebral flow reduction from hypoperfusion or embolization.

We have noted 2 sources of emboli associated with acute intraplaque hemorrhage. Thrombus formation occurring on the vessel wall adjacent to a recent or acute hemorrhage may give rise to platelet/thrombus emboli without the presence of frank ulceration. Minute intimal disruption may have occurred in association with the acute hemorrhagic event, but it was not possible to identify this using light microscopy. It is postulated that the emboli arising from this intimal surface reaction are most likely to produce the fleeting type of transient ischemic attack undergoing rapid dissolution with immediate resolution of symptoms. A second embolic source was seen in association with intimal breakdown and ulceration over intraplaque hemorrhages. Here, clumps of degenerated red blood cells and cholesterol crystals exposed to the blood stream become the source of possible emboli. Retinal artery cholesterol crystal emboli and five frank strokes were identified in association with such lesions. Large clumps of such atheromatous debris may be less inclined to disaggregate in distal cerebral vessels and hence place the patient at greater risk for sustaining a serious neurological deficit.

In this study, the angiographic appearance did not reliably predict the surgical pathology. It was not possible to separate a recent from a remote hemorrhagic lesion on the angiographic appearance. The presence of the ulceration was noted in less than one-third of specimens, although almost two-thirds had an angiographic niche or pit reported as an "ulcer." This pit usually represented the only normal part of the vessel wall with hemorrhage causing protrusion of the lumen on either side. The majority of true ulcers occurred in the intimal surfaces over protruding mounds of hemorrhage. Ulceration at a similar site was produced following protrusion of the intima into the lumen caused by a balloon constrictor in the canine model. This intimal breakdown may be a result of stretching over the hemorrhage, shearing forces from altered blood flow and local pressure necrosis. Evidence of intimal healing was seen in several patients operated on some weeks after the onset of symptoms. A large hemorrhagic lesion, however, usually remained beneath the healing surface.

The varying results from trials using aspirin antiplatelet therapy in stroke prophylaxis[36,37] can possibly be explained in terms of the carotid plaque pathology. Aspirin may be effective in reducing platelet aggregation on the luminal surface over a recent subintimal hemorrhage, thus preventing the production of emboli and subsequent transient ischemia. This will not always be so as half the patients with luminal thrombus formation in this study were on aspirin. Aspirin can have little effect in preventing the breakdown of the luminal surface over a protruding subintimal hemorrhage and may, in fact, inhibit the platelet-plugging response to injury, leaving the underlying atheromatous debris in contact with the bloodstream and at risk of embolization. Nor is aspirin likely to alter the mechanical stresses or prevent further intraplaque hemorrhage. In fact, 13 patients in this study who continued to have symptoms on aspirin had evidence of multiple hemorrhages, and 7 had intimal ulceration. Aspirin, in inhibiting the minor platelet embolic events, may mask the symptoms of disease progression secondary to intraplaque hemorrhages in some patients, denying them the opportunity of seeking further medical assessment.

This study has shown the variable vessel wall characteristics associated with the development of transient cerebral ischemia. It has shown the presence of friable tissues and fragile new vessels which, when subjected to additional mechanical stress, may lead to luminal disruption or further intraplaque hemorrhages. Hypertension, which is the most potent risk factor for stroke, may play an important role by adding to the stress applied to such lesions. The increased risk associated with asymptomatic patients with hemodynamically significant lesions may also be explained in terms of the vessel wall pathology.

The observations in this study offer possible explanations for the variable outcomes and responses to treatment following the onset of TIAs, as well as the mechanism of sudden disease progression.

REFERENCES

1. Whisnant JP: A population study of stroke and TIA: Rochester, Minnesota, in Gillingham FJ, Mawdsley C, Williams AE (eds): Stroke, New York, Churchill Livingstone, 1976, p. 21
2. Lusby RJ, Ferrell LD, Stoney RJ, et al: The role of intraplaque hemorrhage in the development of cerebro vascular disease. Arch Surg 1982 (in press)
3. Lusby, RJ, Woodcock JP, Machleder HI, et al: Transient ischemic attacks: The static and dynamic morphology of the carotid artery bifurcation. Brit J Surg 1982 (in press)
4. Chiari H: Uber das Verhalten des Teilungs Winkels der Carotis Communis bei der Endarterutig Chronica deformans. Verh. Dtsch. Ges. Pathol. 9:326, 1905
5. Hunt JR: The role of the carotid arteries in the causation of vascular lesions of the brain, with remarks on certain special features of symptomatology. Am J Med Sci 147:704, 1914
6. Fisher M: Transient monocular blindness associated with hemiplegia. Arch Opthalmol 47:167, 1952
7. Fisher M: Occlusion of the carotid arteries. Further experience. Arch Neurol Psychol 72:187, 1954
8. Fisher M: Concerning recurrent transcerebral ischemic attacks. Can Med Assoc J 86:1091, 1962
9. Millikan CH, Siekert RG, Shick RM: Studies in cerebro vascular disease V. the use of anticoagulant drugs in the treatment of intermittent insufficiency of the internal carotid arterial system. Proc Mayo Clin 30:578, 1955
10. Russell RWR: Observations on the retinal blood vessels in monocular blindness. Lancet 2:1422, 1961
11. Gunning AJ, Pickering GW, Robb-Smith AHT, et al: Mural thrombosis of the internal carotid artery and subsequent embolization. Quarterly Journal of Medicine 33:155, 1964
12. McBrien DJ, Bradley RN, Ashton N: The nature of retinal emboli in stenosis of the internal carotid artery. Lancet 1:697, 1963
13. Denny-Brown D: Recurrent cerebrovascular episodes. Arch Neurol 2:194, 1960
14. Witmer R, Schmid A: Cholesterinkristal als retinaler arterieller Embolus. Ophthalomologica (Basel). 135:432, 1958
15. Hollenhorst RW: Significance of bright plaques in the retinal arterioles JAMA 178:23, 1961
16. Ehrenfeld WK, Hoyt WF, Wylie EJ: Embolization and transient blindness from carotid atheroma. Arch Surg 93:787, 1966
17. Meyer JS, Leiderman H, Denny-Brown, D: Electroencephalographic study of insufficiency of the basilar and carotid arteries in man. Neurology 6:455, 1956
18. Schwartz CJ, Mitchell JRA: Atheroma of the carotid and vertebral arterial systems. Brit Med J ii:1057, 1961
19. Hutchinson EC, Yates PO: Carotid vertebral stenosis. Lancet 1:2, 1957
20. Martin MJ, Whisnant JP, Sayre GP: Occlusive vascular disease in the extracranial cerebral circulation. Arch Neurol 3:530, 1960
21. Whisnant JP, Martin MJ, Sayre GP: Atherosclerotic stenosis of cervical arteries: Clinical significance. Arch Neurol 5:429, 1961
22. Busuttil RW, Baker JD, Davidson RK, et al: Carotid artery stenosis-hemodynamic significance and clinical course. JAMA 245:1438, 1981

23. Batacharji SK, Hutchinson EC, McCall. Stenosis and occlusion of vessels in cerebral infarction. Brit Med J iii:270, 1967
24. McDonald DA: Blood Flow in Arteries (ed 2). London, Edward Arnold; Baltimore, Williams & Wilkins, 1974, p. 55
25. Bougner DR, Roach MR: Effect of low frequency vibration on arterial wall. Circulation Res 29:136, 1973
26. Gersten JW: Relation of ultrasound effects to orientation of tendon in ultrasound field. Arch Phys Med Rehabil 37:201, 1956
27. Heath D, Smith P, Harris P, et al: The atherosclerotic human carotid sinus. J Path 110:49, 1973
28. Lusby RJ, Machleder HI, Jeans W, et al: Vessel wall and blood flow dynamics in arterial disease. Phil Trans R Soc B 294:231, 1981
29. Gonza ER, Mason WF, Marble AE, et al: Necessity for elastic properties in synthetic arterial grafts. Can J Surg 17:1, 1974
30. Glagov S: Hemodynamic risk factors: mechanical stress, mural architecture, mural nutrition and the vulnerability of arteries to atherosclerosis, in The Pathogenesis of Atherosclerosis. Ed. Wissler, R. W. and Greer, J.C. Baltimore: Williams & Wilkins Co., pp. 164–199, 1972
31. Born GVR: Arterial thrombosis and its prevention, in Proc. VIII World Congress of Cardiology Tokyo. Hayase S, Murao S: (eds) p. 81, Amsterdam, Oxford & Princeton: Excerpta Medica. 1978
32. Pessin MS, Hinton RC, Davis KR, et al: Mechanisms of acute carotid stroke. Ann Neurol 6:245, 1979
33. Thompson JE, Patman DE, Talkington CM: Asymptomatic carotid bruit: Longterm outcome of patients having endarterectomy compared with unoperated controls. Ann Surg 188:308, 1978
34. Kartchner MM, McRae LP: Non-invasive evaluation and management of the asymptomatic carotid bruit. Surgery 82:840, 1977
35. Javid H, Ostermiller WE, Henge JW, et al: Carotid endarterectomy for asymptomatic patients. Arch Surg 102:389, 1971
36. The Canadian Cooperative Study Group: A randomized trial of aspirin and sulfinpyrazone in threatened stroke. N Engl J Med 299:53, 1978.
37. Fields WS, Lemak NA: Controlled trial of aspirin in cerebral ischemia. Stroke 8:301, 1977

Mark L. Dyken

5

Evaluation of Cerebral Ischemia: Transient, Focal, Lateralizing, and Nonhemispheric Ischemic Attacks

Transient ischemic attacks (TIAs) do not cause permanent dysfunction and are usually brief and do not greatly interfere with life. Their major importance is that they are markers for increased risk for stroke and death. Therefore, early diagnosis permits an opportunity for medical and surgical intervention to reduce this likelihood. In addition, failure to make a correct diagnosis can lead to inappropriate studies and incorrect treatment.

TIAs are widely defined as episodes of temporary focal cerebral dysfunction of vascular origin. Unfortunately, this definition is too broad and requires further clarification. The term "transient" must be further defined and conditions, such as migraine or migraine-equivalent disease states, which would answer this definition, must be excluded. In addition, focal seizures may occur in response to vascular lesions. Also, transient global ischemia of the brain associated with drops in blood pressure or reduced cardiac output answer the definition but have different implications. The definition used by the "Cooperative Study of Hospital Frequency and Character of Transient Ischemic Attacks"[1] is more precise: "transient (less than *24 hours hypofunction* of the nervous system thought to be related to ischemia in the recognized *distribution* of the carotid or vertebral arterial systems without residual from that attack [migraine or migraine equivalents excluded])."

As people with TIAs can only be identified and treated after they enter the medical system, this communication will refer often to the data from the Cooperative Study of Hospital Frequency [1-8] which was designed to do the following: (1) identify all inpatients and outpatients with complaints and diagnosis of TIA in six participating institutions representing known variations in geography, referral pattern, and socioeconomic status, (2) establish the reliability of the diagnosis, (3) determine the usual diagnostic procedures, (4) determine the types, effects, and complications of therapy, and (5) determine the frequency of changes in diagnoses, new vascular events, and intercurrent disease during a follow-up period. The six participating centers included the following: Indiana University School of Medicine, Indianapolis; The Institute of Medical Sciences, San Francisco; University of Maryland, Baltimore; Massachusetts General Hospital, Boston; University of Mississippi, Jackson; and University of Washington Hospitals (University Harbor View Medical Center, Veterans Administration, U.S. Public Health Service, Group Health Cooperative of Puget Sound, and The Virginia Mason Hospital), Seattle. They had the following: (1) competent neurologists with special interests in cerebral vascular diseases, (2) established methods for identifying all patients with complaints or diagnosis of TIA, (3) an adequate number of patients, and (4) personnel who could guarantee meticulous reporting of pertinent information. Together, they represented different geographic distributions of the incidence of cerebral vascular disease, variations in referral patterns, and both private and public institutions.

ETIOLOGY

As TIAs have a high degree of association with atherosclerosis, it has been logically assumed that they commonly were associated with decreased blood flow or pressure distal to an atherosclerotic stenosis of an artery. A review of the literature and prospective studies comparing occlusion versus dynamically insignificant lesions fails to reveal any quantitative correlation between the stenosis and clinical manifestations of cerebral vascular disease.[9] In fact, with adequate collaterals, complete occlusion of both internal carotid and vertebral arteries is possible without symptoms and without objective neurological deficit.[9] In addition, some studies indicate that as high as 3 percent of people over 50 years of age may have asymptomatic complete or near-complete internal carotid artery stenosis.[10] The Hospital Frequency Study also failed to show any good correlation between the degree of the angiographically demonstrated lesions and clinical symptoms[2] or prognosis[8]. For these reasons, one must assume that in the usual case, TIAs are not precipitated by dynamic obstruction at the site of the atherosclerotic plaque but that it is more likely that the lesion may act as a trigger for some type of embolic phenomenon. As early as 1959, C. Miller Fisher described a patient with transient episodes of monocular blindness accompanied by white microemboli slowly advancing in the retinal arteries, and he suggested that these might be platelet fibrin emboli.[11] Hollenhorst[12] described shiny yellow cholesterol emboli in retinal arteries in 27 out of 235 patients with carotid artery disease. In addition to these established embolic phenomena, H.J.M. Barnett has noted in a summary that artery-to-artery emboli, cardiac emboli, hemodynamic factors, altered coagulability, lacunar infarction, nonarteriosclerotic vasculopathies, extracranial mechanical interference with arteries, and primary thrombocytosis could all act as mechanisms and could be potentiated by hemodynamic mechanisms.[13] Nevertheless, it does appear that the dynamic causes must occur rarely and not be a major factor and that it is much more likely that the common event is an artery-to-artery embolus to the point that the material blocks an artery distal to its collateral supply. In the event of a friable embolus, such as that composed of platelet-fibrin, this would be temporary. Further evidence to support this hypothesis is obtained from some of the clinical studies using anticoagulant, surgical, and antiplatelet aggregating agent therapy.

In the older literature before the strict criteria for focal distribution of the symptomatology were required, transient ischemic attacks were commonly attributed to general drops in blood pressure, cardiac arrhythmias, and decreased cardiac output. The Hospital Frequency Study gave no support for this concept. In fact, cardiac arrhythmia and ischemic heart disease had a lower percentage frequency in the definite carotid artery system TIA group than in the other groups. This might be easily explained as cardiac output problems were more likely to produce symptoms of other disease or vertebral basilar disease symptomatology. In addition, during the study, 79 patients with the diagnosis of TIA were examined during an attack. All cardiac arrhythmias present during an attack were still present after the attack. Thus, there was no evidence for a causal relationship of transient arrhythmia to the attack.

PATIENT DESCRIPTION

The average age of onset for patients at entry was about 63 years, with a range of from 26 to 97 years. Attacks occurred at a younger age in men than in women. Men had TIAs twice as frequently as women, they occurred more commonly in whites than nonwhites, and a person was more likely to be seen medically if the area of ischemia was in the dominant hemisphere. The attacks averaged 14 minutes in the anterior circulation and 8 minutes in the posterior. Common associated diseases included hypertension (52 percent), ischemic heart disease (36 percent), cardiac arrhythmia (19 percent), diabetes mellitus (18 percent), gastrointestinal tract ulceration (18 percent), and peripheral vascular disease (17 percent). These common associated diseases were not significantly different between those who turned out to definitely have transient ischemic attacks and those who turned out not to have them. As the attacks are brief and there is no dysfunction between attacks, diagnosis is almost always made by history.

THE ATTACK BY HISTORY

Despite the usually accepted 24-hour upper limit for duration of a transient ischemic attack, when one reviews the large studies each attack tends to be quite brief. In the carotid artery system, the attacks average 14 minutes, and 90 percent are less than 6 hours. In the vertebral-basilar system, they average 8 minutes, and 90 percent are less than 2 hours.[1] Therefore, the diagnosis is usually made by history, and the clinician must depend on the symptoms and their interpretation to make the diagnosis. The onset of symptoms is usually rapid, within a few minutes, as is the resolution of each attack. When attacks are multiple, they are stereotyped in 75 to 83 percent of cases.[2]

The Hospital Frequency Study reported detailed analyses of all common symptoms associated with carotid artery and vertebral-basilar transient ischemic attacks. Before these are reviewed, the clinician should be aware that it is impossible and of little value simply to memorize symptom complexes. For example, at least 27 symptoms and all recognized factors that qualified these symptoms were analyzed for the study. The mathematical possibilities for combinations are virtually incomprehensible. To diagnose any type of cerebral vascular disease, particularly transient ischemic attacks, one must have a concept of basic neuroanatomy and the usual distribution of arteries. This will enable the clinician to diagnose a single attack. Although certain symptom complexes might be typical for transient ischemic attacks, they might also occur in other disease states and a memorizer would miss the diagnosis. Table 5-1, taken from the fifth paper of the Cooperative Study, summarizes those symptoms that occur commonly among TIA diagnoses.

When single symptoms were analyzed, it was noted that ipsilateral monocular visual loss or contralateral sensory and motor complaints were most common for carotid artery system TIAs. In the vertebral-basilar system, ataxia and dizziness were common single symptoms, but they were also common for patients who did not have transient ischemic attacks; therefore, when they occurred alone they were of little value in diagnosis. Similarly, dysarthria was seen commonly in both systems but uncommonly in the control group. When a patient presented with the complaint of loss of consciousness or confusion as part of the attack, further workup usually established the diagnosis to be something other than TIA. Of all symptoms, the clearest diagnostic relationship was monocular loss of vision to ipsilateral carotid artery system TIA. In the left carotid system, a combination of speech disturbance with any of the other common symptoms had a high diagnostic

Table 5–1
Distribution (%) of Common Symptoms Among TIA Diagnoses*

Symptom	R CAS	L CAS	VBS	Not TIA	No of Cases
Dizziness	10	5	41	42	98
Ataxia	3	0	63	34	88
Diplopia	6	4	73	16	49
Dysarthria	29	30	22	18	115
Dysphasia	5	79	1	15	96
Confusion	8	24	13	54	71
Loss of consciousness	4	8	20	68	84
Bilateral					
Leg W	3	9	32	58	31
Arm W	0	13	40	47	15
Vision (loss or blur)	5	8	49	30	84
Face					
WR	0	82	4	14	50
WL	81	0	5	12	42
SR	0	74	10	13	39
SL	76	0	6	17	54
Leg					
WR	0	74	9	15	54
WL	71	0	7	21	68
SR	0	74	5	18	38
SL	74	0	7	19	54
Arm					
WR	0	83	4	11	113
WL	74	1	5	18	94
SR	0	82	5	11	92
SL	75	0	8	16	100
Vision					
Loss R	88	0	5	5	43
Loss L	0	92	0	5	37
Blur R	60	7	0	27	15
Blur L	10	80	0	10	10

*TIA indicates transient ischemic attack; R, right; L, left; CAS, carotid artery system; VBS, vertebral-basilar artery system; S, any sensory complaint; and W, weakness.

value. In the vertebral-basilar system, single symptoms were of little value unless combined with other symptoms of brain stem dysfunction. All of these symptom analyses were dependent upon an adequate history and the interpretation of the history by the examiner.

THE ATTACK BY EXAMINATION

During the time of the study, 79 patients were examined during a transient ischemic attack, and an additional 42 were examined during an attack that was proved to be a condition other than TIA.[6] These examinations revealed some unexpected findings. Although a definite diagnosis was more likely to be established when a patient was examined during an attack, this was not always true. In addition, those examined during an attack had much longer attacks than the average for all patients. For those 49 patients with carotid artery system TIAs, the mean duration was 6 hours compared to 14 minutes for all patients with this diagnosis. This suggested that this group might be atypical. More visual deficits were identified by examination than were recognized by the patient. The most common neurological finding supporting the patient's history was weakness of an arm or side of the face. It was uncommon to find muscle stretch reflex changes unless there was accompanying weakness. Retinal emboli were observed in only 2.5 percent. Although patients frequently complained of symptoms such as paresthesias or numbness, seldom were objective sensory deficits elicited. In no instance was a cardiac arrhythmia identified that seemed to have a causal relationship to the attack. All cardiac arrhythmias noted during the attack continued after the attack had ceased. There was thus no evidence for a causal relationship of transient arrhythmia to the attack.

DIAGNOSTIC WORKUP

Routine Laboratory Evaluation

Although we have presented data establishing that the diagnosis of TIA is made primarily by history and suggested that there is no quantitative relationship to degree of atherosclerosis, a number of laboratory studies are indicated. The Hospital Frequency Study reviewed 30 tests commonly performed on patients with complaints suggesting transient ischemic attacks.[7] Twenty-three tests were performed at least 10 percent of the time. Those tests most commonly abnormal included the electrocardiogram, chest radiograph, BUN, urinalyses, fasting and 2 hour postprandial blood sugar, cholesterol, electroencephalogram, serum triglycerides, dynamic brain scan, and supraorbital Doppler. A number of studies that were abnormal in a smaller percentage of cases are easily done and have high enough yield that they are probably indicated. These include thyroid function studies, cerebral spinal fluid analysis, serum electrolytes, serology, and dynamic brain scan. These abnormalities were not confined to the TIA group but were commonly seen in those patients who turned out not to have TIA. In fact, in most instances the group without TIA had the highest frequency. While these abnormalities contributed to the establishment of a diagnosis other than TIA as the cause of the symptoms of those not having TIA, their relatively high frequency in patients with TIA indicated an association of TIA with other diseases that produced abnormal laboratory findings. This might be a reflection of age (median 63 years), the high prevalence of arteriosclerotic cardiovascular disease, glucose intolerance in the overall group, or other unrecognized similar factors. These tests frequently led to the establishment of a diagnosis other than TIA for patients who presented with TIA-like symptoms or to the recognition of associated conditions when TIA is present. Therefore, although these tests are not diagnostic, they are of value in aiding the physician in determining possible causes of TIA, in detecting risk factors for associated conditions, in ruling out alternative diagnoses, and in assessing the patient's ability to tolerate different types of therapy.

Indirect Measurements of Flow

Indirect measurements of flow included ophthalmodynamometry, dynamic brain scan, Doppler ultrasound method, thermography, and carotid artery bruit.

The presence of a bruit over a carotid artery indicated stenosis of the underlying carotid artery in about half of the patients who had angiography. A substantial number of bruits (20 percent) were reported in the patients who were not found to have a stenotic lesion. In another series,[14] ipsilateral carotid arteries were normal in 15 percent of the cases when an ipsilateral carotid bruit was heard. As loudness and precise location were not recorded, it was not clear whether these were different from those associated with stenotic carotid vessels. Also, in the Hospital Frequency Study, 19 to 27 percent of the patients who had notable stenotic lesions were reported not to have bruits. Presence or absence of a bruit did not, therefore, appear to be a good criterion to indicate angiography on a patient suspected of having carotid artery stenosis.

Ultrasonic flow studies have a fairly high correlation to angiography but are far from perfect. A review of the Hospital Frequency Study and a review of the literature indicates that false positive results occur in about 10 percent and false negative results in 20 percent.[15] Although these will be discussed later during this symposium, the possibility that the relatively innocuous digital venous subtraction angiography technique will replace these procedures must be considered. Dynamic brain scan had poor correlation to angiography, and thermography was done so infrequently that an adequate analysis could not be performed.

Angiography

When angiography was carried out, arterial lesions were seen frequently, but the lesions could not always be correlated with the patient's clinical symptoms. For example, 57 percent of the patients who had vertebral-basilar system TIAs were found to have unilateral or bilateral carotid artery lesions. The best correlation was in patients who definitely had carotid artery system TIAs. However, here it was more common for angiographic lesions in the carotid artery to be bilateral rather than unilateral, as was also found in the Joint Study of Extracranial Vascular Occlusion.[16]

In the past, the author performed four-vessel angiography on virtually all patients not having a definite contraindication to this procedure. The reasons were two-fold: first, to rule out other treatable diseases that mask as TIA; and second, to identify potentially treatable surgically accessible vascular lesions. Although angiography is still performed, it is done much less frequently than in the past. The change in philosophy is related to the introduction of computerized tomography and the suggestion that antiplatelet aggregating agents may be of therapeutic value.[17-20] At the present time, if a patient gives a classic history for attacks, the neurological history and examination are classically normal and not suggestive of any other process, and if computerized tomography of the head, with and without contrast, reveals no treatable lesion, then a therapeutic trial will be initiated on antiplatelet aggregating agents. If the patient continues to have attacks with good antiplatelet aggregating effect or if follow-up history and examinations are questionable, the patient is then readmitted for four-vessel angiography with visualization of the vessels extracranially and intracranially. In this instance, if an appropriate surgically accessible lesion is present, we recommend that it be surgically removed. The advent of digital venous subtraction angiography is changing this philosophy. Currently and in the future, we intend to have the arch and neck vessels studied by this technique on all patients with any complaints suggestive of cerebral vascular disease. If the patient has good kidney function, we will also have intracranial vessels studied.

DIAGNOSTIC RELIABILITY

The inability of diagnostic tests, including angiography, to confirm or make a diagnosis necessitates that the reliability of the clinical diagnosis as made by history be tested. This was done in the Hospital Frequency Study[4] in

3 ways: (1) the independent diagnosis of the institutional investigator was compared to that of the principal investigator at the central registry, (2) a total of 42 entry forms were selected randomly from the first 485 cases entered into the study and each center's principal investigator reviewed these cases and made a diagnosis, and the diagnostic impressions were compared, and (3) a separate blind review of all entry forms and narrative summaries on all patients was made by two independent referees with special expertise in cerebral vascular disease, Drs. Raymond Bauer and Arthur Klassen. The 42 randomly selected cases resulted in 84 percent agreement for all subgroups and 93 percent for the definite TIAs. The independent referees agreed in 88 percent of the total cases and in 93 percent for those who were considered to be definitely TIA. This agreement was much better than was expected from previous studies of independent interpretations of other data.[21,22] Therefore, although one can never be assured that there will be agreement in the individual case, one would expect in large series that competent neurologists trained in cerebral vascular disease would have the same degree of diagnostic correlation.

FACTORS AFFECTING PROGNOSIS

In order to better assess the risk for further TIAs, stroke, and death, the Hospital Frequency Study identified 180 variables of which 60 could be studied in detail. Analyses used were Chi^2, regression and factor analysis for risk factors, and if a combination of risk factors was associated with outcome, these were multifactorially analyzed. In addition, the type of treatment was analyzed as a risk factor. History of multiple TIAs was a significant predictor of further TIAs, and a single TIA placed the patient at greater risk for early infarction. Older age, male sex, and unreliability to take dangerous medication were found to be risk factors for cerebral infarction. Anticoagulant therapy, older age, male sex, diabetes mellitus, heart disease, abnormal ECG, and poor surgical risk were factors for death. The increased mortality associated with anticoagulants was confined to the older age group. While white patients treated with antiplatelet aggregating agents had a lower mortality than those treated otherwise, this was not true among black patients. The type of TIA, whether vertebral-basilar or carotid artery, did not appear to affect the prognosis. The most surprising observation was that hypertension did not turn out to be a risk factor for further TIAs, infarction, or death. This is assumed to be related to the good treatment of recognized hypertension at the participating institutions.

One must conclude because of the large number of risk factors that can affect the prognosis of patients with TIAs, one cannot seriously consider any study of therapy that is not prospective, randomly selected, controlled, and double blind. For example, although the death rate each year was 6 percent, if one selects a group with normal ECGs, this can be decreased to 2 percent each year. Or if a group is composed of patients with diabetes mellitus or who are poor surgical risks, the death rate will increase to 13 percent each year. If one knows the risk factors, one can affect the prognosis considerably by combining just two virulent risk factors or two protective factors. The expected mortality can be changed from 1 percent to 30 percent each year. With these facts in mind, one must be extremely suspicious of studies describing therapeutic results where factors are not randomly distributed. Such properly designed studies are extremely rare, and this accounts for a great deal of the controversy concerning ideal therapy.[23] For instance, a large number of anecdotal studies described excellent results with long-term anticoagulants, but only four small, well-controlled studies have ever been reported.[24-27] Results of these studies combined suggest that although anticoagulants do decrease the likelihood of having further TIAs, they do not decrease the risk for infarction and very likely increase the likelihood for death. Many anecdotal studies concerning endarterectomy have been reported, but only one random double blind prospective study, and its results are inconclusive.[28] One must give more credence to the three prospectively designed, random, double blind studies that indicate that aspirin is associated with decreased TIA, death, and infarction in males, but not in females.[17-19] It is not the charge of this presentation to discuss these therapeutic approaches as this will be done in greater detail later in the symposium. Nevertheless, these data should raise some caution in interpretation of anecdotal studies, regardless of how large.

Despite controversies concerning the types of therapies, overwhelming evidence is available that in the last decade there has been a significant decrease in mortality due to stroke and heart disease in the United States.[29] Epidemiologists are convinced that the decrease is real but are not as convinced as to why. Possible explanations include better diagnosis and treatment of hypertension, heart disease, and other diseases that act as risk factors. Changes in diet, routine exercise programs, and many other changes in society may also contribute. Even though the reason for this decrease is not known, it would be appropriate that the risk factors in patients with transient ischemic attacks be treated vigorously. In addition, as part of specific therapy, the patient should be followed at close intervals and monitored for the development of risk factors such as high blood pressure, cardiac disease, obesity, cigarette smoking, sedentary life style, and hyperlipedemia so that these could be recognized early and treated vigorously when they occur.

Some paragraphs were published in Comprehensive Therapy, November 1981, Volume 7, pages 6 to 11. Permission to use this material has been obtained from the editor.

REFERENCES

1. Dyken ML, Conneally PM, Haerer AF, et al: Cooperative study of hospital frequency and character of transient ischemic attacks: I. Background organization and clinical survey. JAMA 237:882, 1977
2. Swanson PD, Calanchini PR, Dyken ML, et al: Cooperative study of hospital frequency and character of transient ischemic attacks: II. Performance of angiography among six centers. JAMA 237:2202, 1977
3. Haerer AF, Gotshall RA, Conneally PM, et al: Cooperative study of hospital frequency and character of transient ischemic attacks: III. Variation in treatment. JAMA 238:142, 1977
4. Calanchini PR, Swanson PD, Gotshall RA, et al: Cooperative study of hospital frequency and character of transient ischemic attacks. IV. The reliability of diagnosis. JAMA 238:2029, 1977
5. Futty DE, Conneally PM, Dyken ML, et al: Cooperative study of hospital frequency and character of transient ischemic attacks: V. Symptom analysis. JAMA 238:2386, 1977
6. Price TR, Gotshall RA, Poskanzer DC, et al: Cooperative study of hospital frequency and character of transient ischemic attacks. VI. Patients examined during an attack. JAMA 238: 2512, 1977
7. Gotshall RA, Price TR, Haerer AF, et al: Cooperative study of hospital frequency and character of transient ischemic attacks: VII. Initial diagnostic evaluation. JAMA 239:2001, 1978
8. Conneally PM, Dyken ML, Futty DE, et al: Cooperative study of hospital frequency and character of transient ischemic attacks: VIII. Risk factors. JAMA 240:742, 1978
9. Dyken ML, Klatte E, Kolar OJ, et al: Complete occlusion of common or internal carotid arteries. Archives of Neurology, 30:342, 1974
10. Dyken ML, Doepker JF, Kiovsky R, et al: Asymptomatic occlusion of an internal carotid in a hospital population: Determined by directional Doppler ophthalmosonometry. Stroke 5:714, 1974
11. Fisher CM: Observations of the fundus oculi in transient monocular blindness. Neurol 9:333, 1959
12. Hollenhorst RW: Significance of Bright plaques in the retinal arteriole. JAMA 178:23, 1961
13. Barnett HJM: "Platelet Antiaggregants—An Update", Deuxiemes Conferences De La Salpetriere, Maladies Vasculaires Cerebrales Cerebrovascular Disease, April, 1979, 257. Publisher: J.B. Balliere, 1980
14. Ramirez-Lassepas M, Sandok BA, Burton RE: Clinical indications of extracranial carotid artery disease in patients with transient symptoms. Stroke 4:537, 1973
15. Dyken ML: Ultrasonic flow studies: A critical review, in Moossy J, Reinmuth OM (eds): Cerebrovascular Diseases, Twelfth Research (Princeton) Conference, 115, 1981
16. Gomensoro JB, Maslenikov V, Azambuja N, et al: Joint study of extracranial arterial occlusion: VIII. Clinical-radiographic correlation of carotid bifurcation lesions in 177 patients with transient cerebral ischemic attacks. JAMA 224:985, 1973
17. Fields WS, Lemak NA, Frankowski RF, et al: Controlled trial of aspirin in cerebral ischemia. Stroke 8:301, 1977
18. Canadian Cooperative Study Group: Randomized trial of aspirin and sulfinpyrazone in threatened stroke. New Eng J Med 299:53, 1978
19. Reuther R, Dorndorf W: Aspirin in patients with cerebral ischemia and normal angiograms or non-surgical lesions: Results of a doubleblind trial, in Breddin K, Dorndorf W, Loew D, et al. (eds): Acetylsalicylic Acid in Cerebral Ischemia and Coronary Heart Disease, Stuttgart, New York, F.K. Schattauer Verlag 1978, p. 97

20. Dyken ML: Antiplatelet aggregating agents in transient ischemic attacks and the relationship of risk factors: (Total experience of six medical centers). V. Colfarit Symposium, Mainz, West Germany, 1980 (in press)
21. Koran LM: The reliability of clinical methods, data and judgments (part 2). N Engl J Med 293:695, 1975
22. Sisk C, Ziegler DK, Zileli T: Discrepancies in recorded results from duplicate neurological history and examination in patients studied for prognosis in cerebrovascular disease. Stroke 1:14, 1970
23. Dyken ML, Jones FA: Transient ischemic attacks. Comprehensive Therapy 7:6, 1981
24. Report of Veterans Administration Cooperative Study of Atherosclerosis, Neurology Section: An evaluation of anticoagulant therapy in the treatment of cerebrovascular disease. Neurology 11:132, 1961
25. Baker RN, et al: Anticoagulant therapy in cerebral infarction. Neurology 16:841, 1962
26. Pearce JMS, Gubbay SS, Walton, JN: Long-term anticoagulant therapy in transient cerebral ischemic attacks. Lancet 1:6, 1965
27. Baker RN, Schwartz WS, Rose AS: Transient ischemic strokes: A report of a study of anticoagulant therapy. Neurology 16:841, 1966
28. Fields WS, Maslenikov V, Meyer JS et al: Joint study of extracranial arterial occlusion. V. Progress report of prognosis following surgery or nonsurgical treatment for transient cerebral ischemic attacks and cervical carotid artery lesions. JAMA 211:1993, 1970
29. Dyken ML, Calhoun RA: Changes in stroke mortality that have an effect on evaluating and predicting outcome for therapeutic studies, Raven Press (Presented at Cerebrovascular Diseases Thirteenth Research (Princeton) Conference, Williamsburg, Virginia, March 1, 1982).

William S. Fields

6

Medical Treatment for Patients with Transient Ischemic Attacks

In order to understand the rationale for antiplatelet therapy in cerebrovascular disease, one must take into consideration the pathogenesis of transient ischemic attacks and of ischemic infarction. These considerations are essentially the same as those which underlie the selection of patients for arterial reconstructive surgery of the extracranial carotid arteries.[1] Serial arteriographic studies of extracranial atherosclerotic lesions have demonstrated clearly that the majority of such lesions remain remarkably stable, while a small but significant number demonstrate changes which occur quite abruptly.[2] This dynamic transformation of the extracranial lesion almost certainly underlies certain alterations in cerebral function and as many neurologists concede, provides an explanation of the pathogenesis of cerebral ischemic events. Unlike most surgeons who tend to be guided by the hemodynamic concept of the origin of cerebral ischemia, neurologists for the most part tend to adhere to the thromboembolic theory. In other words, strategically situated extracranial and intracranial complicated atherosclerotic lesions are important not because they produce stenosis but rather because they are the site from which downstream embolization occurs.[3,4] The surface of atherosclerotic plaques may become irregular as a result of being denuded of epithelium, progress to ulceration, and then be the source of small emboli which propagate into the distal branches of the middle cerebral artery.[5] Such ulceration in carotid plaques may occur not only in the presence of high-grade stenosis but also where the lumen is minimally compromised and there is no distal reduction in flow and pressure.[6]

This report, therefore, begins with consideration of platelet adhesion and aggregation on an irregular or ulcerated extracranial arterial lesion. Fibrinoplatelet material which is adherent to such a lesion becomes detached and embolizes downstream. When embolization of fibrinoplatelet aggregates occurs into the ophthalmic artery and its branches in the retina, "white bodies" may be seen moving through these vessels in a pulsatile manner.[7] Moreover, when the plaque itself breaks down it may discharge its contents, and emboli consisting of cholesterol crystals can be observed in the retinal arterioles. These "bright plaques" appear as refractile emboli permanently lodged at points of bifurcation without completely obstructing the flow of blood.[8] Considerable evidence may be found to support the hypothesis that change in the surface of extracranial atherosclerotic lesions along with secondary platelet aggregation and arterial-arterial embolism and/or occlusive thrombosis is the most common but by no means the only pathogenetic mechanism for ischemic stroke signs and symptoms in many patients. This concept has led neurologists and others to look for therapeutic methods that might modify or eliminate ischemic events in the brain. In properly selected cases, carotid endarterectomy has proven effective in diminishing the frequency of recurrent TIAs and completed stroke in the territory of the operated carotid artery.[9] In some communities where these surgical procedures are not done frequently, however, the operative mortality and morbidity may be unacceptably high and neurologists and other physicians have felt that antiplatelet therapy might offer a safer and more rational prophylactic approach to this problem by preventing platelet adhesion and aggregation on an ulcerated plaque and diminishing the likelihood of the production of fibrinoplatelet emboli or thrombus.

In the late 1960s, when reports appeared that aspirin was an active inhibitor of collagen-induced platelet aggregation, it seemed worthwhile to review the available data and plan clinical trials of aspirin for the prophylactic management of ischemic stroke syndromes.[10,11]

The conduct of clinical trials of antiplatelet drugs poses unusual problems for the physician. Aspirin, which thus far has been shown to be the most effective drug, is so widely used and easily available in North America that it is difficult to conduct a properly controlled trial without the risk of either inadvertent aspirin ingestion or an ability on the part of the individual to break the double-blind. Moreover, the old adage, "Go home, take two aspirin, go to bed, and call me in the morning," has become so much a part of medical folklore that it is difficult for a physician to convince his patient that recently discovered virtues of such a commonplace medication may have an important influence on the management of a serious health problem. In spite of these dilemmas, there was remarkable compliance with the prescribed treatment by the subjects enrolled in both the American and Canadian antiplatelet drug trials so that the investigators had every reason to be confident of the validity of their results. The subjects who stuck with the investigators through a long follow-up period and came regularly for visits must be considered the real heroes of this saga.

An interesting but seldom mentioned fact is that in both the Canadian and American trials of patients with transient ischemic attacks there was a rather remarkable reduction or cessation of such attacks with aspirin in both male and female patients.[12] These findings supported observations made previously in clinical practice and reported in the medical literature. More important, however, was the demonstration by the Canadian stroke trial of a reduction in stroke morbidity and overall mortality of 31 percent.[13] Unfortunately, when the male and female populations were analyzed independently, the efficacy appeared to be confined to the male subjects in whom there was a reduction of stroke morbidity and mortality of 48 percent. This benefit was not noted among the females. This observation suggests a difference in pathogenesis of TIAs and cerebral infarction. The sex difference in response still remains unexplained. However, recently reported experimental work also indicates a sex differential response to aspirin in some animal species as well as in humans.

Since the benefit from aspirin in the prevention of stroke morbidity and mortality is confined to male patients suffering from TIAs, it has been suggested that the combination of aspirin and dipyridamole (Persantine), a phosphodiesterase inhibitor, might prove to be effective in both sexes. For this reason, another clinical trial involving institutions in both the United States and Canada has been underway for nearly 3 years. Aspirin and dipyridamole are being compared with aspirin and a placebo given with a similar dosage schedule. At the time of this report, nearly 800 subjects have been recruited into this clinical trial. No information is available as yet since the trial is double-blinded and the code has not been broken.

At the time that the aforementioned clinical trials with aspirin were planned, very little was known about the role of prostaglandins in vascular disease, particularly with respect to interaction between the platelets in the blood and the endothelial surface of the vessel. Virtually all of the information now available on this subject was accumulated subsequent to the beginning of recruitment of subjects into these trials. As a consequence, the daily dose of 1.3 grams of aspirin was selected for empirical reasons based on prior experience in clinical practice and because of the fact that a maximum inhibition of platelet aggregation had been observed in vitro with 0.5 mM level of aspirin in the blood.[14]

Recently it has been shown, both in experimental models and by in vitro testing, that a much smaller dose of aspirin suffices to produce a significant effect on platelet aggregation. Aspirin appears to interfere with arachidonic acid conversion into thromboxane A_2 in platelets in a dose approximately 1/10 of that necessary to inhibit arachidonic acid conversion into prostaglandin I_2 (prostacyclin) in vascular endothelial cells.[15] Since thromboxane A_2 induces aggregation and prostacyclin inhibits it, one could theorize that it would be advantageous to block the former while sparing the latter. A recent report by Preston, however, demonstrates that this idea is both unsound and unrealistic.[16] This hypothesis is still not universally accepted and has yet to be proven in a clinical trial. There is only one study which has been reported to date in which a single daily dose of only 160 mg of aspirin was compared with a placebo in patients suffering from renal failure who were on dialysis. There was a sharp reduction in the number of thrombi appearing in the dialysis shunts among those receiving this small amount of aspirin.[17] It is hardly fair to deduce from this, however, that low-dose aspirin would be equally effective in vascular disorders associated with atherosclerosis since platelet function is known to be altered in uremia and the thrombi occur on artificial surfaces rather than within human arteries.

A clinical trial in patients with TIAs comparing placebo against two different daily doses of aspirin is now being conducted in the United Kingdom. More than 1200 patients have been recruited into this study, but it will be another 2 years before the results will be available. Investigators hope to be able to determine whether one 325 mg tablet of aspirin daily is equally or more effective than four aspirin tablets and that either one or both regimens is more effective than a placebo.[18]

It is not known to what extent platelet thromboxane A_2 synthesis must be inhibited in order to reduce the risk of thrombosis. It is, however, reasonable to assume that in the clinical trials which employ 1.3 grams of aspirin daily, the inhibition was close to 100 percent. A recent study, using young, healthy adult volunteers, demonstrated that ceiling effect is obtained with a single 2 mg. per kg. dose and that a relatively constant degree of inhibition of greater than 90 percent can be maintained by administering this small dose once every 72 hours.[19] Over a 3-day period, this represents approximately 1/30 of the dose currently recommended by the Food and Drug Administration for clinical use in men suffering from TIAs. It also appears likely that platelets of patients at risk of thrombosis may have a different sensitivity for aspirin when compared with the platelets of healthy, young subjects in whom thromboxane B_2 levels have been measured after low-dose aspirin administration. Moreover, a sex and/or age related change in aspirin sensitivity may only become apparent later in life.

There is no doubt that it would be advantageous to have another trial which utilizes low-dose aspirin to achieve an antithrombotic effect in symptomatic individuals. Quantification would allow a reappraisal of exclusion criteria, increase medication compliance of the subjects who are recruited, and reduce withdrawals by minimizing gastrointestinal complaints. It is to be hoped that another clinical trial using low-dose aspirin will permit us to address both the issues of aspirin dosage and the male/female difference in response. An answer to the latter question may also be forthcoming when the current trial of aspirin and dipyridamole (Persantine) is completed.

REFERENCES

1. Fields WS: Selection of patients with ischemic cerebrovascular disease for arterial surgery. World J Surg 3:147, 1979
2. Bauer RB, Boulos RS, Meyer JS: Natural history and surgical treatment of occlusive cerebrovascular disease evaluated by serial arteriography. Am J Roent 104:1, 1968
3. Fisher CM: Occlusion of the carotid artery: Further experiences. Arch Neurol Psychiat 72:187, 1954
4. Gunning AJ, Pickering GW, Robb-Smith AHT, et al: Mural thrombosis of the internal carotid artery and subsequent embolism. Quart J Med 33:155, 1964
5. Gomensoro JB, Maslenikov V, Azambuja N, et al: Joint study of extracranial arterial occlusion. VIII. Clinical-radiographic correlation of carotid bifurcation lesions in 177 patients with transient cerebral ischemic attacks. JAMA 224:985, 1973
6. Moore WS, Hall AD: Ulcerated atheroma of the carotid artery, a cause of transient cerebral ischemia. Am J Surg 116:237, 1968
7. Fisher CM: Observations of the fundus oculi in transient monocular blindness. Neurology 9:333, 1959
8. Hollenhorst RW: Significance of bright plaques in the retinal arterioles. Trans Am Ophthal Soc 59:252, 1966
9. Fields WS, Maslenikov V, Meyer JS, et al: Joint study of extracranial arterial occlusion. V. Progress report of prognosis following surgery or non-surgical treatment for transient cerebral ischemic attacks and carotid artery lesions. JAMA 211:1993, 1970
10. Weiss HJ, Aledort LM, Kochwa S: The effect of salicylates on the hemostatic properties of platelets in man. J Clin Invest 47:2169, 1968
11. Evans G, Packham MA, Nishizawa EE, et al: The effect of acetylsalicylic acid on platelet function. J Exp Med 128:877, 1968
12. Fields WS, Lemak NA, Frankowski RF, et al: Controlled trial of aspirin in cerebral ischemia. Circ 62 (suppl. V):90, 1980
13. Canadian Cooperative Study Group: A randomized trial of aspirin and sulfinpyrazone in threatened stroke. N Engl J Med 299:53, 1978
14. Levy G, Leonards JR: Absorption, metabolism and excretion of salicylates, in Smith, MJH, Smith PK (eds): The Salicylates, A Critical Biographical Review. New York, Interscience Publishers, Inc., 1966
15. Masotti G, Poggesi L, Galanti G, et al: Differential inhibition of prostacyclin production and platelet aggregation by aspirin. Lancet 1:1213, 1979
16. Preston FE, Shipps S, Jackson CA, et al: Inhibition of prostacyclin and platelet thromboxane A_2 after low-dose aspirin. N Engl J Med 304:76, 1981
17. Harter HR, Burch JW, Majerus PW, et al: Prevention of thrombosis in patients on hemodialysis by low-dose aspirin. N Engl J Med 301:577, 1979
18. Warlow CB: Personal communication, 1981
19. Patrono C, Ciabattoni G, Pinca E, et al: Low dose aspirin and inhibition of thromboxane B_2 production in healthy subjects. Thromb Res 17:317, 1980

PART III

New Radiologic Diagnostic Studies

W.D. Turnipseed

7

The Diagnosis of Carotid Artery Stenosis by Digital Subtraction Angiography

Standard arteriography has played an important role in the diagnosis and management of cerebrovascular disease because of its ability to define the anatomic distribution and severity of arterial lesions. Arteriography has been commonly used to examine patients with symptoms of cerebral ischemia because of the unpredictable relationship between physical findings, the severity of symptoms, and the hemodynamic significance of cranial vascular lesions. Standard angiography, however, has not been widely employed as a method of diagnostic screening in asymptomatic patients because of the invasive nature and the cost of the procedure. The need for arterial catheterization and for hospitalization during standard angiography, in addition to rather poor patient acceptance, has forced clinicians to use standard angiograms as a means of preoperative mapping of cerebrovascular disease in symptomatic patients being considered for surgical management. The restricted use of standard angiography in the day-to-day management of cerebrovascular problems has resulted in a proliferation of noninvasive testing techniques. These procedures have been used as a supplement to clinical examination in order to improve the detection of occult disease and to more objectively evaluate the hemodynamic significance of asymptomatic cervical bruits. These tests (oculodynamometry, oculoplethysmography, phonoangiography, Doppler arterial imaging with spectral analysis, real time ultrasonography) are safe, can be performed on an outpatient basis, have good patient acceptance, are suited for repetitive testing, and have proven to be very accurate in the detection of hemodynamically significant stenoses (greater than 50 percent).[1-8] By definition, however, the noninvasive test techniques are indirect and require the expertise and interpretive skills of a trained technician. The equipment is very specialized and frequently limited to the evaluation of isolated vascular segments such as the carotid bifurcation. Minor stenoses and ulcerated plaques which are of little hemodynamic significance but of considerable clinical importance are frequently missed by these tests. In addition, noninvasive tests do not accurately define the vascular anatomy of the intrathoracic and intracranial segments of the brachiocephalic circulation. A new method of computerized arterial imaging has made it possible to visualize the entire peripheral vascular and much of the cardiopulmonary system by intravenous injection of standard contrast agents (Renografin 76, Conray 400). This technique has been referred to by a variety of terms including intravenous video angiography (IVA), digital video angiography (DVA), digital video subtraction angiography (DVSA), and more recently, digital subtraction angiography (DSA). All of these terms refer to the same method of computerized fluoroscopic enhancement to obtain arterial imaging by intravenous injection of contrast agent.[9-15] Digital subtraction angiography (DSA) seems to hold the middle ground between standard angiography and noninvasive testing. It is safer than the standard cerebral angiography because catheterization can be avoided, along with the risk of hemorrhage, thrombosis, and/or embolization. DSA can be performed as an outpatient study just like noninvasive tests yet it provides more precise anatomic information about the intra- and extracranial circulation than can be obtained by noninvasive techniques.

TECHNIQUE

Digital subtraction angiography (DSA) is the term currently preferred by radiologists when referring to computer augmented intravenous angiography. This method of arteriographic imaging is performed by power injecting standard contrast agent into the peripheral venous system at a rate of 12-15 cc/sec. The power injection of contrast media (40-60 cc) shortens the injection time and gives a more compact bolus of contrast delivery to the right heart. Originally, DSA was performed by placing a short 16 gauge catheter into an antecubital vein, but technical failures occurred in about 5 percent of the studies because of extravasation of contrast or because of sequestration of contrast media in the upper extremity veins. Our technique has been modified and is now performed by threading a #5 French polyethylene catheter through an antecubital vein into the subclavian vein or superior vena cava. If upper extremity access is unavailable, a percutaneous retrograde femoral puncture is made with catheterization of the iliac vein or inferior vena cava. Central placement of this catheter has virtually eliminated the problem of contrast sequestration or extravasation and guarantees a crisp delivery of contrast media to the right heart.[16,17] Contrast agents commonly used for digital subtraction angiography include Conray 400 (400 mg of iodine/ml, in the form of 66 percent sodium iothalamate) and Renografin 76, (which has an iodine concentration of 370 micrograms of iodine/ml, in the form of 66 percent meglumine and 10 percent sodium diatrizoate). Amopaque, which is an experimental nonionic contrast medium, derived from the molecule metrizamide, appears to have a major advantage over the other contrast agents because it does not cause the tearing pain sensation, which elicits involuntary swallowing and patient motion.[18]

There are several factors that can affect the quality of arterial imaging produced by digital subtraction angiography. Perhaps the greatest problem is image quality degradation due to motion. DSA provides the best angiographic images when there is little cardiac or respiratory motion and when assessment of short vascular segments such as the carotid bifurcation is necessary. The field size for current DSA imaging is about 9 inches (22.9 cm). This creates a problem because multiple injections of contrast are frequently needed to completely evaluate the cerebrovascular circulation. Image intensifiers with larger field sizes will significantly reduce this problem. Biplane imaging which is particularly important in the assessment of extracranial vascular lesions is not possible with DSA. Separate contrast injections are required for each projection that is needed. A minimum of 5 injections are currently required to complete a thorough diagnostic study. These include an AP projection of the aortic arch, a right and left lateral, and oblique projections of the intracranial circulation. The total contrast volume required is between 150 and 200 cc and the total radiation exposure for the entire study is between 2 and 4 rads.[17,19]

One potential limitation of digital subtraction angiography in evaluation of the cerebrovascular system is the fact that contrast density and focal resolution of the technique is limited to vessel diameters and anatomic lesions greater than 1 mm in size. This means that it is possible that intravenous digital subtraction angiography will miss band-like stenoses, minor ulcerations and small vessel occlusions or tiny aneurysms in the intracranial circulation.

Digital subtraction angiography uses a time subtraction technique known as mask mode radiography. This is a serial subtraction technique used for imaging static vessels in the cerebrovascular system. A mask image is taken before arrival of contrast and is stored in one of the memory units of the digital processor. As the contrast media is pumped through the heart into the cerebrovascular system, additional static images are taken, summated, and stored in a second memory unit. The mask is subtracted from the summation image resulting in contrast enhanced angiography. The arterial image is stored on a video disk, projected on a TV screen, and converted to hard copy angiography by a standard multiformat camera. The ability to store video images on tape promises to be a significant economic advantage because the

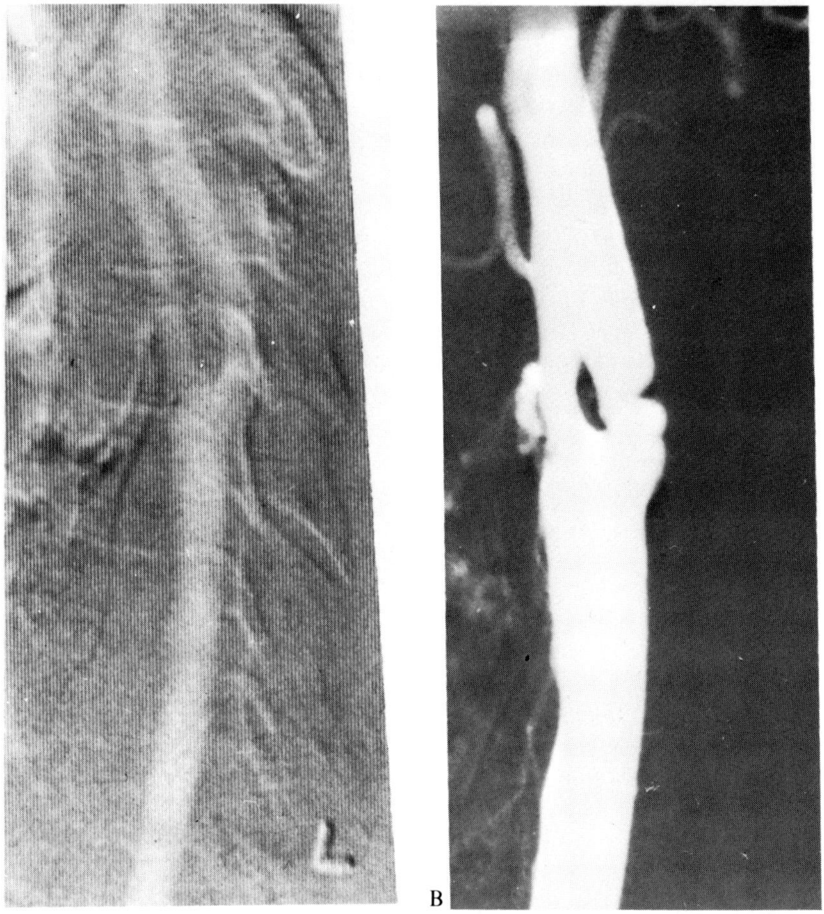

Figure 7-1. (A) Intravenous DSA study showing the left carotid of a patient who had symptoms of left sided amaurosis fugax. This false negative study failed to demonstrate a critical band stenosis just distal to the take off of the internal carotid artery. (B) Intraarterial digital subtraction study clearly shows the band-like stenosis just beyond the origin of the internal carotid artery. Whenever symptomatic patients have normal-appearing intravenous DSA studies, intraarterial DSA or standard angiography should be performed in order to rule out web-like stenoses or small ulcerated plaques.

number of standard x-rays needed can be greatly reduced, thus saving not only storage space but the cost of developing standard x-ray films.[19-22]

Recently computerized imaging techniques have been used in conjunction with intraarterial injection of contrast into the aortic arch. Intraarterial DSA may prove to be an important radiologic technique because it can significantly reduce the volume of contrast needed to obtain arterial imaging of the cerebrovascular system and at the same time can significantly improve contrast resolution and the ability to visualize small vessel pathology (Fig. 7-1A,B). Intraarterial DSA can provide precise arterial imaging of both intra- and extracranial vessels with contrast injection volumes of less than 3 cc for each projection. This means that the total volume of contrast used in a standard cerebrovascular study can be reduced by at least 1/3. This is a major advantage in the assessment of diabetic patients who appear to be more susceptible to the nephrotoxic effects of contrast and patients who have elevated creatinines or known impaired renal function. Another safety factor with intraarterial DSA is that selective catheterization of the vertebral and carotid arteries is not necessary. Intraarterial DSA makes it possible to safely extend the limits of standard angiography and to obtain anatomic information about asymptomatic cervical bruits in patients who are having standard arterial evaluations of the aorta and the distal runoff system for symptoms of peripheral ischemia. In addition, small volume injections in the aortic root can be used to obtain views of the right and left coronary artery origins. This makes it possible to identify potentially threatening mainstem coronary artery lesions in patients preoperatively and to evaluate the patency of aorto-coronary bypass procedures in patients who are being evaluated for overtly symptomatic peripheral vascular disease.[21]

CLINICAL APPLICATIONS

Our greatest clinical experience with digital subtraction angiography has been in the assessment of patients who are at increased risk for stroke because of the physical findings such as a cervical bruit or symptoms suggesting cerebral ischemia. Digital subtraction angiography provides anatomic detail of the brachiocephalic vessels and can identify a variety of clinically significant lesions including minor stenoses, ulcerated plaques, aneurysms, severe stenoses, and occlusions (Figs. 7-2-5). In a recent study, we compared the results of intravenous DSA with those obtained from standard angiography in a group of patients with symptoms of cerebral ischemia. Standard angiography was used to define the anatomical status of carotid and vertebral arteries in 36 patients with cerebrovascular symptoms. Five anatomic categories were defined. Group 1 consisted of 13 anatomically normal carotids; Group 2 consisted of 14 carotids with plaqueing or minor stenosis. In Group 3, there were 12 carotids with moderate-grade stenosis ranging from 50–75 percent reduction of transverse lumen diameter. In Group 4 there were 15 carotids with severe stenosis which was greater than 75 percent reduction in transverse lumen diameter. In Group 5, there were 18 complete internal carotid artery occlusions. Digital subtraction angiography correctly identified all of the normal carotid arteries in Group 1. Twelve of 14 carotids with minor

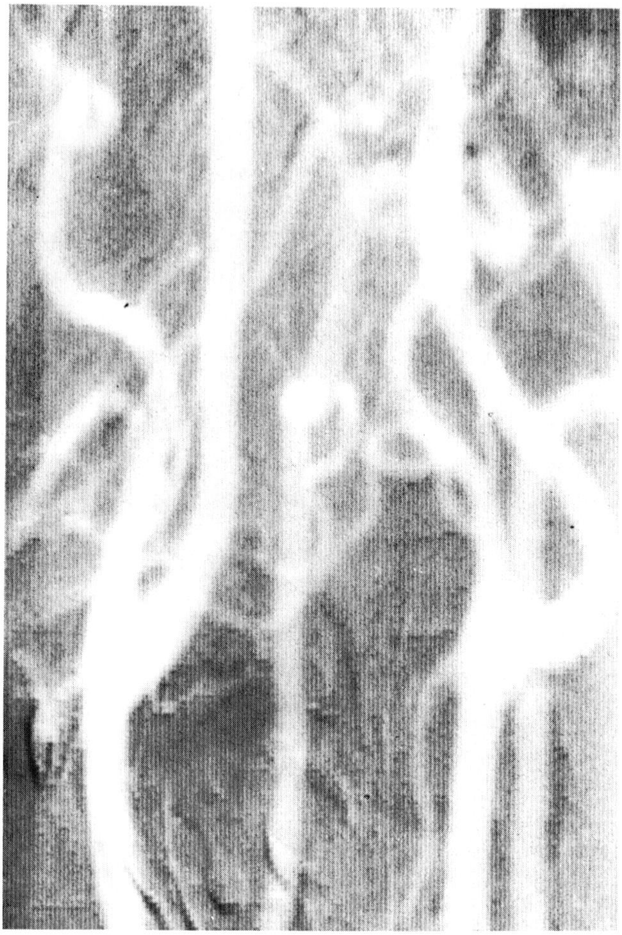

Figure 7–2. Intravenous DSA showing normal bilateral carotid bifurcations. The posterior vertebral arteries are visualized as well.

plaqueing or stenosis in Group 2 were correctly identified, but two minor stenoses were missed resulting in a false negative error rate of 14 percent. Only 3 of 9 ulcerated plaques in this group (33 percent) were correctly identified by digital angiography. Digital subtraction angiography correctly identified 26 of the 27 stenotic lesions in Groups 3 and 4, and 11 of 12 ulcerated lesions in these 2 groups. DSA correctly identified all complete internal carotid artery occlusions.

Preliminary comparisons between standard and intravenous digital subtraction angiography of the extracranial carotid suggest that standard

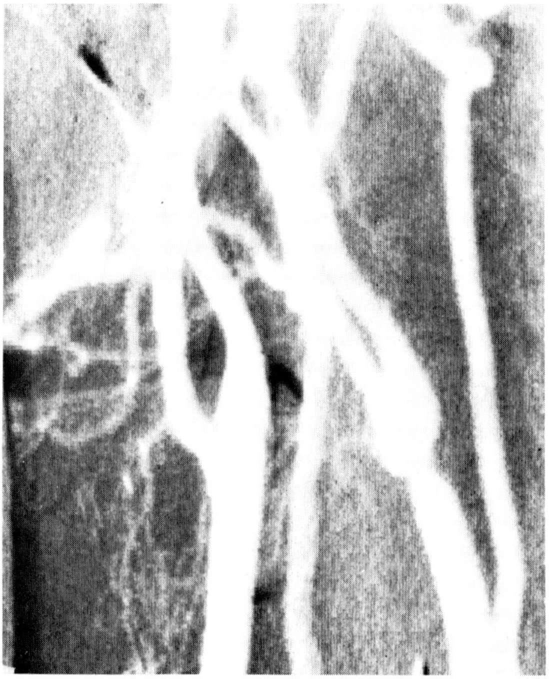

Figure 7-3. Intravenous DSA shows a moderate grade stenosis of the left carotid bifurcation. The right carotid bifurcation is normal. The posterior vertebral arteries are widely patent.

angiography is more accurate in the ability to define minor stenoses and small ulcerated plaques. DSA is as accurate as standard angiography when it comes to the identification of stenotic lesions which are greater than 50 percent of the transverse lumen diameter. In addition, ulcerated lesions associated with moderate or severe stenoses can be identified by either technique with great accuracy. Complete occlusions have not been missed by standard or digital subtraction angiography.[20] More recent comparisons between intraarterial DSA studies of the extracranial vessels and standard angios show that there is no significant difference in image quality and that even small ulcerations and band stenoses can be correctly identified. Intraarterial DSA can be performed with less than 1/3 the contrast required for standard angios (Fig. 7-6A,B).

Intravenous DSA has been of more limited value in the assessment of intracranial circulation. It can identify major occlusions in the carotid siphons and large ulcerations or aneurysms in the proximal branches of the circle of Willis. This ability to define the location and anatomical status of the cavernous portion of the internal carotids has made it possible to eliminate standard cerebral angiography as a preoperative study in patients who require

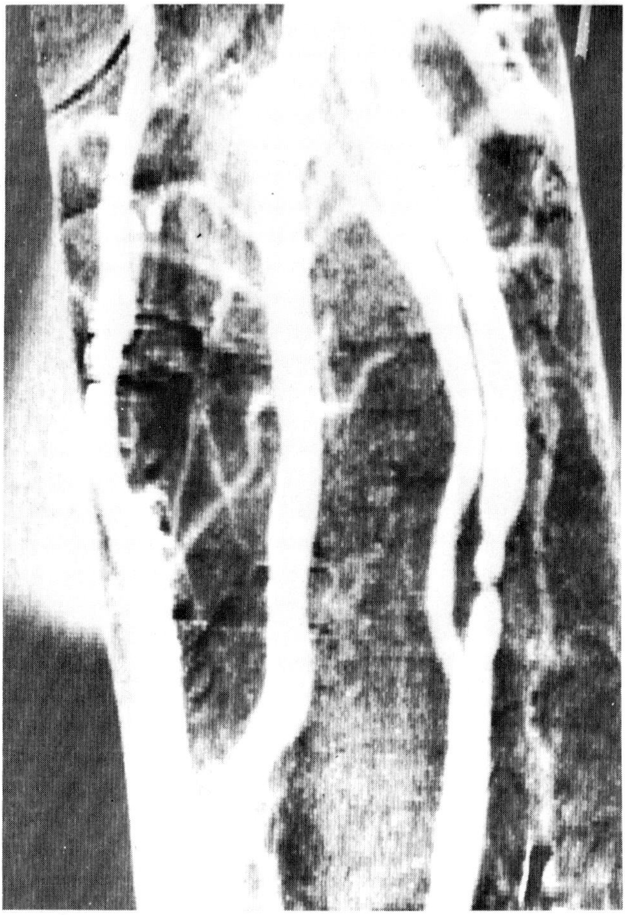

Figure 7-4. This demonstrates a preocclusive stenosis of the internal carotid artery on the left side (arrow). The vertebral artery to the right of the bifurcation is widely patent.

transsphenoidal hypophysectomy. Intravenous DSA can be used to diagnose and locate aneurysms at the base of the brain. Small lesions in the peripheral vessels of the cerebral cortex are difficult to evaluate because of limitations in spatial resolution and vascular superimposition caused by simultaneous opacification of all the intracranial vasculature. For this reason, intravenous DSA has not yet been used to plan surgical correction of intracranial aneurysms. Intraarterial DSA images of the intracranial circulation, however, are comparable to images obtained by standard injection techniques and can be used for this purpose (Fig. 7-7A,B).

The advent of digital subtraction angiography has generated tremendous enthusiasm among clinicians who must diagnose and treat patients with

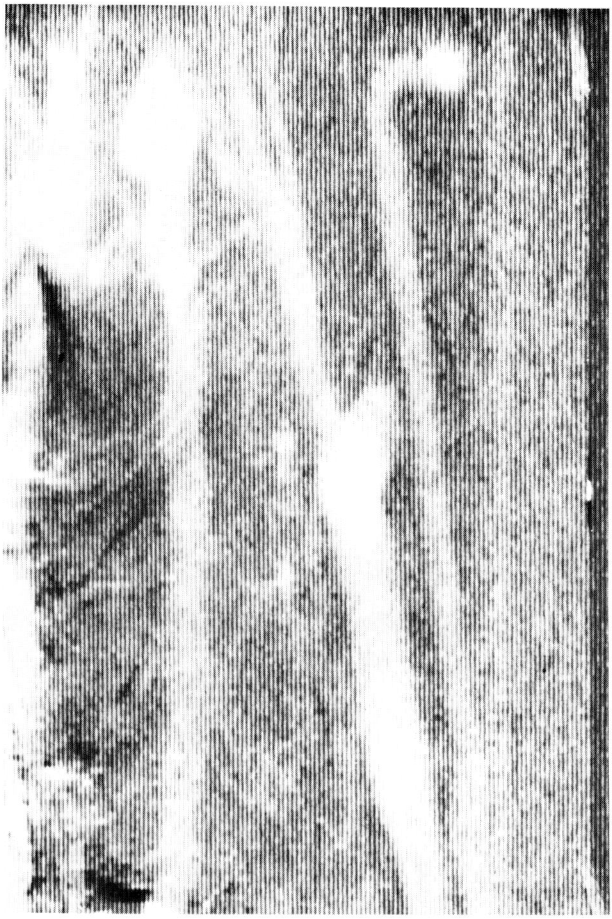

Figure 7-5. This intravenous DSA shows complete occlusion of the internal carotid artery origin. The external carotid is widely patent. The vertebral arteries are visualized on either side of the carotid artery.

cerebrovascular disease. It is not entirely clear what the ultimate role of this new diagnostic technique will be. Many have questioned how it will affect the use of standard angiography and how it will interface with widely used noninvasive diagnostic methods. At present, these questions cannot be precisely answered. Early clinical experience with cerebrovascular DSA suggests that because of the ease and safety of this procedure, the indications for obtaining angiograms will be much more liberal than before. Intravenous DSA will not eliminate the need for noninvasive diagnostic screening methods. In fact, DSA can be used to supplement information obtained from noninvasive screening tests. Most of these procedures, including oculodyna-

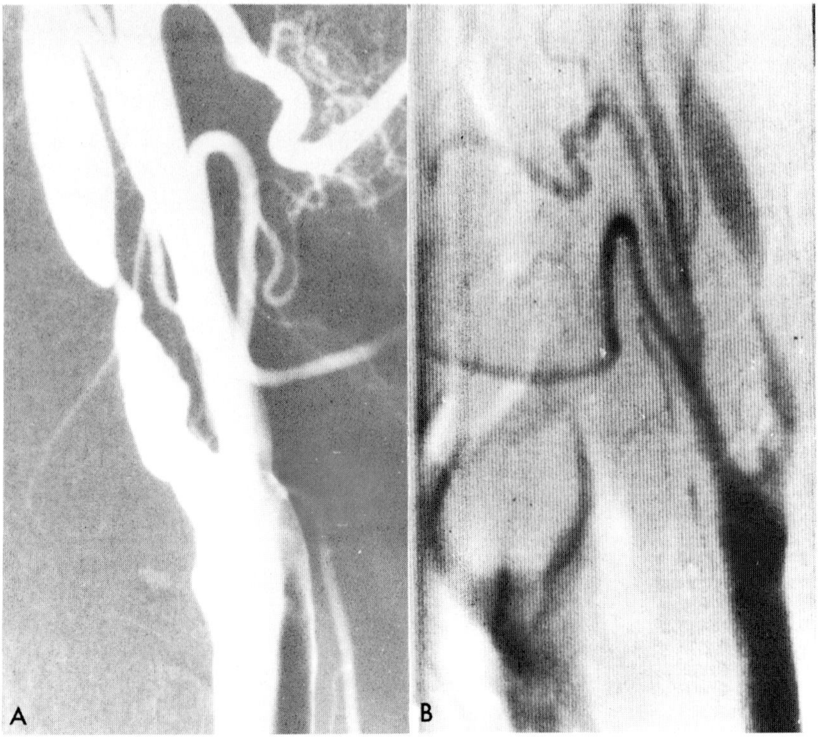

Figure 7-6A. This is a standard angiogram of a carotid artery with a preocclusive stenosis of the internal carotid branch. This arteriogram is obtained by selectively injecting 10 cc of contrast into the common carotid origin. (B) Intraarterial DSA showing the same carotid stenosis. This arteriogram was obtained by injecting 1 cc of contrast into the aortic arch near the origin of the common carotid.

Figure 7-7A. This is an intravenous DSA showing the intracranial circulation of a patient who has complete occlusion of the right internal carotid artery. The left carotid siphon is widely patent. Both hemispheres are supplied by the left internal carotid artery. Although the carotid siphon is clearly visible, the fine detail of the more peripheral intracerebral vessels is obscured because of limitations in spatial resolution. This intravenous DSA required 40 cc of contrast. (B) This is an intraarterial DSA which was performed with 2 cc of contrast injected into the aortic arch. Note the fine definition and excellent spatial resolution obtained by computerized enhanced nonselective injection of contrast material. Much more detailed evaluation of the smaller intracranial vessels is possible with intraarterial DSA.

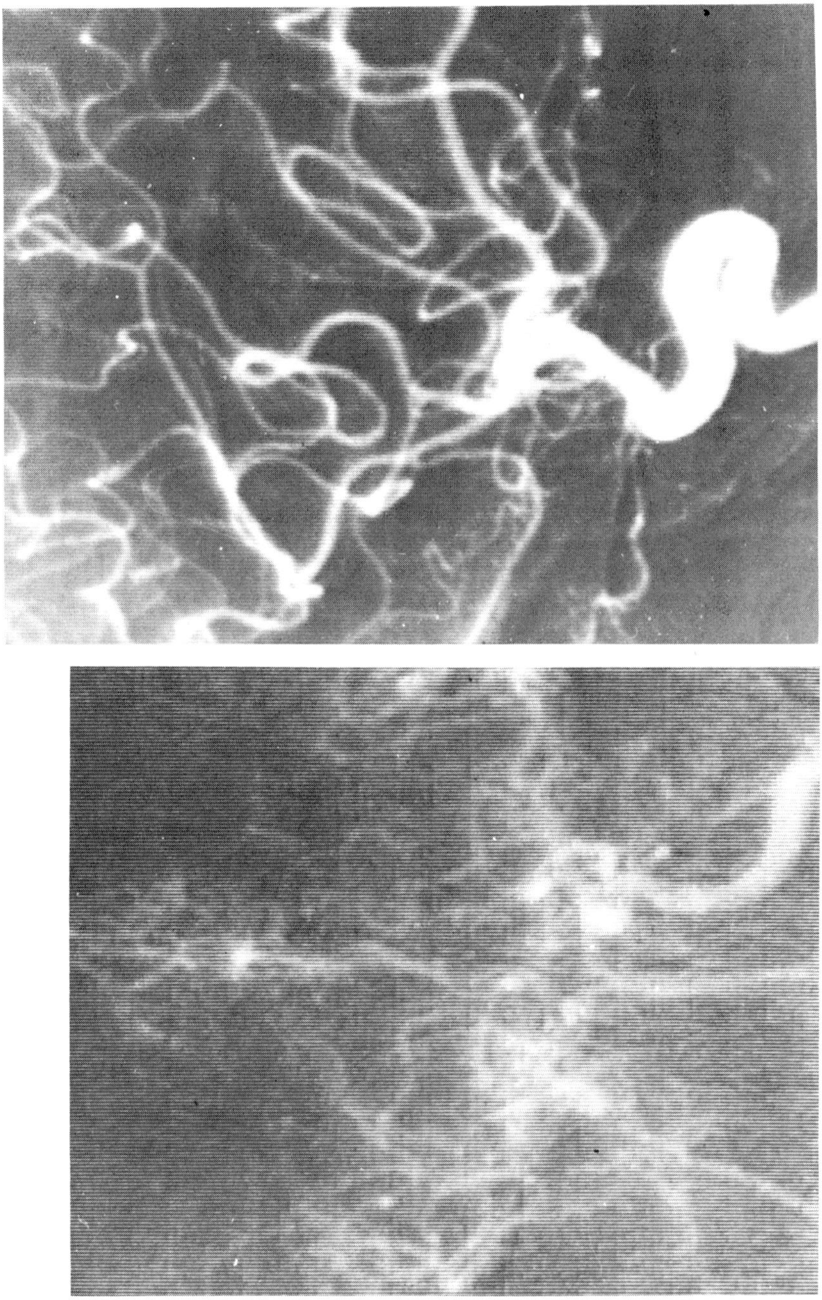

B

A

mometry, oculoplethysmography, phonoangiography and Doppler imaging with spectral analysis, are very good at identifying lesions which reduce the transverse lumen diameter of the carotids by 50 percent or more. Minor-grade stenoses, ulcerated plaques, and occasionally complete internal carotid artery occlusion are commonly missed by these diagnostic procedures. Real-time ultrasonography has been of some value in identifying ulcerated plaques. Intravenous cerebral DSA studies can more accurately identify these problem lesions than can most noninvasive procedures. In addition, DSA can provide important information about patency and anatomic status of the vertebral arteries and the major vessels in the intracranial circulation. The combined use of noninvasive diagnostic techniques and cerebrovascular DSA will be commonly employed in the evaluation of patients who have diffuse neurological symptoms suggesting cerebral ischemia. DSA will be of some value in more precisely defining suspected intracranial mass lesions identified by CAT scan and in clarifying equivocal noninvasive cerebrovascular tests. There are also occasions when the noninvasive tests may be helpful in clarifying equivocal DSA studies. This is particularly true in the assessment of patients with asymptomatic cervical bruits. We have found that DSA will occasionally miss a critical band stenosis which was easily identified by the noninvasive tests. Whenever there is a conflict between DSA and noninvasive test findings, standard angiography or intraarterial DSA should be performed.

Intravenous DSA is currently being used as the first diagnostic test in the assessment of patients with symptoms suggesting cerebrovascular insufficiency. We request the radiologist to examine not only the carotid bifurcation, but the origin of the carotid and vertebral vessels and the intracranial circulation in all symptomatic patients. When an isolated lesion can be defined at the level of the carotid bifurcation in the absence of major intracranial or proximal brachial cephalic occlusive disease, management decisions are based on the results of this test alone. If intravenous digital subtraction angiography cannot clearly identify a lesion in the carotid system, then standard angiography or intraarterial DSA must be performed in order to rule out minor ulcerations or narrow web stenoses which can be missed because of spatial resolution limitations of the intravenous technique. We are currently using DSA to evaluate patients who are being considered for cardiac or peripheral vascular reconstructive procedures when noninvasive screening tests are positive for significant brachiocephalic occlusive lesions (Fig. 7-8). Intraarterial DSA of the cerebrovascular system can be combined with coronary artery or peripheral angiography to obtain additional information about the cerebral circulation. It is safer than standard angiographic methods because complications associated with selective arterial catheterization of the brachiocephalic arteries and the effects of excess contrast load on the kidneys can be avoided. DSA has been used for diagnostic purposes in the evaluation of patients with absent cervical bruits and symptoms of cerebral insufficiency,

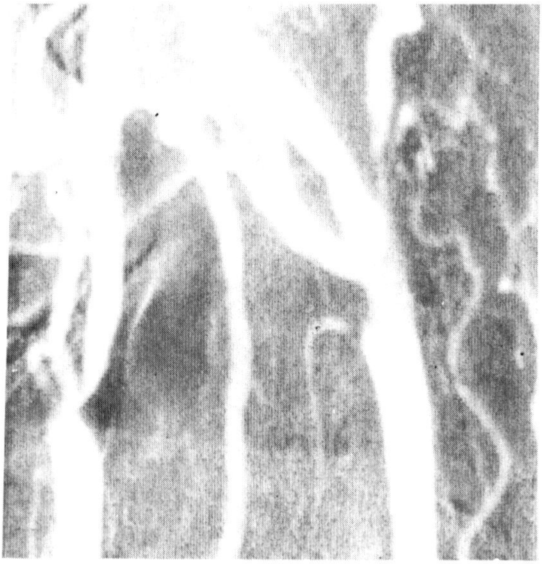

Figure 7-8. This is an intravenous DSA performed on a patient who is being prepared for aortofemoral bypass surgery. Noninvasive tests performed to evaluate asymptomatic carotid bruits were positive for high grade stenosis. DSA shows bilateral stenotic lesions in the carotid bifurcations. The right is more severe than the left.

in the assessment of completed or acute strokes, and for the evaluation of nonspecific neurologic symptoms and vertebral-basilar type TIAs. Patients with normal or occluded cervical or intracranial carotid arteries can often be spared the risks of standard angiography. Anatomic detail of the vertebral-basilar system can be accurately defined by DSA, and space-occupying lesions identified by CAT scan can be identified as vascular or solid in nature without additional risk to the patient (Figs. 7-9,10). DSA can also be used to clarify equivocal noninvasive tests in patients with symptoms of cerebrovascular ischemia, particularly when there is a question of minor stenosis, ulceration, aneurysm, or occlusion (Fig. 7-11). At present, we feel that noninvasive testing is inessential in the evaluation of patients with cerebrovascular-type symptoms in view of the fact that vascular reconstructive procedures of the brachiocephalic system cannot safely be performed without angiographic definition of arterial anatomy in this area.

We routinely use noninvasive testing, however, in the assessment of asymptomatic cervical bruits. Noninvasive tests are completely safe and are cheaper than DSA for purposes of diagnostic screening and can be used to identify patients who may need more precise anatomic definition of their

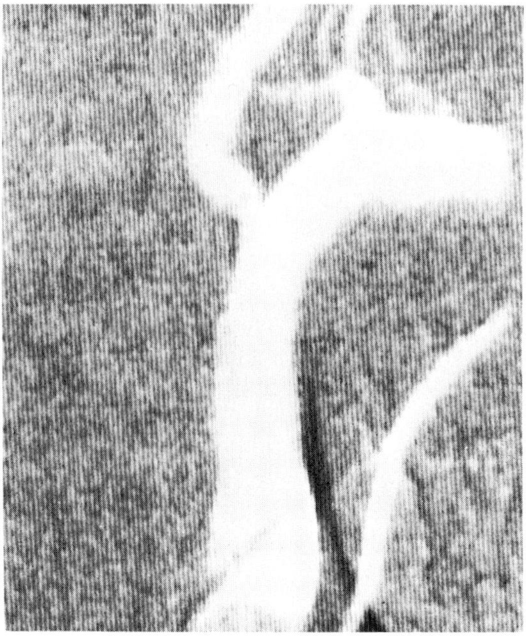

Figure 7-9. This is an intravenous DSA showing the vertebral artery origin in a patient who had symptoms suggesting vertebral basilar insufficiency. There is no evidence of obstructive disease at the origin of the vertebral artery.

carotid or brachiocephalic disease. Our noninvasive tests for cerebrovascular disease include Doppler arterial imaging with spectral analysis of the carotid flow and the Barnes technique of periorbital Doppler assessment. This combination of noninvasive cerebrovascular tests, in our experience, has proven to be as useful as phonoangiography or oculoplethysmography in identification of moderate and high-grade stenoses and is actually more accurate in identification of obstructive internal carotid disease. We have also used the noninvasive tests as a routine method of postoperative follow-up in patients who have had previous carotid endarterectomy. Although the noninvasive tests are very accurate in identifying recurrent stenoses, they will occasionally miss a complete occlusion and will usually miss an intimal dissection or pseudoaneurysm. Early postoperative assessment is a particular problem for noninvasive techniques that directly evaluate the carotid bifurcation. It is difficult to do an accurate examination of the carotid when there is a fresh operative wound with edema and possibly hematoma in the area. We have found that DSA is a much more practical method of early postoperative assessment because it provides direct anatomic detail of the

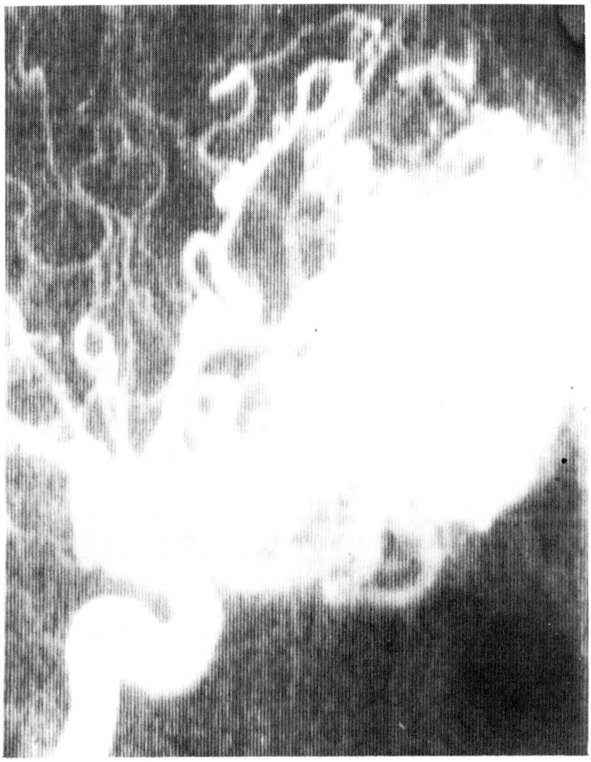

Figure 7-10. This demonstrates an arterio-venous fistula in a patient who had diffuse neurological symptoms and a positive CAT scan suggesting a tumor-like mass posteriorly.

carotid bifurcation and surgical area. We also use DSA to provide supplemental information obtained in noninvasive tests when there is a question about vertebral artery involvement or when the minor ulcerations and stenoses must be ruled out.

Digital subtraction angiograpy should also simplify the diagnosis of cervical and brachiocephalic vascular injuries in patients evaluated for trauma. DSA can be performed rapidly by using intravenous catheters placed for resuscitation purposes, and the technique should be particularly useful in detecting penetration injuries of major branches of the aortic arch or to the cervical carotid vessels. Although standard angiography can accurately identify most vascular injuries, the time required to set it up is a major problem in the management of severely injured patients. DSA may help reduce the number of surgical explorations for suspected vascular trauma in the thorax and the cervical regions.

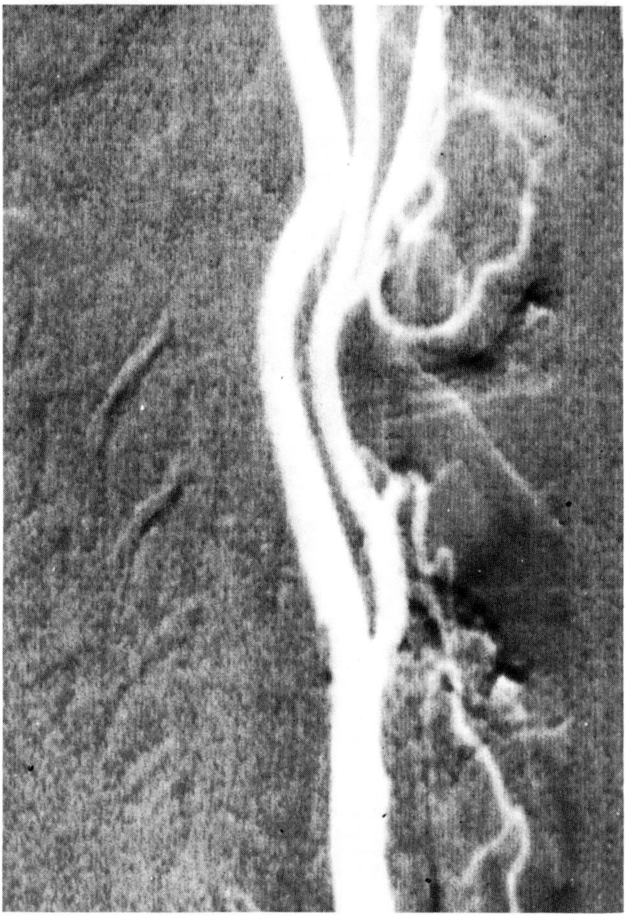

Figure 7-11. This intravenous DSA was performed to rule out possible ulcerative disease in this patient who had recurrent episodes of transient cerebral ischemia. The arrow demonstrates a small nonstenotic ulcerated plaque at the origin of the internal carotid artery.

In conclusion, it is apparent that digital subtraction angiography will expand the role of arteriography and alter our dependence on noninvasive testing. This method of arterial imaging probably will be used to evaluate segments of the vascular system which cannot be accurately appraised by noninvasive tests and to eliminate the need for standard angiography in many clinical situations. This method of arterial imaging promises to make the diagnosis and management of brachiocephalic disease simpler, safer, and less traumatic for the patient.

REFERENCES

1. Barnes RW: Noninvasive diagnostic techniques in peripheral vascular disease. Am Heart J 79:241, 1979
2. Bone GE, Slaymaker EE, Barnes RW: Noninvasive assessment of collateral blood flow of the cerebral hemisphere by Doppler ultrasound. Surg Gynecol Obstet 145:873, 1977
3. Gee W, Oller DW, Amundsen DG: The asymptomatic carotid bruit and oculoplethysmography. Arch Surg 112:1381, 1977
4. Satiani B, Cooperman M, Clark M, et al: An assessment of carotid phonoangiography and oculoplethysmography in detection of carotid artery stenosis. Am J Surg 136:618, 1978
5. Blackshear WM, Thiele BL, Harley JD: A prospective evaluation of carotid oculoplethysmography and carotid phonoangiography. Surg Gynecol Obstet 148:201, 1979
6. Turnipseed WD, Berkoff HA, Barriga P: Echo Doppler scanning and spectral frequency analysis: A screening procedure for carotid artery disease. Trans Am Neurol Assoc 102:28, 1977
7. Crummy AB, Zweibel WJ, Barriga P: Doppler evaluation of extracranial cerebrovascular disease. AJR 132:91, 1979
8. Cooperberg PA, Robertson WD, Fry P: High resolution real time ultrasound of the carotid bifurcation. JCU 7:13, 1979
9. Mistretta CA: Digital videoangiography. Diagnostic Imaging 14, 1981
10. Kruger RA, Mistretta CA: Computerized fluoroscopy techniques for noninvasive imaging of the cardiovascular system. Radiology 130:49, 1979
11. Kruger RA, Mistretta CA, Riederer SJ: Computerized fluoroscopy techniques for noninvasive study of cardiac patients. Investigative Radiology 14:279, 1979
12. Ergun DL, Mistretta CA, Krueger RA: A hybrid computerized fluoroscopy technique for noninvasive cardiovascular imaging. Radiology 132:739, 1979
13. Meany TF, Weinstein MA, Buonocou P: Digital subtraction angiography of the human cardiovascular system. SPIE 233:272, 1980
14. Ovitt T, Capp MP, Christenson P: Development of a digital video subtraction system for intravenous angiography. SPIE 206:73, 1979
15. Kruger RA, Mistretta CA, Lancaster J: A digital video image processor for real time x-ray subtraction imaging. Optic Engin 17:652, 1978
16. Crummy AB, Strother CM, Lieberman RP: Digital subtraction angiography for evaluation of peripheral vascular disease. Radiology 141:33, 1981
17. Strother CM, Sackett JF, Crummy AB, et al: Clinical application of computerized fluoroscopy: The extracranial carotid artery. Radiology 136 (2):781, 1980
18. Sackett JF, Mann FA: Contrast media for digital subtraction angiography of cerebral arteries. Digital Subtraction Arteriography: An Application of Computerized Fluoroscopy. Chicago, Yearbook Publishers, 1981
19. Myerowitz PD, Turnipseed WD, Shaw CG, et al: Computerized fluoroscopy. Thor Cardiovas Surg 83:65, 1982
20. Turnipseed WD, Sackett JF, Strother CM: Computerized arteriography of the cerebrovascular system: its use with intravenous injection of contrast agent. Arch Surg 116:470, 1981
21. Turnipseed WD, Sackett JF, Strother CM, et al: A comparison of standard cerebral arteriography with noninvasive doppler imaging and intravenous angiography. Arch Surg 117:419, 1982
22. Turnipseed WD, Crummy AB, Strother CM, et al: Computerized intravenous angiography: A technique for visualizing the peripheral vascular system. Surgery 89:118, 1981

Norman R. Hertzer
Michael T. Modic

8

Digital Subtraction Angiography after Extracranial Carotid Reconstruction

Accurate angiography is prerequisite to the appropriate surgical management of cerebrovascular disease. Since ulcerated atheromatous lesions often cannot be detected by either physical examination or noninvasive testing, complete cerebral angiography is essential for patients who have experienced previous transient ischemic attacks (TIA) or completed strokes within the carotid distribution. Noninvasive carotid imaging or hemodynamic assessment may be used to select patients with asymptomatic carotid stenosis for diagnostic angiography, but all noninvasive methods have an irreducible incidence of inaccurate results. Despite its many advantages, however, routine angiography has rarely been performed to determine the technical results of extracranial arterial operations. Because of its inconvenience, expense, and low but measurable risk, postoperative angiography after carotid reconstruction has usually been limited to patients suspected to have surgical complications.

Digital subtraction angiography (DSA) is a recent innovation in computerized arterial imaging that requires only the intravenous injection of contrast medium. DSA presently is especially suitable for imaging of the extracranial circulation, and its safety, convenience, and accuracy in the diagnosis of cerebrovascular disease already have been established.[1-5] Experience with DSA at the Cleveland Clinic indicates that, with the exception of traditional angiography, this procedure also is the best available means to determine the technical results of carotid endarterectomy and other extracranial arterial operations.

TECHNICAL CONSIDERATIONS

Advances in television technology and digital electronics have improved video imaging to the point that its quality is comparable to standard silver halide film. These improvements presently permit visualization of the cardiovascular system after the intravenous injection of a modest volume of contrast medium and have renewed interest in intravenous angiography, a technique that was originally described nearly 50 years ago by Robb and Steinberg[6] but proved to be too cumbersome and time-consuming to supplant traditional angiographic procedures.

As depicted schematically in Figure 8-1, DSA at the Cleveland Clinic is

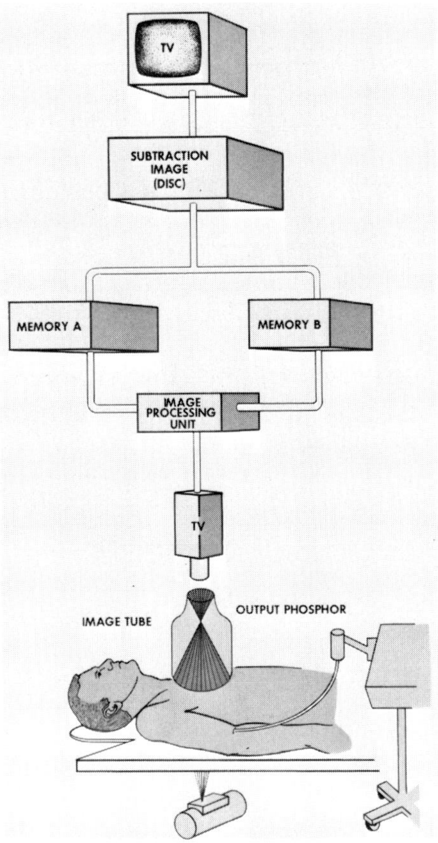

Figure 8-1. Schematic illustration of digital subtraction angiography (DSA).

performed with the DSR-960* equipment utilizing a 512 × 512 matrix. A 16-gauge intravenous catheter is inserted into a suitable vein in the upper extremity, and each DSA view of the cervical vessels is obtained after the pressure injection of 40 cc of Renograffin-76† contrast medium. During an examination of the carotid bifurcations, a 4″ image intensifier field is used for 70° right and left anterior oblique projections. A 35° left anterior oblique view is usually satisfactory for evaluation of the aortic arch and the brachiocephalic vessels. The total volume of contrast medium for a routine examination is customarily limited to 3 cc per kg, but may be further modified in aged patients and in those having impaired renal function.

Following the bolus administration of contrast medium, the initial digital image of the injection sequence is stored in memory "A" (Fig. 8-2). Subsequent digitized radiographic frames are obtained at the rate of one each second and are subtracted from the original, or mask, frame available in memory "A." The difference in image between the two frames represents only the presence of the injected contrast medium and is transmitted to memory "B" for viewing on the console television monitor. This procedure produces a real-time, subtracted image corresponding to the arrival of the contrast medium in the area of clinical interest. Additional frames that precede the appearance of contrast medium may be used as masks to correct motion artifacts, including those commonly caused by inadvertent swallowing.

While intravenous DSA cannot be strictly defined as a noninvasive test, it has several advantages in comparison to either Doppler or B-mode imaging and conventional film screen angiography. It demonstrates arterial anatomy on an outpatient basis with greater clarity and reliability than is possible with any noninvasive technique, while avoiding the risk, expense, and hospitalization required for Seldinger angiography. Furthermore, it is likely that digital data obtained during DSA will eventually be used to quantitate blood flow at the level of an arterial stenosis, thus providing a unique image of arterial disease as well as the simultaneous assessment of its hemodynamic significance.

POSTOPERATIVE DSA AFTER CAROTID ENDARTERECTOMY

Patency of the internal carotid artery is one of the principal objectives of carotid endarterectomy. While neurologic symptoms in some patients who have symptomatic, microembolic lesions within the carotid bifurcation and adequate intracranial circulation might be improved by carotid endarter-

---

*Technicare Corporation, Solon, Ohio.

†Squibb Pharmaceuticals, Princeton, New Jersey.

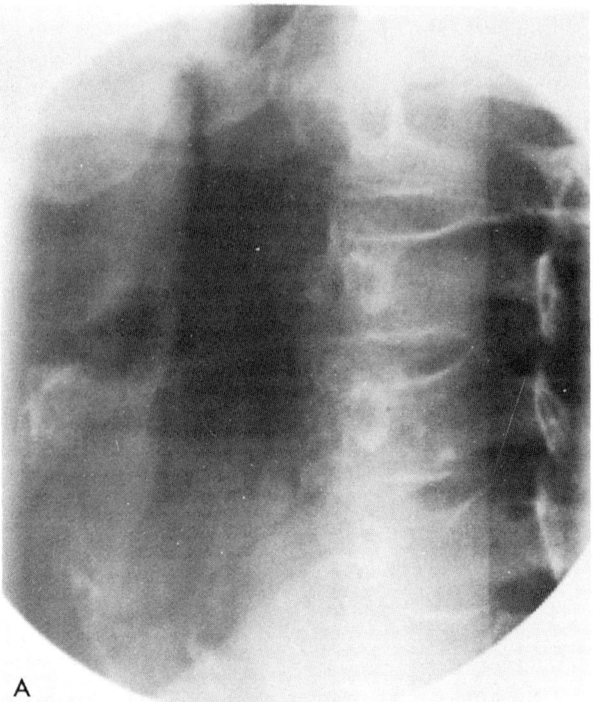

A

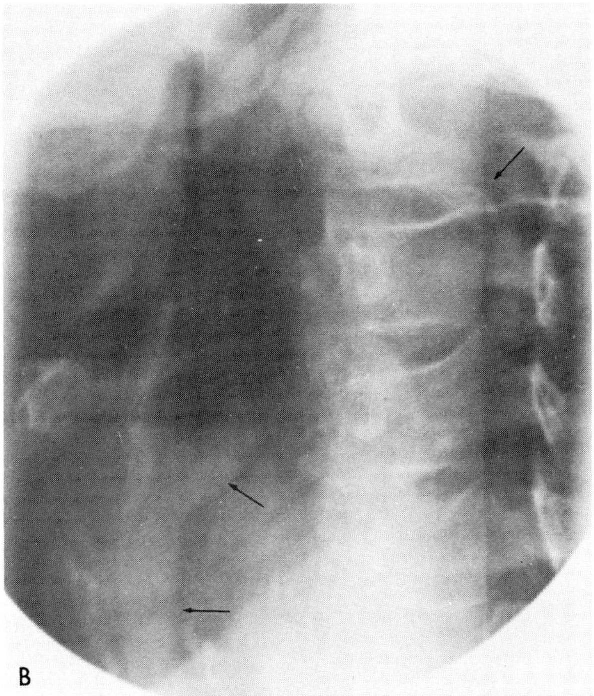

B

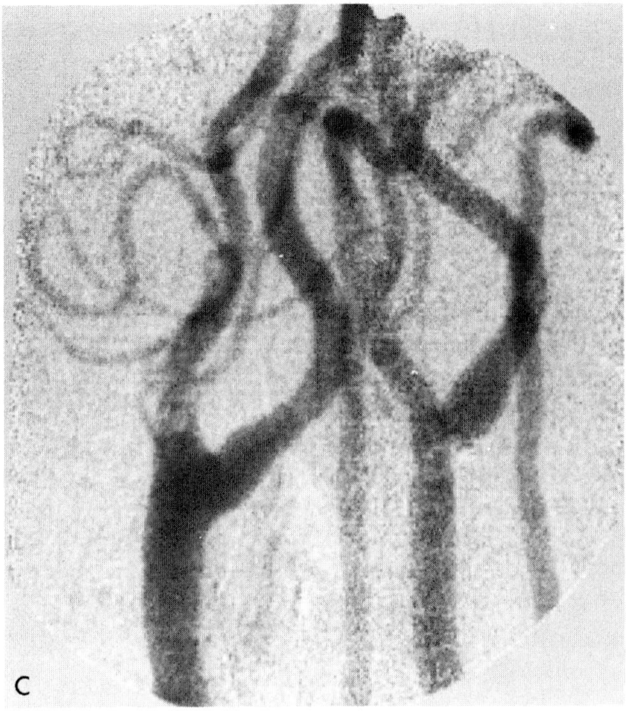

Figure 8-2. (A) Digitized video mask preceding the injection of contrast medium. (B) After intravenous injection, contrast medium is barely perceptible in the carotid arteries (arrows). (C) Digital angiogram after subtraction of image A from image B.

ectomy even if postoperative internal carotid occlusion occurred, restoration of normal internal carotid diameter is critically important for optimal early and late results in the majority of those who require carotid reconstruction. Provided technical failure is adequately reflected by the postoperative neurologic complication rate and by the incidence of recurrent carotid stenosis, the results of previous series from the Cleveland Clinic suggest that occlusion or residual stenosis of the internal carotid artery rarely occurs after endarterectomy.[7,8] Successful clinical results and a palpable carotid pulse, however, do not necessarily imply that the internal carotid artery is normal. While some studies have employed noninvasive carotid testing during the early postoperative period,[9,10] angiography is clearly the most dependable method to determine the status of the internal carotid artery.

In 1967, Blaisdell et al.[11] performed operative angiography after completion of carotid endarterectomy in 100 consecutive patients to define the incidence of correctable technical defects that would otherwise escape detection and could compromise the success of surgical management. In this study, immediate revision of the endarterectomy site was necessary because of internal carotid occlusion in 5 patients and because of unexpected stenosis or thrombus in 21 others. Rosental et al.[12] and Hobson et al.[13] subsequently investigated the value of intraoperative angiography and discovered remedial defects in 3 percent to 4 percent of internal carotid arteries and in 4 percent to 6 percent of external carotid arteries, respectively. Andersen et al.[14] later demonstrated unsuspected internal carotid lesions after endarterectomy in only 1.5 percent of patients and discouraged the use of operative angiography because it was associated with complications in 2.3 percent of the 131 patients in whom it was employed.

During a recent 12-month interval, 265 patients underwent a total of 314 carotid endarterectomies at the Cleveland Clinic.[15] In order to document the postoperative status of the carotid bifurcation, DSA was performed during the same hospital admission following 262 (83 percent) of the 314 operations, involving a study group of 214 (80 percent) of the 265 patients in this series. DSA was not obtained after 52 operations in 51 patients because of relative contraindications to the use of contrast medium, patient reluctance, or a number of other random factors. All patients sustaining postoperative neurologic deficits, however, underwent DSA investigation or reoperation.

Indications for Operation

One hundred twenty-three operations (39 percent) were performed because of TIA caused by carotid artery stenosis or atheromatous ulceration (Fig. 8-3). Thirty-one other procedures (10 percent) were performed after an appropriate recovery period in patients who had sustained previous completed strokes. Severe, asymptomatic carotid stenosis (Fig. 8-4) was the indication for the remaining 160 operations (51 percent). Seven procedures (2.2 percent), bilateral in one patient, were limited to external carotid endarterectomy in order to improve the cerebral collateral circulation or to facilitate subsequent middle cerebral artery bypass in patients with occlusion of the ipsilateral internal carotid artery.

Preoperative carotid angiograms were obtained using the conventional Seldinger approach in 174 (66 percent) of the 265 patients. Another 66 patients (25 percent) underwent ciné carotid angiography at the time of cardiac catheterization. DSA was employed as a screening study in a total of 99 patients (37 percent) and was the only preoperative angiographic procedure performed in 25 (9 percent).

Surgical Management

Dissection of the common carotid, the internal carotid, and the external carotid arteries was performed without manipulation of the carotid bifurcation in an attempt to reduce the incidence of intraoperative embolization. After the systemic administration of 5,000 to 10,000 international units of sodium heparin, an arteriotomy was begun in the proximal common carotid

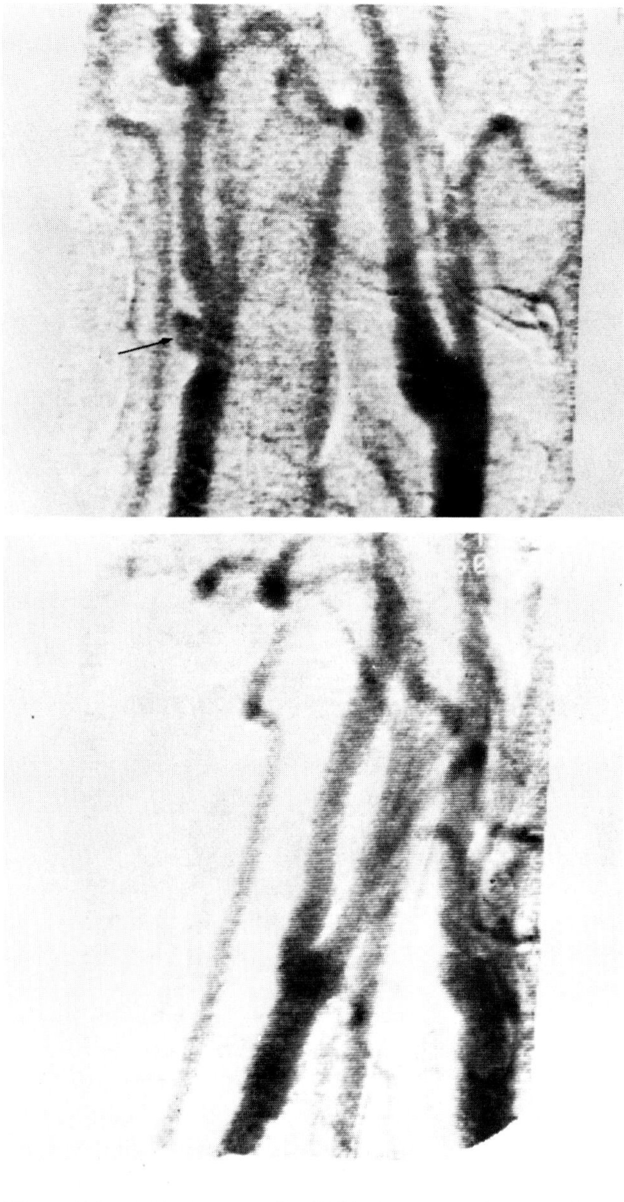

A

B

Figure 8-3. (A) Preoperative DSA demonstrating an atheromatous ulcer (arrow) in the right carotid bifurcation of a patient with previous TIA. (B) Postoperative DSA after carotid endarterectomy.

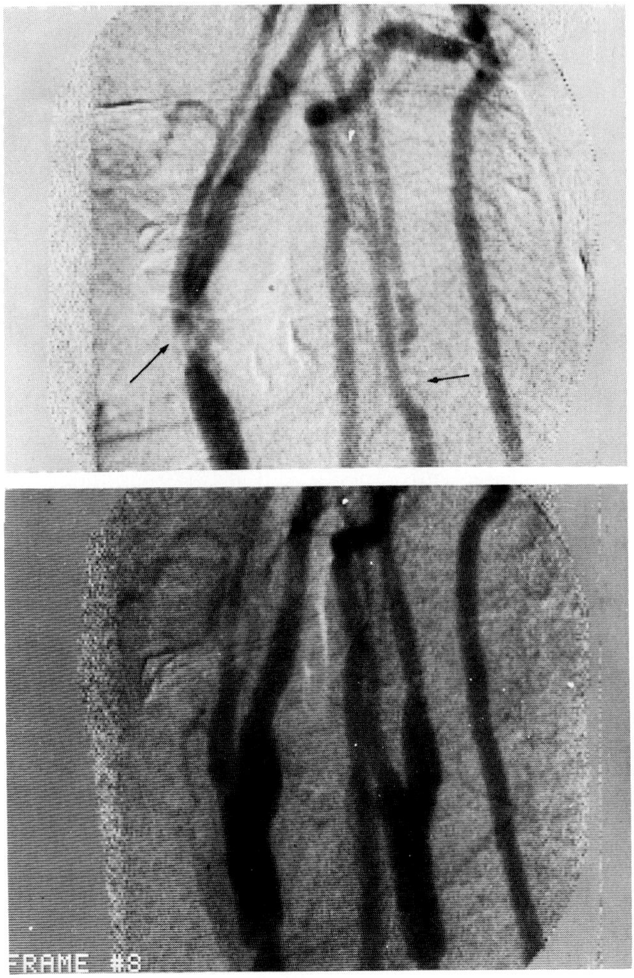

A B

Figure 8-4. (A) Preoperative DSA showing severe, bilateral carotid stenosis (arrows). (B) Postoperative DSA after staged, bilateral carotid endarterectomy.

artery and extended beyond the termination of atheromatous disease in the internal carotid artery. A temporary carotid shunt‡ was inserted during 312 of the 314 operations. Although a separate arteriotomy incision was not performed in the external carotid artery, an attempt was made to maintain patency of the external carotid artery during the endarterectomy procedure.

‡Carotid Loop Shunt, Heyer-Schulte Corporation, Goleta, California.

Unless the transition from the endarterectomy segment to the intima of the distal internal carotid artery was imperceptible, interrupted tacking sutures of 7-0 vascular silk were used to prevent elevation of an intimal flap during the postoperative period. The arteriotomy was closed with a continuous suture of 6-0 vascular material during 285 procedures (91 percent). A patch of autogenous saphenous vein was applied in all 7 patients who required external carotid endarterectomy and in 22 (7 percent) of the remaining 307 standard carotid reconstructions.

Early Results

Three patients died as the direct result of carotid endarterectomy, for a patient mortality of 1.1 percent and a corresponding procedure mortality of 1.0 percent. Postoperative strokes occurred after six (1.9 percent) of the 314 operations in this series. Four patients sustained intraoperative strokes that were discovered at the time they awakened from general anesthesia, and two others experienced sudden neurologic deterioration 12 hours and 24 hours postoperatively. DSA was performed immediately in five of these patients and demonstrated a normal postoperative endarterectomy result in four. One patient was found to have an occlusion of the ipsilateral internal carotid artery on DSA and underwent prompt reoperation for internal carotid thrombectomy. The final patient with a postoperative stroke had urgent carotid exploration without preliminary DSA investigation and also was found to have thrombosis of the internal carotid artery. In summary, unnecessary reoperations were avoided on the basis of normal DSA findings in four of the 6 patients with postoperative strokes.

Postoperative DSA was performed to determine the technical results of a total of 262 operations in 214 patients. Since seven of these operations were limited to external carotid endarterectomy, the results of 255 standard bifurcation procedures were included in the DSA study group and are presented in Table 8-1.

Internal Carotid Artery

The internal carotid artery was entirely normal (Fig. 8-5) after 239 operations (94 percent). A perceptible defect compromising the internal carotid lumen by less than 30 percent was identified on nine postoperative studies (3.6 percent). These minimal defects occurred near the apex of the previous arteriotomy (Fig. 8-6), probably were caused by slight inversion at the site of the apical arteriotomy suture, and should perhaps be considered as normal findings. Two additional DSA studies (0.8 percent) suggested the presence of 30 percent to 50 percent stenosis of the internal carotid artery.

Five patients (1.9 percent) had postoperative internal carotid occlusion. Two of these 5 patients experienced obvious neurologic complications and

Table 8-1
Results of digital subtraction angiography (DSA) after 255 carotid bifurcation endarterectomies.

Postoperative DSA Results	Internal Carotid Artery No.	Internal Carotid Artery %	External Carotid Artery No.	External Carotid Artery %
Normal	239	93.7	238	93.3
Stenosis				
<30%	9	3.6	0	—
30–50%	2	0.8	2	0.8
>50%	0	—	3	1.2
Occlusion	5	1.9	12	4.7
Total	255	100	255	100

underwent immediate reoperations for thrombectomy of the internal carotid artery. Asymptomatic internal carotid occlusion was discovered by DSA after three (1.1 percent) of the 255 bifurcation endarterectomies in the study group. Two of these patients, however, had extensive atherosclerosis and diminutive internal carotid arteries that had nearly escaped detection at the time of

A

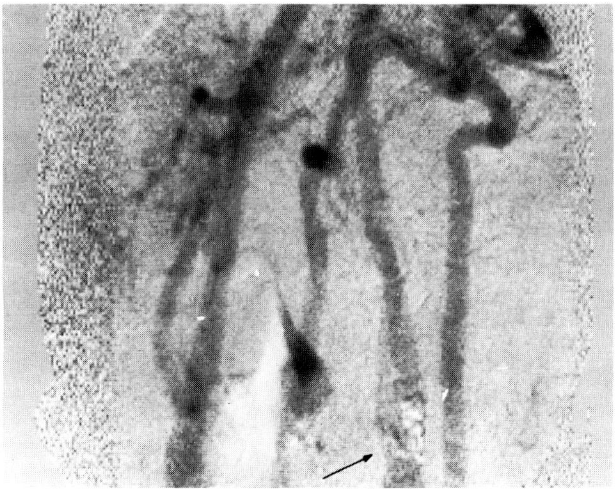

Figure 8-5. (A) Initial DSA view in a patient suspected to have left carotid stenosis. Calcification (arrow) obscures the carotid bifurcation. (B) Another preoperative DSA view in the same patient, demonstrating severe internal carotid artery stenosis (arrow). (C) Normal postoperative DSA after carotid endarterectomy.

preoperative angiography, and each had asymptomatic internal carotid occlusion after a salvage procedure despite the use of an autogenous vein patch for arteriotomy closure. Only one patient in the study group (0.4 percent) sustained asymptomatic internal carotid occlusion postoperatively that was entirely unanticipated.

One patient who required carotid endarterectomy because of severe internal carotid stenosis (Fig. 8-7) developed an asymptomatic arterial infection resulting in a false aneurysm that initially was detected by subsequent DSA studies. Although the routine, postoperative DSA was

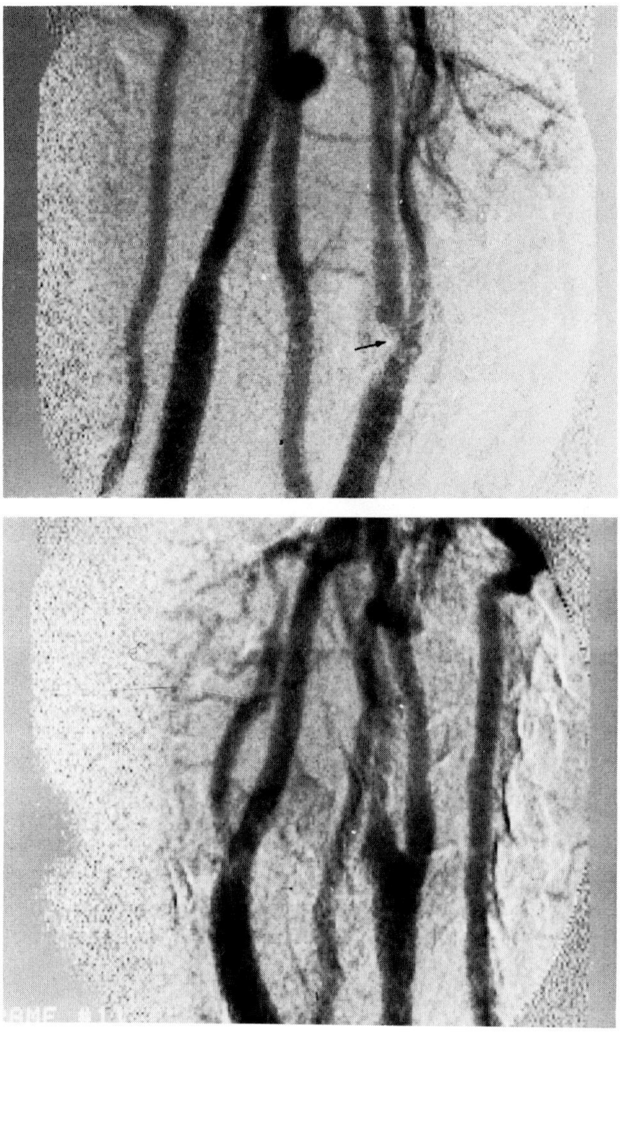

B

C

A

B

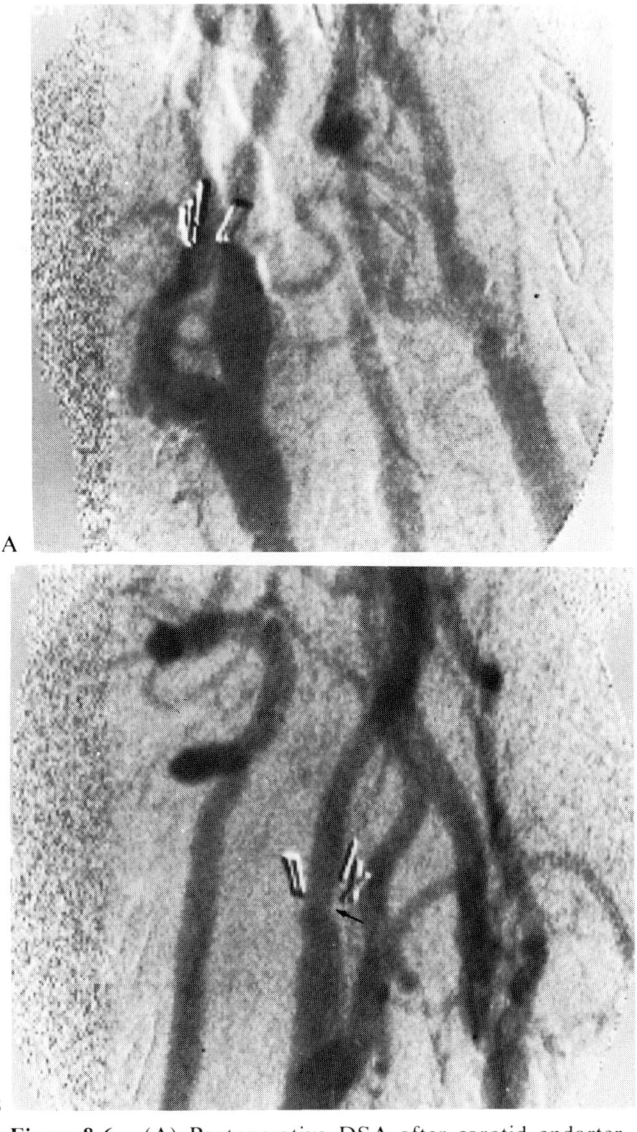

Figure 8-6. (A) Postoperative DSA after carotid endarterectomy. Surgical clips obscure the distal endarterectomy site. (B) Another postoperative DSA view in the same patient, suggesting a minimal intimal defect corresponding to the apical arteriotomy suture (arrow).

normal, this patient was found to have a small, palpable mass in the area of the carotid bifurcation 6 weeks later. This mass was thought to represent a cervical lymph node, but a second postoperative DSA examination demonstrated a false aneurysm involving the internal carotid artery. A staphylococcal infection was confirmed at the time of reoperation, and the carotid artery was ligated. Although direct reconstruction was not feasible, this patient did not experience a postoperative stroke.

External Carotid Artery

The external carotid artery was normal after 238 operations in the study group (93 percent). A total of 5 patients (2 percent) had intimal defects representing as much as 50 percent lumen stenosis, and 12 patients (4.7 percent) had postoperative external carotid occlusion.

Common Carotid Artery

A shelf of atherosclerosis in the common carotid artery proximal to the endarterectomy site was identified on 17 DSA studies (6.5 percent). This type of angiographic lesion is unavoidable in some patients whose disease extends to the level of the aortic arch. One patient with an atherosclerotic shelf in the common carotid artery had another DSA study 4 months postoperatively that demonstrated a smooth transition at the endarterectomy site. This observation suggests that the proximal shelf is eventually remodeled by deposition and organization of mural thrombus.

FUTURE CLINICAL APPLICATIONS OF DSA

Other Cerebrovascular Procedures

DSA is presently used at the Cleveland Clinic for routine postoperative assessment of other extracranial arterial operations in addition to carotid endarterectomy. Since it is difficult, if not impossible, to determine direction of blood flow in the vertebral artery with strictly noninvasive methods, DSA is especially appropriate for documentation of the results of vertebral artery reconstruction after either carotosubclavian bypass (Fig. 8-8) or direct implantation procedures (Fig. 8-9). DSA also provides excellent visualization of the aortic arch after brachiocephalic arterial reconstruction. Finally, Little et al.[2] have demonstrated that DSA may be used to demonstrate the technical results of a variety of intracranial arterial procedures, including middle cerebral artery revascularization.

Late Results and Complications

On the basis of crude clinical criteria limited to the neurologic status and physical examination, recurrent carotid stenosis after endarterectomy has

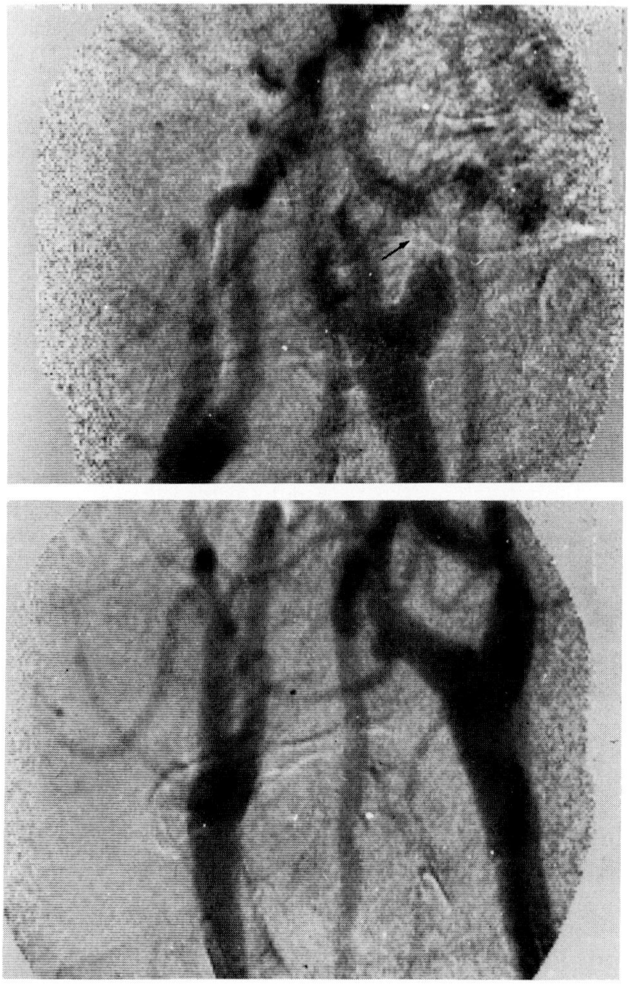

A

B

Figure 8-7. (A) Preoperative DSA demonstrating severe stenosis of the left internal carotid artery (arrow). (B) Normal postoperative DSA 5 days after carotid endarterectomy. (C) Another DSA in the same patient 6 weeks postoperatively. A false aneurysm involves the internal carotid artery.

previously been considered to be an unusual complication.[8] However, Cantelmo et al.[16] and Kremen et al.[17] have suggested that recurrent stenosis may be discovered in as many as 10 percent to 12 percent of patients provided an annual postoperative evaluation with objective noninvasive studies is performed. Considering the safety and convenience of its use on an outpatient basis, DSA will undoubtedly become an important adjunct for the periodic

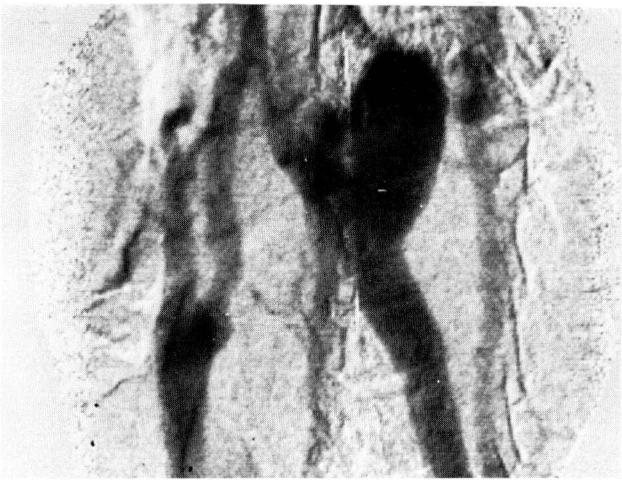

C

evaluation of patients who have previously undergone cerebrovascular arterial procedures. Annual DSA studies presently are obtained following carotid endarterectomy at the Cleveland Clinic and already have been used to establish the diagnosis of recurrent carotid stenosis in patients whose operations were performed during earlier periods of study (Fig. 8-10).

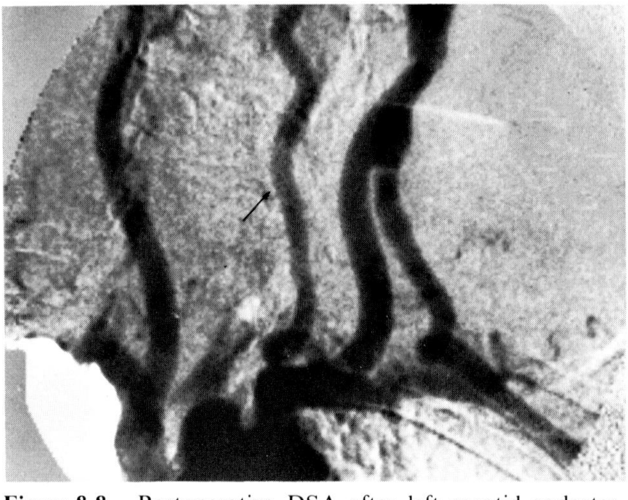

Figure 8-8. Postoperative DSA after left carotid endarterectomy with patch angioplasty and left carotosubclavian bypass in a patient with occlusion of the left subclavian artery at its origin from the aortic arch. Normal perfusion has been restored to the left vertebral artery (arrow).

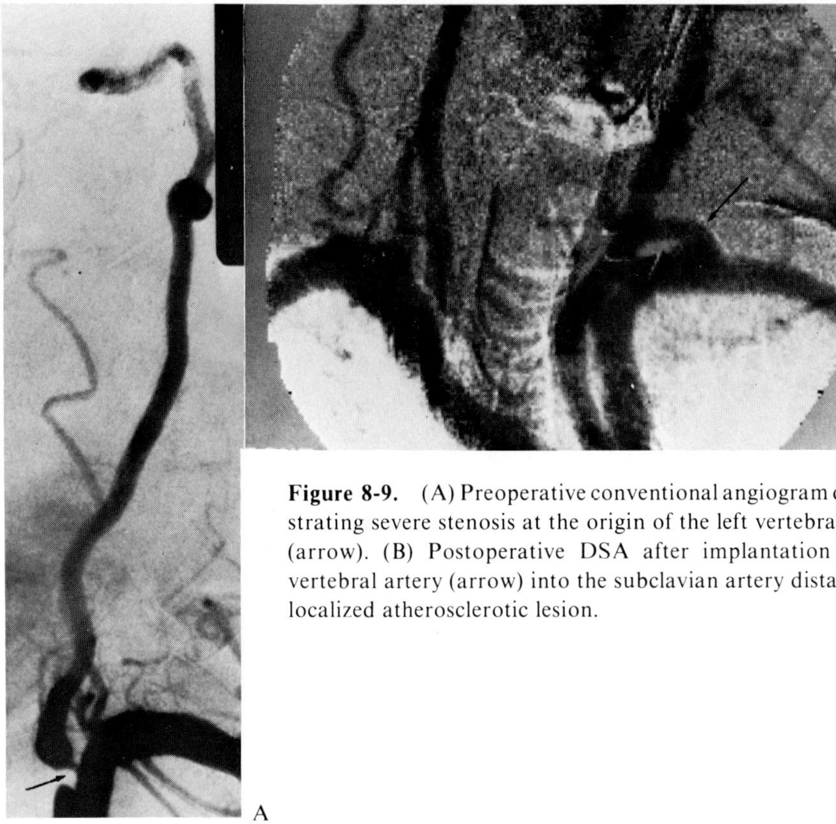

A

B

Figure 8-9. (A) Preoperative conventional angiogram demc strating severe stenosis at the origin of the left vertebral art (arrow). (B) Postoperative DSA after implantation of t vertebral artery (arrow) into the subclavian artery distal to t localized atherosclerotic lesion.

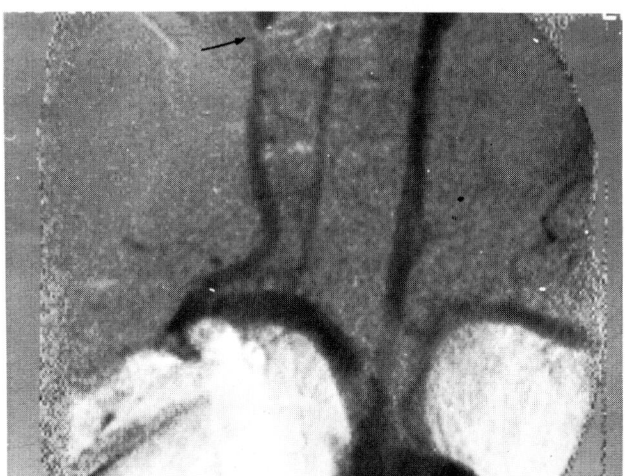

A

CONCLUSIONS

Experience at the Cleveland Clinic confirms that DSA is a safe, convenient, and accurate means to assess the early technical results of extracranial arterial operations and to obtain a reference study for compari-

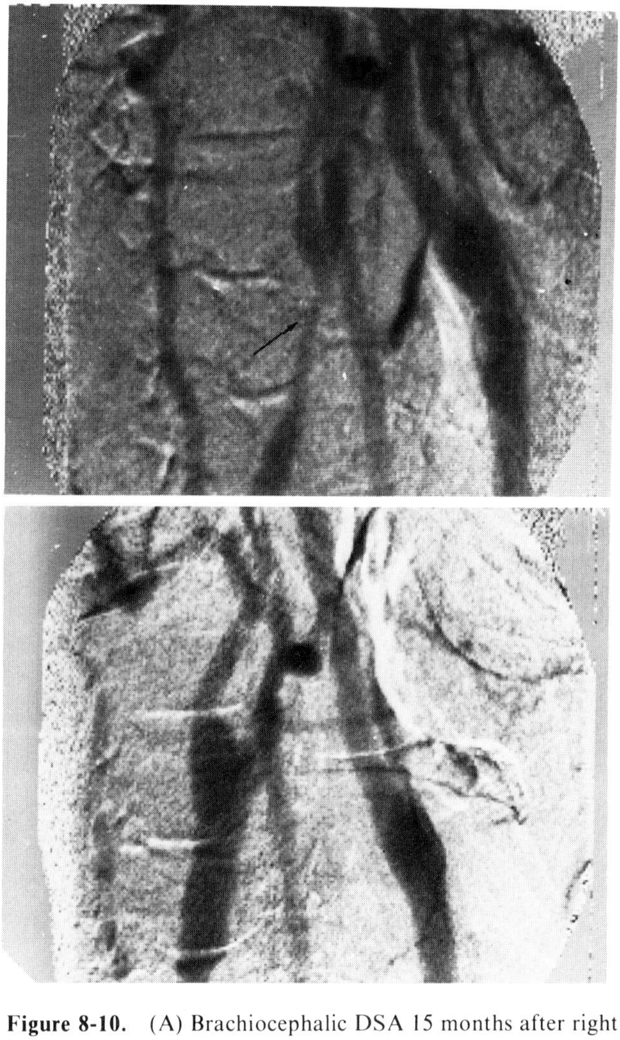

B

C

Figure 8-10. (A) Brachiocephalic DSA 15 months after right carotid endarterectomy and subclavian-carotid saphenous vein bypass. This view suggests the presence of recurrent carotid stenosis near the bifurcation (arrow). (B) Another DSA view confirming the area of recurrent stenosis (arrow). (C) Postoperative DSA after reoperation, carotid endarterectomy, and application of a vein patch.

son during subsequent postoperative examinations. Documentation of immediate technical results has obvious prognostic value and, just as importantly, contributes substantially to the education and subsequent performance of the surgeon. DSA provides an extraordinary opportunity to study the course of cerebrovascular disease as well as the durability of operations performed to correct it.

ACKNOWLEDGEMENT

Miss Linda Maljovec assisted in preparation of the manuscript.

REFERENCES

1. Chilcote WA, Modic MT, Pavlicek WA, et al: Digital subtraction angiography of the carotid arteries: A comparative study in 100 patients. Radiology 139:287, 1981
2. Little JR, Furlan AJ, Modic MT, et al: Intravenous digital subtraction angiography: Application to cerebrovascular surgery. Neurosurgery 9:129, 1981
3. Meaney TF, Weinstein MA, Buonocore E, et al: Digital subtraction angiography of the human cardiovascular system. Am J Roentgenol 135:1153, 1980
4. Mistretta CA, Crummy AB, Strother CM: Digital angiography: A perspective. Radiology 139: 273, 1981
5. Modic MT, Weinstein MA, Chilcote WA, et al: Digital subtraction angiography of the intracranial vascular system: Conparative study in 55 patients. AJNR 2:527, 1981
6. Robb GP, Steinberg I: Visualization of the chambers of the heart, pulmonary circulation, and the great blood vessels in man. Am J Roentgenol 41:1, 1939
7. Hertzer NR, Beven EG: A retrospective comparison of the use of shunts during carotid endarterectomy. Surg Gynecol Obstet 151:81, 1980
8. Hertzer NR, Martinez BD, Beven EG: Recurrent stenosis after carotid endarterectomy. Surg Gynecol Obstet 149:360, 1979
9. Ortega G, Gee W, Kaupp HA, et al: Postendarterectomy carotid occlusion. Surgery 90:1093, 1981
10. Turnipseed WD, Berkoff HA, Crummy A: Postoperative occlusion after carotid endarterectomy. Arch Surg 115:573, 1980
11. Blaisdell FW, Lim R Jr, Hall AD: Technical result of carotid endarterectomy. Arteriographic assessment. Am J Surg 114:239, 1967
12. Rosental JJ, Gaspar MR, Movius HJ: Intraoperative arteriography in carotid thromboendarterectomy. Arch Surg 106:806, 1973
13. Hobson RW II, Rich NM, Wright CB, et al: Operative assessment of carotid endarterectomy: Internal carotid arterial back pressure, carotid arterial blood flow, and carotid arteriography. Am Surgeon 41:603, 1975
14. Anderson CA, Collins GJ Jr, Rich NM: Routine operative arteriography during carotid endarterectomy: A reassessment. Surgery 83:67, 1978
15. Hertzer NR, Beven EG, Modic MT, et al: Early patency of the carotid artery following endarterectomy. Digital subtraction angiography after 262 operations. Surgery (in press)
16. Cantelmo NL, Cutler BS, Wheeler HB, et al: Noninvasive detection of carotid stenosis following endarterectomy. Arch Surg 116:1005, 1981
17. Kremen DE, Gee W, Kaupp HA: Restenosis or occlusion after carotid endarterectomy: A survey with ocular pneumoplethysmography. Arch Surg 114:608, 1979

PART IV

Noninvasive Diagnostic Studies

David S. Sumner
James B. Russell
Richard D. Miles

9

Pulsed-Doppler Arteriography and Computer Assisted Imaging of the Carotid Bifurcation

Pulsed-Doppler imaging of the carotid bifurcation was introduced about a decade ago with the work of Hokanson and his colleagues.[1,2,3] Shortly thereafter, Spencer and Reid employed a continuous wave instrument for the same purpose.[4,5] Over the years, several modifications have been made to improve the quality of the image and to increase diagnostic accuracy, particularly in reference to disease of the carotid bifurcation. Investigators in England have added more gates to the pulsed-Doppler to furnish more input sources;[6,7] White has color-coded the output of a continuous-wave system to provide frequency information reflecting the velocity of blood flow;[8] and Spencer and Reid have incorporated spectral analysis of the Doppler signal to yield additional information regarding flow disturbances.[9,10] All of these have improved the sensitivity of the technique.

In our laboratory, we have found that the image itself has considerable diagnostic value but have noted some errors that relate to the fact that the usual scanning method depicts the bifurcation in only 1 plane.[11,12] It is well recognized that even high-quality roentgenograms of the carotid in one plane, or even two, may miss lesions that would be evident had 3 views been obtained. Concern for this problem prompted us to devise a method capable of producing simultaneous views of the carotid bifurcation in more than one plane, without extending the time required to complete the test.[13,14,15] The pulsed Doppler provides depth information not ordinarily used in the usual scanning procedure. This information can be processed by a microcomputer to produce simultaneous orthogonal views. Even this, however, does not make the most efficient use of the available information. Recently, in our laboratory, we have added a program that constructs a histiogram that shows the cross-sectional area of the carotid bifurcation along its entire length.[16]

By using these modifications in conjunction with spectral analysis of the Doppler signal obtained at selected points along the carotid artery, we hope to improve the overall accuracy of the test. Initial results have been encouraging.

DETECTION OF FLOW WITH THE PULSED-DOPPLER

Pulsed-Dopplers work on a time-gated principle similar to that employed by radar or sonar devices.[17] A short burst of ultrasonic energy lasting about 1.0 μsec is emitted from a single crystal mounted at the end of a probe. The Hokanson pulsed-Doppler emits 15,600 bursts per second, providing a 63 μsec quiescent period between bursts. During this quiescent period, the same crystal that was used to transmit the ultrasound is also used to receive the signals that are backscattered from acoustic interfaces along the path of the sound beam. The crystal is activated for a brief period at a specific time following the transmission burst to provide a "window" or "gate" for receiving the signal. Because the ultrasonic pulse, which travels at about 1.56×10^5 cm/sec through the underlying tissues, is reflected to a variable degree all along the way, only those signals that return when the gate is open will be received. When the sound burst encounters moving red blood cells, its frequency will be shifted according to the Doppler principle. By adjusting the time between the transmission burst and the activation of the gate, one can select the depth at which the flow signals will be detected. Thus, unlike continuous-wave Dopplers, which sense flow at all points along the sound beam, the pulsed-Doppler provides a mechanism for detecting flow at and only at a specific distance from the probe. Multiple gates can be employed, enabling the instrument to pick up flow from various depths simultaneously. Some instruments have as many as 30 gates.

The importance of these features for mapping flow patterns will be discussed later in this chapter.

PULSED-DOPPLER ARTERIOGRAPHY

The Hokanson ultrasonic arteriograph* employs a transducer containing a 4 mm piezoelectric crystal mounted on a position-sensing arm, a 5 MHz directional pulsed-Doppler ultrasonic flow detector with six range gates, and a bistable storage oscilloscope (Fig. 9-1). When flow in the proper direction is

*D.E. Hokanson, Inc., Issaquah, Washington.

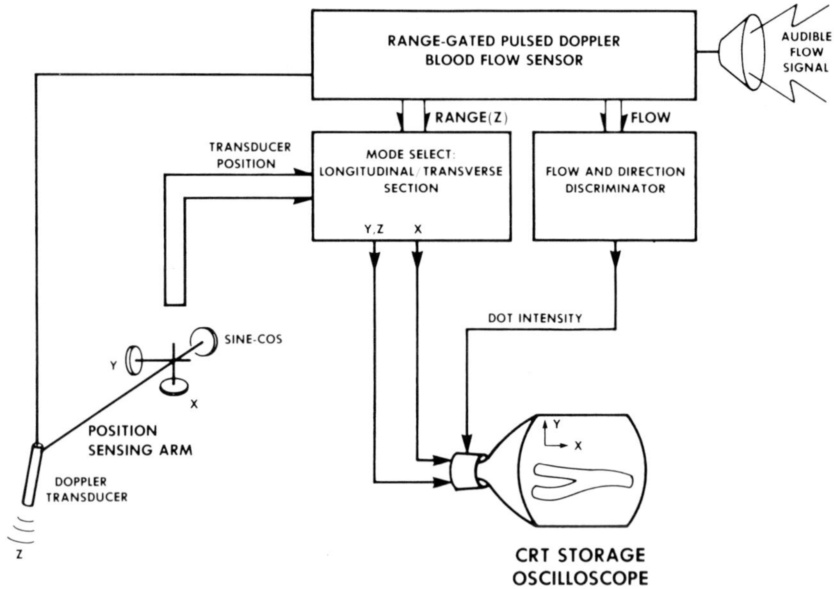

Figure 9-1. Block diagram of Hokanson pulsed-Doppler arteriograph.

detected, a spot appears on the oscilloscope screen, the position of which is determined by the sensing arm. As the probe is moved over the surface of the neck, the individual spots coalesce to create an image of the carotid lumen, which resembles that obtained with conventional contrast arteriography (Fig. 9-2). Guided by the audible output, the examiner first traces the common carotid to the bifurcation, then follows the internal carotid cephalad until further progress is impeded by the mandible, and finally completes the picture by tracing the external carotid caudad to its origin at the bifurcation. At no time are the previously interrogated areas restudied. This would introduce errors due to slight shifts in the position of the carotid artery. It is far better to repeat the entire study than to retrace the arterial lumen. The resulting flow-map corresponds roughly to a lateral projection of the carotid bifurcation.

Accuracy

In our initial study, 209 ultrasonic arteriograms (UAs) from 122 consecutive patients were compared with x-rays of the carotid bifurcation. Independent measurements of the percent diameter reduction of the internal carotid arterial lumina were made from the ultrasonic and x-ray images. When a diameter reduction of 40 percent was selected as the dividing line between positive and negative studies, the UA was shown to have a sensitivity of 87 percent and a specificity of 91 percent.[11]

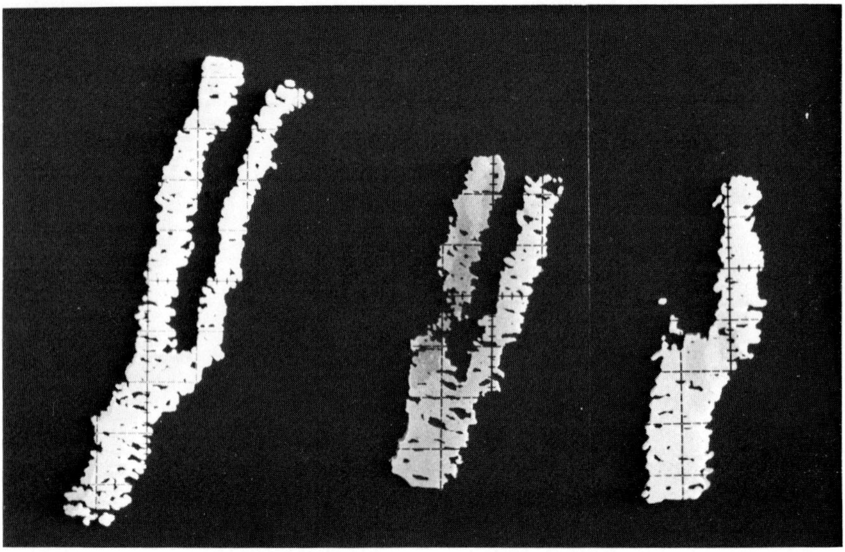

Figure 9-2. Pulsed-Doppler images of the carotid bifurcation (plan views, lateral projection). Shown from left to right are a normal bifurcation, a stenosis of the internal carotid artery, and a total occlusion of the internal carotid artery. In each example, the internal carotid is on the left and the external on the right. (From Sumner DS: Ultrasound, in Kempczinski RF, Yao JST (eds), *Practical Noninvasive Vascular Diagnosis,* Chicago, Year Book Medical Publishers, Inc., 1982 p. 40.

Prior to June, 1981, 1771 patients with suspected extracranial carotid arterial disease had undergone noninvasive studies in our laboratory.[12] At the discretion of the referring physician, 382 (19 percent) of these patients underwent arteriography, providing 604 arteriographic images for comparison. Satisfactory UAs were obtained on 571 (92 percent) of these arteries. The rest were excluded from comparison because of calcification (23 studies, 4 percent), technical inadequacy (20 studies, 3 percent), and equipment malfunction (6 studies, 1 percent). To estimate the degree of stenosis, we relied primarily on measurements of the image; but audible information[11,18] and spectral analyses[12,19,20] of the Doppler signals were used to modify the interpretation,† particularly in instances where calcification was suspected.

Receiver operator characteristic curves were used to assess the accuracy of the UA (Fig. 9-3).[22,23] Because ultrasonic images can be estimated in terms of the degree of stenosis and because different degrees of stenosis visible on roentgenograms can be considered "positive," this statistical device more adequately depicts the accuracy of a test than simply listing sensitivities and

†Angioscan, Unigon Industries, Inc. , Mt. Vernon, New York.

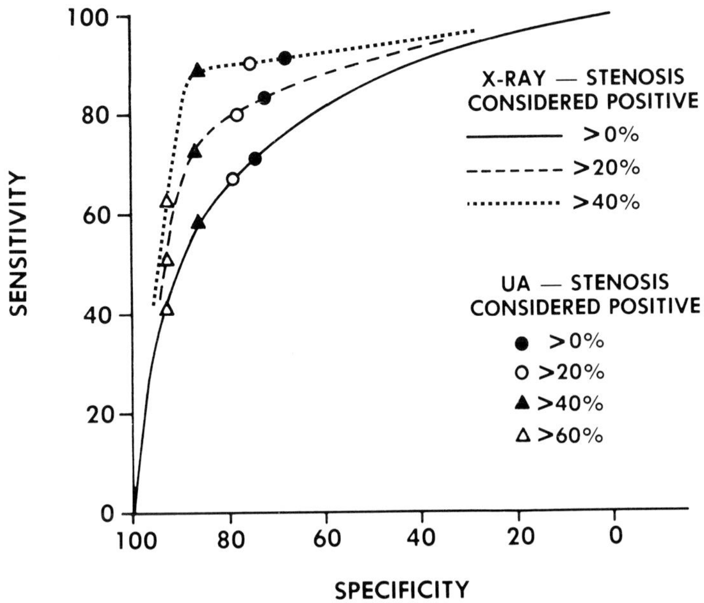

Figure 9-3. Receiver operator characteristic curves comparing the accuracy of pulsed-Doppler imaging with roentgenograms of the internal carotid artery. Symbols (circles or triangles) indicate the degree of stenosis on the UA that was considered positive. (From Sumner DS, Russell JB, Miles RD: Are noninvasive tests sufficiently accurate to identify patients in need of carotid arteriography? Surgery, 1982 [in press.])

specificities. When the criterion for calling an ultrasonic image positive is lax (i.e. any suspected disease), the sensitivity increases, but the specificity declines. Similarly, when only severe disturbances of the ultrasonic image are considered positive, the sensitivity of the test decreases, but its specificity is improved.

Depending upon how strictly the UA was read, its sensitivity for 40 percent diameter stenoses ranged from 63 percent to 91 percent and its specificity from 68 percent to 93 percent. (Dotted line, Fig. 9-3).[12] When any stenosis visible on the UA was considered positive, a maximum sensitivity of 83 percent was observed for stenoses exceeding 20 percent (dashed line) and a maximum sensitivity of 71 percent was observed for any detectable lesion (solid line). Specificities were greatest, about 93 percent, for all 3 curves when the UA was required to demonstrate a 60 percent diameter reduction before being called positive; but the sensitivities were only 41 to 63 percent.

Overall, the best results were obtained when the same criteria were used for both UA and x-ray. As shown in Figure 9-3, these were as follows: any disease (sensitivity 71 percent, specificity 74 percent), diameter stenosis greater than 20 percent (sensitivity 80 percent, specificity 78 percent), and diameter stenosis greater than 40 percent (sensitivity 89 percent, specificity 86 percent). The UA detected 92 percent of internal carotid lesions with a diameter reduction exceeding 60 percent and 72 percent of those with stenoses between 20 and 59 percent.

Table 9-1 lists the accuracy of (Hokanson) pulsed-Doppler ultrasonic arteriography as reported by various investigators.

Identification of Patients with Carotid Disease

Improved selection of patients for carotid arteriography has been proposed as a primary role of noninvasive tests. Since most surgeons do not recommend endarterectomy in patients with asymptomatic bruits or nonhemispheric symptoms unless they have hemodynamically significant carotid disease, tests that reliably detect stenoses that reduce the lumen of the internal carotid artery by more than 40 percent should be sufficiently accurate. On the other hand, localizing symptoms (such as TIAs, strokes, or amaurosis fugax) are often caused by emboli that arise from ulcerated plaques, many of which cause minimal stenosis. Therefore, to avoid overlooking one of these potentially dangerous lesions, the test should be able to detect a high percentage of low-grade stenoses.

As shown in Figure 9-4, the UA identified 86 percent of those patients with nonhemispheric symptoms and 100 percent of those with asymptomatic bruits who had lesions that compromised the internal carotid lumen by more than 40 percent. The UA was positive in 83 percent of the patients with TIAs, 75 percent of those with strokes, and 96 percent of those with amaurosis fugax who had angiographically evident lesions that could have been responsible for the symptoms.[12] Although the specificity was less satisfactory, a low specificity may be an acceptable tradeoff for a high sensitivity in patients with symptomatic disease. Moreover, it is possible that the arteriogram failed to detect some of the disease that was picked up by the UA, accounting for some of the "false positive" studies.

In the patients who ultimately underwent endarterectomy, the UA was positive in 97 percent of those with nonhemispheric symptoms, in 100 percent of those with asymptomatic bruits, in 100 percent of those with TIAs, in 89 percent of those with strokes, and in 100 percent of those with amaurosis fugax.[12] While it would be fallacious to draw too many conclusions from these statistics, it does appear that the UA is capable of identifying most patients who are in need of carotid surgery.

Sources of Error

Probably the single most important cause of poor results is lack of expertise on the part of the technician performing the test. Obtaining a good

Table 9-1
Accuracy of Pulsed-Doppler Imaging

No Disease *vs* Any Disease				N = 1038* Range = 64–571
References		Sensitivity %	Specificity %	Prevalence %
11,12,24,	Range	70–82	74–88	57–88
25,27	Median	73	87	60
	Mean*	72	79	67
Stenosis < 10–25% *vs* ≥ 10–25%				N = 977* Range = 82–571
References		Sensitivity %	Specificity %	Prevalence %
11,12,19,27	Range	78–96	44–88	46–70
	Median	81	73	51
	Mean*	81	78	55
Stenosis < 40–50% *vs* ≥ 40–50%				N = 1544* Range = 67–571
References		Sensitivity %	Specificity %	Prevalence %
11,12,19,23,	Range	48–93	65–94	26–46
24,25,26,27,	Median	89	85	37
28	Mean*	87	83	38
Unoccluded *vs* Total Occlusion				N = 1056* Range = 79–571
References		Sensitivity %	Specificity %	Prevalence %
12,19,25,26,	Range	61–100	95–98	9–22
27	Median	93	96	13
	Mean*	79	97	11

*N represents the total number of unduplicated carotid artery studies. Individual studies that are found in two reports from the same laboratory are included only once in the N value and used only once for calculating mean values.

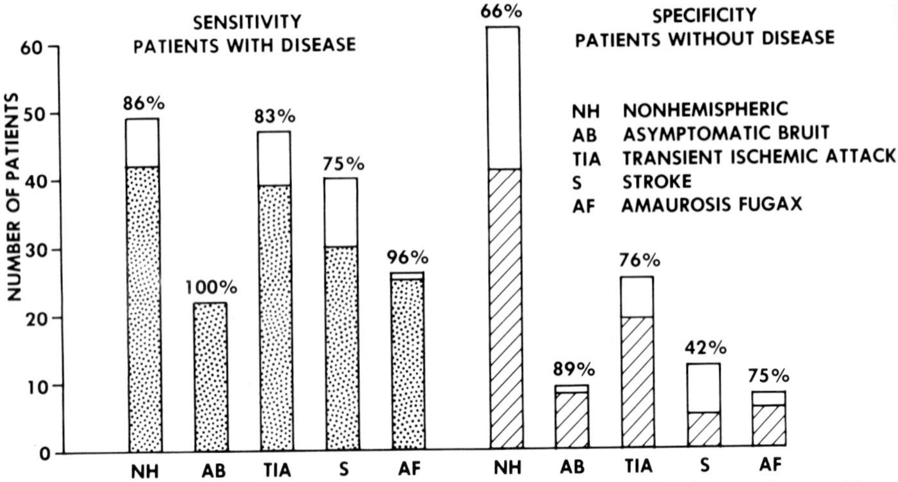

Figure 9-4. Accuracy of pulsed-Doppler imaging for identifying patients with surgically correctable lesions of the internal carotid artery. On the left side of the chart, stippled areas indicate the number of patients with positive studies in the group with disease; and on the right side, cross-hatched areas indicate the number of patients with negative studies in the group without disease. (From Sumner DS, Russell JB, Miles RD: Are noninvasive tests sufficiently accurate to identify patients in need of carotid arteriography? Surgery, 91:700, 1982.

ultrasonic image, interpreting the audible information, and perhaps performing a spectral analysis—all simultaneously—requires skill, concentration, and experience. Accuracy tends to improve as the technician becomes more comfortable with the procedure, learns to recognize anatomical variations, and develops an ear for the Doppler signal.

Calcification of the arterial wall interferes with the transmission of ultrasound, creating an area of sonic opacity, which may mask a stenosis or mimic an occlusion in an otherwise normal vessel. In our experience, calcification interfering with the interpretation of the image is just as common in arteries without evident stenosis as it is in arteries with disease. Finding a normal spectral analysis or hearing a normal signal beyond an area of sonic opacity makes stenosis unlikely; conversely, an abnormal signal or spectral analysis signifies stenosis.[11,23,20] Obtaining views from a different angle will sometimes clarify the situation.[29]

Anatomical variations, including tortuosity of the internal carotid artery, a low or high bifurcation, overlapping vessels, and a reversal of the positions of the internal and external carotid arteries may confuse the examiner, leading to false interpretations.[29,30] Obesity, scar tissue, muscle tension, swallowing, and patient movement all make scanning more difficult. Low cardiac output, stenoses at the origin of the carotid arteries, and fluid overload may not only distort the signal but also may compromise the ability to obtain a good image.[29]

Not infrequently, it is difficult to locate the bifurcation when the internal carotid artery is totally occluded. Lacking this information, the examiner may assume that the external carotid is the internal and fail to recognize the occlusion.[11] Under such circumstances, the external carotid may be as large as the internal and may have a signal that resembles that of a normal internal carotid. Moreover, a large branch of the external carotid (usually the lingual) may be misidentified as the external itself. In our experience, this is a particularly treacherous cause of false negative errors; and although we have long been aware of its existence, we still occasionally make the same mistake. The position of the arteries relative to the angle of the mandible is of some value in their identification, even when one of the arteries is occluded. Ordinarily, the internal carotid artery sweeps away from the bifurcation and is directed posterior to the angle of the mandible. The external carotid is directed anterior to the angle of the mandible.

Projection Errors

Arteriosclerotic plaques are rarely axisymmetric. Surgeons and radiologists have long been aware that the arteriographic appearance of a lesion is often more severe in one view of the carotid bifurcation than it is in another. In fact, a lesion may entirely escape detection in 1 or even 2 projections but be evident in the third. For this reason, most radiologists endeavor to obtain anterior, lateral, and oblique views of each carotid bifurcation.

Pulsed-Doppler ultrasonic arteriography is subject to the same sort of projection errors. When the ultrasonic arteriograph is employed in the usual manner, the long axis of the probe is aligned with the position sensing arm; and the sound beam acts as an extension of the arm. Although several of the gates may be activated simultaneously by flow in the underlying artery, only 1 spot appears on the oscilloscope screen. As the probe is moved over the surface of the neck, the dimensions of the arterial lumen that lie in a plane at right angles to the sound beam are depicted. The resulting image, which is called a "plan" view, ordinarily resembles a lateral arteriogram of the carotid bifurcation. If the major axis of the residual lumen lies at right angles to the sound beam, the stenosis may be underestimated or missed entirely (Fig. 9-5). Some of the false negative errors with the UA are due to projection errors.

AVOIDING PROJECTION ERRORS

In addition to the plan view, the pulsed-Doppler arteriograph is capable of providing longitudinal and transverse cross-sectional views (Fig. 9-6). To obtain these views, the probe must be rotated so that its long axis is

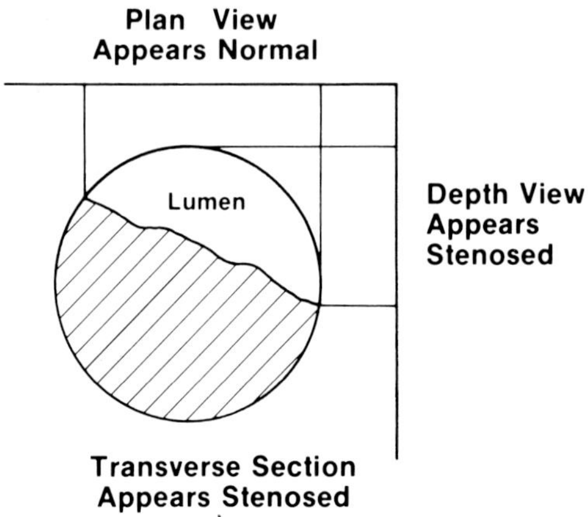

Figure 9-5. Diagram illustrating how the plan view (lateral projection) may overlook lesions that would be evident on the depth view (A-P projection).

perpendicular to the position sensing arm. In this position, a separate spot appears on the oscilloscope screen for each of the gates that are activated by the motion of blood in the underlying artery. When the probe is swept longitudinally along the artery, a longitudinal cross section appears on the screen, providing a projection of the arterial lumen that is orthogonal to the plan view. In other words, the resulting image will resemble an anterior-posterior (AP) arteriographic view. By sweeping the probe across the long axis of the artery, the examiner can also obtain cross sectional views at selected sites.

While this method was employed in most of the original investigative work, it proved to be more difficult than scanning with the probe oriented along the long axis of the position sensing arm.[2,3] Moreover, in order to obtain both a lateral and an AP view, it was necessary to perform two separate studies, thereby increasing the time required for each examination. For these reasons, most laboratories have discarded the cross-sectional view in favor of the plan view. In so doing, they fail to fully exploit all the information continually being produced by the ultrasonic arteriograph and have increased the chance of making projectional errors.

COMPUTER INTERFACE

In order to obtain simultaneous plan (lateral) and depth (A-P) views of the carotid bifurcation, we interfaced the pulsed-Doppler ultrasonic arteriograph to a microcomputer with 48k RAM.[13,14,15] The computer is programmed in BASIC and assembly language to digitize the x-y position of the

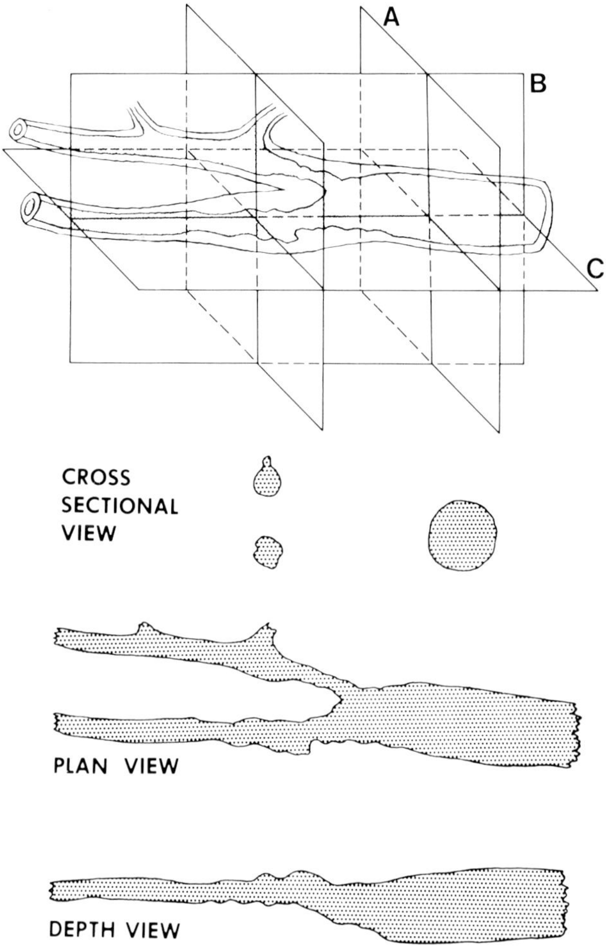

Figure 9-6. Projection planes that can be obtained with the ultrasonic arteriograph: A, transverse cross section; B, plan (lateral) view; C, depth (A-P) view.

transducer, input binary flow signals from the six range gates, and output a signal that controls the depth of the range gates. A 12 button keypad permits the examiner to select imaging routines during the examination (Figs. 9-7 and 9-8).

The six sample gates are used to produce the depth view. A separate dot appears on a video monitor each time one of the gates senses blood flow. When a lesion is encountered in the depth view, fewer gates will be activated.

The procedure is similar to that used for plan view scanning. After the gates have been placed at the proper depth to insonate the entire arterial

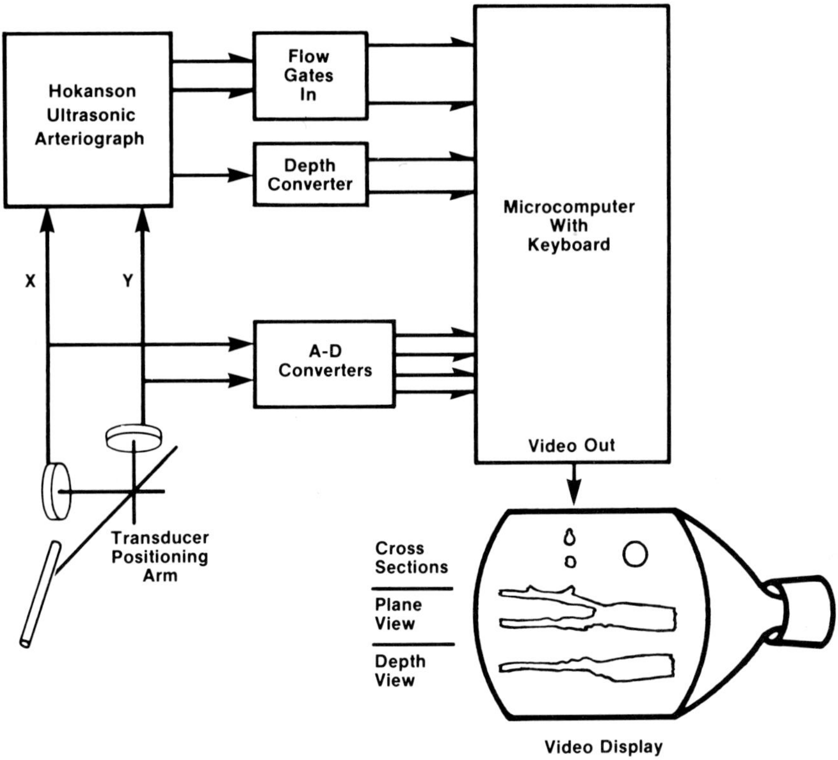

Figure 9-7. Block diagram of the "computerized ultrasonic arteriograph" (CUA). Interconnections between the basic Hokanson instrument and the microcomputer are shown. (From Miles RD, Russell JB, Sumner DS: Computerized ultrasonic arteriography: A new technique for imaging the carotid bifurcation. IEEE Trans Biomed Eng, BME-29: 378–381, 1982.)

lumen, the transducer is moved back and forth over the surface of the skin, beginning at the common carotid artery, progressing up the internal carotid, and then returning to the bifurcation along the external carotid. When the external is scanned, the depth view is turned off by pushing the "lateral-only" button on the keypad. This avoids superimposition of the external carotid and the internal carotid in the A-P view. At any point during the scanning routine, a transverse cross-section can be made by pressing the "transverse" button on the keypad. Once the transverse view has been obtained, the examiner merely presses the "continue" button to return to the simultaneous plan and depth view routine. Because the position of the probe on the position-sensing arm is never changed, the entire examination requires no more time than that ordinarily taken with the unmodified ultrasonic arteriograph—usually about 3 to 5 minutes.

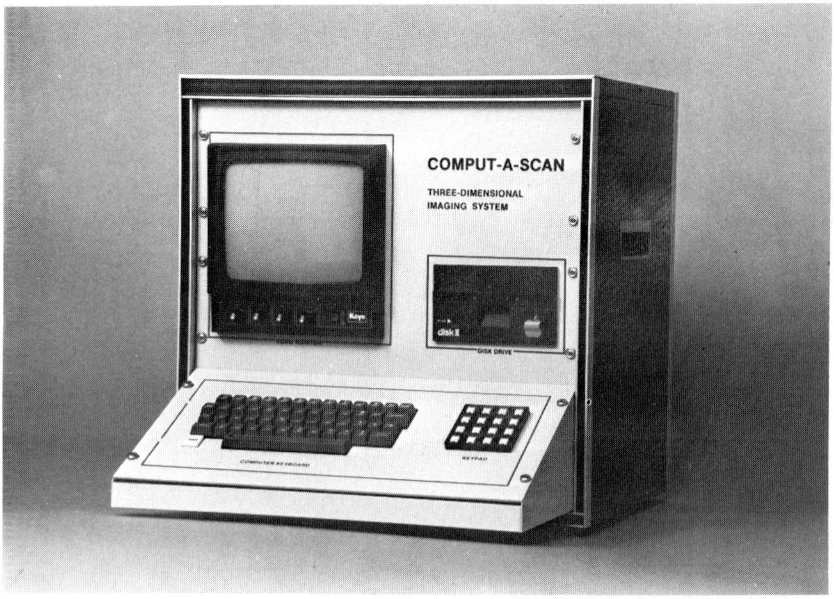

Figure 9-8. Module used for computerized ultrasonic arteriography. Video screen, disk drive, and the keypad (used for selecting special scanning routines) are shown.

The image is permanently stored on floppy diskettes for subsequent retrieval. A hard copy may be obtained by photographing the video screen or by making inexpensive copies with a thermal printer (Fig. 9-9).

Results

The plan and depth views corresponded in 85 percent of 388 internal carotid arteries examined in our laboratory with the computerized ultrasonic arteriograph (CUA). The depth view was positive, however, in 51 (18 percent) of the 286 arteries that were negative on the plan view; and the plan view was positive in 9 (4 percent) of the 244 arteries that were negative on the depth view. Overall, the incidence of positive studies was increased 13 percent (51/388) by obtaining the depth view.

In a series of 66 internal carotid arteries compared with contrast arteriograms, we found that the plan view alone had a sensitivity of 86 percent and a specificity of 90 percent for distinguishing between diameter stenoses greater or less than 40 percent. The combined plan and depth views obtained with the CUA increased the sensitivity to 100 percent, with little decrease in specificity (88 percent). Kleaveland and Judd,[31] using CUA, found a sensitivity of 98 percent and a specificity of 69 percent when any diameter reduction greater than 20 percent was considered to be positive. The

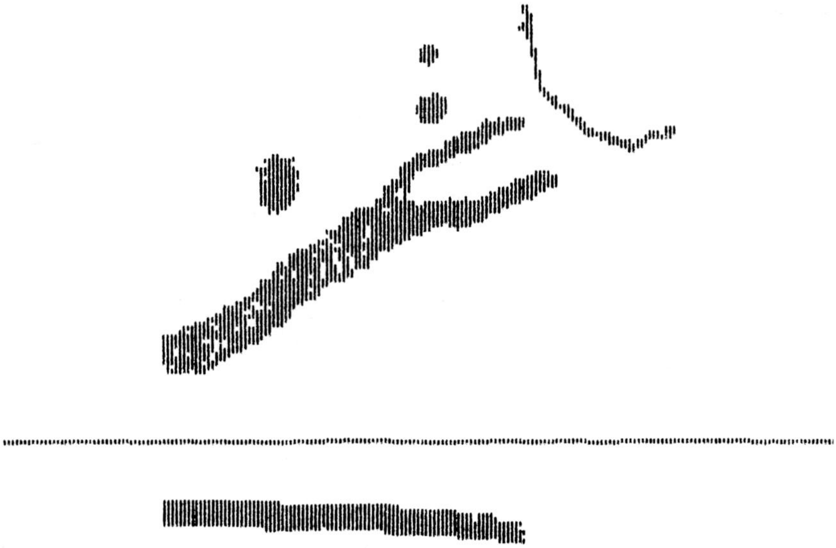

Figure 9-9. Thermal printed image of normal carotid bifurcation, showing the following from top to bottom: transverse cross sections, plan (lateral) view, and depth (A-P) view. The depth view includes only the common and internal carotid arteries. The curved line at the right of the image defines the angle of the mandible. (From Miles RD, Russell JB, Sumner DS: Computerized ultrasonic arteriography: A new technique for imaging the carotid bifurcation. IEEE Trans Biomed Eng, BME–29: 378–381, 1982.)

sensitivity and specificity were 97 percent and 85 percent, respectively, when a 40 percent diameter-reduction criterion was employed.

As one would expect, the additional view tends to increase the sensitivity of the test at the expense of the specificity. This is probably an acceptable compromise when one is surveying a population with a high incidence of carotid disease. High negative predictive values in the range of 96-100 percent insure that few truly positive cases will be overlooked.

ESTIMATING THE LUMEN AREA

Although two orthogonal views decrease the likelihood that a lesion will be missed, they do not entirely eliminate the chance of a false negative error. Moreover, physiologic effects depend on total reduction in cross-sectional area, not on diameter reduction. When the lesion is axisymmetrical, diameter measurements permit an accurate assessment of the lumen area; but when the lesion is asymmetrical, even two orthogonal diameter measurements may not accurately portray the dimensions of the residual lumen.

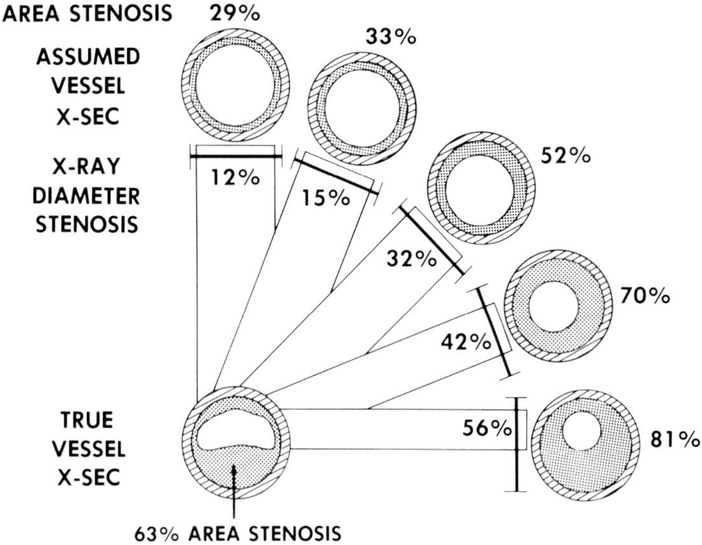

Figure 9-10. Apparent degrees of diameter and area stenosis when an asymmetrical lesion is visualized in different projections.

As shown in Figure 9-10, a 63 percent area reduction in an asymmetrically narrowed vessel could be interpreted on a single view as a 29 percent to 81 percent area reduction, depending upon the angle at which the x-ray or ultrasonic beam intersects the vessel. The potential error when two orthogonal views are available is illustrated in Figure 9-11. When a 40 percent diameter reduction is measured from the projection showing the greater degree of stenosis, the actual area reduction could vary from 38 percent to 82 percent. A precise estimate of area reduction (64 percent) would be obtained only when the lesion was symmetrical. Looking at the graph in the opposite way, one can see that a hemodynamically critical stenosis, that is one with a 75 percent area reduction, could be associated with apparent maximum diameter reductions ranging from 30 percent to 70 percent. In other words, at one end of the scale the measured diameter reductions would seriously underestimate the degree of stenosis while at the other end, it would seriously over-estimate the stenosis.

PLOTTING THE LUMEN AREA

The computer system has now been updated to provide a histiogram that depicts the cross-sectional area of the common and internal carotid arteries at 1.0 mm intervals along the vessel axis.[16] This histiogram appears on the video monitor simultaneously with the plan and depth views. As the ultrasonic

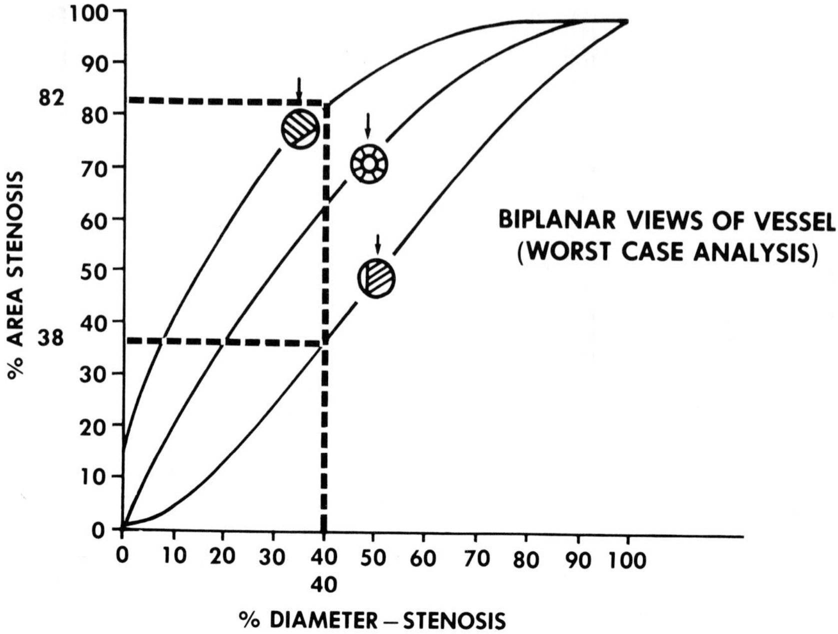

Figure 9-11. Graph showing the relationship between area stenosis and diameter stenosis when the artery is asymmetrically narrowed (upper and lower lines) and when it is symmetrically narrowed (middle line). Two orthogonal projections are assumed. Arrows indicate the direction of the x-ray beam in the projection that shows the greater degree of arterial narrowing. For any given diameter stenosis, the actual area stenosis must lie between the upper and lower lines.

beam is swept across the vessel lumen, the total number of gates activated are added to provide an estimate of the luminal area (Fig. 9-12). After the examination has been completed, the data table which stores the flow coordinates is used to generate a diameter histiogram that is easier to correlate with the x-ray findings. The diameter histiogram represents the square root of the area and therefore depicts the diameter of the vessel as if it were symmetrically narrowed (Fig. 9-13).

Results

Our early data are summarized in Figure 9-14. The percent area stenosis derived from the histiogram is compared with the maximum diameter stenosis obtained from the x-ray arteriogram on a plot that allows for the discrep-

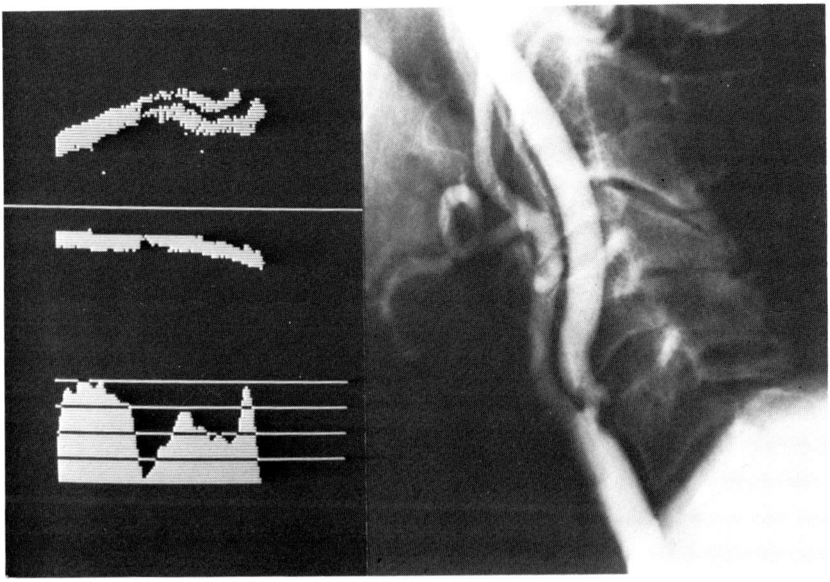

Figure 9-12. Left panel: Computerized ultrasonic arteriogram, showing (from top to bottom) plan (lateral) view, depth (AP) view, and area histiogram. Histiogram indicates an 89 percent area reduction compared to the maximum area of the internal carotid artery. Flat appearance of the top of the AP view is due to the fact that the entire cross section of the artery was not insonated. Right panel: lateral contrast arteriogram of same artery showing a 62 percent diameter reduction and an estimated 86 percent area reduction.

ancies discussed above. Twenty-four of the 27 studies appeared to correlate well. There were one false positive and two false negative errors.

One problem with area plotting that has not been addressed arises from the fact that the ultrasonic beam intersects the lumen of the artery at an angle, which usually approximates 40 to 60 degrees. This has the effect of creating an elliptical cross-section rather than a circular cross-section, causing the residual lumen to appear larger than it actually is. When the internal carotid artery is traced high under the mandible, the area often appears to increase markedly owing to the fact that the angle of incidence of the ultrasonic beam is reduced. A similar distortion occurs when the internal carotid is tortuous and dives away from the sound beam at an acute angle. For these reasons, the area plot is valid only when the arteries describe a moderately straight course and then only within a few centimeters of the bifurcation. In order to obtain optimum accuracy, area histiograms must be interpreted in conjunction with the plan and depth views.

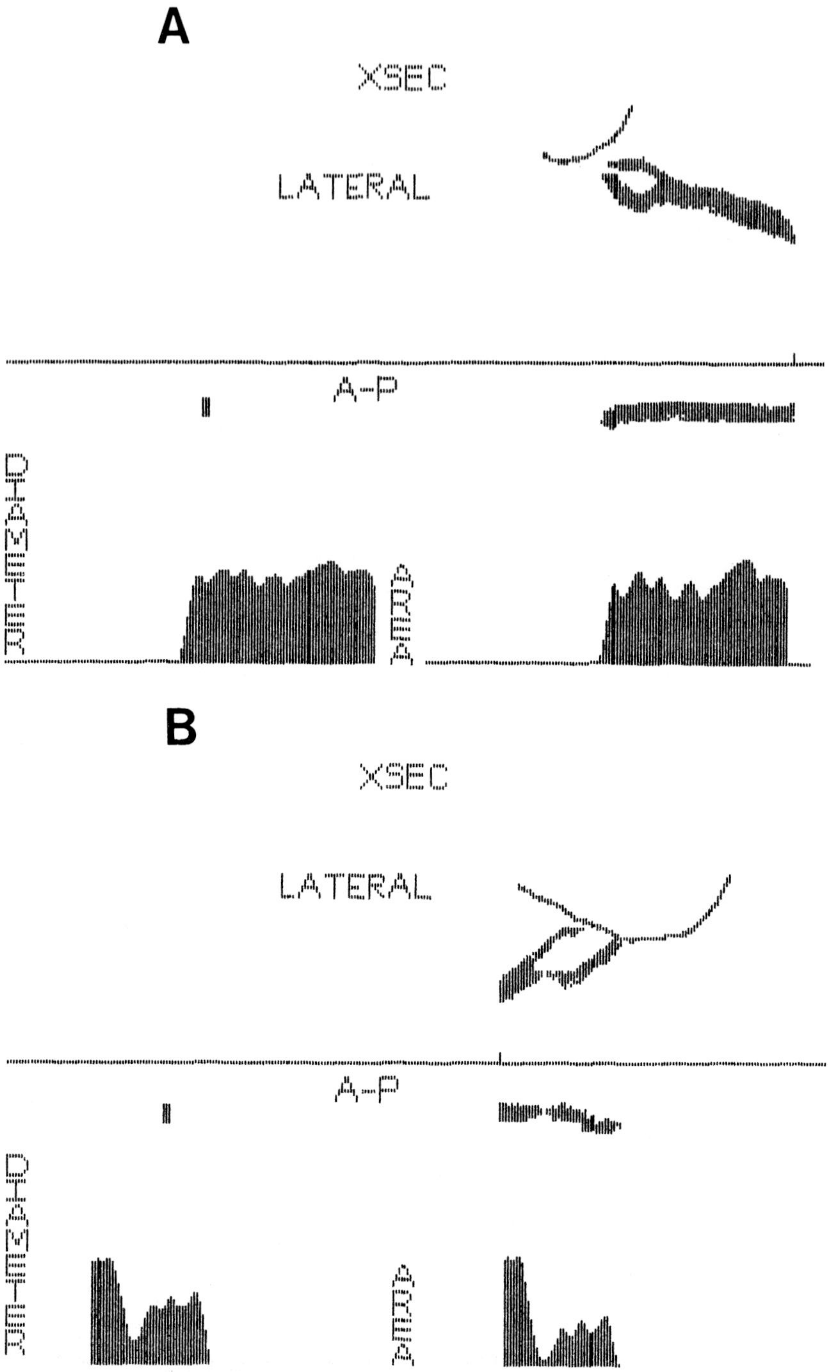

Figure 9-13. Thermal printouts of computerized ultrasonic arteriograms showing area and diameter histiograms. (A) Normal. (B) Stenosis of internal carotid artery.

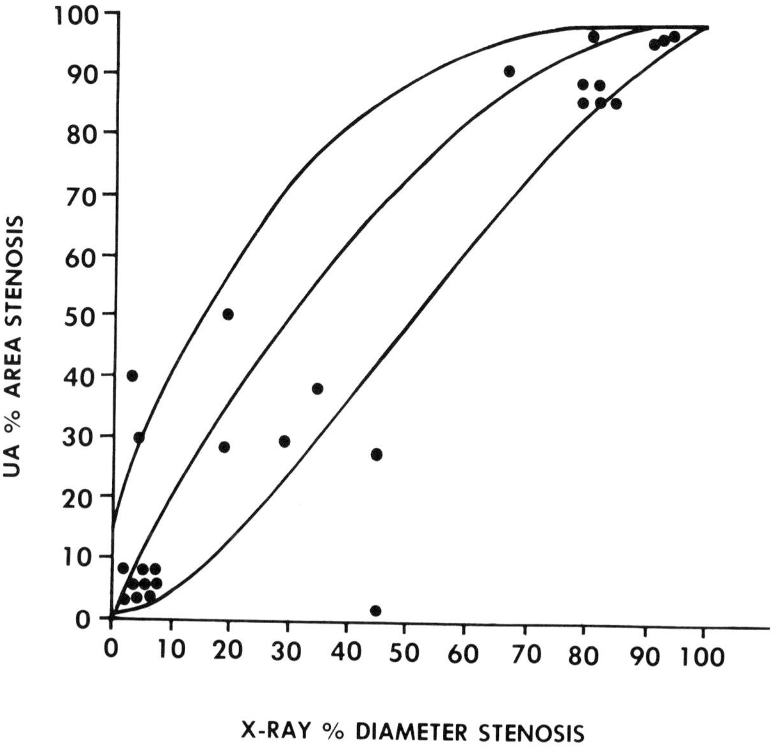

Figure 9-14. Comparison of CUA area histiograms with diameter stenoses measured from the biplanar x-ray view showing the greater degree of stenosis. Upper and lower lines indicate the range of possible areas associated with a given diameter stenosis (see Fig. 9–11).

CONCLUSION

Pulsed-Doppler ultrasonic arteriography has proved to be a rapid, reasonably reliable, and relatively inexpensive method for detecting disease at the carotid bifurcation. In our hands, it has been far more accurate than periorbital Doppler sonography or pulse-delay oculoplethysmography.[11,12] The addition of spectral analysis has increased the sensitivity of the test, albeit with some loss of specificity.[20] Although the ultimate value of computerized scans has not been firmly established, our early results with the orthogonal views and the area histiograms have been encouraging.[14,16] Perhaps the biggest impediment to further progress has been the relatively large volume sampled by each gate, which impairs the resolution of the instrument. With the current instrument, lesions less than 1.0 mm in size cannot be detected reliably. Also, for computerized applications, an increase in the number of gates would significantly improve the accuracy of the depth view and the area histiogram. With continued research, these problems may soon be solved.

REFERENCES

1. Hokanson DE, Mozersky DJ, Sumner DS, et al: Ultrasonic arteriography: A new approach to arterial visualization. Biomed Eng 6:420, 1971
2. Mozersky DJ, Hokanson DE, Baker DW, et al: Ultrasonic arteriography. Arch Surg 103:663, 1971
3. Mozersky DJ, Hokanson DE, Sumner DS, et al: Ultrasonic visualization of the arterial lumen. Surgery 72:253, 1972
4. Reid JM, Spencer MP: Ultrasonic Doppler technique for imaging blood vessels. Science 176:1235, 1972
5. Spencer MP, Reid JM, Davis DI, et al: Cervical carotid imaging with a continuous-wave Doppler flowmeter. Stroke, 5:145, 1974
6. Fish PJ: Multichannel, direction-resolving Doppler angiography, in Proc. 2nd European Congress on Ultrasonics in Medicine, Munich, 1975, Amsterdam, Oxford, Excepta Medica, 1975, p 153
7. Warlow CP, Fish PJ: Pulsed Doppler imaging of the carotid artery. J Neurol Sci 45:135, 1980
8. White DN, Curry GR: A comparison of 424 carotid bifurcations examined by angiography and the Doppler echoflow, in White D, Lyons EA (eds): Ultrasound in Medicine vol. 4, New York, Plenum Publishing Corporation, 1978, p 363
9. Spencer MP, Reid JM: Quantitation of carotid stenosis with continuous-wave (C-W) Doppler ultrasound. Stroke 10:326, 1979
10. Reneman RS, Spencer MP: Local Doppler audio spectra in normal and stenosed carotid arteries in man. Ultrasound Med Biol 5:1, 1979
11. Sumner DS, Russell JB, Ramsey DE, et al: Noninvasive diagnosis of extracranial carotid arterial disease. Arch Surg 114:1222, 1979
12. Sumner DS, Russell JB, Miles RD: Are noninvasive tests sufficiently accurate to identify patients in need of carotid arteriography? Surgery 91:700, 1982
13. Miles RD, Sumner DS, Russell JB, et al: Computerized ultrasonic arteriography, in Guyote MF (ed): Biomedical Sciences Instrumentation, vol. 116, Research Triangle Park, Instrument Society of America, 1980, p 81
14. Russell JB, Miles RD, Sumner DS: Computerized ultrasonic arteriography: A noninvasive technique for producing multiplanar images of the carotid bifurcation. Bruit 4:27 (Sept.), 1980
15. Miles RD, Russell JB, Sumner DS: Computerized ultrasonic arteriography: A new technique for imaging the carotid bifurcation. IEEE Trans Biomed Eng BME-29:378, 1982
16. Miles RD, Sievers BE, Russell JB, et al: Plotting the cross-sectional area of the internal carotid artery in real time. Stroke 13:121 (abs 36), 1982
17. Baker DW: Pulsed ultrasonic Doppler blood-flow sensing. IEEE Trans Sonics and Ultrasonics, SU-17:170, 1970
18. Nix ML, Barnes RW, Rittgers SE, et al: Direct carotid Doppler examination: Technique and results. Bruit 3:13 (Sept.), 1979
19. Barnes RW, Rittgers SE, Putney WW: Real-time Doppler spectrum analysis. Arch Surg 117:52, 1982
20. Russell JB, Miles RD, Sumner DS: Pulsed-Doppler ultrasonic arteriography with sound spectral analysis for evaluation of the carotid bifurcation. Bruit 6:23 (March), 1982

21. Metz CE: Basic principles of ROC analysis. Semin Nucl Med 8:283, 1978
22. O'Donnell TF Jr, Pauker SG, Callow AD, et al: The relative value of carotid noninvasive testing as determined by receiver operator characteristic curves. Surgery 87:9, 1980
23. Barnes RW, Bone GE, Reinertson J, et al: Noninvasive ultrasonic carotid arteriography: Prospective validation by contrast arteriography. Surgery 80:328, 1976
24. Blackshear WM Jr., Phillips DJ, Thiele BL, et al: Detection of carotid occlusive disease by ultrasonic imaging and pulsed Doppler spectrum analysis. Surgery 86:698, 1979
25. Hobson RW II, Berry SM, Katocs AS Jr, et al: Comparison of pulsed Doppler and real-time B-mode echo arteriography for noninvasive imaging of the extracranial carotid arteries. Surgery 87:286, 1980
26. Hobson RW II, Berry SM, Jamil Z, et al: Oculoplethysmography and pulsed Doppler ultrasonic imaging in diagnosis of carotid occlusive disease. Surg Gynecol Obstet 152:433, 1981
27. Cardullo PA, Cutler BS, Wheeler HB, et al: Noninvasive detection of carotid disease: An evaluation of oculoplethysmography, carotid phonoangiography, and pulsed Doppler ultrasonic arteriography. Bruit 5:26 (Dec), 1981
28. Wolf EA Jr: Discussion of Sumner, D.S. et al: Noninvasive diagnosis of extracranial carotid arterial disease. Arch Surg 114:1229, 1979
29. Godsey J, Nybro J, Koch P, et al: Technique of ultrasonic arteriography. Bruit 4:16 (June), 1980
30. Prendes JL, McKinney WM, Buonanno FS, et al: Anatomic variations of the carotid bifurcation affecting Doppler scan interpretation. J Clin Ultrasound 8:147, 1980
31. Kleaveland RN, Judd MA: (426 Medical Center Building, Spokane, Washington 99204): Personal communication, 1982

R. Eugene Zierler
Ghislaine O. Roederer
D. Eugene Strandness, Jr.

10

The Use of Frequency Spectral Analysis in Carotid Artery Surgery

INTRODUCTION TO DOPPLER SIGNAL ANALYSIS

Of all the noninvasive methods for the diagnosis of vascular disorders, Doppler ultrasound is the most widely used and thoroughly evaluated.[1] While simple auditory analysis of Doppler flow signals by an experienced examiner is generally adequate for the study of peripheral arterial and venous disease, the diagnosis of cerebrovascular disease presents unique problems. The carotid bifurcation, which is the principal site for extracranial carotid artery disease, is easily accessible to ultrasound, allowing a direct examination of the flow patterns in the diseased segment. It is also known that neurologic symptoms may be associated with a variety of carotid lesions, including all grades of stenosis with or without ulceration and total occlusion.[2] Therefore, an ideal diagnostic test would be capable of detecting a wide range of disease states. Auditory analysis of Doppler flow signals from the common carotid artery and its branches may identify the harsh, high-frequency sounds produced by high-grade stenoses. Although the flow disturbances associated with minor stenoses are not audible, experimental work has shown that abnormal flow patterns can be detected in the vicinity of such lesions.[3,4]

Two basic analytic methods have been developed in an effort to extract more information from the Doppler signal: zero-crosser systems and spectral analysis. The zero-crossing detector uses a frequency-to-voltage converter which measures the number of zero-crossings in the Doppler signal and produces a voltage output to drive a strip-chart recorder. An analog waveform is generated which gives an estimate of the change in Doppler frequency with respect to time. While the zero-crosser is relatively inexpensive and easy to use, it may be affected by errors and artifacts related to signal-to-noise ratio, amplitude dependency, and transient response.[5] In spite of these theoretical difficulties, Rutherford and associates examined common carotid analog waveforms and used discriminant analysis to separate normal, less than 50 percent stenotic, greater than 50 percent stenotic, and occluded arteries with 95 percent accuracy.[6] The accuracy of their method in distinguishing between less than and greater than 50 percent stenosis was 82 percent, although further estimation of percent stenosis was not attempted.

Spectral analysis is a method that discriminates between the true waveform and noise or artifact. A spectrum analyzer determines the amplitude of all frequencies present in a Doppler signal. The amplitude of a particular frequency is proportional to the number of red blood cells moving through the Doppler beam which produce that particular frequency shift at a point in time. Spectral information is usually presented graphically with frequency on the vertical axis, time on the horizontal axis, and amplitude indicated by the intensity of the gray-scale. Unlike the analog waveform, which reduces the Doppler signal to a single line, a spectrum analyzer continuously displays the complete frequency and amplitude content of the Doppler signal.

METHODS AND INSTRUMENTATION FOR SPECTRAL ANALYSIS

The first spectrum analyzers operated off-line using a relatively slow process. Instruments are now available that can perform on-line spectral analysis in real time. Techniques for real time spectral analysis include parallel filter systems,[7] time compression analysis,[8] and fast Fourier transform.[9] The spectrum analyzer used in the studies to be described employs a digital fast Fourier transform (FFT). This method provides a wide dynamic range and operates on-line to give a continuous display of frequency and amplitude. The analyzer outputs 100 bits of frequency data every 2.5 milliseconds, thus providing 400 spectra per second with a total frequency display of 10 KHz and frequency resolution of 100 Hz. Hard copy records are produced on light-sensitive paper with the zero flow baseline shifted to allow 7 KHz for forward and 3 KHz for reverse velocity components.

Spectral analysis of carotid artery velocity patterns has been performed using both continuous wave[10,11] and pulsed Doppler[12,13,14,15,16] systems. These devices also incorporate some type of ultrasonic imaging to assist in locating the arteries to be studied. Imaging techniques include flow visualization with the ultrasonic arteriograph[12,13] and tissue imaging with the B-mode component of the Duplex scanner.[14,15,16] Although useful data have been obtained with both continuous wave and pulsed Dopplers, the use of pulsed

Doppler signals for spectral analysis has several theoretical and practical advantages. Since a continuous wave Doppler detects flow at any point along the sound beam, the flow signals from several vessels may be superimposed. Even within a single artery, the flow profile at a particular point in time may contain a wide range of blood cell velocities. Continuous wave Doppler spectra thus tend to be complex and difficult to interpret. The pulsed Doppler detects flow at a discrete point in tissue referred to as the sample volume. Pulsed Doppler systems avoid the problem of superimposed vessels and, if the sample volume is smaller than the artery being studied, they permit examination of flow patterns at specific points across the arterial lumen. Generally, sampling from the center of the flow stream is preferred, since the laminar flow pattern normally present at that site can be distinguished from the turbulent patterns produced by arterial disease.[14]

The criteria for spectral interpretation and the analysis results described in the next sections are, except where noted, based on data obtained with the Duplex scanner.[14,15,16] This device combines a single-gated directional 5 MHz pulsed Doppler and a real time B-mode imaging system. The B-mode image is used to locate the common carotid artery and its branches and facilitate placement of the Doppler sample volume in the center of the flow stream. Both the Doppler angle and sample volume depth can be adjusted to allow flow detection at any point in the B-mode image. The Doppler sample volume is 3 cubic millimeters at a focal point of 2 cm. The pulse repetition frequency of the Doppler is 19.2 KHz which allows accurate detection of Doppler shifts up to 9.6 KHz. For all Doppler flow measurements, an angle of approximately 60 degrees was maintained between the ultrasound beam and the long axis of the artery.

INTERPRETATION OF SPECTRAL DATA

Studies in Experimental Models

The use of spectral analysis in the diagnosis of carotid artery disease is based on the supposition that certain disease states give rise to characteristic flow patterns. Clinical experience[14,15,16] and data from experimental models[4,17,18] both indicate that this is indeed the case. Centerstream flow in a normal artery during systole is laminar with all the red blood cells moving with nearly the same speed and direction. In this situation, the spectrum shows a narrow band of frequencies during the systolic phase of the cardiac cycle. During diastole the flow pattern is less uniform, and the spectrum shows a relative increase in the width of the frequency band. Stenoses and irregularities of the arterial lumen, such as those caused by atherosclerotic plaques, interfere with laminar flow, and the speed and direction of the red blood cells become random. The resulting disturbed flow patterns produce spectra with a wider range of frequencies and amplitudes, and this increase in the width of the frequency band is referred to as spectral broadening.

Pulsed Doppler studies of centerstream flow in the dog thoracic aorta have characterized the spectral changes occurring distal to graded stenoses.[4,18] With minor nonpressure-reducing stenoses producing as little as 10 percent diameter reduction, spectral broadening was noted only in late systole and early diastole. As the severity of stenosis was increased, spectral broadening occurred earlier in systole, and with high-grade pressure-reducing stenoses spectral broadening was present throughout the cardiac cycle. Another important finding in these studies was that the flow disturbances were observed only in close proximity to the stenoses. Spectral changes produced by nonpressure-reducing stenoses were evident one vessel diameter distal to the stenosis but had dissipated by the three diameter downstream position. The spectral changes distal to pressure-reducing stenoses were propagated farther downstream, although they also tended to disappear by the three diameter site. Increases in flow velocity, as indicated by increased spectral frequencies, have also been associated with graded stenoses.[4,17] The velocity changes are maximal within or immediately distal to the stenosis. These observations emphasize that, in order to detect carotid artery disease with Doppler ultrasound and spectral analysis, data must be obtained directly from the diseased segment.

Sources of Error and Artifacts

Since interpretation of Doppler spectra is based on peak systolic frequency and spectral width, it is important to recognize the changes in these parameters which can result from artifacts or variations in examination technique. As previously mentioned, the pulsed Doppler sample volume should be placed in the center of the flow stream. Even in normal arteries, significant velocity gradients can be present near the arterial wall, and spectral broadening may be observed when the sample volume is not located in the centerstream. This is illustrated in Figure 10-1 for a common carotid artery with the sample volume placed in the mid-stream, near the vessel wall, and between the artery and adjacent internal jugular vein. The mid-stream spectrum is narrow throughout systole, while the spectrum obtained near the wall is markedly broadened. A band of frequencies below the zero line (reverse flow) represents flow in the jugular vein.

Doppler sample volume size is also an important consideration, since a sample volume which is large compared to the vessel being examined will detect the velocity gradients near the arterial wall even when it is positioned in the center of the stream. This will result in spectral broadening as shown in Figure 10-1 and tends to overestimate the amount of disease present.

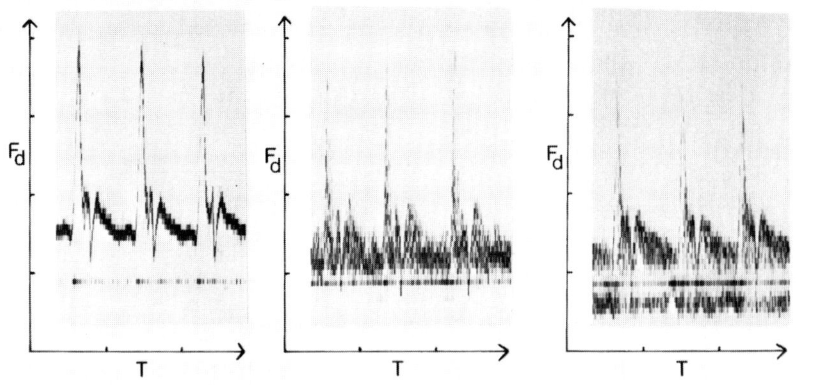

Figure 10-1. Effect of sample volume placement on common carotid artery (CCA) spectra. Sample volume was placed in the midstream, near the vessel wall, and between the artery and internal jugular vein. F_d: Doppler frequency shift; T: time.

The factors which influence the Doppler frequency shift are given by the equation:

$$F_d = \frac{F_o \, 2V \cos \theta}{C}$$

where F_d is the frequency shift, F_o is the Doppler transmitting frequency, V is the blood cell velocity, θ is the angle between the ultrasound beam and the direction of blood flow, and C is the velocity of sound in tissue. It is evident that the variables that determine Doppler shift are blood cell velocity and the angle θ. The effect of variations in θ on the Doppler frequency shift is shown in Figure 10-2. As the angle θ is increased, the frequency shift decreases.

In order to use the Doppler frequency shift as a measure of blood cell velocity, the angle θ must either be known or kept constant. With the Duplex scanner, the position of the Doppler beam and sample volume are indicated by cursors superimposed on the B-mode image, and the angle θ can be measured directly. Knowledge of the Doppler angle is particularly important when unusual anatomic configurations, such as internal carotid artery kinks, are encountered.

Another potential source for error in spectral analysis is incorrect identification of vessels. At the time of Duplex scanning, imaged vessels are identified by their anatomic location and the characteristics of their Doppler flow signals. The relatively low vascular resistance of the cerebral circulation normally produces a quasi-steady internal carotid artery flow pattern which

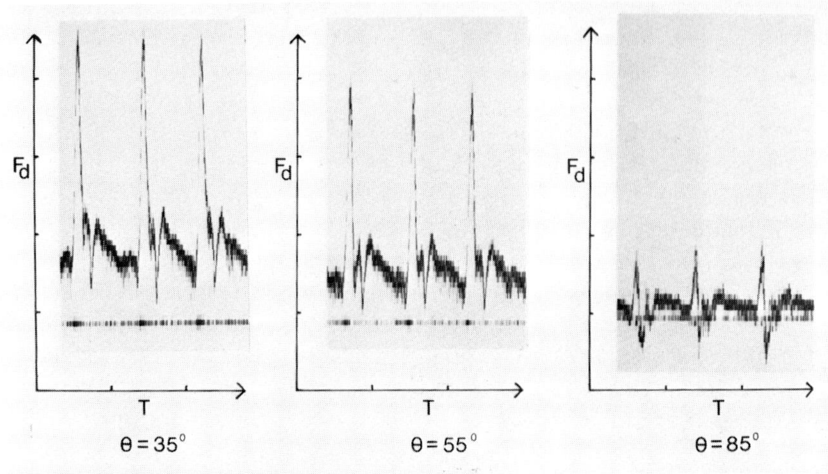

Figure 10-2. Effect of variations in the angle θ between the ultrasound beam and the direction of blood flow on common carotid artery spectra. F_d: Doppler frequency shift; T: time; k: constant factors in the Doppler equation.

remains above zero throughout the cardiac cycle. In the normal external carotid, the flow pattern goes to zero or reverses in diastole, similar to any other peripheral artery. The common carotid flow pattern usually resembles that of the internal carotid. The presence of carotid artery disease causes predictable alterations in these flow patterns. When the internal carotid is occluded, the common carotid flow pattern reflects the high vascular resistance of the external carotid and goes to zero in diastole. If the external carotid is providing collateral flow to the intracranial circulation, the vascular resistance may become low enough to produce quasi-steady flow similar to that normally present in the internal carotid. Examples of spectra will be used to illustrate some of these normal and abnormal flow patterns.

Criteria for Qualitative Interpretation of Spectra

Over the past 5 years, a series of comparisons have been made between certain spectral characteristics and the degree of carotid artery narrowing as determined by contrast arteriography.[14,15,16] In order to obtain an indication of the agreement between spectral analysis and arteriography, the Kappa value (K) was computed for each comparison. Kappa is a technique of statistical evaluation that measures agreement corrected for chance in two way tables of categorical data.[19,20] The value of Kappa is zero when the observed agreement is equivalent to that expected from chance alone. A maximum value of +1.0 indicates perfect agreement, and an inverse correlation results in a negative value. When a diagnostic test is evaluated by comparison to some standard test, Kappa is a measure of accuracy. If Kappa is computed for repetitions of the same test, it is a measure of precision. The Kappa value is expressed as $K \pm SE(K)$.

The most recent set of spectral criteria for classification of internal carotid artery disease is shown in Table 10-1.

These criteria are derived from visual inspection of the hard copy spectrum analyzer output. Using a 5 MHz pulsed Doppler and an angle (θ) of approximately 60 degrees, normal peak systolic frequencies are in the range of 2 KHz to 3 KHz, while high-grade stenoses are associated with peak frequencies above 4 KHz. Normal arteries and those with less than 50 percent diameter reduction are classified according to an estimate of the extent of spectral broadening. Stenoses of greater than 50 percent diameter reduction show elevated peak systolic frequencies as well as extensive spectral broadening. Internal carotid artery occlusion is indicated by failure to obtain a flow signal from the imaged vessel and flow to zero during diastole in the common carotid. In the following examples of spectra, Doppler shift frequency (KHz) is on the vertical axis, time (seconds) is on the horizontal axis, and amplitude is represented as shades of gray. Forward flow is indicated by a positive and reverse flow by a negative Doppler shift.

A normal common carotid artery spectrum is shown in Figure 10-3. The systolic upstroke is narrow and the peak is sharp. Although there is some spectral broadening in the deceleration phase of systole, the area under the systolic peak is clear. Flow remains above zero throughout the cardiac cycle.

Figure 10-4 shows the common carotid artery spectrum in the presence of ipsilateral internal carotid occlusion. The systolic pattern is similar to that in

Table 10-1
Arteriographic and spectral criteria for classification of internal carotid artery disease.

Arteriographic Criteria	Spectral Criteria
Normal (0% diameter reduction)	Peak systolic frequency up to 4 KHz; no spectral broadening.
5–15% diameter reduction	Peak systolic frequency up to 4 KHz; spectral broadening in deceleration phase of systole.
16–49% diameter reduction	Peak systolic frequency up to 4 KHz; spectral broadening throughout systole.
50–99% diameter reduction	Peak systolic frequency above 4 KHz; spectral broadening throughout systole; increased diastolic frequencies.
Occlusion (100% diameter reduction)	No internal carotid flow signal; flow to zero during diastole in common carotid artery.

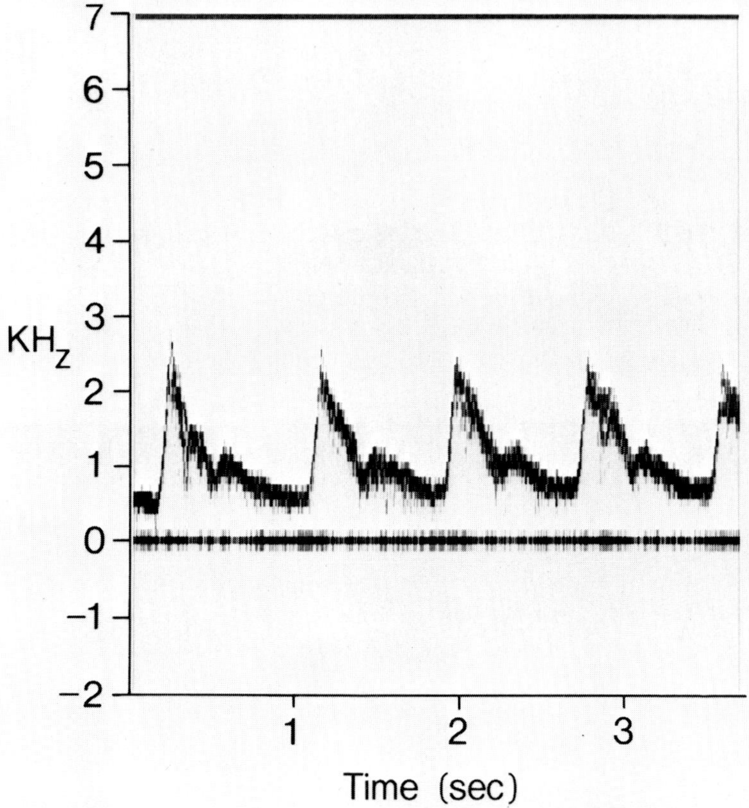

Figure 10-3. Spectrum from a normal common carotid artery.

Figure 10-3; however, there is a brief phase of flow reversal in early diastole, and diastolic flow remains near zero.

The normal internal carotid artery spectrum (Fig. 10-5) is similar to the common carotid with a narrow band of frequencies during the systolic upstroke and deceleration phases, a sharp systolic peak, and flow above zero throughout the cycle.

A lesion reducing the internal carotid diameter by 5 to 15 percent is associated with spectral broadening in the deceleration phase of systole (Fig. 10-6).

When a lesion reduces the internal carotid diameter by 16 to 49 percent, spectral broadening extends throughout systole, and the clear area under the systolic peak is filled in (Fig. 10-7).

High-grade stenoses which reduce the internal carotid diameter by 50 to 99 percent are associated with peak systolic frequencies above 4 KHz, spectral

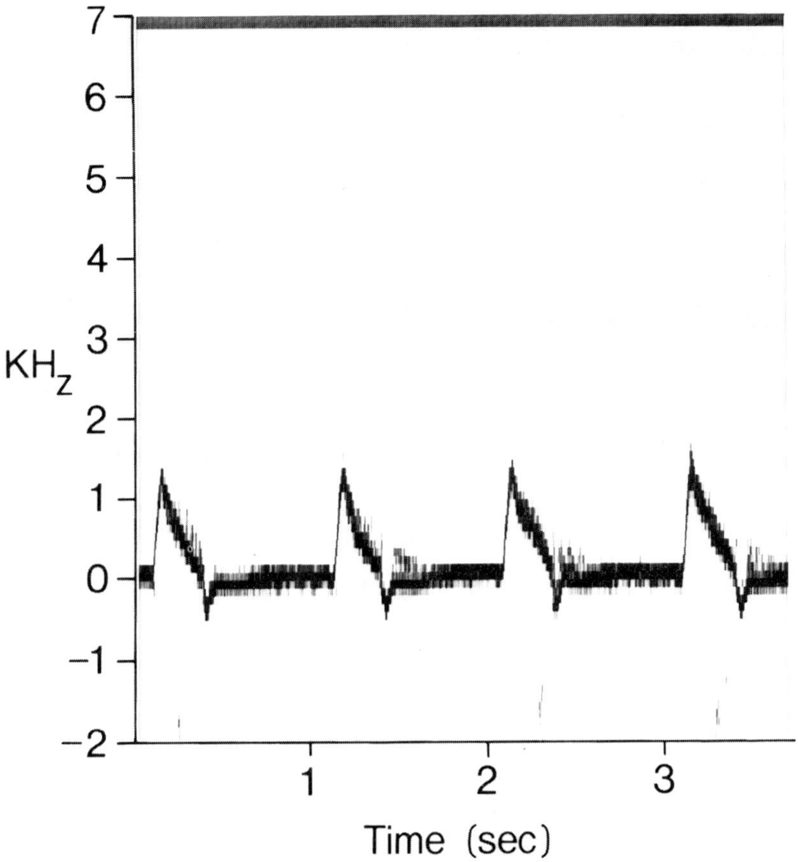

Figure 10-4. Common carotid artery spectrum in the presence of ipsilateral internal carotid occlusion.

broadening throughout systole, and increased diastolic frequencies, as shown in Figure 10-8.

A normal external carotid artery spectrum shows the triphasic flow pattern characteristic of peripheral arteries (Fig. 10-9). The prominent systolic forward flow phase is followed by a brief phase of flow reversal in early diastole and a final smaller phase of forward flow. The pattern is similar to that observed in the common carotid artery when the internal carotid is occluded (see Fig. 10-4).

Quantitative Spectral Analysis

Experience with the qualitative spectral criteria described in the last section suggested that, in the presence of carotid disease, the internal carotid

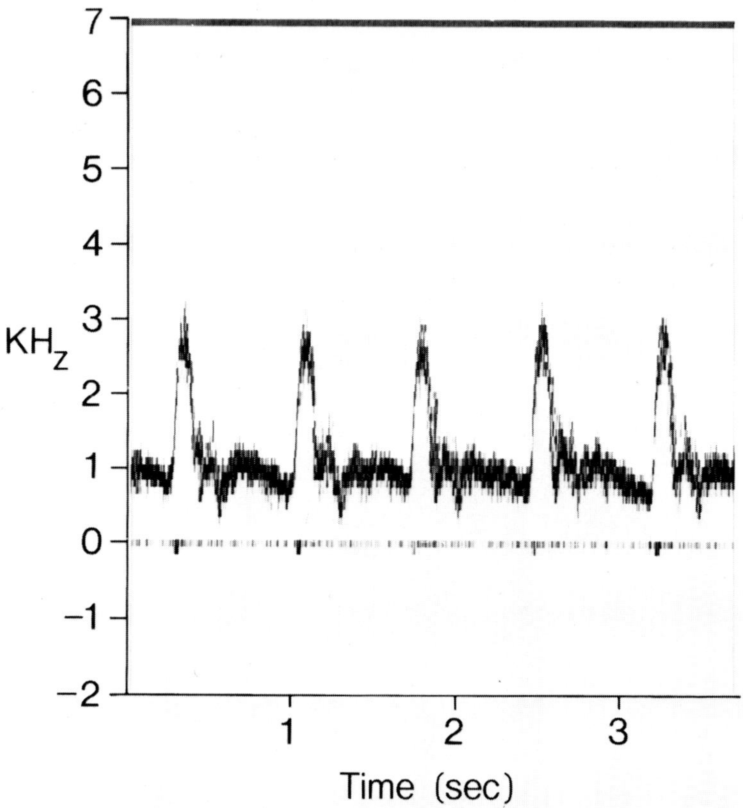

Figure 10-5. Spectrum from a normal (0 percent diameter reduction) internal carotid artery.

flow velocity tended to increase, while the common carotid flow velocity tended to decrease. This observation led to the use of velocity ratios as indices of carotid artery disease. Flow velocity at any point in the cardiac cycle can be calculated using the Doppler equation after obtaining frequency shift from the spectrum analyzer and Doppler angle θ from the B-mode image of the Duplex scanner. The ratio of mean peak internal carotid velocity to mean peak common carotid velocity at systole would be expected to increase with increasing degrees of disease. Accordingly, this ratio was found to be less than 0.8 in all 36 normal arteries studied and greater than 1.5 in all 21 stenoses of 60 percent or greater diameter reduction.[21] Another study used the ratio of peak systolic internal carotid velocity to end diastolic common carotid velocity.[22] With this ratio, it was possible to classify diameter reducing stenoses as 60

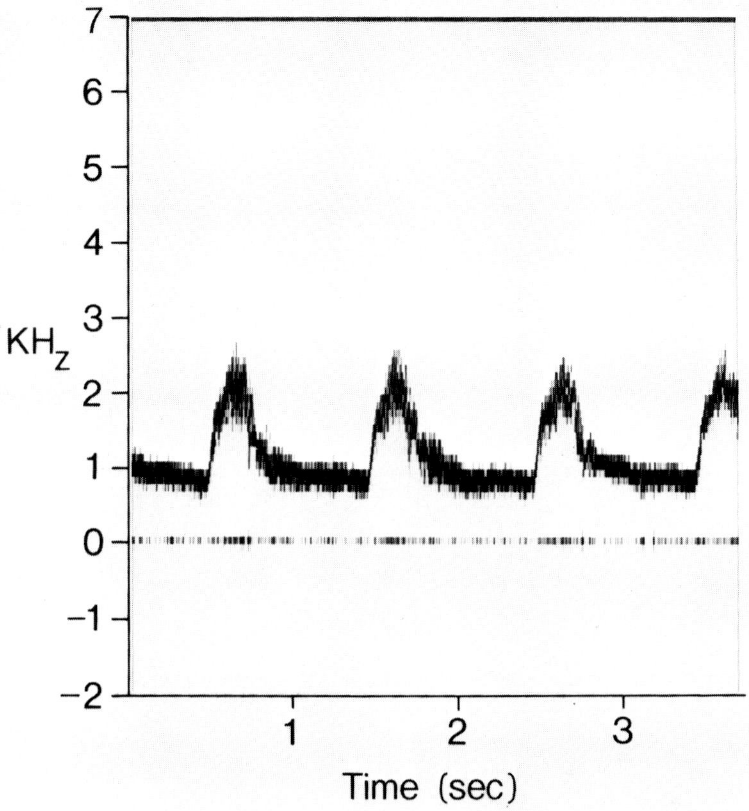

Figure 10-6. Internal carotid artery spectrum associated with a 5–15% diameter reducing stenosis.

percent or greater with 95 percent accuracy, 65 percent or greater with 97 percent accuracy, and 90 percent or greater with 100 percent accuracy. While these ratios will identify high-grade carotid stenoses, they are relatively insensitive to less severe lesions. In order to expand the diagnostic capabilities of quantitative spectral analysis, a computer based pattern recognition method is being developed.[23,24]

The pattern recognition process involves identification of recurring patterns in the spectral and temporal characteristics of the Doppler signal. This approach relies on data representing known degrees of disease as determined by contrast arteriography to develop decision rules that will eventually be used to classify unknown data. The data used to "train" the classification scheme are referred to as the "training set." Training set data

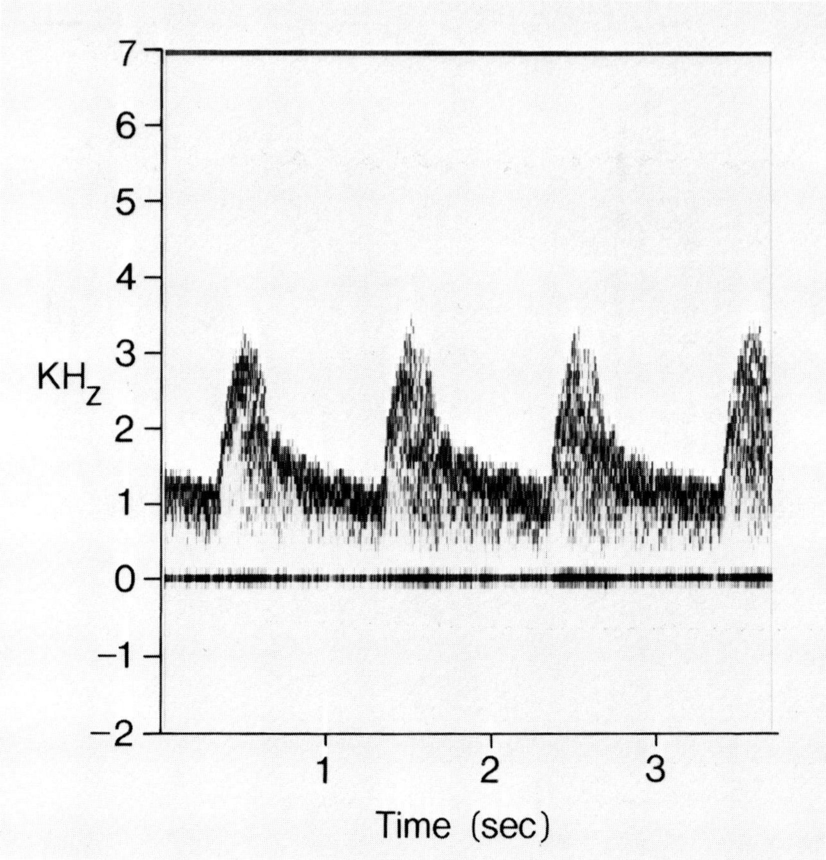

Figure 10-7. Internal carotid artery spectrum associated with a 16–49% diameter reducing stenosis.

consist of Doppler signal spectra obtained with the Duplex scanner from sites in the common and internal carotid arteries. The Doppler signals are recorded on audio tape together with an electrocardiographic R-wave signal which is used as a point of reference for timing.

Prior to entry into the pattern recognition program, the Doppler signals are processed by the FFT spectrum analyzer, and spectra from 20 regular cardiac cycles are used to create an ensemble averaged waveform. Ensemble averaging minimizes the effect of random, non-periodic components of the spectrum which result from variations in pulse rate and cardiac output. An algorithm is then used to find the mode (maximum amplitude) frequency and the 3 dB and 9 dB amplitude levels on either side of the mode frequency for

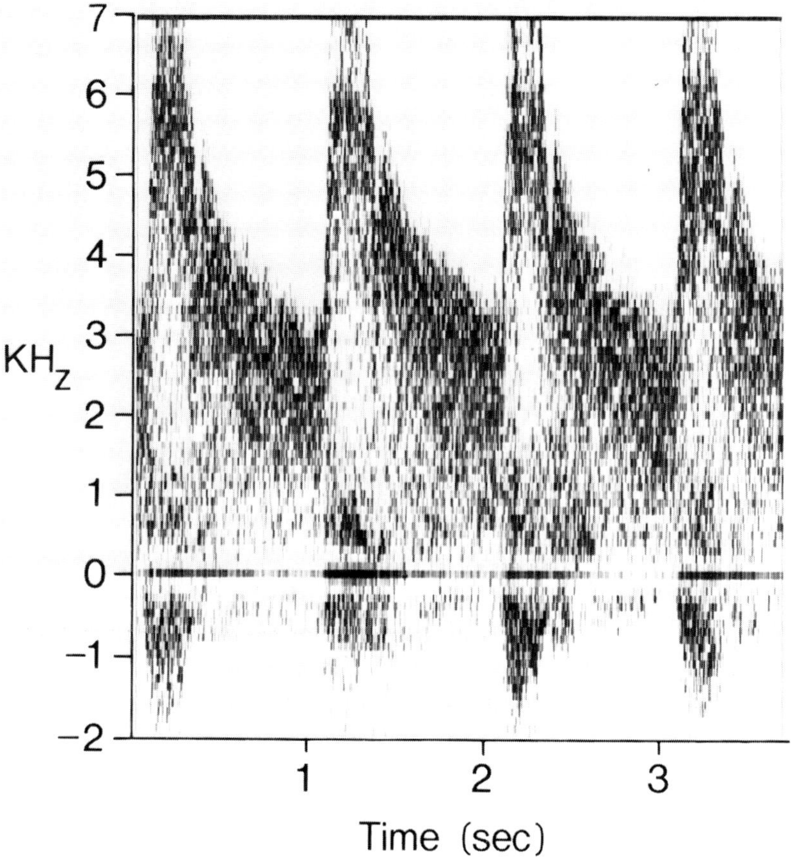

Figure 10-8. Spectrum from a high-grade (50–99 percent diameter reduction) internal carotid artery stenosis.

each point in the spectrum. This results in a contour plot of five lines which represents spectral data in compressed form. Further analysis is performed on this compressed data.

The details of the pattern recognition process have been described by Greene and associates.[23] Briefly, a number of features are extracted from the spectral data based on time relationships and spectral width measurements. The features are then classified by the computer and weighted according to their degree of correlation to the known disease states. A series of three separate binary decisions are used to classify the data: (1) Decide normal vs. diseased; (2) If diseased, then decide greater vs. less than 50 percent stenosis; and (3) If less than 50 percent stenosis, then decide greater vs. less than 20

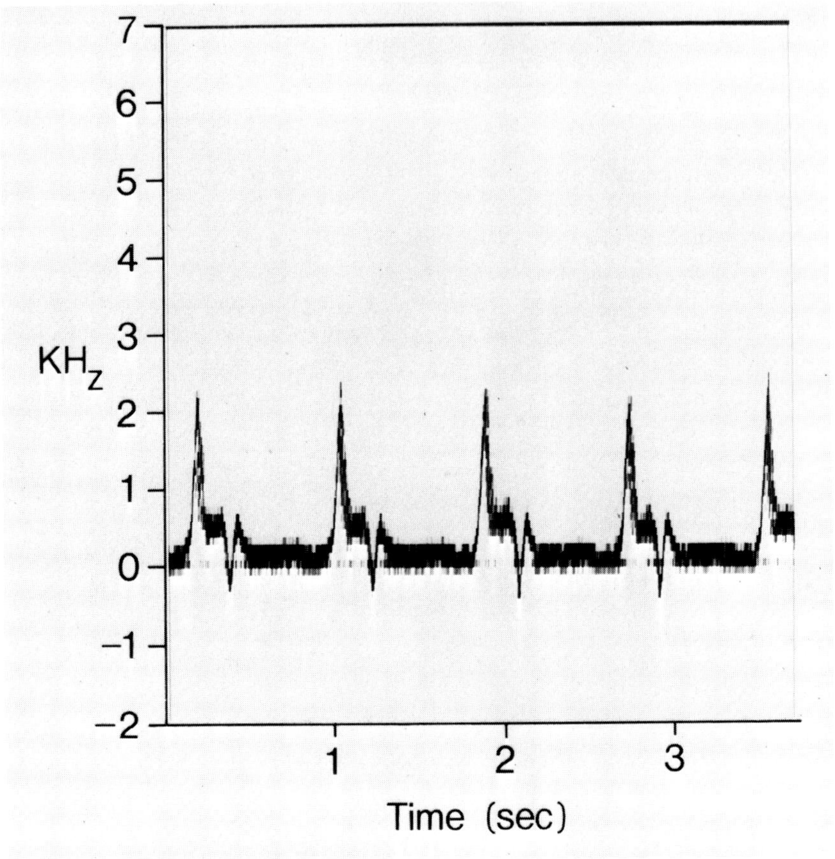

Figure 10-9. Normal external carotid artery spectrum.

percent stenosis. The subset of features selected by the program for the first decision are all based on common carotid data, while those for the second and third decisions include both common and internal carotid data.

The accuracy of the decision rules in classifying the training set data was assessed by a cross-validation technique. This gives an estimate of accuracy in classifying unknown data, assuming that the training set is representative of the actual distribution of unknowns. The results of cross-validation follow. (1) Normal vs. diseased, 97.5 percent correct; (2) Greater vs. less than 50 percent stenosis, 98.2 percent correct; and (3) Greater vs. less than 20 percent stenosis, 85.9 percent correct.

A set of 105 carotid sides was used as "unknown data" to test the accuracy of the pattern recognition program.[24] This set included 22 presumed normal sides from 11 asymptomatic normotensive volunteers and 83 sides with arteriographic confirmation of the extent of disease. In addition to the 3 binary decisions already described, an "undecided" category was used when the classification score failed to exceed a preselected threshold. A comparison between the pattern recognition classification and contrast arteriography is shown in Table 10-2.

A definite decision was reached in 83 carotid sides, leaving 22 in the undecided category. Of the 24 normal arteries, 18 were correctly classified, and 3 were undecided. For the 10 arteries with less than 20 percent diameter reduction, 7 were identified correctly, and 2 were undecided. In 39 arteries with 20 to 50 percent diameter reduction, 19 were correctly classified, and 10 were undecided. Of the 32 greater than 50 percent diameter stenoses, 22 were identified correctly and 7 were undecided. The Kappa value for this comparison is 0.721 ± 0.059. A review of the sides in the undecided group showed that they tended to lie near the borderlines of the arteriographic stenosis categories. This illustrates that there is some overlap between the features of adjacent disease categories. The problem of classifying borderline lesions is made more difficult by the variability in the arteriographic estimation of percent stenosis.[25]

Although this experience is still preliminary, it appears promising.

Table 10-2
Comparison of pattern recognition program classification with contrast arteriography. Data for the internal carotid artery (ICA) on 83 sides.

		Pattern Recognition Program				
	ICA Stenosis	Normal	Less than 20%	20–50%	Greater than 50%	Total
ARTERIOGRAPHY	Normal*	18	2	1		21
	Less than 20%		7	1		8
	20–50%		7	19	3	29
	Greater than 50%			3	22	25
	Total	18	16	24	25	83

*Includes presumed normal arteries.
K ± SE(K) = 0.721 ± 0.059

Pattern recognition may be particularly useful for the identification of normals and minor stenoses, since the accuracy of qualitative spectral analysis in detecting lesser degrees of disease is still relatively low. If this is the case, computerized pattern recognition will be suitable for documenting disease progression, both before and after carotid endarterectomy.

THE PREOPERATIVE EVALUATION

The Role of Noninvasive Testing in Patient Management

The role of noninvasive tests, such as Duplex scanning and spectral analysis, in the evaluation of patients prior to carotid artery surgery, is determined largely by the therapeutic approach of the individual surgeon. For those who believe that only patients with definite hemispheric or ocular symptoms should undergo arteriography and carotid endarterectomy, non-invasive tests will have little effect on clinical decisions. If, on the other hand, it is thought that asymptomatic carotid disease requires operative treatment, then noninvasive tests provide a practical means for screening patients.

In practice, a significant number of patients present with vague or atypical neurologic symptoms, and it is in this group that noninvasive tests can be of most value. If these patients are shown to have normal carotid arteries, then arteriography might be avoided. Patients with total occlusion of the internal carotid artery are generally not candidates for endarterectomy, and if this condition were detected noninvasively, many of these patients could also be spared arteriography. In one study, 25 percent of patients with fixed neurologic deficits had internal carotid occlusion.[2] The reasons for Duplex scanning and spectral analysis in 491 patients examined during a single year were as follows: focal symptoms lasting less than 24 hours (156), focal symptoms lasting more than 24 hours (107), non-focal symptoms (147), and asymptomatic bruits (81). In all 4 groups of patients, there was a significant relationship between the reporting of a high-grade internal carotid stenosis and the performance of arteriography and surgery. Therefore, the finding of significant carotid artery disease by noninvasive testing appears to be an important factor in the decision to proceed with arteriography.

Clinical Applications and Results

Several studies comparing the results of Duplex scanning and spectral analysis with contrast arteriography have been reported.[14,15,16] Over the past few years, the Duplex scanner has undergone numerous modifications, both in the design of the Doppler system and in the procedure for Doppler signal analysis. In January, 1980, the research prototype system was replaced by a commercially available unit, the ATL Mark V Duplex Scanner.* Initially, a "medium focus" Doppler transducer with a 4 cm focal length and sample volume of 24 cubic millimeters was used. When the importance of sample volume size became apparent, this was replaced by a "short focus" Doppler transducer having a 2 cm focal length and sample volume of 3 cubic millimeters. Doppler signal processing was performed by a Honeywell research prototype digital FFT spectrum analyzer with hard copy output from an ATL 130A Line Scan Recorder.

Between January, 1980 and October, 1980, 85 patients (169 carotid sides) were evaluated by Duplex scanning with the medium focus Doppler and contrast arteriography. Subsequently, between November, 1980 and May, 1981, 39 patients (77 carotid sides) were examined using the short focus Doppler and contrast arteriography. The results in these two patient groups for the internal carotid artery are shown in Tables 10-3 and 10-4.[15]

In these studies, test results are based on spectral analysis according to the criteria listed in Table 10-1. The B-mode image was used for vessel identification and sample volume placement and, although arterial wall

*Advanced Technology Laboratories, Inc., Bellevue, Washington.

Table 10-3
Comparison of spectral analysis using the medium focus Doppler transducer with contrast arteriography.
Data for the internal carotid artery (ICA) on 169 sides.

	Spectral Analysis					
ARTERIOGRAPHY: ICA Stenosis	0%	5–15%	16–49%	50–99%	100%	Total
0%	1	6	4	1		12
5–15%	1	19	15	2		37
16–49%	2	10	24	5		41
50–99%		1	2	61	1	65
100%				1	13	14
Total	4	36	45	70	14	169

$K \pm SE(K) = 0.581 \pm 0.046$

Table 10-4
Comparison of spectral analysis using the short focus Doppler transducer with contrast arteriography. Data for the internal carotid artery (ICA) on 77 sides.

		Spectral Analysis					
	ICA Stenosis	0%	5–15%	16–49%	50–99%	100%	Total
A							
R	0%	4	4				8
T							
E	5–15%	1	9	3			13
R							
I	16–49%		4	16	3		23
O							
G	50–99%		1	2	25		28
R							
A	100%					5	5
P							
H	Total	5	18	21	28	5	77
Y							

K ± SE(K) = 0.682 ± 0.064

calcification was often noted, no attempt was made to estimate the degree of stenosis from the image alone. The experience of others using B-mode imaging to grade carotid artery disease has shown relatively low sensitivities, particularly for severe stenoses and total occlusions.[26]

In the medium focus Doppler group (Table 10-3), only one of 12 arteriographically normal internal carotid arteries was correctly identified, resulting in a specificity of 8 percent (1/12). The overall sensitivity for detecting any degree of disease was 98 percent (154/157). For the individual disease categories the sensitivities were as follows: 5-15 percent diameter reduction 51 percent (19/37); 16-49 percent diameter reduction 59 percent (24/41); 50-99 percent diameter reduction 94 percent (61/65); and total occlusion 93 percent (13/14). For this comparison, K ± SE(K) = 0.581 ± 0.046.

The overall specificity and sensitivity in the short focus Doppler group were 50 percent (4/8) and 99 percent (68/69), respectively (Table 10-4). In the individual disease categories the sensitivities were as follows: 5-15 percent diameter reduction 69 percent (9/13); 16-49 percent diameter reduction 70 percent (16/23); 50-99 percent diameter reduction 89 percent (25/28); and total occlusion 100 percent (5/5). The value for Kappa in this comparison is 0.682 ± 0.064.

The results in normal arteries and those with less than 50 percent diameter reduction were significantly better using the short focus Doppler. In that group, all four incorrectly classified normal vessels were placed in the category with the least amount of disease. The importance of sample volume size has been discussed, and these data indicate that the smaller sample volume improves accuracy for identification of normals and minor stenoses while maintaining the high level of accuracy established for severe stenoses and occlusions. The diagnostic accuracy for internal carotid occlusion has been improved by recognizing the importance of the ipsilateral common carotid artery spectrum.[27]

When noninvasive tests are compared to a standard such as contrast arteriography, the variability of the standard test must be considered. The precision of arteriographic interpretation was determined by Chikos and associates in a study of 128 multiview carotid arteriograms read by three radiologists.[25] When the same radiologist interpreted the same arteriogram on different occasions (intraobserver agreement), the agreement rate was 75 percent for normal internal carotid arteries and 90 percent for a 50 percent or greater diameter reduction. The rate of agreement between radiologists (interobserver agreement) for normal internal carotid arteries was 57 percent, and for a 50 percent or greater diameter stenosis it was 85 percent. Both intra- and interobserver agreement for total internal carotid occlusion were 97 percent. Thus, the agreement rate is lowest for normal arteries, and it tends to increase with increasing degrees of carotid disease. In this study, the Kappa value for intraobserver agreement is 0.711 ± 0.054, and for interobserver agreement it is 0.568 ± 0.058. The Kappa values for comparisons between spectral analysis and arteriography are similar to those for intra- and interobserver comparisons of arteriographic interpretation. When arteriography is used as the standard, this variability limits the accuracy which can be achieved with noninvasive tests.

An asymptomatic cervical bruit is a common reason for referral to the vascular laboratory. Although the presence of a bruit correlates with a higher risk of stroke in males, the site of the bruit and the side of the stroke are not consistently related.[28] It has also been shown that not all bruits are associated with significant carotid artery disease.[29] Of 100 patients with 165 asymptomatic cervical bruits evaluated with Duplex scanning and spectral analysis[30] 12 (7.3 percent) were normal, 83 (50 percent) had stenoses of less than 50 percent diameter reduction, 61 (37 percent) had 50-99 percent diameter reducing stenoses, and 9 (5.5 percent) had total occlusions of the internal carotid artery. The management of patients with asymptomatic cervical bruits and asymptomatic carotid stenoses remains controversial; however, if a high-grade stenosis is considered an indication for arteriography and surgery, then 37 percent of these patients would require further investigation.

Another controversial area in carotid artery surgery is the role of noninvasive testing in screening for cerebrovascular disease prior to major surgical procedures. Duplex scanning and spectral analysis were used to evaluate 102 patients undergoing coronary artery bypass operations.[31] Of 24 patients with either a bruit or previous neurologic symptoms, 13 (54 percent) had unilateral or bilateral internal carotid lesions of more than 50 percent diameter reduction. In the 78 patients without symptoms or signs, only 5 (6 percent) had unilateral or bilateral internal carotid stenoses of more than 50 percent diameter reduction. One stroke and one transient ischemic attack occurred postoperatively in two separate patients. Both of these patients were without symptoms or signs, and neither had a high-grade stenosis.

Although the presence of a bruit or a history of neurologic symptoms are more likely to be associated with a high-grade internal carotid stenosis, these factors do not appear to increase the risk of postoperative neurologic complications. These results are consistent with other reports[32,33] that failed to relate the incidence of perioperative stroke to the presence of high-grade stenosis. Thus, the available data do not support "prophylactic" carotid endarterectomy as an adjunct to cardiac or other major surgery.

INTRAOPERATIVE ASSESSMENT

The methods available for intraoperative assessment of carotid endarterectomy include operative arteriography,[34] supraorbital Doppler studies, and auditory analysis of continuous wave Doppler flow signals.[35] While operative arteriography is the standard method for detecting technical error during carotid endarterectomy, it has several disadvantages: it allows only a single plane view of the artery; it does not provide data on the flow patterns through the endarterectomized segment; and it exposes patients to the risks of arterial puncture and injection of radiographic contrast. Although complications due to operative arteriography are rare, their occurrence has led some surgeons to stop using this technique routinely.[34]

A new method for intraoperative assessment has been developed which employs a 20 MHz pulsed Doppler and an FFT spectrum analyzer.[36] The Doppler probe contains a small ultrasonic transducer mounted at the end of a 16 gauge needle which produces a sample volume of approximately 0.2 cubic millimeters. During use, the transducer is placed directly on the external surface of the artery and acoustically coupled with saline. The sample volume is positioned in the center of the flow stream by adjustment of the range control, and an angle of approximately 60 degrees is maintained between the transducer and the long axis of the artery. The spectrum analyzer is used to visually monitor the arterial flow patterns, and the Doppler signals are also recorded on tape for subsequent analysis and review. Flow patterns are examined at several sites along the common carotid, carotid bulb, external carotid, and internal carotid arteries. These sites are examined twice during each operation: once after exposure of the arteries but prior to endarterectomy (pre-TEA), and once immediately following endarterectomy and restoration of arterial flow (post-TEA).

The criteria for interpretation of intraoperative spectra were based on the principles previously described for the 5 MHz pulsed Doppler of the Duplex scanner. Since the 5 MHz and 20 MHz Doppler systems have different transmitting frequencies and sample volume sizes. However, their spectra cannot be compared directly with each other. For the intraoperative studies, corresponding pre-TEA and post-TEA spectra were compared, and the flow disturbances were classified as mild, moderate, or severe, depending on the extent of spectral broadening and the presence of increased peak systolic frequencies. No attempt was made to estimate actual percent stenosis from the intraoperative spectra.

Intraoperative studies were performed during 45 carotid endarterectomies.[36] In all cases, an indwelling silastic shunt was used to maintain ipsilateral internal carotid artery perfusion, and the arteriotomy was closed with continuous 6-0 Prolene suture under 2.5 × magnification. Operative arteriography was performed at the conclusion of each procedure. The pre-TEA internal carotid spectra showed flow disturbances which were mild in 6 arteries and moderate to severe in 39 arteries. On the post-TEA spectra, all 6 mild flow disturbances remained in that category, while 35 of the remaining 39 arteries showed a definite improvement in the degree of flow disturbance. Four arteries with moderate to severe flow disturbances did not change significantly. In one case, the initial post-TEA spectrum showed increased spectral broadening, and the operative arteriogram revealed a stenosis due to technical error at the distal end of the arteriotomy. After a vein patch angioplasty, the spectrum was improved, and arteriography showed a widely patent internal carotid artery. No other significant technical errors were noted on operative arteriography, although some irregularity of the lumen in the endarterectomized segment was often present. There was no perioperative neurologic morbidity or mortality in any patient studied. A normal operative arteriogram with its corresponding post-TEA spectra is shown in Figure 10-10.

Although the present experience with intraoperative pulsed Doppler assessment is limited, several conclusions can be made. The technique offers advantages over operative arteriography in terms of safety, speed, and provision of physiologic data. Of the cases with significant spectral abnormalities prior to endarterectomy, the majority show improvement after endarterectomy, although some flow disturbance often persists. A lack of improvement or deterioration in spectra after endarterectomy may indicate a technical problem and could be used to select patients for operative arteriography. Technical factors are apparently not a major cause of flow disturbances after

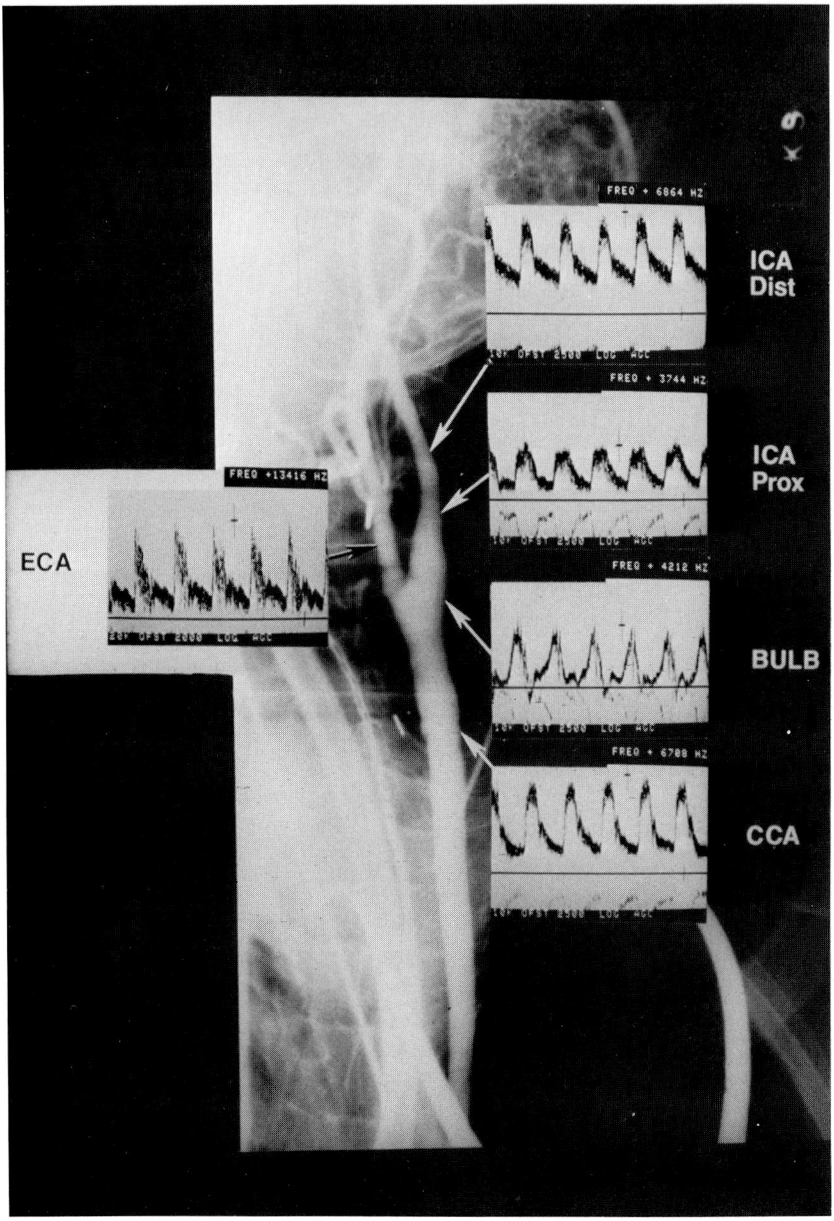

Figure 10-10. Normal operative arteriogram with intraoperative spectra obtained after endarterectomy. Spectra from the CCA, Bulb, and ICA all represent mild flow disturbances, while the ECA spectrum shows moderate spectral broadening. CCA: common carotid artery; ICA: internal carotid artery; ECA: external carotid artery; Prox: proximal; Dist: distal.

endarterectomy. Any relationship between these residual flow disturbances and recurrent carotid stenosis must be determined by prospective long-term follow-up. Intraoperative spectra provide important baseline data for such long-term studies, since the flow disturbances due to progression of disease at the carotid bifurcation must be distinguished from those directly attributable to endarterectomy.

POSTOPERATIVE FOLLOW-UP

Most reported estimates for the incidence of recurrent stenosis at the site of a previous carotid endarterectomy are less than 5 percent.[37,38,39,40] These estimates, however, are based almost entirely on patients who presented with recurrent neurologic symptoms which prompted repeat investigations including arteriography. Since the majority of patients who remained asymptomatic are not considered, it is likely that the true incidence of recurrent carotid stenosis has been underestimated. Although arteriography is not suitable for routine postoperative follow-up, noninvasive methods can be used to document recurrent stenosis in asymptomatic patients.[41]

Thirty-six patients were evaluated after carotid endarterectomy using both Duplex scanning with spectral analysis and arteriography.[42] Forty-four operated sides were available for comparison after a mean postoperative follow-up interval of 28 months. Recurrent focal symptoms prompted arteriography in 27 patients. In 14 of these patients, symptoms were appropriate to the previously operated side, while in the remaining 13 patients they were related to the contralateral non-operated side. Only one of the 44 sides was considered normal by arteriography, and this was interpreted as a 16-49 percent diameter stenosis on spectral analysis. The overall sensitivity for detecting any degree of disease was 100 percent (43/43); that is, no diseased arteries were classified as normal by spectral analysis. In the individual disease categories, the sensitivities were as follows: 5-15 percent diameter reduction 60 percent (3/5); 16-49 percent diameter reduction 76 percent (16/21); 50-99 percent diameter reduction 93 percent (14/15); and total occlusion 100 percent (2/2). The Kappa value for this comparison is 0.675 ± 0.096. This value is similar to those previously given for preoperative spectral analysis compared to arteriography and comparisons of arteriographic interpretation. These results indicate that the criteria used for spectral analysis preoperatively can also be applied to the postoperative carotid artery.

In a separate study, Duplex scanning with spectral analysis was used to evaluate 76 patients undergoing 89 carotid endarterectomies.[43] In all cases, operative arteriography was performed to document the status of the endarterectomized segment. The mean duration of postoperative follow-up was 16 months. Indications for operation were transient ischemic attacks or amaurosis fugax in 57, completed stroke in 19, nonhemispheric symptoms in 5, and asymptomatic stenosis in 8. Preoperative evaluation of the internal carotid artery (ICA) showed stenosis of greater than 50 percent diameter reduction in 76 and less than 50 percent diameter reduction in 13.

Postoperatively, spectral changes indicating an ICA stenosis of 50 to 99 percent diameter reduction were observed in 32 of the 89 sides. Of these 32 high-grade stenoses, 12 persisted on serial examinations, 8 reverted to less than 50 percent diameter reduction, one became occluded, and 11 had only a single follow-up study. The estimated incidence of persistent high-grade stenosis, based on the serial studies, was 20 percent. All but three of the high-grade stenoses were noted during the first postoperative year. Eight patients experienced recurrent symptoms which were appropriate to the operated side; of these, 3 had less than 50 percent stenosis, 4 had greater than 50 percent stenosis, and one had ICA occlusion.

The incidence of recurrent carotid stenosis in this study is higher than estimates based on patients with neurologic symptoms. There appear to be two kinds of lesions that occur following carotid endarterectomy: an early lesion consisting of myointimal cell proliferation and a late-developing lesion of typical atherosclerotic plaque.[37,38] The firm, smooth, non-ulcerated early lesion may be a manifestation of the reparative process following arterial injury. During serial follow-up, some of the high-grade stenoses which were noted in the early postoperative period became less severe. This observation is consistent with proliferation and regression of myointimal lesions. Technical factors have been suggested as a cause of recurrent stenosis;[40] however, operative arteriography did not show any abnormalities that would account for the observed spectral changes.

The majority of recurrent high-grade stenoses in this study were not associated with neurologic symptoms, presumably because of their smooth surfaces and the abundant collateral blood supply to each cerebral hemisphere. If this high incidence of recurrent carotid stenosis is corroborated by other studies, issues such as prophylactic endarterectomy for asymptomatic carotid disease will have to be re-evaluated. The effect of antiplatelet drugs on the response to endarterectomy will also require investigation. Studies are in progress that will provide quantitative analysis of spectral patterns following endarterectomy and relate intraoperative and subsequent flow disturbances to the development of recurrent carotid stenosis.

CONCLUSIONS

Spectral analysis of Doppler velocity signals is a direct noninvasive technique which is ideally suited for the diagnosis of carotid bifurcation disease. Although qualitative analysis of spectra has been emphasized in recent studies, new techniques for quantitative spectral analysis, such as computerized pattern recognition, have shown great potential for improving diagnostic accuracy. An important advantage of the quantitative approach is that it avoids the subjective evaluations which appear to limit the accuracy of qualitative spectral analysis.

Clinical application of spectral analysis has been facilitated by combining pulsed Doppler and B-mode imaging in one system. Up to now, the main purpose of the B-mode image has been to orient the Doppler beam; however, continued improvement in the quality of B-mode images may increase their diagnostic value. It seems logical to use imaging techniques for demonstrating arterial wall anatomy and pulsed Doppler to obtain physiologic data on adjacent flow patterns. A variety of instruments are commercially available, both for Doppler flow detection and spectral analysis. Since these devices differ in features such as Doppler mode (continuous wave or pulsed), transmitting frequency, sample volume size, dynamic range, and display characteristics, the specific criteria for spectral analysis will vary from one laboratory to another. Nevertheless, the basic principles relating flow disturbances to carotid artery disease should remain the same.

At present, spectral analysis plays two general roles. In the clinical setting, it can determine the location and extent of carotid artery disease, and, at least in some patients, it appears to influence subsequent investigation and treatment. As a research tool, it provides a means for documenting the natural history of carotid artery lesions, both before and after endarterectomy. It is to be hoped that when this information is related to neurologic symptoms and specific risk factors, it will promote a more rational approach to the treatment of carotid artery disease.

REFERENCES

1. Kempczinski RF, Rutherford RB: Current status of the vascular diagnostic laboratory. Advances in Surgery 12:1, 1978
2. Thiele BL, Young JV, Chikos PM, et al: Correlation of arteriographic findings and symptoms in cerebrovascular disease. Neurology 30:1041, 1980
3. Giddens DP, Mabon RF, Cassanova RA: Measurements of disordered flows distal to subtotal vascular stenoses in the thoracic aorta of dogs. Circ Res 39:112, 1976
4. Thiele BL, Hutchison RJ, Greene FM, et al: Pulsed Doppler waveform patterns produced by smooth stenosis in the dog thoracic aorta. Blood Flow Theory and Practice (in press)
5. Johnston KW, Maruzzo BC, Cobbold RSC: Errors and artifacts of Doppler flowmeters and their solution. Arch Surg 112:1335, 1977.
6. Rutherford RB, Hiatt WR, Kreutzer EW: The use of velocity waveform analysis on the diagnosis of carotid artery occlusive disease. Surgery 82:695, 1977.
7. Yao JST, Needham TN: Frequency analysis of Doppler-shift blood flow signals by a band-pass filter: Preliminary report. Biomed Eng 5:438, 1970.

8. Coghlan BA, Taylor MG, King DH: On-line display of Doppler shift spectra by a new time compression analyser, in Reneman RS (ed): Cardiovascular Applications of Ultrasound, Amsterdam, North-Holland Publishing Company, 1974
9. Cooley JW, Tukey JW: An algorithm for the machine calculation of complex Fourier series. Math Comp 19:297, 1965
10. Lewis RR, Beasley MG, Hyams DE, et al: Imaging the carotid bifurcation using continuous-wave Doppler-shift ultrasound and spectral analysis. Stroke 9:465, 1978
11. Spencer MP, Reid JM: Quantitation of carotid stenosis with continuous-wave (C-W) Doppler ultrasound. Stroke 10:326, 1979
12. Barnes RW, Bone GE, Reinertson J, et al: Noninvasive ultrasonic carotid angiography: Prospective validation by contrast arteriography. Surgery 80:328, 1976
13. Russell JB, Miles RD, Sumner DS: Pulsed-Doppler ultrasonic arteriography with sound spectral analysis for evaluation of the carotid bifurcation. Bruit 6:23, 1982
14. Blackshear WM, Phillips DJ, Thiele BL, et al: Detection of carotid occlusive disease by ultrasonic imaging and pulsed Doppler spectrum analysis. Surgery 86:698, 1979
15. Breslau PJ, Knox RA, Phillips DJ, et al: The accuracy of ultrasonic Duplex scanning as compared with contrast arteriography in extracranial carotid artery disease. Vascular Diagnosis and Therapy (in press)
16. Fell G, Phillips DJ, Chikos PM, et al: Ultrasonic duplex scanning for disease of the carotid artery. Circulation 64:1191, 1981
17. Hutchison KJ, Thiele BL, Greene FM, et al: Radial variation of disturbed flow downstream of artificial stenoses in the dog thoracic aorta. (submitted to Atherosclerosis)
18. Hutchison KJ, Thiele BL, Greene FM, et al: Detection of disturbed flow produced by artificially created stenoses in the canine thoracic aorta by computer processing of pulsed Doppler spectra. (submitted to J Surg Res)
19. Cohen J: A coefficient of agreement for nominal scales. Educational and Psychological Measurement 20:37, 1960
20. Langlois Y, Roederer GO, Chan A, et al: Evaluating carotid artery disease: The concordance between pulsed Doppler/spectrum analysis and angiography. Ultrasound Med Bio (in press)
21. Blackshear WM, Phillips DJ, Chikos PM, et al: Carotid artery velocity patterns in normal and stenotic vessels. Stroke 11:67, 1980
22. Knox RA, Breslau PJ, Strandness DE Jr: A simple parameter for accurate detection of severe carotid disease. Brit J Surg (in press)
23. Greene FM, Beach KW, Strandness DE Jr, et al: Computer based pattern recognition of carotid arterial disease using pulsed Doppler ultrasound. Ultrasound Med Bio 8:161, 1982
24. Knox RA, Greene FM, Beach KW, et al: Computer based classification of carotid arterial disease: A prospective assessment. (submitted to Stroke)
25. Chilos PM, Fischer L, Hirsch JH, et al: Observer variability in evaluating extracranial carotid artery disease (submitted to Stroke)
26. Comerata AJ, Cranley JJ, Cook SE: Real-time B-mode carotid imaging in diagnosis of cerebrovascular disease. Surgery 89:718, 1981
27. Breslau PJ, Fell G, Phillips DJ, et al: Evaluation of carotid bifurcation disease. The role of common carotid artery velocity patterns. Arch Surg 117:58, 1982
28. Heyman A, Wilkinson WE, Heyden S, et al: Risk of stroke in asymptomatic persons with cervical arterial bruits. N Engl J Med 302:838, 1980
29. David TE, Humphries AW, Young TR, et al: A correlation of neck bruits and arteriosclerotic carotid arteries. Arch Surg 107:729, 1973
30. Fell G, Breslau P, Knox RA, et al: Importance of noninvasive ultrasonic Doppler testing in the evaluation of patients with asymptomatic carotid bruits. Am Heart J 102:221, 1981
31. Breslau PJ, Fell G, Ivey TD, et al: Carotid arterial disease in patients undergoing coronary artery bypass operations. J Thor Cardiovasc Surg 82:765, 1981

32. Barnes RW, Marszalek PB: Asymptomatic carotid disease in the cardiovascular surgical patient: Is prophylactic endarterectomy necessary? Stroke 12:497, 1981
33. Turnipseed WD, Berkoff MA, Belzer FO: Postoperative stroke in cardiac and peripheral vascular disease. Ann Surg 192:365, 1980
34. Anderson CE, Collins GJ, Rich NM: Routine operative arteriography during carotid endarterectomy: A reassessment. Surgery 83:67, 1978
35. Barnes RW, Garrett WF: Intraoperative assessment of arterial reconstruction by Doppler ultrasound. Surg Gynecol Obstet 146:896, 1978
36. Zierler RE, Bandyk DF, Berni GA, et al: Intraoperative pulsed Doppler assessment of carotid endarterectomy. Ultrasound Med Bio (in press)
37. Stoney RJ, String TS: Recurrent carotid stenosis. Surgery 80:705, 1976
38. Cossman D, Callow AD, Stein A, et al: Early restenosis after carotid endarterectomy. Arch Surg 113:275, 1978
39. Hertzer NR, Martinez BD, Bevan EG: Recurrent stenosis after carotid endarterectomy. Surg Gynecol Obstet 149:360, 1979
40. French BN, Rewcastle NB: Recurrent stenosis at site of carotid endarterectomy. Stroke 8:597, 1977
41. Bodily KC, Zierler RE, Marinelli MR, et al: Flow disturbances following carotid endarterectomy. Surg Gynecol Obstet 151:77, 1980
42. Roederer GO, Langlois Y, Chan A, et al: Post-endarterectomy carotid ultrasonic duplex scanning: Concordance with contrast arteriography. Ultrasound Med Bio (in press)
43. Zierler RE, Bandyk DF, Thiele BL, et al: Carotid artery stenosis following endarterectomy. (manuscript in preparation)

Robert W. Hobson II
Silvia M. Berry
Thomas G. Lynch

11

Applications of B-Mode Ultrasonography and Ocular Pneumoplethysmography in the Diagnosis of Carotid Occlusive Disease

Atherosclerotic carotid occlusive disease is a three dimensional process that can be visualized angiographically in only two planes. Noninvasively, it may be characterized indirectly in terms of hemodynamic significance or directly, as a flow dependent or real-time image. Despite its biplanar character, arteriography is the current diagnostic standard, while the clinical role of noninvasive diagnostic testing remains controversial.

In our clinical practice, we have evaluated oculoplethysmography[1,2,3] and ocular pneumoplethysmography[3,4] as well as pulsed Doppler[1,2,3,5] and real-time B-mode imaging.[6,7,8] Subsequently, we have employed a combination of real-time B-mode ultrasonography and ocular pneumoplethysmography in the noninvasive diagnosis of carotid occlusive disease. This chapter reviews the development, technique, and accuracy of these 2 methods as well as the rationale for their combinate use.

REAL-TIME B-MODE ULTRASONOGRAPHY

Our clinical experience with real-time B-mode ultrasonography began in 1977 with the use of a prototype instrument developed by engineers at the New York Institute of Technology's Science and Technology Research Center in Dania, Florida.[6] This was a 6.0 MHz system, which provided gray-scale images of the cervical carotid arteries with lateral resolution of 0.5 mm at a fixed focal length of 2.5 cm. The transducer with its self-contained water bath (Fig. 11-1A), consisted of an emitting and receiving piezoelectric crystal with a

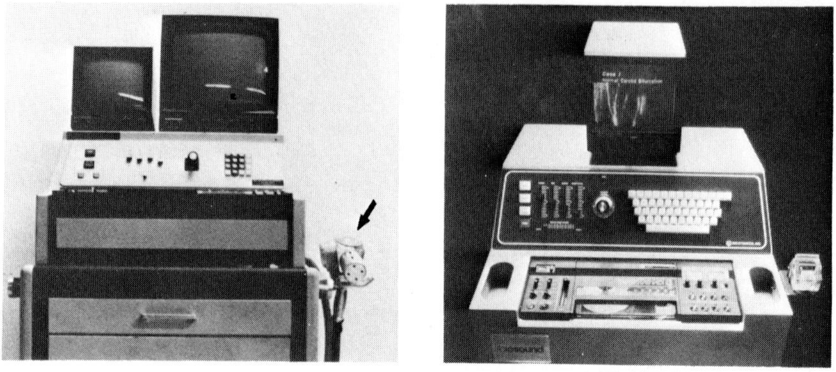

A B

Figure 11-1. The prototype unit (A) with its cumbersome transducer (arrow) is seen, while a smaller more manageable transducer (B) is currently available.

high speed mechanical deflecting system. Images were monitored for immediate evaluation, and videotapes were made for later analysis. In 1980, we began use of a modified system, which has since become available commercially.* This 8 MHz instrument has an improved transducer with a variable focal length of 1.0-3.0 cm, and a lateral resolution of 0.3 mm. A reduction in transducer size (Fig. 11-1B) also permits easier scanning. In addition, an 8 MHz pulsed Doppler circuit was added to the imaging system, thereby allowing the examiner to assess flow velocity characteristics as well as permitting the subsequent use of sound spectrum analysis. It is this combination of imaging and pulsed Doppler ultrasonography, or duplex capability, which has resulted in an improved diagnostic accuracy.

In an initial report,[7] we compared pulsed Doppler ultrasonic imaging with real-time B-mode ultrasonography. These data are presented in Table 11-1. Although both techniques were equally specific in the identification of normal carotid arteries, B-mode ultrasonography was more sensitive to stenotic lesions. Real-time ultrasonography was inaccurate, however, in the diagnosis of internal carotid occlusion. Data reported recently by Comerota and associates[9] have confirmed these conclusions. Since the problem of differentiation between high-grade stenosis and occlusion is important clinically, increased usage of the B-mode technique awaited availability of a pulsed Doppler circuit. With this technical modification, the predictive accuracy for carotid occlusion has increased (Table 11-2).

---

*Biosound®, Bio-Dynamics, Indianapolis, Indiana.

Table 11-1
Comparison of results with pulsed Doppler and B-mode echo arteriography in 43 patients (84 arteries).

	Pulsed Doppler*						B-mode†					
Arteriogram	Normal	<50%	>50%	Occlusion	Echo-free	Accuracy (%)	Normal	<50%	>50%	Occlusion	Shadows	Accuracy (%)
Normal (n = 37)	30	2	2	0	3	81	30	2	1	0	4	81
<50% (n = 18)	8	9	1	0	0	50	3	14	0	0	1	78
>50% (n = 12)	0	2	5	3	2	42	1	2	7	0	2	58
Occlusion (n = 17)	0	0	0	17	0	100	2	4	2	3	6	18

(Taken from Hobson RW, et al: Surgery 87:286, 1980.)
*False positive, six of 55, or 11%; false negative, four of 29, or 14%.
†False positive, six of 55, or 11%; false negative, 17 of 29, or 59%.

Table 11-2
Comparison of angiographically normal and occluded internal carotid arteries with real-time B-mode ultrasonography.

Angiogram	No. Images Correct	Accuracy
Normal (n = 44)	39	89%
Occluded (n = 6)	6	100%

Technical Considerations and Interpretation

Patients are examined in a supine position with the neck slightly extended and rotated away from the side of examination. The transducer is coupled to the skin with an acoustic gel and moved both anterior and posterior to the sternomastoid muscle from the level of the clavicle to the angle of the mandible. Two longitudinal scans are obtained in planes lateral and posterior to the carotid artery. The transducer is then rotated 180 degrees for cross-sectional visualization. Measurement of any reduction in luminal diameter is facilitated with the aid of 2 mm graticules.

The capabilities and limitations of real-time B-mode ultrasonography are best demonstrated by illustrative examples of the technique. Figure 11-2 is representative of a normal carotid bifurcation, seen in longitudinal and cross-sectional views. The examiner must be aware of adjacent anatomical structures as well as the orientation of the carotid artery relative to the transducer. In the longitudinal plane, the sternomastoid muscle and jugular vein are superficial to the artery. On cross-section, identification of the medially placed thyroid gland will facilitate identification of the internal and external carotid arteries.

Carotid visualization and interpretation are also dependent upon the relationship of the transducer to the carotid artery. When the transducer can be positioned so that the scanning plane includes the internal and external carotid arteries, an image (Fig. 11-2) demonstrating the bifurcation and its branches is obtained. In 70 percent of cases, however,[10] the probe must be moved laterally from the bifurcation to visualize the internal carotid artery or medially toward the thyroid gland to visualize the external carotid artery. The spatial relationship of the bifurcation to the external and internal carotid arteries is presented in Figure 11-3.

Evaluation of the Doppler signals which are recorded from the common, internal, and external carotid arteries is also an important part of the examination. The external carotid signal is biphasic with minimal diastolic flow secondary to a high resistance run-off. The internal carotid signal is monophasic and characterized by increased diastolic flow into the low resistance cerebral circulation. Common carotid flow has characteristics of

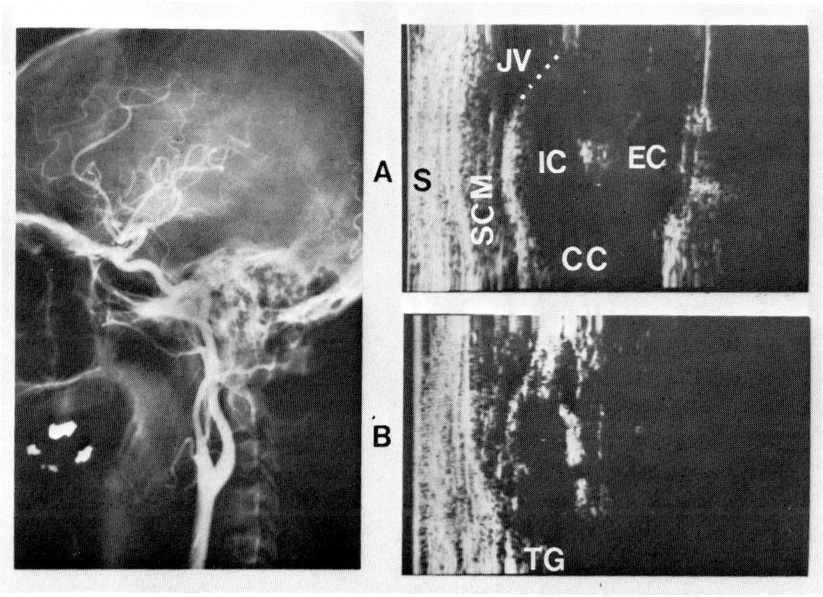

Figure 11-2. Normal contrast arteriogram (left) with corresponding longitudinal (A) and cross-sectional (B) images, skin(s), sternocleidomastoid muscle (scm), and jugular vein (JV) are seen anterior to the carotid artery. The common carotid (CC), internal carotid (IC), and external carotid (EC) arteries are demonstrated. Location of thyroid gland (TG) is indicated.

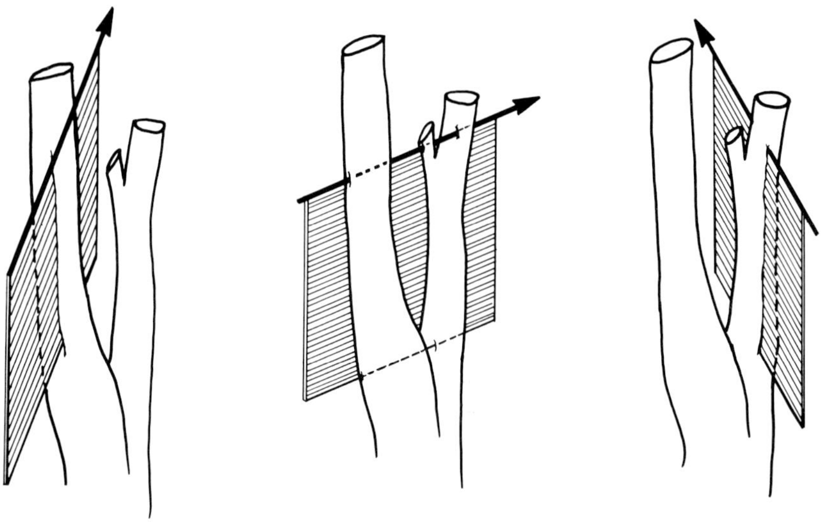

Figure 11-3. Spatial relationships are relevant to the appearance of real-time images. An artist's conception of various anatomical examples.

both, being biphasic in nature but with a greater diastolic component than the external carotid artery. A knowledge of these characteristics is valuable in the identification of the internal and external carotid arteries as well as confirmation of their patency.

Figures 11-4 and 11-5 illustrate characteristics of internal carotid occlusion. While the presence of intraluminal reflectivity (Fig. 11-4) and the absence of arterial pulsatility are consistent with internal carotid occlusion, a recent thrombosis (Fig. 11-5) may not be sufficiently organized to confirm the diagnosis without use of flow detecting pulsed Doppler circuitry.

Minimal atherosclerotic changes, occasionally not seen on contrast arteriograms, are demonstrated in Figures 11-6 and 11-7. The appearance of intimal thickening (Fig. 11-6) is the first ultrasonic evidence of early atherosclerotic change. Smaller ulcerative lesions (Fig. 11-7) can also be associated with normal contrast arteriography.

The identification of highly stenotic lesions may be complicated by the presence of calcification which results in "shadowing" (Fig. 11-8). Nonetheless, the technique is often of value in the diagnosis of moderate and severe stenosis (Fig. 11-9). The common carotid stenosis seen in Figure 11-9 demon-

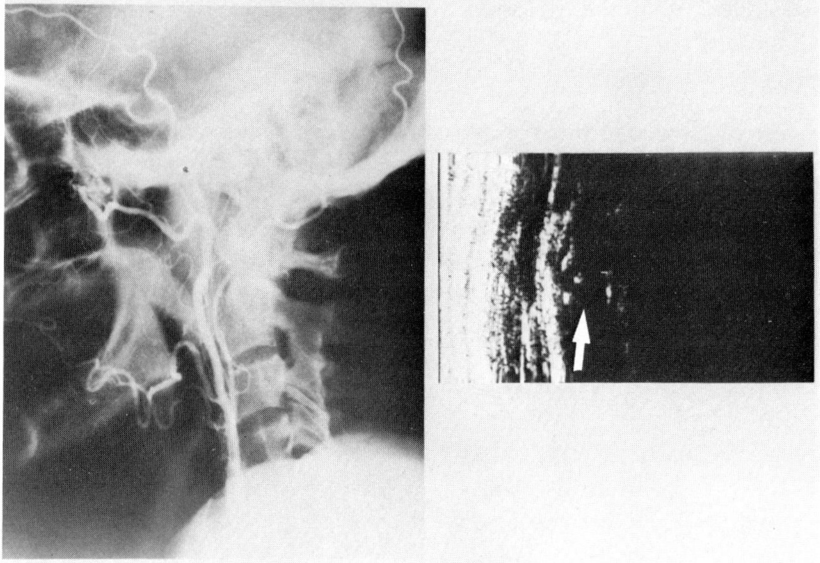

Figure 11-4. Contrast arteriogram (left) demonstrates occlusion of the internal carotid artery. Multiple reflective densities (arrow) within the proximal internal carotid artery of the corresponding image (right) suggested occlusion of the internal carotid artery.

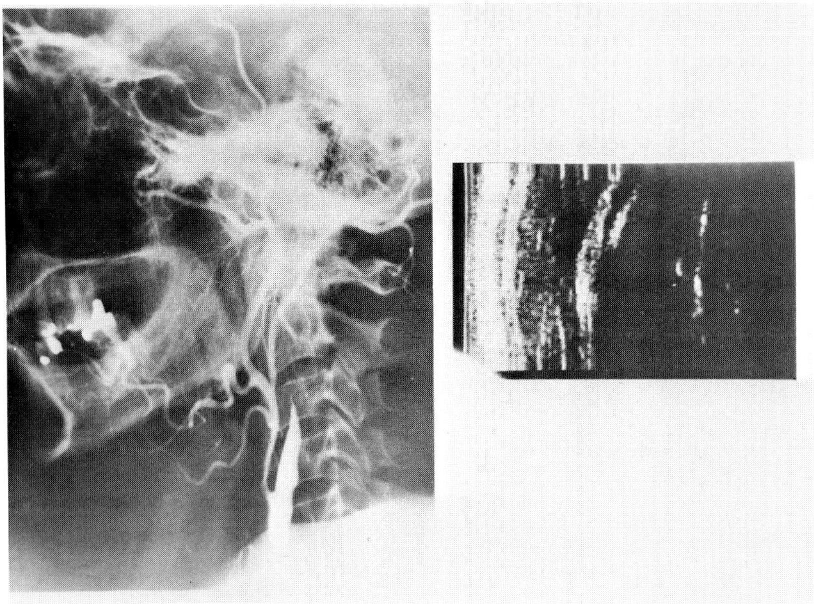

Figure 11-5. Contrast arteriogram (left) demonstrates an acutely occluded internal carotid artery. The ultrasonogram (right) suggested a patent internal carotid artery. However, the real-time display and pulsed Doppler ultrasound confirmed occlusion.

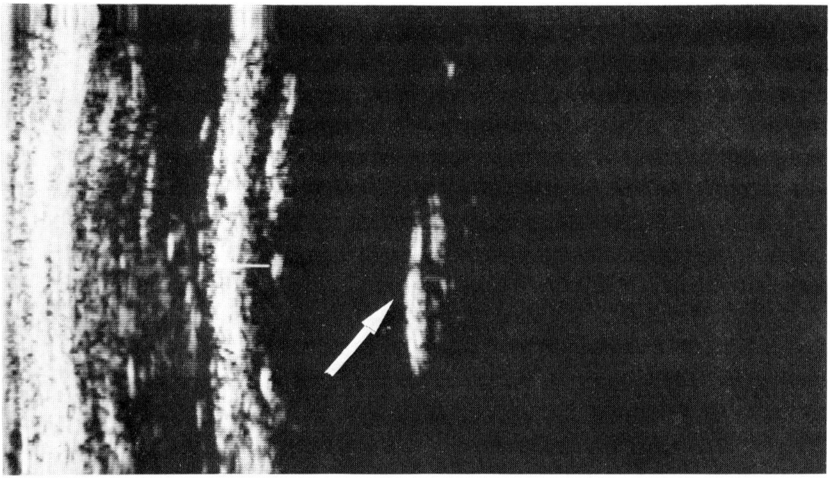

Figure 11-6. Image demonstrating intimal thickening (arrow) along the arterial wall (Lynch TG, et al: The role of real-time, B-mode ultrasonography and ocular pneumoplethysmography following carotid endarterectomy. Am Surg in press, 1982.)

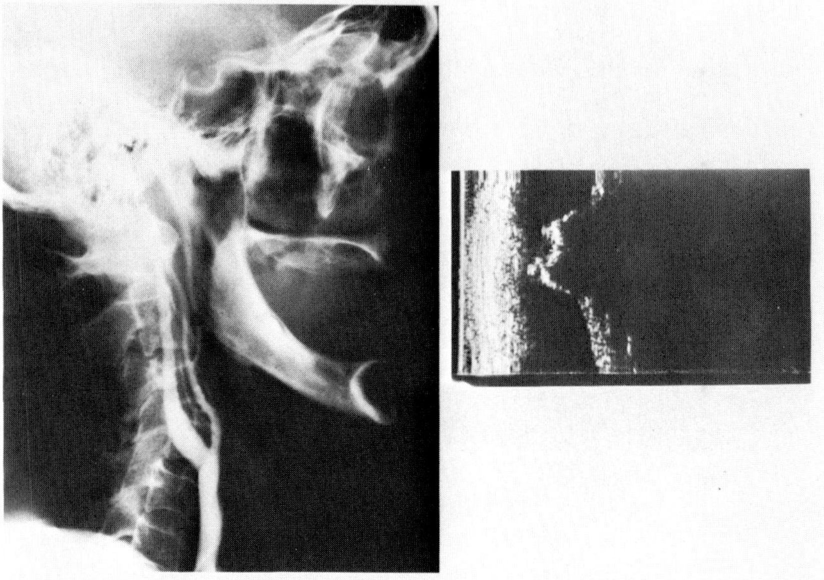

Figure 11-7. Normal contrast arteriogram (left) and accompanying scan (right) demonstrates an ulcerative lesion.

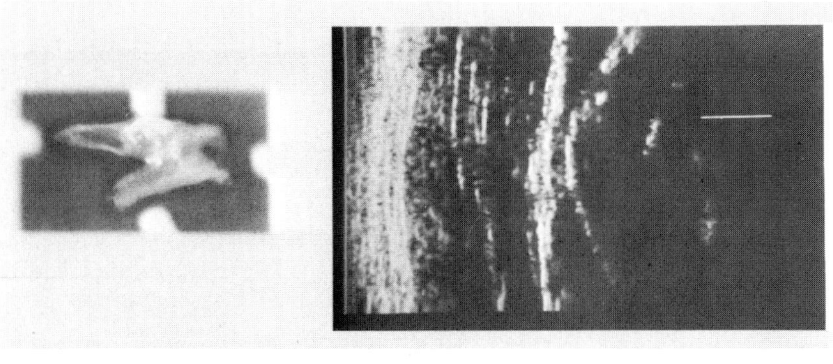

Figure 11-8. Image (right) of a 50 percent stenosis within the internal carotid artery. The marker demonstrates the area of "shadowing" caused by calcification. A roentgenogram (left) of the operative specimen confirmed the presence of calcium.

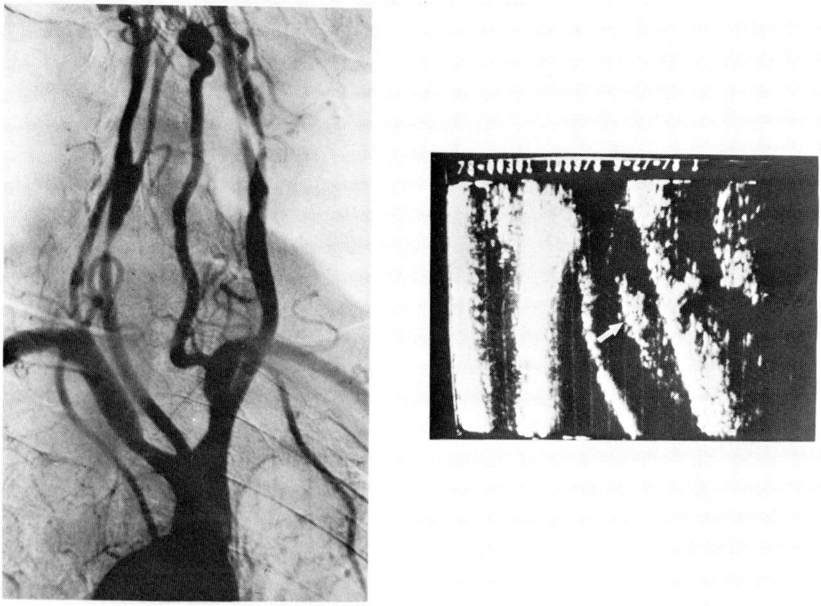

Figure 11-9. This arch arteriogram (left) demonstrates a significant common carotid stenosis proximal to the carotid bifurcation. The accompanying B-mode image (right) demonstrates the ultrasonic morphology of the plaque (arrow) within the common carotid artery (Modified from Hobson RW, et al: Comparison of pulsed-Doppler and real time echoarteriography for noninvasive imaging of the extracranial carotid arteries. Surgery 87:286, 1980.)

strates the relationship between the variable densities within an atherosclerotic plaque and the arterial wall.

OCULAR PNEUMOPLETHYSMOGRAPHY

The technique of ocular pneumoplethysmography (OPG-G) was described by Gee,[11] while the details of its use have been reported from this and other institutions.[3,8,12,13,14] It provides a simultaneous measurement of ophthalmic artery pressures and is a reflection of the internal carotid artery pressure. In the presence of a hemodynamically significant carotid obstruction (>50 percent of the arterial diameter) the ophthalmic artery pressure will be less than two-thirds of the brachial systolic pressure, and/or the difference between ophthalmic artery pressures will be 5 mm Hg or greater.

In comparison with the oculoplethysmographic technique (OPG-K) of Kartchner,[15] we have reported that ocular pneumoplethysmography is more sensitive to hemodynamically significant carotid occlusive disease.[3] Of 66 patients evaluated with both techniques, the sensitivity and specificity relative to hemodynamically significant disease were 98 percent and 92 percent, respectively, with the OPG-G and 70 percent and 83 percent, respectively, with the OPG-K. This difference in sensitivity was significant ($p < 0.05$).

Kartchner and co-workers,[15] in their original report, noted a sensitivity of 76 percent when the technique was used without carotid phonoangiography. Of their 24 false negative studies, 15 were associated with significant contralateral disease. Blackshear and co-workers[16] suggested that the bilateral presence of hemodynamically significant disease adversely affected the accuracy of the Kartchner technique. In our study,[3] 14 patients were identified with bilaterally significant lesions. The false negative results in this group of 28 arteries accounted for 59 percent of the false negative OPG-K examinations. Of the remaining false negative studies, three (18 percent) were associated with 50-70 percent stenosis, three (18 percent) with 71-99 percent stenosis, and one (6 percent) with occlusion. Using the OPG-G, there was only one false negative study (98 percent sensitivity) and this was in a patient with bilateral disease in whom a 50 percent stenosis was misdiagnosed.

In a subsequent series[4] from this institution, 147 patients (294 arteries) were evaluated with the OPG-G. There was a 24 percent incidence of false negative studies with 50-70 percent stenoses, a 15 percent incidence associated with 71-99 percent stenoses, and 6 percent incidence with carotid occlusion. In addition, the presence of bilateral disease was associated with 88 percent of the false negative studies in this larger series. Nonetheless, sensitivity to hemodynamically significant disease was an acceptable 85 percent.

Despite the diagnostic inaccuracies associated with bilaterally significant occlusive disease, we continue to prefer the OPG-G technique. Furthermore, time required for testing was significantly less with the OPG-G method as compared with the OPG-K.[3] The supine position used to perform the OPG-G testing also was more acceptable to our patients than the upright, forward sitting position required for the OPG-K technique. As a result, we use OPG-G as a primary screening tool to identify hemodynamically significant carotid occlusive disease.

DISCUSSION

We currently employ both ocular pneumoplethysmography and real-time B-mode ultrasonography in our noninvasive carotid evaluation. Ocular pneumoplethysmography has become our preferred screening technique for hemodynamically significant carotid occlusive disease in patients with asymptomatic carotid bruits, patients with symptoms of cerebrovascular insufficiency which are not characteristic of carotid circulation ischemia, in those patients with major risk factors associated with generalized atherosclerotic occlusive disease, and in those patients who are candidates for major vascular reconstructive procedures. We reviewed[13] the incidence of asymptomatic carotid stenosis at our institution in patients scheduled for general and vascular surgical procedures. The incidence of asymptomatic disease in the general surgical population over age 40 without evidence of vascular disease was only 0.5 percent and does not justify routine screening. The 10 percent incidence of disease among patients scheduled for vascular reconstruction emphasizes the potential need for preoperative screening in this population. Fifty percent of the patients with hemodynamically significant stenosis did not have carotid bruits, further emphasizing the need for preoperative evaluation.

We continue to recommend contrast arteriography in patients with lateralizing neurological symptoms. Under these circumstances, noninvasive testing is used for purposes of registration and baseline measurements. Ocular pneumoplethysmography permits the noninvasive measurement of ophthalmic artery back pressure yielding an index of cerebral collateral perfusion.[17,18] In selected patients, this can be helpful in planning the sequence of staged bilateral procedures, as well as the timing of carotid endarterectomy in high risk patients. Kremen and associates[19] have recently reported the value of preoperative and immediate postoperative ocular pneumoplethysmography to insure the adequacy of carotid endarterectomy. Their data suggest that 5 percent of carotid endarterectomies occlude in the perioperative period, frequently unassociated with neurological symptoms.

Unfortunately, the indirect noninvasive techniques such as ocular pneumoplethysmography cannot distinguish stenosis from occlusion and are not capable of identifying ulcerative lesions in the absence of significant stenosis. Real-time B-mode ultrasonography with its current duplex capability, however, distinguishes stenosis from occlusion with a demonstrated accuracy approaching 100 percent. In the asymptomatic patient or the individual with nonlateralizing symptomtology, documentation of carotid occlusion would in many instances obviate the need for contrast arteriography. The identification of hemodynamically insignificant disease including ulcerative plaques also underscores the value of B-mode ultrasonography. It has the capability of accurately identifying lesser stenoses which can be important clinically in the etiology of atheroembolic phenomena. Stenoses of less than 50 percent were identified accurately in 78 percent of cases.[7]

Of additional significance is the application of B-mode ultrasonography during the operative and postoperative management of vascular surgical cases. Sigel and colleagues[20] have recommended operative use of B-mode imaging to evaluate the adequacy of carotid endarterectomy and to assess the presence of unsuspected technical errors. Lynch and associates[8] have utilized B-mode imaging and ocular pneumoplethysmography in a clinical follow-up of 41 patients (54 arteries) following carotid endarterectomy. Recurrent stenosis was observed in three (6 percent), postoperative occlusion in three (6 percent), and external carotid occlusion in one patient resulting in lateralizing neurological symptoms secondary to atheroembolism.

Only two of these 7 patients were symptomatic and three of the seven had hemodynamically insignificant stenoses. B-mode ultrasonography also permitted the identification of several characteristic postoperative findings. An intimal shelf was observed frequently at the proximal limit of the endarterectomy. Thickening of the arterial wall was observed in 74 percent of cases and calcifications were observed in the area of endarterectomy in 45 percent.

The combinate use of these noninvasive techniques is important in our evaluation of carotid occlusive disease. In the asymptomatic patient, the ocular pneumoplethysmograph provides the means with which to screen for hemodynamically significant carotid occlusive disease. When used in combination with real-time B-mode ultrasonography, it has the potential to noninvasively distinguish carotid stenosis from occlusion, thereby obviating the need for angiography in these asymptomatic patients. Preoperative B-mode ultrasonography in the symptomatic individual without evidence of hemodynamically significant disease may provide the physician with evidence of minimal and/or ulcerative disease prior to angiography. Postoperatively, we have found this combination of noninvasive studies to be valuable in assessing the immediate and continued patency of the carotid endarterectomy. The addition of real-time B-mode ultrasonography has been useful in the identification of early hemodynamically insignificant recurrence and the evaluation of patients with associated intracranial pathology resulting in a positive oculoplethysmographic study.

REFERENCES

1. Ghosh A, Abou-Samra S, Berry SM, et al: Evaluation of extracranial carotid occlusive disease with directional Doppler, fluid-filled oculoplethysmography, carotid phonoangiography and pulsed Doppler ultrasonic imaging. Current Surgery 37:129, 1980
2. Hobson RW, Berry SM, Jamil Z., et al: Oculoplethysmography and pulsed Doppler ultrasonic imaging in the diagnosis of carotid arterial disease. Surg Gyn & Obstet 152:433, 1981
3. Hobson RW, Berry SM, Lynch TG, et al: Prospective comparison of ultrasonic imaging and two oculoplethysmographic techniques in carotid occlusive disease. (submitted to Arch Surg, 1982)
4. Lynch TG, Berry SM, Hobson RW: (unpublished data)
5. Berry SM, O'Donnell JA, Hobson RW: Capabilities and limitations of pulsed Doppler ultrasonography in carotid imaging. J Clinical Ultrasound 8:405, 1980
6. Hobson RW, Lipp JA, O'Donnell JA: Real-time ultrasonic arteriography of the extracranial carotid artery, in Dietrich EB (ed): Noninvasive Cardiovascular Diagnosis: Current Concepts. Baltimore, University Park Press, 1978

7. Hobson RW, Berry SM, Katocs AS, et al: Comparison of pulsed Doppler and real-time B-mode echo arteriography for noninvasive imaging of the extracranial carotid arteries. Surgery 87:286, 1980
8. Lynch TG, Hobson RW, Berry SM: The role of real-time B-mode ultrasonography and ocular pneumoplethysmography following carotid endarterectomy. Am Surg (in press, 1982)
9. Comerota AJ, Cranley JJ, Cook SE: Real-time B-mode carotid imaging in the diagnosis of cerebrovascular disease. Surgery 98:718, 1981
10. Prendes JL, McKinney WM, Buonanno FS, et al: Anatomic variations of the carotid bifurcation affecting Doppler scan interpretation. J Clinical Ultrasound 8:147, 1980
11. Gee W, Oller DW, Wylie EJ: Non-invasive diagnosis of carotid occlusion by ocular pneumoplethysmography. Stroke 7:18, 1976
12. Lynch TG, Wright CB, Miller EV, et al: Evaluation of cerebrovascular Doppler examination and oculopneumoplethysmography in a clinical perspective. Stroke 12:325, 1981
13. Jain KM, Hobson RW, Jamil Z, et al: Clinical screening of preoperative patients for carotid occlusive disease by oculoplethysmography. Am Surg 46:679, 1980
14. McDonald PT, Rich NM, Collins GJ, et al: Doppler cerebrovascular examination, oculoplethysmography, and oculopneumoplethysmography. Use in detection of carotid disease: A prospective study. Arch Surg 113:1341, 1978
15. Kartchner MM, McRae LP, Morrison FD: Non-invasive detection and evaluation of carotid occlusive disease. Arch Surg 106:528, 1973
16. Blackshear WM, Thiele BL, Harley JD, et al: A prospective evaluation of oculoplethysmography and CPA. Surg Gyn & Obstet 148:201, 1979
17. Baker JD, Barker WF, Machleder HI: Evaluation of extracranial cerebrovascular disease with ocular pneumoplethysmography. Am J Surg 136:206, 1978
18. Gee W, Mehigan JT, Wylie EJ: Measurement of collateral hemispheric blood pressure by ocular pneumoplethysmography. Am J Surg 130:121, 1965
19. Kremen JE, Gee W, Kaupp HA, et al: Restenosis or occlusion after carotid endarterectomy: A survey with ocular pneumoplethysmography. Arch Surg 114:608, 1979
20. Sigel B, Coelho JCU, Flanigan DP, et al: Detection of vascular defects during operation by imaging ultrasound. Am Surg (in press, 1982)

William H. Pearce Donna Blackburn
Jean-Baptiste Ricco Richard G. Considine
James S.T. Yao

12

Direct and Indirect Tests for Carotid Artery Lesions

During the last decade, there has been a steady growth in the development of noninvasive tests in the detection of extracranial carotid artery stenosis. The development is based on the fact that, no matter how small the risk of cerebral arteriography, it still carries discomfort and the possibility of a stroke. Further, it is hoped that an accurate noninvasive test, if available, would be useful for screening or epidemiology studies. For vascular surgeons, such a test would be helpful to determine the significance of a carotid bruit and, more importantly, to assess the result of carotid endarterectomy objectively.

Noninvasive methods for evaluation of carotid artery disease have been designated as either indirect or direct. The indirect methods rely on hemodynamic alterations in the orbital and supraorbital circulation. It is generally acknowledged that the ophthalmic artery is the terminal branch of the internal carotid artery, and any changes in the flow in this artery would reflect disease in the carotid artery. Indirect tests, however, require a significant stenosis of the internal carotid artery (>50 percent) to detect hemodynamic changes. Any lesser degree of stenosis will have no effect on the distal circulation. Like the ankle/brachial index in the lower extremity, indirect tests are not specific to the carotid artery bifurcation, but may reflect any stenotic lesion from the aortic valve to the terminal branches of the ophthalmic artery. Lastly, cross-over circulation from the circle of Willis may compensate completely for an occluded internal carotid artery.

The direct tests examine the carotid artery bifurcation and accessible portions of the extracranial vessels transcutaneously by ultrasound. The information may be anatomic or physiologic, or both. Since these tests do not depend upon hemodynamic alterations in the distal vascular bed, the methods

Table 12-1
Direct and Indirect Tests for Carotid Artery Stenosis

I. Indirect Tests
  A. Superficial orbital circulation
    1. Thermography
    2. Forehead skin blood pressure
    3. Supraorbital or periorbital Doppler examination
    4. Supraorbital plethysmography
  B. Deep orbital circulation
    1. Ophthalmodynamometry (ODM)
    2. Oculoplethysmography (OPG)

II. Direct Tests
  A. Real-time B-mode scan
  B. Duplex scan and frequency spectral analysis
  C. Flow imaging (ultrasonic arteriography)
    1. Continuous-wave Doppler
    2. Pulsed Doppler
  D. Frequency analysis
    1. Spectral analysis (sonogram)
    2. Phonoangiography
  E. Flow velocity waveform analysis
  F. Flow velocity profiles

can detect a broad spectrum of milder changes in the artery. Direct tests, however, will not detect carotid siphon or ophthalmic artery stenosis, nor will they determine the state of collateral circulation.

Table 12-1 outlines the direct and indirect tests currently available for diagnostic use. The purpose of this chapter is to review each of these testing techniques and their application in clinical practice.

INDIRECT TESTS

Superficial Orbital Circulation

Thermography

Both the supraorbital and frontal arteries, distal branches of the ophthalmic artery which exit from each orbit, supply the skin over each inferior medial quadrant of the forehead. This region receives no contribution of blood flow from the external carotid artery. Such a discrete skin area, therefore, is useful for skin temperature determination. In 1966, Wood and Hull[1] first described asymmetrical supraorbital skin temperatures in a patient with internal carotid artery occlusion. With a cutaneous thermistor, Austin and Sajid[2] were able to identify correctly internal carotid artery occlusions in 10 patients. Later, Shapiro found that, with varying degrees of stenosis, the sensitivity of the skin temperature examination was only 75 percent.[3] In the late 1960s, thermography using the infrared principle was introduced to display graphically the skin temperature in humans. Using this technique, Capistrant and Gumnit[4] reported a sensitivity of 57 percent in the detection of internal carotid artery stenosis. The sensitivity increased to 83 percent if temporal artery compression was added as a diagnostic maneuver. Even with temporal artery compression, however, the test was insensitive to lesser degrees of stenosis, and accuracy was only 36 percent. Bilateral occlusions caused diagnostic problems, and only two-thirds of patients with bilateral disease were detected with this technique. Because of the low sensitivity of the test and the cumbersome instrumentation, thermography has now vanished from the diagnostic laboratory for detection of carotid artery stenosis.

Nevertheless, measurement of skin temperature of the forehead remains a simple screening technique. Recently, Hofferberth and his co-workers[5] have introduced the plate thermography technique. This technique uses a foil coated with specific cholesterol esters to indicate differences in temperature by changes in color. The foil is applied to the forehead and the skin temperature measured is related to the perfusion supplying the skin of the forehead. In normal individuals, both sides are equal in color. In the presence of occlusion or stenosis, a different color is displayed on the corresponding side. The results obtained by this technique were found to be comparable to periorbital Doppler examination.[5]

Forehead Skin Blood Pressure

Using a Xenon technique, Nielsen et al. have succeeded in recording the skin blood pressure in the forehead and have related its changes to carotid artery occlusion. Similar to other indirect tests to assess superficial circulation of the orbit, the technique lacks sensitivity and is of limited use in bilateral occlusive disease.

Supraorbital or Periorbital Doppler Examination (Doppler Ultrasonography)

The technique of supraorbital Doppler examination was first introduced by Brockenbrough.[7] Since then, many modifications of the technique have been suggested. These include compression of the facial artery and the common carotid artery,[8] directional flow detection,[9] and supraorbital blood pressure measurements.[10] The technique is simple in concept but requires considerable skill to perform. Also, a positive result is obtained only when a stenosis is hemodynamically significant, or when there is total occlusion. The technique is, however, superior to auscultation of the carotid artery by stethoscope alone, and it is of particular value in patients who do not have a carotid bruit.[11] The diagnostic accuracy of the technique has been documented by many investigators.[12-19] The technique, when compared to oculoplethysmography, is less accurate.[20-22] Since the introduction of oculoplethysmography, we no longer employ supraorbital Doppler examination in our diagnostic laboratory, and others have also abandoned the technique in favor of other testing methods.[23]

Supraorbital Photoplethysmography

The simple technique to record flow dynamics in the frontal and supraorbital arteries was first described by Barnes and his colleagues.[24,25] An infrared photosensor is used to detect pulse in the arteries in the forehead and observe its changes after compression maneuvers (facial, carotid, and temporal arteries). The technique is similar in principle to that of Doppler supraorbital flow detection, except that a photosensor is used. The main advantage of the technique is simplicity of performance, and exact positioning of the sensor is less critical than with the supraorbital Doppler examination. The technique, however, is less accurate when compared to oculoplethysmography and supraorbital Doppler examination,[20-23] and it is seldom used in vascular laboratories.

In addition to its diagnostic value, supraorbital photoplethysmography has been found to be a useful technique to monitor the patency of a shunt during carotid endarterectomy.[26]

Deep Orbital Circulation

Assessment of orbital pulse or pressure by direct examination of the eye globe represents an indirect technique based on the status of the deep orbital circulation. In this examination, the ophthalmic artery, the terminal branch of the internal carotid artery, is examined. Ophthalmodynamometry and oculoplethysmography are the tests most commonly used. We have no experience with ophthalmic tonometry and, hence, will not discuss this technique here.

Ophthalmodynamometry (ODM)

This time-honored technique, first described by Bailliart in 1917,[27] is somewhat like oscillography to peripheral vascular surgeons, and has rapidly disappeared from the noninvasive vascular laboratory. The technique is found mostly in the hands of neuro-ophthalmologists. In principle, the procedure is designed to detect flow in the internal carotid artery by measuring the pressure indirectly in the ophthalmic artery.

Two types of ophthalmodynamometry are available: the compression type and the suction type. Both types require the use of medication to dilate the pupil for examination. The compression type requires two persons to perform the test, the fundus being examined by one observer while the other applies the instrument to the sclera and records results. Both diastolic and systolic values are recorded.

Suction ophthalmodynamometry uses the identical technical approach of the compression type, except that application of pressure to the eye is delivered using a vacuum scleral suction cup, and only one person is needed to perform the test. The endpoint of the pressure is determined by the return of pulsation in the fundus arteries, while the suction cup is deflated. The test is simple to perform but it is not reliable nor reproducible. When correlated with arteriography, the sensitivity in detection of stenoses greater than 50 percent ranged from 70 to 80 percent, with a high false-negative rate of 20 to 30 percent.[28,29] The technique is useful in total occlusion of the internal carotid artery.[30] Nearly one-half of the patients with bilateral disease will have a negative test. Further, the test is not applicable in patients with glaucoma or other eye diseases. The technique, therefore, is not widely used. Ophthalmodynamometry, however, did emphasize the importance of ocular circulation in carotid artery disease and was the forerunner of oculoplethysmography.

Oculoplethysmography

In principle, oculoplethysmography is similar to ophthalmodynamometry, except that the endpoint of measurement is determined by a more sophisticated instrument and not by human eyes. The technique was first introduced by Brockenbrough in 1967.[31] Currently, two types of oculoplethysmography are available, the pulse-delay technique popularized by Kartchner, McRae, and Morrison[32] and the pressure technique introduced by Gee, Oller, and Wylie,[33] better known as oculopneumoplethysmography. Both techniques involve orbital volume changes with each cardiac cycle. The pulse-delay technique measures pulse arrival in the ophthalmic vessels and compares this to the pulse arrival in the ear. A delay of eye pulse arrival in reference to the ear is considered diagnostic for carotid artery stenosis. This delay may be expressed graphically by the fluid-filled oculoplethysmograph, or in digital display of millisecond delay by an air-filled plethysmograph.[34]

Since the introduction of this instrument, numerous investigators have reported the value of the technique.[23,32,34,35,36,37,38] With either device, the sensitivity for significant stenosis is from 61 to 73 percent, with a specificity of 90 to 97 percent. The OPG will detect 75 to 87 percent of total occlusions. A major failure of this test is in the detection of equal degrees of bilateral stenosis. In view of the common ocurrence of bilateral carotid artery stenosis, Blackshear and his colleagues have abandoned the technique as a routine laboratory test.[37]

Instead of measuring pulse arrival delays, ophthalmic artery pressure can be determined by applying suction to the sclera to a point at which the pulse volume waveform disappears. As the suction is released, the reappearance of the signal indicates the ophthalmic artery pressure, and this technique, pioneered by Gee,[33] is another form of oculoplethysmography. As with the pulse-delay technique, the sensitivity of this type of OPG is high for stenosis greater than 60 percent, and it is insensitive to lesser degrees of stenosis. The technique is not useful in hypertensive patients. Although higher suction apparatus is available to overcome this shortcoming, it is doubtful that the new instrument would make any difference. Also, bilateral, equal stenoses may cause diagnostic problems.

The Gee-OPG measures pressure, and such a finding helps to determine the adequacy of collateral circulation by compression of the ipsilateral common carotid artery. A normal OPG-Gee test, however, is no assurance of normal carotid anatomy. Nevertheless, Busuttil and his colleagues have demonstrated that patients with hemodynamically significant stenosis determined by OPG-Gee have a greater risk of cerebrovascular death, stroke, or TIA when treated nonoperatively than do patients treated with surgery.[40]

Regardless of the type of oculoplethysmograph used, this indirect technique suffers from the same limitations as ophthalmodynamometry, in that a high-grade stenosis is needed to produce predictive results. A normal test does not rule out the presence of carotid artery stenosis. The oculoplethysmograph, when compared with direct carotid tests, is definitely inferior, with high false-negative rates of 40 to 54 percent reported by Keagy et al.[41] and Cardullo et al.[42]

DIRECT TESTS

Direct tests consist of various imaging techniques and frequency analysis of carotid bruits. These two techniques are often used in combination. Imaging techniques currently available are the pulsed or continuous-wave Doppler to image flow within the artery, or anatomical display of the lumen by B-mode ultrasound scan.

Real-time B-mode Scan or Duplex Scan

This technique represents a new generation in ultrasonic imaging systems and offers promise in refinement of diagnostic accuracy.[43] The details of the scan are well-described in Chapter 11 (Hobson, et al.) and in Chapter 12 (Zierler, Roederer and Strandness) and will not be discussed here. Currently, pulsed Doppler sound signal analysis is added to the B-mode scan in an attempt to provide hemodynamic information, especially in differentiation between high-grade stenosis and total occlusion. In an analysis of 584 arteriograms, Cranley[23] concluded that the major value of this technique is its sensitivity in normal or nearly normal vessels. B-mode scan is also able to detect small ulcerating plaques, a feature not provided by flow imaging techniques. The diagnostic accuracy of B-mode scan reported by Cranley is shown in Table 12-2.

Table 12-2
B-mode Scanning Correlated with 584 Arteriograms Reported by Cranley[23]

	Numbers	(%)
Sensitivity		
40%–60% stenosis	63/84	(75)
70%–100% stenosis	57/92	(62)
Positive predictive value > 40% stenosis	120/175	(68)
Specificity		
0%–39% stenosis	353/408	(87)
Negative predictive value	353/409	(86)

Imaging of Flow by Pulsed Doppler or Continuous-Wave Doppler

Imaging of arterial flow by the pulsed Doppler was first introduced by Hokanson and associates in 1971.[44] With the aid of a computer, Sumner et al.[45] have upgraded the technique to provide bi-plane projections. This technique of computer-assisted imaging is described in detail by Sumner and his co-workers in Chapter 13.

Instead of the pulsed Doppler, other investigators, including Spencer et al.[46] and White,[47] have introduced continuous-wave Doppler imaging. In the technique reported by Reid and Spencer, spectral frequency analysis was also used to add diagnostic value. The continuous-wave Doppler technique of White uses a color-coded system to provide frequency information in relation to velocity. Both systems enjoy a respectable diagnostic accuracy.

Frequency Spectral Analysis of Carotid Bruits

Phonoangiography. Two techniques are currently available to analyze carotid bruits. Phonoangiography used in combination with oculoplethysmography, developed by Kartchner, McRae and Morrison[32] displays the audio signal as intensity versus time. The spectral phonoangiograph, a more sophisticated technique, was first introduced by Lees and Dewey,[48] and analyzes the bruit as intensity versus frequency.

The use of Kartchner/McRae phonoangiography is not reliable and, in our experience, it is accurate in only 50 percent of the cases. Cardullo et al.[42] reported a sensitivity of 82 percent for significant carotid stenosis but an accuracy of only 17 percent when total occlusion was present. For stenosis less than 50 percent, Kempczinski was unable to detect 40 percent of the cases.[49] The technique is not diagnostic in transmitted bruit, and external carotid artery stenosis may be confused with internal carotid artery stenosis. Because of these problems, we no longer employ phonoangiography as a diagnostic test in our laboratory.

The spectral phonoangiograph has now been refined with the introduction of a microprocessor.[50,51] This technique is designed to analyze bruit against the residual lumen diameter of a stenosed artery. By calculating the "breakpoint" frequency, Kistler and his colleagues have been able to extrapolate the diameter of the residual lumen. In 31 of 33 cases studied, the spectral phonoangiogram predicted the residual lumen diameter to within 0.5 mm of the measured value. The technique, however, is not without problems. First, a low-intensity bruit may be too low to give an accurate spectrum for analysis. Second, the technique depends on the relationship of peak systolic linear flow velocity in the carotid artery, which may be influenced by blood pressure, heart rate, and partial pressures of carbon dioxide. Finally, external carotid artery stenosis may mimic the findings in internal carotid lesions.

Frequency Spectral Analysis. Frequency spectral analysis is now a popular technique, and it is often used in combination with B-mode scanning or ultrasonic arteriography. The use of B-mode scanning or ultrasonic arteriography allows the examiner to interrogate the flow velocity from a definitive area or an area where disease is suspected. The technique of frequency spectral analysis is described in the chapter by Zierler et al. and, hence, will not be discussed here.

Although frequency spectral analysis provides an objective technique to interpret disturbed flow, the use of audible signals, when correlated with scan and imaging techniques by a skilled technician, is the single most reliable noninvasive technique to detect carotid stenosis. Barnes and his colleagues[52] have emphasized the importance of audible interpretation of carotid Doppler signals. In their study, the sensitivity in detecting severe (≥50 percent or greater) stenosis or occlusion was 92 percent. Further, the audible signal is helpful when a calcified arterial wall is present. Because of calcification, imaging may show no graphic display, and the presence of audible signals helps in interpretation of this finding.

Flow Velocity Waveform Analysis. Pulse waveforms recorded from the common carotid artery by the pulsed Doppler or continuous-wave Doppler, when subjected to analysis, may yield diagnostic information. The waveform may be used for spectral frequency analysis, as described in Chapter 10, or it may be analyzed by resistance index (RI), as suggested by Pourcelot,[53] or multidiscriminant analysis, as proposed by Rutherford et al.[54] Also, the use of the pulsed Doppler may allow the determination of blood velocity and volume flow in the carotid artery.

The resistance index is defined as the relationship between the peak systolic flow velocity level and the diastolic flow velocity level; this is then calculated by dividing the difference between peak systolic and diastolic levels by the peak systolic level. In normal individuals, the resistance index ranges from 0.55 to 0.75. If the ratio is greater than 0.9, it is very likely that a high-grade stenosis or occlusion is present. The calculation of the resistance index in the common carotid artery, when combined with the supraorbital resistance index and the temporal artery occlusion test, gives the best sensitivity and specificity for detection of both severe and minor carotid bifurcation disease.[55]

Multidiscriminant analysis, described by Rutherford and associates, involves the use of a computer to perform nine-dimensional analysis of the waveform. In 75 patients studied, the accuracy rate in separating normal, stenosed, and occluded carotid arteries was 100 percent. The sensitivity in distinguishing critical from non-critical stenosis was 82 percent.

With the pulsed Doppler technique, it is possible to calculate volume flow from velocity and diameter determined by the Doppler echo-tracking technique.[56] In 50 normal common carotid arteries, the mean volume was found by Fitzgerald, O'Shaughnessy, and Keaveny[56] to be 536 ± 104 cm^3min^{-1}, with a range of 326 to 755 cm^3min^{-1}. In patients with carotid artery disease, the mean volume was 324 ± 139 cm^3min^{-1}, with a range of 61 to 601 cm^3min^{-1}. Of interest is the ability of the technique to determine the hemodynamic significance of a lesion when a contralateral lesion co-exists. Also, in unilateral lesions, high flow through the contralateral artery is often observed, and this finding suggests the presence of a significant lesion. The technique offers new supplementary information in the evaluation of arteriographically demonstrated stenotic lesions.

Frequency Velocity Profiles. It is generally known that flow through an artery is always streamlined in laminar profile and that the presence of an atherosclerotic plaque may cause a disturbed flow profile or, in severe stenosis, turbulence. Despite this vital physiologic information, the use of the flow profile in clinical practice was not reported until the introduction of the pulsed Doppler to record velocity profiles transcutaneously. The technique was introduced by Peronneau et al.[57] and subsequently, Keller and his associates[58] applied it to humans in the detection of carotid artery stenosis. They used a 14-channel pulsed Doppler instrument, and the Doppler-shift frequency was calculated simultaneously for 14 target streamlines. The technique can also estimate blood flow volume in ml per minute. Measurements can be performed with an accuracy of about ±20 percent under clinical conditions. In healthy subjects, the common carotid artery flow was found to be 300 to 480 ml/min; whereas, in carotid artery stenosis, the flow value was often less than 180 ml/min.

COMBINED TESTING TECHNIQUES

Recognizing that no single diagnostic test is totally accurate, some investigators have advocated the use of two or more tests to improve diagnostic accuracy.[42,43,55,59,60,61] If two or more tests measure the same physical parameter, then adding one test to another will not increase the overall accuracy. On the other hand, if two or more tests are totally independent, such as an indirect and a direct test, then combining these two could enhance diagnostic accuracy. Combination of more than three tests is not cost-effective, and it may cause a problem in deciding which test results to rely upon. If multiple tests are used, Sumner[62] has suggested that the overall result be considered positive if any one test is positive and negative only if all tests are negative. Such an approach would increase sensitivity at the expense of specificity but probably is an acceptable compromise when the population being studied has a high incidence of disease. Multiple tests also are subject to biased opinions and often, the result of one test will influence the reading of another. Inevitably, the interpreter of the tests would choose one test over the other, rendering subjective rather than objective reporting of the results. In a strict statistical sense, multiple tests are difficult to interpret and probably are not scientific. Nevertheless, combination of two tests based on different principles appears to be a compromise approach to increase diagnostic accuracy.

THE NORTHWESTERN UNIVERSITY EXPERIENCE

Since the establishment of a vascular laboratory at Northwestern University Medical Center, oculoplethysmography of the Kartchner-McRae type has been used as a diagnostic test for carotid disease. Our early publications suggested that the technique is accurate when stenosis exceeds 75 percent. In stenosis less than 50 percent, there was a high false-negative rate, both in unilateral and in bilateral lesions.[63] In bilateral disease, the test could be normal because of balanced lesions. Also, we found that phonoangiography is useless and adds no supplementary information to oculoplethysmography.

Because oculoplethysmography is an indirect test, we decided to use a direct test to improve the diagnostic ability in our laboratory. The Hokanson unit, modified by Sumner by means of a computer, together with sound interpretation by the technician, is now an integral part of our carotid artery examination. In order to evaluate the results of the direct and indirect tests, 46 patients who had oculoplethysmography, ultrasonic arteriography, and sound analysis were evaluated. All these patients also underwent arteriography. Ninety-one arteriograms were considered to be of good quality for measurement of the degree of stenosis. The technique for determination of the degree of stenosis has been described previously.[64] Positive and negative results of each test were analyzed against arteriographic evidence of stenosis greater than 50 percent, or less than 50 percent, and subjected to statistical analysis by the method of Griner et al.[65] Tables 12-3, 12-4, and 12-5

Table 12-3
Analysis of OPG/Kartchner versus Arteriographic Findings (N = 91)

	Arteriographic Findings	
	Stenosis >50%	Normal or Stenosis <50%
OPG +	20	10
OPG –	16	45
Sensitivity	55%	
Specificity	82%	
False-negative	44%	
False-positive	18%	
Positive predictive value*	66%	
Negative predictive value†	74%	

*Probability that the disease is present when the test is positive
†Probability that the disease is not present when the test is negative

demonstrate the results of these three tests, respectively. Table 12-6 summarizes the results of combined scan and audible interpretation.

Oculoplethysmography, as suspected, had a high false-negative rate of 44 percent, with a sensitivity of 55 percent. The result is similar to that reported by others.[37,41,42] In contrast, the false-negative rate by scan and sound analysis was ten percent and six percent, respectively. The sensitivity of the Hokanson scan and sound analysis of 94 percent was much better than that of oculoplethysmography. The combination of ultrasonic imaging and audible sound interpretation by the technician appears to offer the best diagnostic information.

Table 12-4
Analysis of Ultrasonic Arteriography (Hokanson Scan) versus Arteriography (N = 61)

	Arteriographic Findings	
	Stenosis > 50%	Normal or Stenosis <50%
Ultrasonic Arteriography +	26	7
Ultrasonic Arteriography –	3	25
Sensitivity	90%	
Specificity	78%	
False-negative	10%	
False-positive	21%	
Positive predictive value	79%	
Negative predictive value	89%	

Table 12-5
Analysis of Sound Interpretation versus Arteriography (N = 73)

	Arteriographic Findings	
	Stenosis >50%	Normal or Stenosis <50%
Sound interpretation +	30	12
Sound interpretation −	2	29
Sensitivity	94 %	
Specificity	71 %	
False-negative	6 %	
False-positive	2.9%	
Positive predictive value	71 %	
Negative predictive value	93 %	

COMMENTS

The proliferation of noninvasive tests for carotid artery disease requires clarification on the usefulness of each technique. In the 1970s, indirect testing was popular, especially oculoplethysmography. Our experience, as well as that of others, has suggested that this type of indirect test is far from ideal.[37,41] As demonstrated in our analysis, oculoplethysmography has a high false-negative rate and low sensitivity. Because of this, Keagy et al.[41] and Blackshear et al.[37] have abandoned this technique in their laboratories. In addition to the ability to detect siphon (intracranial) stenosis, the indirect test is simple to use. Unfortunately, simplicity does not substitute for accuracy,

Table 12-6
Analysis of Combined Ultrasonic Arteriography and Audible Sound Interpretation versus Arteriography (N = 73)

	Arteriographic Findings	
	Stenosis >50%	Normal or Stenosis <50%
Combined Test +	33	9
Combined Test −	2	29
Sensitivity	94%	
Specificity	76%	
False-negative	6%	
False-positive	24%	
Positive predictive value	79%	
Negative predictive value	94%	

and all indirect tests, though easy to use, are inaccurate unless the stenotic lesion exceeds 75 percent reduction in diameter of the lumen. Of all indirect tests reviewed, oculoplethysmography is probably the choice for indirect examination.

The need for direct testing is apparent. Two types of direct tests are now in use, flow imaging by pulsed Doppler (ultrasonic arteriography) and anatomical display by B-mode scan. Most B-mode scanners are equipped with a pulsed Doppler for sound analysis. This adds hemodynamic information to the anatomical display. Each test has its merits, and the diagnostic accuracy is clearly superior to the indirect tests. For direct testing, however, a skillful operator is needed to achieve good results. Also, the testing time is longer.

One of the main advantages of the B-mode scan, or duplex scan is the ability to detect ulcerating plaques. Small ulcerating plaques, not visualized on conventional bi-plane arteriography, may be detected by B-mode scan, and Cranley has reported four such cases. All 4 patients had B-mode scan findings corresponding to appropriate hemispheric TIAs, and all had plaques found at operation. Although it is premature to advocate the use of B-mode scan rather than arteriography prior to surgical intervention, such findings did emphasize the inaccuracy of arteriography in detection of small ulcerating plaques. The inability of arteriography to detect such plaques has been stressed by several investigators.[66,67] Thus, B-mode scan is helpful to evaluate patients with typical symptoms who have had normal arteriograms.

Valuable information may also be extracted from common carotid artery flow waveform analysis. Calculation of the resistance index and flow waveform inspection are simple and may yield hemodynamic information. Both flow calculation and velocity profile studies are newer techniques, and further study is needed to establish the diagnostic value of these tests.

At present, we believe that a vascular laboratory should be equipped with both direct and indirect testing instruments. The use of these two tests may complement each other, or it may improve diagnostic accuracy. For patients with symptoms of cerebrovascular insufficiency, we believe the use of direct and indirect tests as outlined below is appropriate:

1. Patients with typical ischemic attacks (monocular blindness or hemispheric attacks) and who are otherwise healthy should have cerebral arteriography regardless of noninvasive findings. Direct and indirect tests are used when the patient becomes a candidate for surgery or when the physician wishes to have a baseline study. In the event of a normal arteriogram, a B-mode scan should be done to search for ulcerating plaques.
2. Direct tests should be done in patients suspected to have carotid artery disease and in whom there is a risk for arteriography. This applies to patients who have had a recent stroke (complete or incomplete) and to patients in acute renal failure. Direct testing must be used in these patients

because of its high sensitivity rate. Identification of carotid artery disease helps to establish a definitive diagnosis and allows proper timing for eventual arteriographic examination.

3. In patients with equivocal symptoms, the use of the direct test in combination with an indirect test helps to rule out the need for arteriography.
4. Direct testing should be used to evaluate patients with posterior fossa symptoms. A positive test helps to rule in arteriography and, at the same time, assess the contribution of carotid stenosis to the patient's problems. A normal direct test does not rule out vertebral artery stenosis or occlusion. In view of a low stroke rate in vertebral artery stenosis, the need for arteriography depends upon the disability of the patient and the number of previous attacks.
5. Patients with asymptomatic bruit, especially bilateral bruits, should be assessed by a direct technique. Oculoplethysmography is not advised because of its high false-negative rate and its limitation in bilateral disease. A positive test indicates the need for arteriography. Once arteriography is done, oculoplethysmography may be used to provide hemodynamic information. Patients with hemodynamically significant lesions should proceed to surgery prior to other major surgical procedures. Likewise, candidates for coronary bypass surgery should be evaluated in a similar manner. Simultaneous carotid and coronary surgery is indicated when there is an hemodynamically significant carotid artery stenosis and a heart with poor reserve.
6. Oculoplethysmography should be used to evaluate angiographic evidence of siphon disease. Also, it helps to choose the side for carotid endarterectomy in patients with bilateral carotid stenosis and in whom the presenting symptoms were non-lateralizing. Here, hemodynamic measurement supplements arteriographic estimation of the degree of stenosis.
7. Enough evidence has now documented the value of noninvasive tests (direct and indirect) in patients after carotid endarterectomy.[68–70] Therefore, a direct or indirect test must be used prior to surgery and repeated during the postoperative period. During the immediate postoperative period, the indirect test is preferred because of its simplicity and because the neck wound may prevent an adequate study by the direct test. Late follow-up by noninvasive testing helps to detect recurrent stenosis.
8. B-mode scanning provides a more reliable way to evaluate the efficacy of antiplatelet drugs in ulcerating carotid plaques discovered on arteriography on the contralateral, asymptomatic side or in those patients who are not candidates for surgery. Evidence of progressive asymptomatic carotid stenosis is better assessed by noninvasive techniques than by clinical examination.

Noninvasive testing for carotid artery disease must be included as an integral part of evaluation by vascular surgeons. These tests are not designed to replace arteriography. Direct and indirect tests complement each other and a combination is used in selected instances. For indirect testing, the Gee and Kartchner oculoplethysmographs yield similar diagnostic accuracy, but the Gee instrument is preferred because it provides pressure readings. The B-mode scan with pulsed Doppler flow interrogation is an intriguing technique and appears to be ideal because it gives both anatomical and hemodynamic information. But, further study is needed to show that this technique is superior to flow imaging by pulsed or continuous-wave Doppler. The B-mode scan with sound analysis is now undergoing a comparative study in our laboratory.

REFERENCES

1. Wood EH, Hull RP: Thermography in the diagnosis of cerebrovascular disease. Acta Radiol (Stockholm) 15:961, 1966
2. Austin JH, Sajid MH: Direct thermometry in ophthalmic-internal carotid blood flow. Arch Neurol 15:376, 1966
3. Shapiro HM, et al: Direct thermometry, ophthalmodynamometry, auscultation, and palpation in extracranial cerebrovascular disease. Stroke 1:205, 1970
4. Capistrant TD, Gunmit JR: Detecting carotid occlusive disease by thermography. Stroke 4:57, 1973
5. Hofferberth B, Gottschaldt M, Dykan S: Comparison of Doppler sonography and plate thermography for detection of carotid artery stenosis. Stroke 11:27, 1980
6. Nielsen PE, Hubke P, Poulsen HL: Skin blood pressure in the forehead in patients with internal carotid lesions. Stroke 6:58, 1975
7. Brockenbrough EC: Screening for the Prevention of Stroke: Use of a Doppler Flowmeter. Washington/Alaska Regional Medical Program, Information and Education Resource Support Unit, 1969
8. Barnes RW, Bone GE, et al: Noninvasive ultrasonic carotid angiography: Prospective validation by contrast arteriography. Surgery 80:328, 1970
9. Muller HR: Directional Doppler sonography. A new technique to demonstrate flow reversal in the ophthalmic artery. Neuroradiol 5:91, 1973
10. Wyatt AP, Ratnavel K, Loxton GE: The technique and possible application of supra-orbital artery blood-pressure estimation. Br J Surg 60:741, 1973
11. Moore WS, Bean B, Burton R, et al: The use of ophthalmosonometry in the diagnosis of carotid artery stenosis. Surgery 82:107, 1977
12. Prichard DR, Martin TRP, Sherriff SB: Assessment of directional Doppler ultrasound techniques in the diagnosis of carotid artery diseases. J Neurol, Neurosurg, Psychiat 42:563, 1979
13. LoGerfo FW, Mason GR: Directional Doppler studies of supraorbital artery flow in internal carotid stenosis and occlusion. Surgery 76:723, 1974
14. Machleder HI, Barker WF: Stroke on the wrong side. Use of the Doppler opthalmic test in cerebral vascular screening. Arch Surg 105:943, 1972

15. Maroon JC, Pieroni DW, Campbell RL: Ophthalmosonometry. An ultrasonic method for assessing carotid blood flow. J Neurosurg 30:238, 1969
16. Baker WH, Barnes RW: The cerebrovascular Doppler examination in patients with nonhemispheric symptoms. Ann Surg 186:190, 1977
17. Bone GE, Barnes RW: Limitations of the Doppler cerebrovascular examination in hemispheric cerebral ischemia. Surgery 79:577, 1976
18. Towne JB, Salles-Cunha S, Bernhard VM: Periorbital ultrasound findings. Hemodynamics in patients with cerebral vascular disease. Arch Surg 114:158, 1979
19. Bone GE, Slaymaker EE, Barnes RW: Noninvasive assessment of collateral blood flow of the cerebral hemisphere by Doppler ultrasound. Surg Gynecol Obstet 145:873, 1977
20. Lynch TG, Wright CB, Miller EV: Oculopneumoplethysmography, Doppler examination, and supraorbital photoplethysmography. A comparison of hemodynamic techniques in assessing cerebrovascular occlusive disease. Ann Surg 194:731, 1981
21. Bone GE, Dickinson D, Pomajzl MJ: A prospective evaluation of indirect methods for detecting carotid atherosclerosis. Surg Gynecol Obstet 152:587, 1981
22. Malone JM, Bean B, Laguna J, et al: Diagnosis of carotid artery stenosis. Comparison of oculoplethysmography and Doppler supraorbital examination. Ann Surg 191:347, 1980
23. Cranley JJ: Midwestern Vascular Surgical Society Presidential Address: Stroke—A perspective. Surgery 91:537, 1982
24. Barnes R, Garrett W, Slaymaker E, et al: Doppler ultrasound and supraorbital photoplethysmography for noninvasive screening of carotid occlusive disease. Am J Surg 134:183, 1977
25. Barnes RW, Clayton JM, Bone GE et al: Supraorbital photoplethysmography. Simple, accurate screening for carotid occlusive disease. J Surg Res 22:319, 1977
26. Pearce HJ, Becchetti JJ, Brown HJ: Supraorbital photoplethysmographic monitoring during carotid endarterectomy with the use of an internal shunt: An added dimension of safety. Surgery 87:339, 1980
27. Bailliart P: La pression arterielle dans les branches de l'artere centrale de la retine: Nouvelle technique pour la determiner. Ann Oculistique 154:648, 1917
28. Sanborn GE, Miller NR, McGuire M, et al: Clinical-angiographic correlation of ophthalmodynamometry in patients with suspected carotid artery disease: A prospective study. Stroke 12: 770, 1981
29. Yuson CP, Toole JF: Bruits, ophthalmodynamometry and rectilinear scanning in transient ischemic attacks. Stroke 7:541, 1976
30. Paulson OB: Ophthalmodynamometry in internal carotid artery occlusion. Stroke 7:564, 1976
31. Brockenbrough EC, et al: Ocular plethysmography: A new technique for the evaluation of carotid obstructive disease. Rev Surg 24:299, 1967
32. Kartchner M, McRae L, Morrison F: Noninvasive detection and evaluation of carotid occlusive disease. Arch Surg 106:528, 1973
33. Gee W, Oller D, Wylie EJ: Noninvasive diagnosis of carotid occlusion by ocular pneumoplethysmography. Stroke 7:18, 1976
34. String ST: Zira oculoplethysmography, in Kempczinski RF, Yao JST (eds): Practical Noninvasive Vascular Diagnosis, Chicago, Year Book Medical Publishers, 1982, p 203
35. Kartchner M, McRae L: Noninvasive evaluation and management of the "asymptomatic" carotid bruit. Surgery 82:842, 1977
36. Satiani B, Cooperman M, Clark M, et al: An assessment of carotid phonoangiography and oculoplethysmography in the detection of carotid artery stenosis. Am J Surg 136:618, 1978
37. O'Hara PJ, Brewster DC, Darling RC, et al: Oculopneumoplethysmography. Its relationship to intraoperative cerebrovascular hemodynamics. Arch Surg 115:1156, 1980
38. Martinez SA, Oller DW, Gee W, et al: Elective carotid artery resection. Arch Otolaryngol 101:744, 1975

39. Blackshear WM, Thiele BL, Harley JD, et al: A prospective evaluation of oculoplethysmography and carotid phonoangiography. Surg Gynecol Obstet 148:201, 1979
40. Busuttil RW, Baker JD, Davidson RK, et al: Carotid artery stenosis—Hemodynamic significance and clinical course. JAMA 245:1438, 1981
41. Keagy BA, Pharr WF, Thomas D, et al: Comparison of oculoplethysmography/carotid phonoangiography with duplex scan/spectral analysis in the detection of carotid artery stenosis. Stroke 13:43, 1982
42. Cardullo PA, Cutler BS, Wheeler HB, et al: Noninvasive detection of carotid disease: An evaluation of oculoplethysmography, carotid phonoangiography and pulsed Doppler ultrasonic arteriography. Bruit 5:26, 1981
43. Comerota AJ, Cranley JJ, Cook SE: Real-time B-mode carotid imaging in diagnosis of cerebrovascular disease. Surgery 89:718, 1981
44. Hobson RW, Berry SM, et al: Comparison of pulsed Doppler and real-time B-mode echo arteriography for noninvasive imaging of the extracranial carotid arteries. Surgery 87:286, 1980
45. Sumner DS, Russell JB, Ramsey DE, et al: Noninvasive diagnosis of extracranial carotid arterial disease. Arch Surg 114:1222, 1979
46. Spencer MP, Reid JM, Davis DL, et al: Cervical carotid imaging with a continuous-wave Doppler flowmeter. Stroke 5:145, 1974
47. White DN: Color-coded Doppler carotid imaging, in Bernstein EF (ed): Noninvasive Diagnostic Techniques in Vascular Surgery. St. Louis, C.V. Mosby Co., 1982, p 258
48. Lees RS, Dewey CF, Jr: Phonoangiography: A new noninvasive diagnostic method for studying arterial disease. Proc Natl Acad Sci, U.S.A. 67:935, 1970
49. Kempczinski RF: A combined approach to the noninvasive diagnosis of carotid artery occlusive disease. Surgery 85:689, 1979
50. Kistler JP, Lees RS, Miller A, et al: Correlation of spectral phonoangiography and carotid angiography with gross pathology in carotid stenosis. N Engl J Med 305:417, 1981
51. Miller A, Lees RS, Kistler JP, et al: Spectral analysis of arterial bruits (phonoangiography): Experimental validation. Circulation 61:515, 1980
52. Barnes RW, Nix L, Rittgers SE: Audible interpretation of carotid Doppler signals. An improved technique to define carotid artery disease. Arch Surg 116:1185, 1981
53. Pourcelot L: Applications clinique de l'examen Doppler transcutane. Sem Technol Tech Chirug, Hospital Broussais, 1974
54. Rutherford RB, Hiatt WR, Kreutzer EW: The use of velocity wave form analysis in the diagnosis of carotid artery occlusive disease. Surgery 82:695, 1977
55. Padayachee TS, Lewis RR, Gosling RG: Detection of carotid bifurcation disease: Comparison of ultrasound tests with angiography. Br J Surg 69:218, 1982
56. Fitzgerald DE, O'Shaughnessy AM, Keaveny V: Pulsed Doppler: Determination of blood velocity and volume flow in normal and diseased common carotid arteries in man. Cardiovas Res 16:220, 1982
57. Peronneau PA, Bugnon A, Bournat JP, et al: Instantaneous bidimensional blood velocity profiles in the major vessels by pulsed ultrasonic Doppler velocimeter, in de Vlieger M, White DV, McCready, VR (eds): Ultrasonics in Medicine, Proc. 2nd World Congress, 1973. New York, American Elsevier Publishing Co., 1974, pp 259
58. Keller H, Meier W, Yonekawa Y, et al: Noninvasive angiography for the diagnosis of carotid artery disease using Doppler ultrasound (carotid artery Doppler). Stroke 7:354, 1976
59. Humber PR, Leopold GR, Wickbom IG, et al: Ultrasonic imaging of the carotid artery system. Am J Surg 140:199, 1980
60. O'Donnell TF Jr, Pauker SG, Callow AD, et al: The relative value of carotid noninvasive testing as determined by receiver operator characteristic curves. Surgery 87:9, 1980
61. Hobson RW II, Berry SM, Lynch TG: Applications of B-mode ultrasonography and ocular

pneumoplethysmography in the diagnosis of carotid occlusive disease, in Bergan JJ, Yao JST (eds): Cerebrovascular Insufficiency. New York, Grune & Stratton, Inc., 1982, p 165
62. Sumner DS: Editorial: Noninvasive tests: The more the better? Vasc Diagnos Ther 3:6, 1982
63. Flinn WR, Goodreau JJ, Queral LA, et al: Oculoplethysmography. An assessment of its correlation with angiography, in Diethrich EB (ed): Noninvasive Cardiovascular Diagnosis, 2nd Edition. Littleton, Ma., PSG Publishing Co., 1981, p 107
64. Gross WS, Verta MJ Jr, van Bellen B, et al: Comparison of noninvasive diagnostic techniques in carotid artery occlusive disease. Surgery 82:271, 1977
65. Griner P, Mayewski RJ, Muslin AI, et al: Selection and interpretation of diagnostic tests and procedures, principles and applications. Ann Intern Med 94:571, 1981
66. Croft RJ, Ellam LD, Harrison MJG: Accuracy of carotid angiography in the assessment of atheroma of the internal carotid artery. Lancet 1:997, 1980
67. Edwards JH, Kricheff I, Riles T, et al: Angiographically undetected ulceration of the carotid bifurcation as a cause of embolic stroke. Radiology 132:369, 1979
68. Cantelmo NL, Cutler BS, Wheeler HB, et al: Noninvasive detection of carotid stenosis following endarterectomy. Arch Surg 116:1005, 1981
69. Bodily KC, Zierler RE, Marinelli MR, et al: Flow disturbances following carotid endarterectomy. Surg Gynecol Obstet 151:77, 1980
70. Aukland A, Hurlow RA, Hamer JD: Carotid artery occlusion following endarterectomy: Evaluation by spectral analysis of Doppler ultrasound signals. Br J Surg 69:45, 1982

PART V

Surgery for the Atherosclerotic Carotid Artery

Wesley S. Moore

13

Surgical Significance and Management of the Ulcerated Carotid Plaque

The objective of carotid endarterectomy is to prevent stroke. To the extent that ulcerated atheromatous plaques of the carotid bifurcation, with or without hemodynamically significant stenosis, are involved in the pathogenesis of transient ischemic attack or stroke, surgical removal can be justified.

The objectives of this chapter are to review the pathogenesis of transient cerebral ischemia and stroke relating to ulcerative atheromatous plaques, to explore the dynamics of plaque ulceration with primary and secondary embolic phenomenon, to outline the criteria and limitations of diagnosis, and to present evidence that justifies an aggressive approach for correcting both symptomatic and large asymptomatic ulcerative lesions.

RELATIONSHIP OF ATHEROMATOUS ULCERATION TO TIA AND STROKE

In the early 1950s when the relationship between extracranial cerebral vascular disease and stroke was first being recognized, it was generally assumed that transient ischemic attacks were related to the flow-reducing characteristics of lesions found at the origin of the internal carotid artery. These lesions presumably produced intermittent drops in hemispheric blood flow below a critical threshold which resulted in hemispheric dysfunction.[1-4] When the stenosis compromised the lumen to the point of producing critically low flow, cerebral infarction occurred as a consequence of internal carotid artery thrombosis. This thesis led to the clinical approach of angiographically searching for high-grade stenosis and then carrying out surgical repair with the objective of increasing cerebral hemispheric blood flow. The cessation of transient ischemic attacks and apparent stroke prevention following operation appeared to justify this approach.[5-7]

As more experience was accumulated, several observations were made that were inconsistent with the hemodynamic concept of reduced arterial blood flow producing transient ischemic attacks and stroke. First, measurements of hemispheric cerebral blood flow before and after carotid bifurcation endarterectomy failed to demonstrate any improvement. This suggested that operations simply redistributed flow from collateral to primary anatomic sources.[8] Direct measurement of blood flow through the internal carotid artery with progressive arterial constriction was studied in order to establish a definition for critical arterial stenosis. There was no flow reduction through the internal carotid artery until 90 percent stenosis was accomplished,[1] yet patients were relieved of transient ischemic attacks by removing lesions considerably less than 90 percent occlusive. The transient nature of ischemic attacks has been difficult to reconcile in the face of relatively constant cerebral blood flow demand and a fixed stenosis. Suggestions that drops in cardiac output or systemic blood pressure in the presence of an isolated stenosis might result in transient hemispheric dysfunction[2] could not be validated in experimental studies of patients with TIAs in whom the ischemic events could not be reproduced by deliberate dropping of systemic blood pressure within physiologic ranges.[9-10] There have been many instances observed in which patients suffering from TIAs stopped having symptoms after the internal carotid artery went on to occlusion.[11,12] While it is true that some patients will experience a major stroke as a consequence of internal carotid artery thrombosis, there are many instances of progression to occlusion without symptoms. Finally, it was observed that TIAs would diminish in frequency during the administration of anticoagulants which, in and of themselves, have no effect on improving blood flow.[13,14] These inconsistencies in the hemodynamic theory led investigators to look for alternative explanations for transient ischemic attacks and stroke.

Currently, the theory of emboli originating from atheromatous plaques in the extracranial arterial system is well-established and becoming universally accepted. Retrospective reviews of the older literature will uncover many references that yielded clues as to the potential for atherosclerotic plaques to release emboli to the brain, yet several recent publications stand out in their importance for influencing contemporary thought. In 1961, Hollenhorst[15] observed the presence of "bright plaques" in retinal vessels during a funduscopic examination. He suggested that these were cholesterol crystals originating from eroded atheromatous plaques. That same year, Ross-Russell[16] observed 2 patients who presented with transient monocular blindness and postulated that these symptoms were due to retinal emboli. In 1963, Julian and colleagues[17] reported on a series of patients in whom ulceration was noted in the atheromatous plaques removed from the carotid bifurcation at the time of endarterectomy. They suggested the possibility of a relationship between the patient's symptoms and the embolic material originating from the ulcerative lesions. In 1964, Gunning and colleagues[18] reviewed a series of patients with monocular or hemispheric transient dysfunction associated with mural thrombus adherent to carotid bifurcation plaques. They noted the following: "One of the most important conclusions to emerge is that many instances of transient retinal and cerebral ischemia are due to emboli arising from mural thrombi in the internal carotid artery, as may also be some instances of isolated central retinal artery occlusion and of persistent hemiparesis. These emboli may be so unstable that they disintegrate, thus restoring the circulation, or they may lodge more permanently." Ehrenfeld and colleagues[19] reported a series of patients with transient monocular blindness associated with stenotic ulcerative atheromatous lesions who stopped having symptoms following carotid endarterectomy, presumably from removing an embolic source.

As the evidence began to mount for emboli of carotid origin being responsible for retinal and hemispheric ischemia, it was still difficult to prove this relationship since carotid bifurcation endarterectomy removed not only a potentially embolic source but also a stenotic (presumably flow-reducing) lesion. This dilemma was resolved by a report in 1968 from my group[20] in which 12 patients with monocular and hemispheric ischemic events were found to have ulcerative lesions in association with minimal (non-hemodynamically significant) plaques. Ulceration was proven at operation. Following removal of these ulcerative plaques, symptoms ceased. Since these lesions clearly had no effect on flow, the only basis for symptomatic resolution was the removal of an embolic source. I updated these observations in 1970 with a larger series and longer follow-up substantiating these same conclusions.[21]

MORPHOLOGY AND DYNAMICS OF ATHEROMATOUS ULCERATION AND EMBOLIZATION

Embolic material from atheromatous plaques can consist of cholesterol crystal debris, platelet aggregates, or thrombotic material, depending upon the stage of plaque evolution or degeneration. As long as the endothelial layer covering the atheromatous plaque remains intact and smooth, it is unlikely that any embolic activity will occur. The center of an atheromatous plaque, however, may undergo degeneration, softening and expansion. These changes can lead to rupture of the endothelial lining with discharge of atheromatous debris into the arterial lumen resulting in atheromatous embolization (Fig.

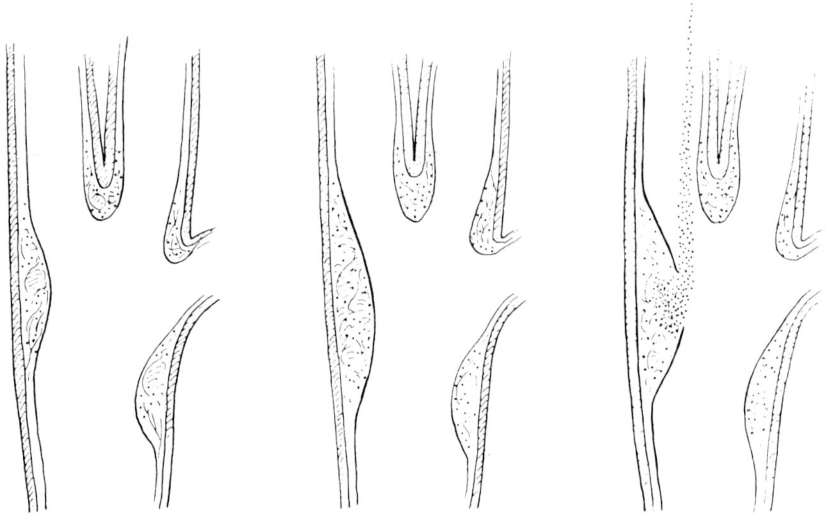

Figure 13-1. This is the artist's concept of an atheromatous plaque involving the carotid bifurcation.
Center: With time, the plaque becomes bulkier and expands into the lumen.
Right: When the plaque expands, the surface endothelium may rupture, allowing loose atheromatous debris to escape into the lumen and be swept by the blood stream up the internal carotid artery to the brain.

13-1). Following plaque rupture, a significant defect in the plaque is left behind which can be grossly identified as an ulcer crater (Figs. 13-2 and 13-3). If a carotid angiogram is obtained in the appropriate projection, the ulcer crater will be identified as an excrescence from the normal lumen (Fig. 13-4). Another mechanism for sudden plaque enlargement leading to rupture is hemorrhage into the substance of the plaque[22] (Fig. 13-5).

After the initial disgorgement of plaque contents, the ruptured plaque may continue to be a source for further atheromatous embolization (Fig. 13-6), or its surface may re-endothelialize leaving a defect with a relatively smooth base. The defect with a smooth base, however, will become an area of relative stasis with eddy currents that are conducive to platelet aggregation and may result in secondary embolization (Fig. 13-7).

It would appear more likely that bulky atheromatous lesions would proceed to rupture and embolization. This suggests that plaques large enough to produce hemodynamically significant stenosis may also be more prone to rupture and embolize. Low profile lesions, however, have been shown to ulcerate and lead to primary embolization. Following plaque rupture, an ulcer crater is left in this low profile plaque which can be a site for a secondary embolization (Fig. 13-8). An even more insidious problem has recently been

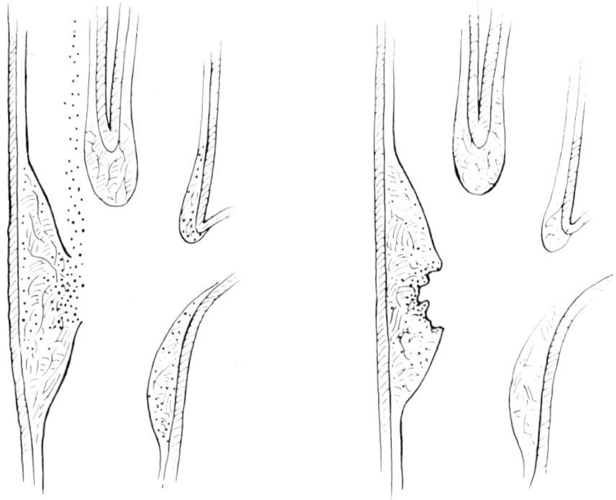

Figure 13-2. Left: When the plaque ruptures, atheromatous contents are released into the lumen, permitting the development of a central defect.
Right: The appearance of the central defect (ulcer) following disgorgement of contents.

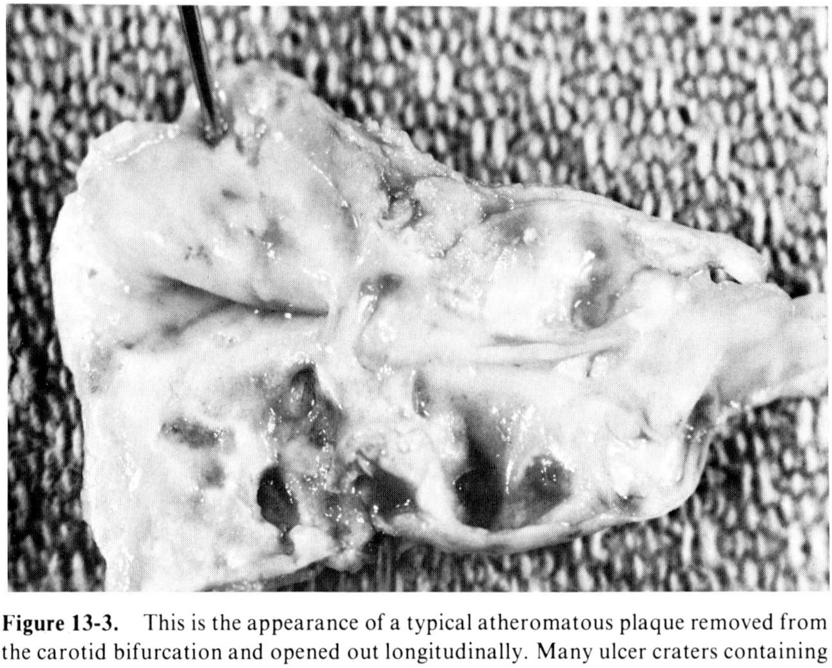

Figure 13-3. This is the appearance of a typical atheromatous plaque removed from the carotid bifurcation and opened out longitudinally. Many ulcer craters containing clot or raw atheromatous surface are seen.

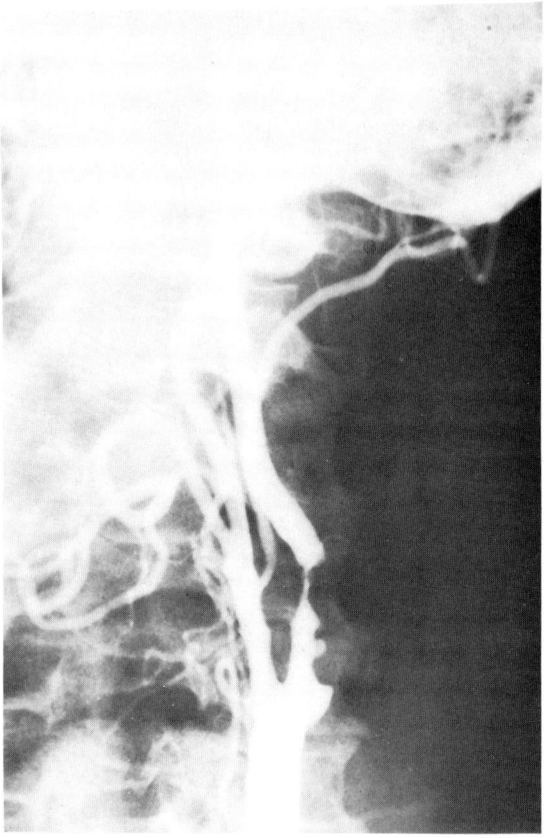

Figure 13-4. This is a left carotid arteriogram seen in a patient who was having left hemisphere transient ischemic attacks. In addition to the high-grade carotid artery stenosis, at least two areas of ulceration are seen on the posterior aspect of the internal carotid artery.

identified which is the process of micro-ulceration. Several authors have done scanning electron microscopy studies of plaque surfaces from specimens removed at the time of carotid endarterectomy. These studies have shown areas of endothelial denudation with exposure of raw cholesterol plaque or subendothelial collagen in the absence of gross ulceration. Platelet aggregate material will loosely adhere to these rough surfaces and then secondarily embolize.[23-26] This may represent an explanation of why patients presenting with transient ischemic attacks or cerebral infarction may fail to show macro-ulceration by angiography or at the time of surgical exploration.

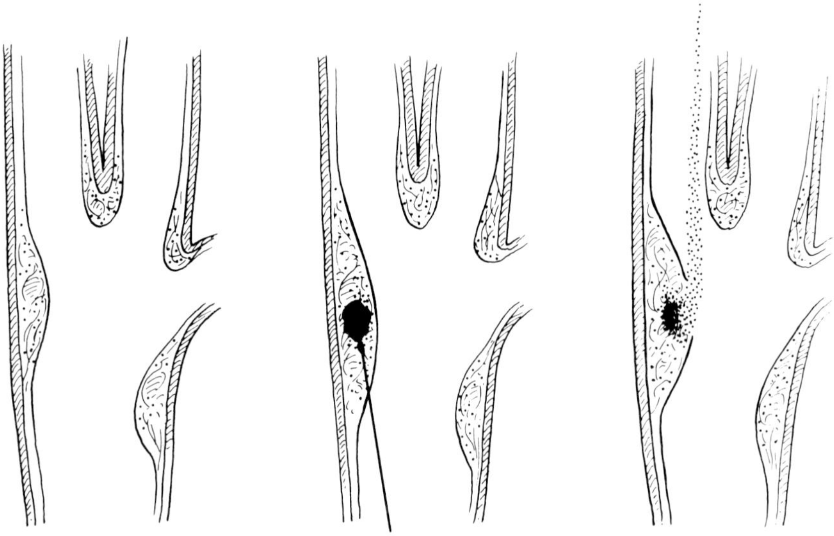

Figure 13-5. Left: An atheromatous plaque at the carotid bifurcation is depicted. Center: Hemorrhage can develop within the center of an atheromatous plaque producing acute expansion.
Right: With acute expansion of the plaque, the endothelial lining can rupture, permitting disgorgement of hemorrhagic atheromatous contents into the lumen of the internal carotid artery.

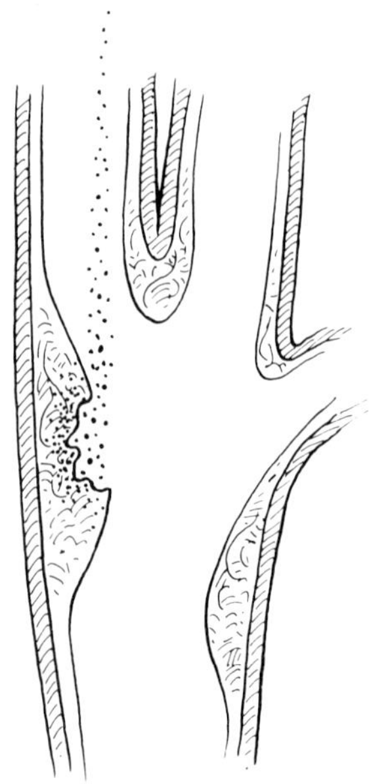

Figure 13-6. As long as the central ulceration within an atheromatous plaque exposes atheromatous debris to the arterial lumen, atheromatous material can continue to flake off and embolize up the internal carotid artery.

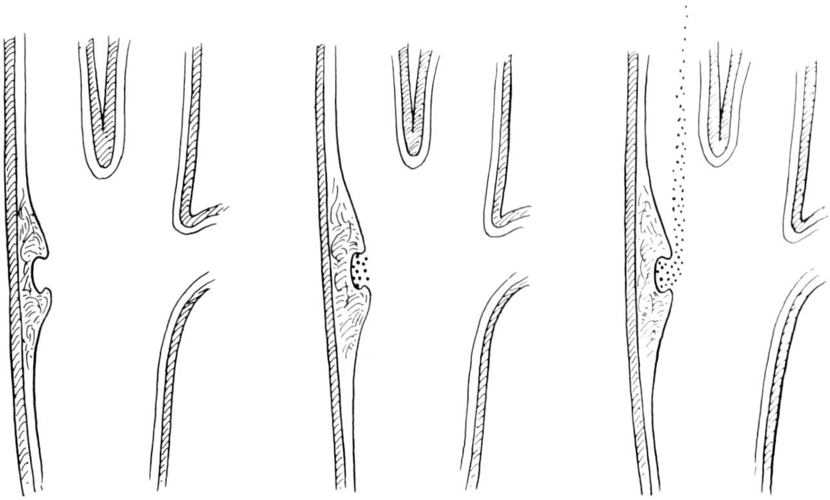

Figure 13-7. Left: This demonstrates the artist's concept of endothelial resurfacing of the central ulcer within an atheromatous plaque.
Center: The ulcer, in spite of its new surface, becomes a site of stasis and potential platelet aggregation.
Right: The platelet aggregates can then secondarily be swept into the arterial stream and embolize up the internal carotid artery.

ANGIOGRAPHIC DIAGNOSIS

The visualization of an ulcerative lesion by angiogram is dependent upon three factors: (1) the angiographic projection must be such that the ulcer is seen in profile; (2) the ulcer crypt must be deep enough to be distinguished from the adjacent plaque; and (3) the ulcer crypt must be empty of blood clot or other debris so as to permit contrast material to fill the cavity and be recognized. Failure in any of these three areas will prevent the angiographic demonstration of ulceration. The accuracy of identification of macroulceration by angiography is reported to range from 60 to 86 percent, depending upon how strict the interpretive criteria.[24,27,28] This diagnostic limitation is further compounded by the fact that relatively superficial ulcers, surface denudation, and microscopic ulceration are all potential sources for platelet aggregation and embolization. Under these conditions, the interpolative skills of the clinicians are called into play and require that the clinical history as well as subtle angiographic findings be combined and placed in perspective for diagnosis. For example, when a patient presents with multiple hemispheric or monocular transient ischemic attacks, and the angiogram fails to demonstrate overt ulceration on multiple views but does demonstrate an irregular plaque at the carotid bifurcation, a decision must be made as to

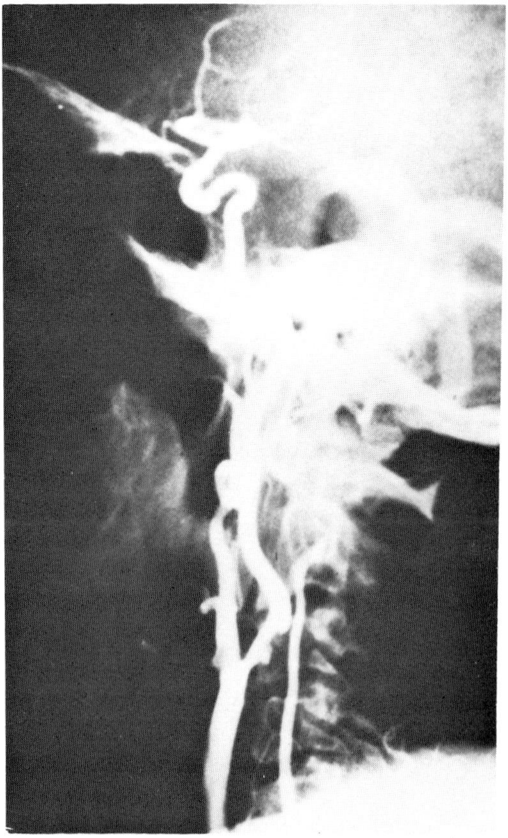

Figure 13-8. This is a right carotid arteriogram obtained in a patient who was experiencing multiple episodes of right-sided transient monocular blindness. Note the ulcerative lesion on the posterior wall of the internal carotid artery in the absence of hemodynamically significant stenosis.

whether this is a shallow ulcer, an ulcer filled with clot, or a condition unrelated to embolization from carotid plaque origin. Obviously, the stronger the clinical history in combination with quality extra-cranial and intra-cranial angiograms which fail to identify a focus other than the carotid bifurcation, the more likely the diagnosis of embolization of carotid origin and the safer the recommendation for carotid endarterectomy.

The size of the ulcer crater, particularly in patients who are currently asymptomatic, appears to have some prognostic significance for future neurologic consequences. While it is not possible to strictly quantitate ulcer size, a scheme for qualitative description of ulcer size has been proposed and found to be quite helpful.[29] Thus a small ulcer niche is described as an "A" ulcer; a moderately large ulcer is described as a "B" ulcer, and a very large, compound, or cavernous ulcer is described as a "C" ulcer.

INDICATIONS FOR OPERATION

Symptomatic Ulceration

The patients who present with transient or permanent focal deficits consistent with embolic events in association with ulcerative lesions are candidates for carotid endarterectomy. It makes no difference whether the ulcerative lesion occurs in a stenotic or a low profile plaque. Thiele and colleagues noted in a series of 66 patients with transient ischemic attacks that potentially embolic lesions were seen no more frequently than lesions producing a hemodynamically significant stenosis (84 percent vs. 50 percent).[30] Transient monocular blindness and focal motor, sensory, or mixed hemispheric deficits can all occur with intermittent embolization originating from a focal source and passing by laminar flow to the same terminal vascular bed. Larger embolic fragments, particularly cholesterol emboli, are more likely to remain intact and produce cerebral infarction rather than break up, pass through the microcirculation, and provide for a return of neurologic function. Patients who present with non-focal or global ischemic events in the absence of hemodynamically significant lesions should not be considered symptomatic from an unidentified ulcerative lesion in and of itself. Decision to operate under these circumstances would depend upon ulcer size and would come under the same considerations as an asymptomatic, non-stenotic ulceration.

Asymptomatic Ulceration

The asymptomatic ulcerative lesion in association with a preocclusive stenosis may be considered for prophylactic carotid endarterectomy. The evidence for preemptive carotid endarterectomy is controversial, but generally can be justified in good risk patients in the hands of a surgeon whose personal combined stroke morbidity and mortality is less than 2 percent.

The natural history of non-stenotic asymptomatic ulceration was recently reported by our group in a retrospective review of patients found to have ulcerative lesions present in a contralateral asymptomatic artery and followed without operation.[31] The incidence of stroke in the small, category "A" ulceration was negligible. On the other hand, the average stroke rate for patients with the larger "B" and "C" ulcers was 12 percent each year of follow-up. This is almost double the expected stroke incidence of patients with hemispheric TIAs (an uncontroversial indication for operation). Our report was challenged by another retrospective review, which failed to demonstrate the same stroke risk.[32] That series, however, lacked patients with the large "C" ulcers. We recently carried out another retrospective review of the experience at UCLA and combined data with our original studies so that sufficient patients were available for analysis in each of the three ulcer categories. Group "A" ulcers continued to have a benign prognosis. Group "B" ulcers had an average stroke incidence of 4.5 percent each year; and group "C" ulcers had a stroke incidence of 7.5 percent each year.[33] Of considerable concern was the fact that the patients who developed stroke from a previously asymptomatic, non-stenotic ulcer, failed to have antecedent TIAs and therefore presented with no warning signs. The exact nature of the lesions at the time of the stroke was unknown. Conceivably, the lesion may have progressed in size and become a stenotic lesion, or it may have remained ulcerated with a reharvesting of embolic debris. In any event, the presence of a "B" or "C" ulcer on angiography represents an important marker indicating a grave prognosis. Our current recommendation is to operate on the large "B" or "C" ulcers with the same caveats expressed for indication of operation on the asymptomatic stenosis.

RESULTS

While there are many reports documenting the early morbidity and mortality for carotid endarterectomy, there are few that studied the late follow-up with respect to stroke prevention and only one report that reviewed the late results of the carotid endarterectomy for symptomatic, non-stenotic ulcerations. Our series[31] looked at the late follow-up up to 96 months for patients presenting with symptomatic ulceration as an indication for operation. Results demonstrated that there was a negligible stroke incidence in these patients, which was in marked contrast to an expected stroke rate of 6 percent each year, or a cumulative stroke incidence of 48 percent had patients not been treated by operation. This presents compelling support for an aggressive approach to the problem.

SUMMARY

1. Emboli from ulcerative lesions of the carotid artery represent a major cause of transient cerebral ischemia and stroke.
2. Emboli may be released from ulcerative lesions in the absence of hemodynamically significant stenosis.

3. Embolic material may consist of atheromatous debris released primarily at the time of plaque rupture or as a continual release from raw, exposed plaque.
4. Secondary emboli may originate from platelet or thrombus aggregates in a residual, lined, ulcer niche.
5. Large ulcerative lesions, currently asymptomatic, carry 5 to 8 percent per year risk of stroke if left untreated.
6. Carotid endarterectomy virtually eliminates stroke risk on follow-up extending to 96 months.
7. An aggressive surgical approach to symptomatic ulcers and large asymptomatic ulcers is justified in good risk patients and in the hands of a surgeon whose overall operative morbidity and mortality is less than 2 percent.

REFERENCES

1. Brice JG, Dowsett DJ, Low RD: Hemodynamic effects of carotid artery stenosis. Br Med J, 3:1363, 1964
2. Corday E, Rothenberg S, Weiner SM: Cerebral vascular insufficency: An explanation of the transient stroke. Arch Intern Med, 98:683, 1956
3. Crawford ES, DeBakey ME, Blaisdell FW, et al: Hemodynamic alterations in patients with cerebral arterial insufficiency before and after operation. Surgery 48:76, 1960
4. Landolt AM, Millakan CH: Pathogenesis of cerebral infarction secondary to mechanical carotid artery occlusion. Stroke 1:52, 1970
5. DeBakey ME, Crawford ES, Fields WS: Surgical treatment of patients with cerebral arterial insufficiency associated with extracranial arterial occlusive lesions. Neurology 11:145, 1961
6. DeBakey ME, Crawford ES, Cooley DA, et al: Cerebral arterial insufficiency: One to 11-year results following arterial reconstructive operation. Annals of Surgery 161:921, 1965
7. Hohf RP: The clinical evaluation and surgery of internal carotid insufficiency. Surg Clin, North Am 47:1, 1967
8. Adams JE, Smith MC, Wylie EJ: Cerebral blood flow and hemodynamics in extracranial vascular disease: Effect of endarterectomy. Surgery 53:449, 1963
9. Fazekas JF, Alman RW: The role of hypotension in transitory focal cerebral ischemia. Am J Med Sci 248:567, 1964
10. Kendall RE, Marshall J: Role of hypotension in the genesis of transient focal cerebral ischemic attacks. Br Med J 2:344, 1963
11. Drake WE Jr, Drake MAL: Clinical and angiographic correlates of cerebrovascular insufficiency. Am J Med 45:253, 1968
12. Russell RW, Cranstone WI: Ophthalmodynamometry in carotid artery disease. J Neurol, Neurosurg & Psychiat 24:281, 1961
13. Fisher CM: The use of anticoagulants in cerebral thrombosis. Neurology 8:311, 1958
14. Millakan CH, Siekert RG, Shick RM: Studies in cerebrovascular disease. V. The use of anticoagulant drugs in the treatment of intermittent insufficiency of the internal carotid arterial system. Proc Staff Meeting Mayo Clin 30:578, 1955
15. Hollenhorst RW: Significance of bright plaques in the retinal arterioles JAMA, 178:23, 1961

16. Russell RWR: Observations on the retinal blood-vessels in monocular blindness. Lancet 2:1422, 1961
17. Julian OC, Dye WS, Javid H, et al: Ulcerative lesions of the carotid artery bifurcation. Arch Surg 86:803, 1963
18. Gunning AJ, Pickering GW, Robb-Smith AHT, et al: Mural thrombosis of the internal carotid artery and subsequent embolism. QJ Med 33:155, 1964
19. Ehrenfeld WK, Hoyt WF, Wylie EJ: Embolization and transient blindness from carotid atheroma. Surgical considerations. Arch Surg 93:787, 1966
20. Moore WS, Hall AD: Ulcerated atheroma of the carotid artery. A cause of transient cerebral ischemia. Am J Surg 116:237, 1968
21. Moore WS, Hall AD: Importance of emboli from carotid bifurcation in pathogenesis of cerebral ischemic attacks. Arch Surg 101:708, 1970
22. Imparato AM, Riles TS, Gorstein F: The carotid bifurcation plaque: Pathologic findings associated with cerebral ischemia. Stroke 10:238, 1979
23. Dujovny M, Kossovsky N, Loubeau JM, et al: Scanning electron microscopic and x-ray energy spectrographic analysis of the inner surface of human atherosclerotic carotid plaques. Neurosurgery 8:60, 1981
24. Edwards JH, Kricheff II, Riles T, et al: Angiographically undetected ulceration of the carotid bifurcation as a cause of embolic stroke. Neuroradiology 132:369, 1979
25. Hertzer NR, Beven EG, Benjamin S: Ultramicroscopic ulcerations and thrombi of the carotid bifurcation. Arch Surg 112:1394, 1977
26. Smith RR, Russell WF, Percy ML: Ultrastructure of carotid plaques. Surg Neurol 14:145, 1980
27. Maddison FE, Moore WS: Ulcerated atheroma of the carotid artery: Arteriographic appearance. American Journal of Roentgenology, Radium Therapy and Nuclear Medicine, 107:530, 1969
28. Blaisdell FW, Glickman M, Trunkey DD: Ulcerated atheroma of the carotid artery. Arch Surg 108:491, 1974
29. Eisenberg RL, Nemzek WR, Moore WS, et al: Relationship of transient ischemic attacks and angiographically demonstrable lesions of the carotid artery. Stroke 8:483, 1977
30. Thiele BL, Young JV, Chikos PM, et al: Correlation of arteriographic findings and symptoms in cerebrovascular disease. Neurology 30:1041, 1980
31. Moore WS, Boren C, Malone JM, et al: Natural history of nonstenotic asymptomatic ulcerative lesions of the carotid artery. Arch Surg 113:1352, 1978
32. Kroener JM, Dorn PL, Shoor PM, et al: Prognosis of asymptomatic ulcerating carotid lesions. Arch Surg 115:1387, 1980
33. Dixon S, Pais O, Raviola C, et al: Natural history of non-stenotic asymptomatic ulcerative lesions of the carotid artery: A further analysis. Arch Surg 1982. (in press)

Kenneth E. McIntyre, Jr.
Jerry Goldstone

14

Carotid Surgery for Crescendo TIA and Stroke in Evolution

Several years have passed since our first report on emergency carotid artery surgery for neurologically unstable patients.[1] At the time of that report, operative intervention in patients with either crescendo transient ischemic attacks or strokes in evolution was considered controversial. Since then, however, other reports have appeared attesting to the efficacy of emergency carotid artery surgery in a highly selected group of patients,[2-4] so that at the present time, the topic of emergency carotid artery surgery is not so controversial. A recent update of the results of emergency carotid endarterectomy for acute neurologic deficits, however, has brought some new evidence to light. This chapter will review these data and suggest a method for evaluation that will select those patients who will benefit from an aggressive surgical approach.

CLINICAL MATERIAL AND METHODS

During the preceding 3 years, 20 patients with acute unstable neurologic deficits underwent evaluation and surgical treatment on an emergency basis at the University of Arizona Health Sciences Center and Veterans Administration Medical Center at Tucson. Fourteen of these patients presented with crescendo transient ischemic attacks (hemispheric or monocular). The other six had stroke in evolution but with neurologic deficits of only mild to moderate degree. None of the patients in this report had an acute, severe, fixed, neurologic deficit or depressed levels of consciousness. As in our previous reports, the following definitions have been used:

Crescendo Transient Ischemic Attacks

Cerebral hemispheric or monocular episodes of transient ischemia, usually lasting a few minutes to a few hours, leaving no residual signs and symptoms between attacks, with the attacks abruptly increasing in frequency to at least several each day.[5]

Stroke in Evolution

Several symptom patterns can be included in this term, which is also known as progressing stroke or incomplete stroke.[5] An acute neurologic deficit of modest degree may, within hours or days of the initial event, progress in a sequential series of acute exacerbations to a major stroke. Alternatively, after the initial episode, the neurologic deficit may improve temporarily only to reappear later, often with more widespread involvement, leading to a pattern of *waxing and waning* of signs and symptoms that occurs over hours to days, with an incomplete recovery.

Due to the nature of their clinical manifestations, these patients were evaluated on an urgent basis. Each patient except the one described below was evaluated by the neurology as well as the vascular surgery service. This team approach insures that the workup proceeds in an orderly and timely fashion. Each patient underwent computed axial tomography (CT scan) of the brain without identifying any who had acute cerebral infarction, intracerebral or subarachnoid hemorrhage, brain tumor, or other pathologic process that could be responsible for the symptoms. Craniocerebral angiography was then obtained without delay. Some of the patients were anticoagulated with intravenous heparin once the CT scan assured the absence of a contraindication to its use. The other patients were heparinized immediately following their arteriograms.

ANGIOGRAPHIC MANAGEMENT

Most patients underwent selective bilateral carotid arteriography by the transfemoral route using the Seldinger technique. In some patients, an incomplete study was done in that the procedure was terminated after a critical arterial lesion was identified. In such circumstances, only the carotid artery appropriate to the symptoms was examined, but in all cases there were at least two projections of the neck and ipsilateral intracranial vessels.

Recently, the technique of digital video subtraction angiography (DVSA or IV angiography) has been employed in selected patients with excellent definition of the arterial lesions.[6,7] Patients who were uncooperative or who exhibited a diminished cardiac output were excluded from this technique because it has been our experience that the quality of the images obtained under these circumstances is not acceptable. Since larger amounts of contrast media are often required for DVSA, we have also avoided its use in patients with renal dysfunction.

As in our previous reports, a *critical arterial lesion* is defined as one producing at least a 95 percent reduction in the diameter of the internal carotid artery or one that is associated with a thrombus seen on the arteriograms to be within the lumen of the vessel, either freely floating or attached to the wall. These preocclusive and thrombotic lesions are believed to be *unstable* due to their propensity to become totally occlusive or to embolize. Fifteen of the 20 patients in the present series had such a critical or unstable arterial lesion appropriate to the side of the cerebral symptoms. They were immediately heparinized and taken to the operating room as soon as possible. The other 5 patients, all in the crescendo TIA group, had non-stenotic ulcerated atheromata at the appropriate carotid bifurcation (one of these patients did not undergo arteriography, the lesion being identified at the time of operation).

SURGICAL MANAGEMENT

Each patient underwent emergency carotid thromboendarterectomy as soon as possible following his arteriogram, the maximum interval being 6 hours. All of these emergency operations were performed under general endotracheal anesthesia, with maintenance of a normal arterial pCO_2. Intraoperative blood pressure was maintained at or near preoperative ward levels. The need for an internal shunt was determined by the carotid back pressure as well as by the presence of a previous infarction of the symptomatic cerebral hemisphere. These criteria have previously been described elsewhere.[8] A shunt was also used in all of the patients who had stroke in evolution, because of concern for the possibility of early cerebral infarction. At the completion of the procedure, an intraoperative arteriogram was performed to ensure an adequate technical result.

CASE REPORTS

Several case histories will be described, each one selected as a typical example of the kinds of patients in this series.

Case 1

A 70-year-old female was admitted to the hospital with a history of right leg and right arm weakness, beginning the evening prior to admission, and lasting for a short time. On the following morning, she sustained five or six similar attacks, each lasting

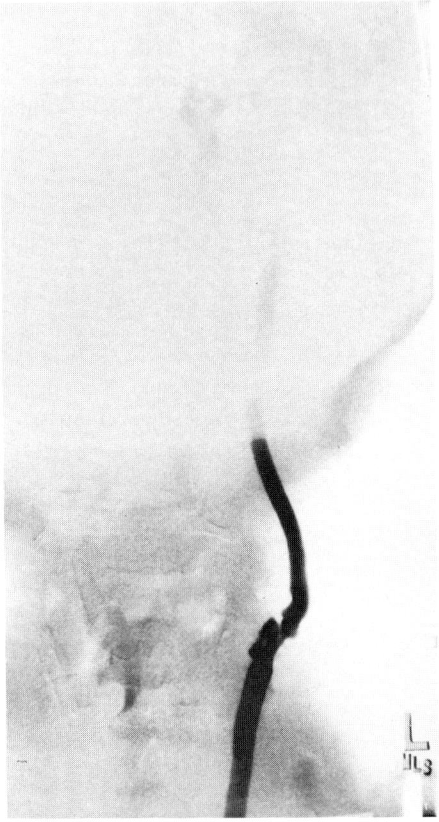

Figure 14-1. Left carotid arteriogram, case 1, showing severe ulceration without stenosis of left internal carotid artery. Note occlusion of external carotid artery.

approximately 10 minutes. She gave no history of previous stroke, transient ischemic attack, or hypertension. Due to the increasing frequency of attacks, an emergency evaluation was initiated. Physical exam revealed a normotensive, white female who was well-oriented. Carotid pulses were normal bilaterally, and there were no neck bruits. There was a central seventh cranial nerve weakness and decreased strength in the right arm and leg.

An initial CT scan was done, and this was interpreted as being normal. The patient then underwent emergency cerebral angiography which demonstrated a non-stenotic but severely ulcerated carotid plaque in the left internal carotid artery (Fig.14-1). Following the angiogram, she was taken immediately to the operating room and underwent an uncomplicated left carotid thromboendarterectomy. She had a smooth postoperative course and was discharged without neurologic deficit.

Comment

This patient was one of the few in this series with a non-stenotic ulcerated plaque as the etiology of her crescendo transient ischemic attacks. Because of the instability in her clinical course, emergent operation was undertaken.

Case 2

A 75-year-old female sustained 4 episodes of left hand and left leg weakness over a 4 hour interval, each lasting a few minutes, with complete resolution. She gave no history of previous cerebrovascular symptoms. She did, however, have a history of mild longstanding hypertension. Due to the rapid decline in her clinical course, with increasing number of left sided TIAs, a right carotid exploration was undertaken emergently. There was no preoperative CT scan or angiogram performed due to technical problems with the equipment. A non-stenotic multiply ulcerated lesion was found in the carotid bifurcation and was removed by carotid endarterectomy. She remained mildly hemiparetic postoperatively. A postoperative CT scan demonstrated only an acute small infarction in the posterior limb of the right internal capsule consistent with lacunar infarction (Fig.14-2).

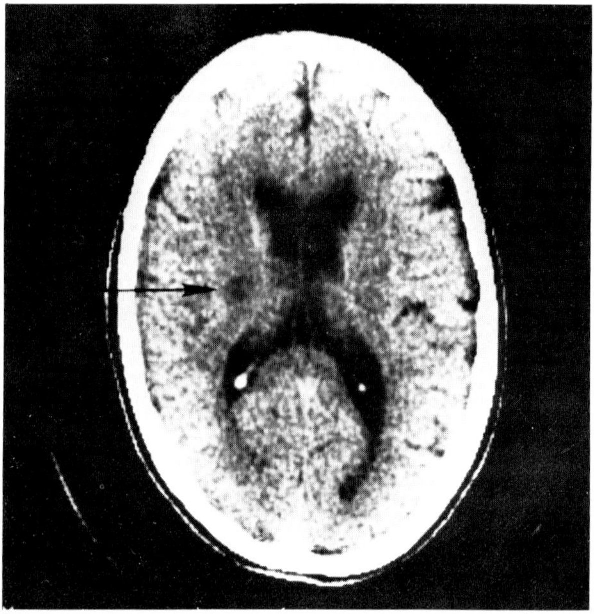

Figure 14-2. Computerized axial tomographic scan, case 2, showing lacunar infarct (arrow) in posterior limb of internal capsule on right side.

Comment

This case history demonstrates the value of a preoperative CT scan in the neurologically unstable patient. Lacunar infarction, subdural hematoma, subarachnoid hemorrhage, and intracerebral hematoma can cause symptoms very similar to those of transient cerebral ischemia. In this patient, a lacunar infarction in the posterior limb of the right internal capsule was the cause of her transient motor hemiparesis. If we had seen this lesion on a preoperative CT scan, we would not have performed carotid endarterectomy. Carotid endarterectomy did not interrupt the natural history of her disease process even though an ulcerated, non-stenotic atheroma was found and removed from her carotid bifurcation.

Case 3

A 68-year-old male presented with a history of two attacks of left hand and leg weakness and numbness lasting approximately 5 minutes. These attacks occurred approximately 2 hours apart. On the following day, he noted progressive weakness and numbness of his left hand, arm, and leg. For this reason, he sought medical attention. This cleared again within a short time, but his left sided hemiparesis became progressively worse over the next several hours. With this waxing and waning course, an emergency arteriogram was undertaken. This demonstrated a 99 percent stenosis of the right internal carotid artery with a free intraluminal thrombus above the stenosis (Fig. 14-3). He was immediately heparinized and taken to surgery. A right carotid endarterectomy was performed. Fresh clot lying within the lumen directly above the carotid stenosis was encountered. His deficit totally resolved immediately post-operatively.

Comment

This case demonstrates the waxing and waning course of a stroke in evolution. Had emergency evaluation with arteriography and subsequent operative intervention not taken place, his carotid artery probably would have totally occluded, and he would likely have suffered a major right hemispheric stroke.

Case 4

A 61-year-old male presented with several attacks of left hand numbness and weakness associated with loss of vision in the right eye on the morning of admission. He had had a previous left hemispheric stroke several years ago with no residual deficit. During the afternoon of his evaluation, he noted four more attacks of right monocular blindness and left arm weakness lasting but a few minutes. An emergency CT scan demonstrated an old left hemispheric infarct. There was no evidence, however, of any right hemispheric pathology. The patient then underwent an emergency carotid arteriogram which demonstrated a critical stenosis of the right internal carotid artery (Fig. 14-4). He was immediately heparinized and taken to the operating room

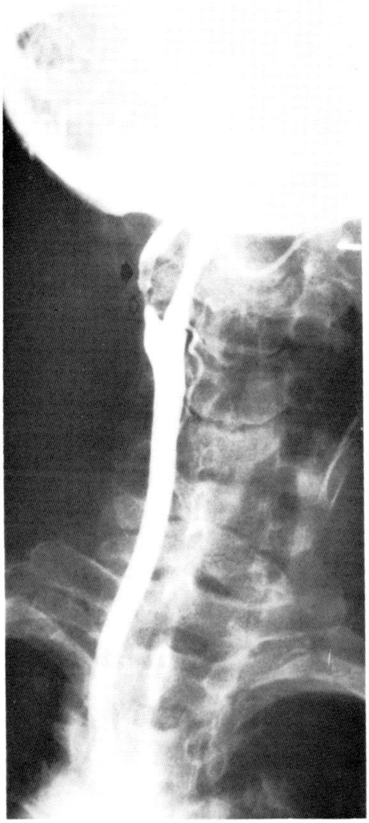

Figure 14-3. Right carotid arteriogram, case 3, showing unstable arterial lesion, with high grade stenosis (open arrow) and intraluminal thrombus (solid arrow) in internal carotid artery.

where a right carotid endarterectomy was performed. Postoperatively, he had complete resolution of his symptoms.

Comment

This is another example of crescendo TIAs originating from a critical stenosis of the internal carotid artery. We assume that he was embolizing small fragments from an ulcerated plaque in the vicinity of the stenosis.

RESULTS

There was no morbidity or mortality related to the angiographic procedures. All of the patients had dramatic, prompt, and complete relief of

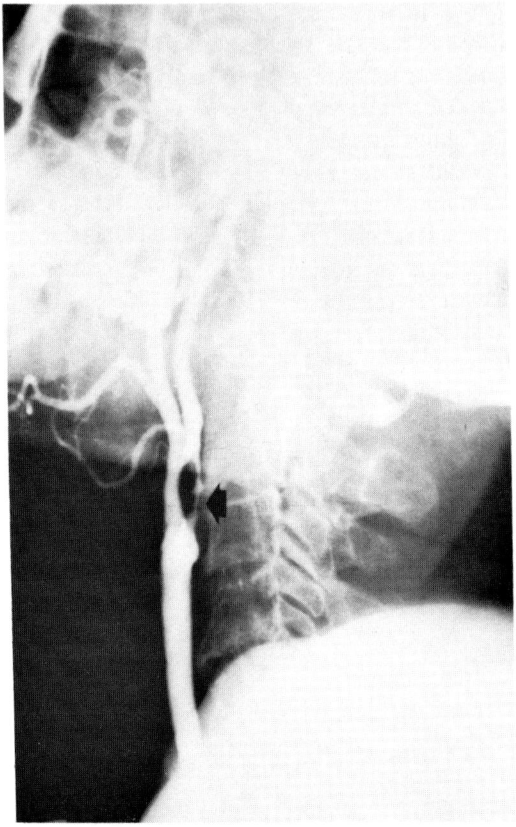

Figure 14-4. Right carotid arteriogram, case 4, showing critical stenosis with ulceration (arrow) of internal carotid artery.

their neurologic deficit following carotid endarterectomy except for the patient in whom preoperative arteriography and CT scan were omitted. This patient's crescendo transient ischemic attacks resulted in a mild, fixed deficit subsequently attributed to a lacunar infarction in the internal capsule (Fig. 14-2). None of the patients were treated with anticoagulants during the postoperative period, but all were given aspirin.

DISCUSSION

In the nearly thirty years since the first report of carotid endarterectomy, this procedure has become an accepted, if not the best, method of preventing strokes in patients with cerebral hemispheric or monocular transient ischemic attacks. Among the factors that determine its success and safety, the neurologic condition of the patient at the time of surgery and the experience and skill of the operating team are the most important. The results vary from institution to institution but appear to be best in patients who are neurologically intact and stable at the time of operation, and in patients with asymptomatic carotid stenosis who are operated upon prophylactically. Thompson, for example, reported a mortality of 4.2 percent for carotid operations performed within the first few days after an acute stroke, compared to 0.8 percent for patients with transient ischemic attacks and 0 percent for those with asymptomatic carotid bruit.[9] Furthermore, the surgical mortality when these operations are performed to restore flow to a totally occluded carotid artery during an acute, severe stroke, as reported by the Cooperative Study on Extracranial Arterial Occlusive Disease (EAO), is 42 percent.[10]

The fourteen patients in the present series with crescendo transient ischemic attacks, although neurologically unstable by virtue of an abrupt increase in frequency of symptoms, can be included in the group in which negligible morbidity and mortality can be expected from carotid endarterectomy. All of these patients, plus the ten reported in a previous publication,[3] had an excellent result except for the one described above who was having lacunar rather than hemispheric events. Carotid endarterectomy could not and did not influence her disease process.

The natural history of what we have called crescendo transient ischemic attacks is impossible to establish from perusal of the scientific literature. Mentzer et al. have recently described 12 patients with this clinical pattern. Seven were operated upon emergently with complete recovery, but five were treated nonoperatively with only one total recovery, three moderately to severely impaired, and one death.[2] In a recent review, Millikan and McDowell referred to patients with "a cluster of frequent carotid TIAs" and recommended emergency evaluation, anticoagulant treatment, and surgery.[11] Thus, while there is little hard data concerning patients with this type of clinical presentation, there appears to be good justification for and little controversy about an aggressive diagnostic and surgical approach.

Contrariwise, the natural history of stroke in evolution has been studied in some detail. Millikan reported a series of 204 consecutive patients in 1972.[12] Fourteen days after the onset of symptoms, 69 percent of this group were hemiparetic, 5 percent monoparetic, 14 percent had died, and only 12 percent had returned to normal. The results of several other series are equally grim. Anticoagulant therapy results in fewer patients having progression of neurologic symptoms but still leaves a large percentage with neurologic deficits. The excellent results obtained in the 5 patients in the present series and in the 18 patients in our previous series indicate that the natural history of selected patients with stroke in evolution can be altered favorably by emergency carotid endarterectomy. Mentzer et al. collated the published results of carotid endarterectomy for stroke in evolution from several series, including his own.[2] Out of a total of 217 patients so treated, 117 (56.5 percent) were improved, 52 (25.1 percent) were unchanged, 13 (8.7 percent) were worse, and only 20 (9.7 percent) died. These data stand in sharp contrast to the natural history data described above. The primary objective of treatment in these patients is prevention of cerebral infarction or the worsening of infarction after the pathologic process has begun. There is no known treatment to date that will reverse infarction once it occurs. Therefore, the timing of surgical intervention, when appropriate, is of utmost importance since the very nature of progressing stroke allows only a limited amount of time in which to make the initial observations and start treatment.

The reluctance of many, perhaps most, surgeons to recommend emergency carotid endarterectomy for patients with progressing stroke is based on data from the EAO Study, as well as the reports of Wylie et al.,[13] Breutman et al.,[14] and Gonzales and Lewis,[15] all of which indicate that carotid surgery is contraindicated for acute severe stroke. It has been postulated that the disastrous result following an apparently successful endarterectomy in this situation is due to restoration of flow and pressure into an area of ischemic brain, thereby converting an anemic into a hemorrhagic infarct and eventually into a massive hemorrhage into the area of infarction. Although experimental studies support the relationship of hemorrhagic infarction to revascularization, the evidence that it is reperfusion per se that produces the damage is not incontrovertible. Experimentally, it is possible to produce hemorrhagic infarction by reestablishing flow in an occluded middle cerebral artery, but hemorrhagic infarcts can also be produced by arterial occlusion alone. In both situations, hypertension appears to play a significant if not essential role. In fact, Fisher, whose early work on mechanisms of cerebral infarction is widely quoted in discussions of this subject, believes that these patients bleed from hypertension, and the idea that operation (reperfusion) converts a pale infarction into a hemorrhagic one "is a myth."[16]

Hemorrhagic cerebral infarction can also be caused by cerebral embolization with or without operation. Of 66 patients with hemorrhagic infarction described by Fisher and Adams, most were shown to have embolic occlusion of cerebral arteries.[17] Most of the patients reported by Wylie et al., Bruetman et al., and Gonzalez and Lewis had fresh, soft thrombus present at the carotid artery bifurcation that could easily have dislodged and traveled downstream during the performance of an operation. This may have been a more significant factor than restoration of flow in the production of the hemorrhagic infarctions in their patients. In addition, most of the patients in whom it occurred had acute, profound neurologic deficits, totally occluded internal carotid arteries, and at least some degree of hypertension. Our patients differ in that the neurologic deficits were only mild to moderate, and the arteries operated upon were not completely occluded. In addition, we have carefully monitored and controlled arterial blood pressure in the perioperative period.

Most of the operative deaths in the joint EAO study were in patients with preoperative severe neurologic deficits. The pathologic correlate of acute stroke is acute cerebral infarction, and, in general, the more extensive the infarction, the worse the clinical stroke. Except for the single patient who had a lacunar infarction, we do not know the pathologic process responsible for the symptoms in any of our patients. The fluctuating deficits preoperatively and their prompt and complete resolution postoperatively suggest that infarction had not occurred, or if it had, it was small.

The most important question that must be answered before making the decision to operate on these patients is whether acute cerebral infarction has occurred. Clinically, it is often very difficult to decide because of the fluctuating neurologic deficits. There are no laboratory tests that provide useful information and the electroencephalogram adds little of significance. Even though the CT scan is usually normal in the first hours following cerebral infarction unless the infarction is hemorrhagic, it is an important part of the early workup in patients like those in this series.[18] It may identify pathologic causes of the symptoms other than extracranial arterial disease, such as intracerebral hematoma, brain tumor, etc. Lacunar infarctions can also be frequently seen[19] (Fig. 14-2). These findings have an important influence on the decision to administer anticoagulants and to proceed with angiography and surgery.

In patients who manifest crescendo transient ischemic attacks or stroke in evolution and whose neurologic deficits cannot be explained by the findings on CT scan, arteriography must be the next diagnostic step. Although many clinicians are reluctant to subject neurologically unstable patients to arteriography for fear of exacerbating the neurologic deficit, we have seen no angiographic complications in this situation. Current arteriographic technique in our institution involves transfemoral retrograde catheterization and selective carotid injections, using small catheters and small amounts of contrast medium. Vertebral artery and aortic arch injections are not done routinely. The availability of intravenous (digital video subtraction) angiography offers an alternative method of obtaining images of the carotid arteries of diagnostic quality and may be especially useful in patients with severe peripheral vascular disease (Fig. 14-5).[7]

In our previous reports, all of the patients had fluctuating neurologic deficits and critical arterial lesions. This was also true in the patients operated upon by Sundt.[20,21] In the present series, although all of the stroke in evolution patients had critical arterial lesions, 4 patients with crescendo TIAs had lesions that were not as severe, yet their clinical presentation and response to surgery were equally dramatic.

Based upon our experience and that reported by others, we continue to

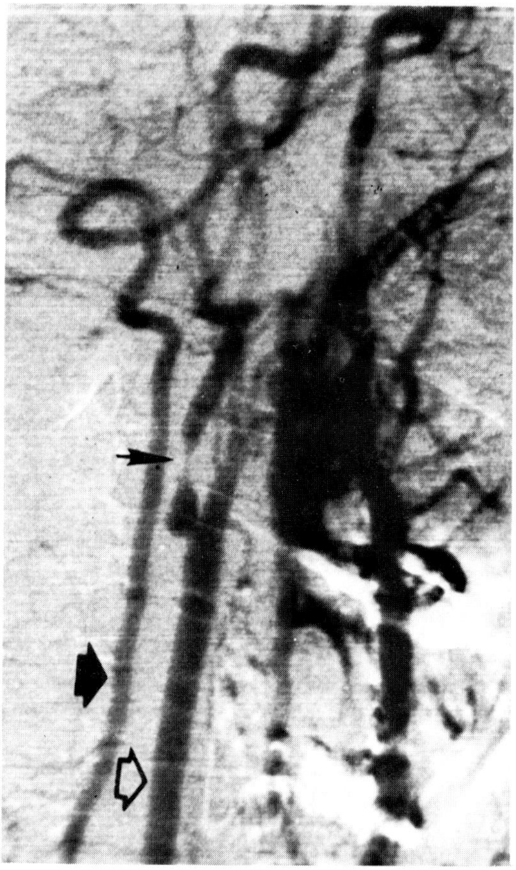

Figure 14-5. Digital video subtraction angiogram showing right common carotid artery (dark arrow), right vertebral artery (clear arrow), and critical stenosis (small dark arrow) in right internal carotid artery.

advocate an aggressive diagnostic and surgical approach to patients with acute unstable neurologic deficits. The workup of such patients should proceed as quickly as possible. Time will usually be saved if the neurologist and surgeon work together from the beginning. Figure 14-6 outlines our algorithm for this evaluation. A CT scan should be done early, primarily to exclude other diagnoses which may mimic transient ischemic attacks and for which anticoagulation may be dangerous.[19,22] The CT scan may not be entirely normal, but if it does not reveal an abnormality that corresponds to the clinical setting, arteriography should be performed as soon as possible. Heparin anticoagulation should be instituted after the CT scan, while the remainder of the clinical evaluation is in progress. If a critical arterial lesion is identified that corresponds to the patient's symptoms, emergency carotid

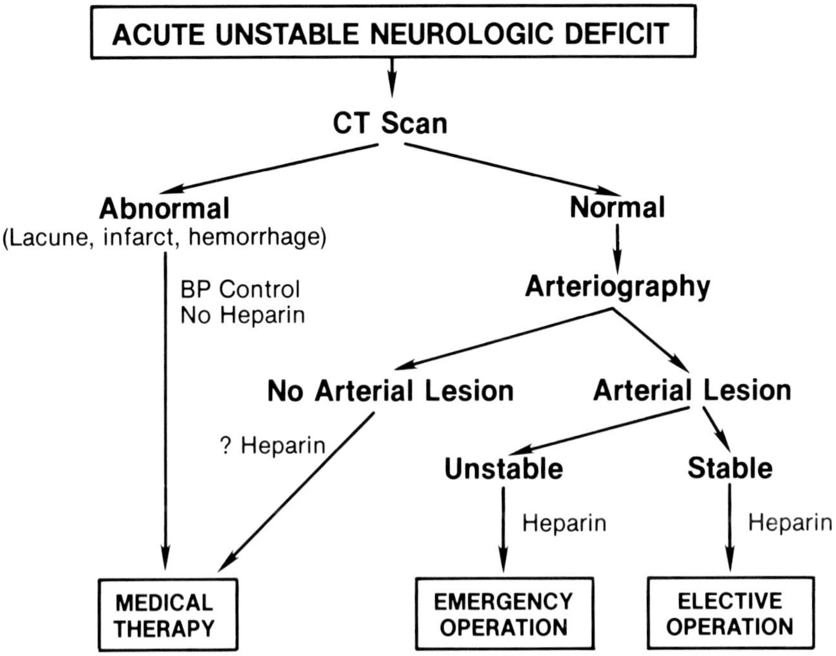

Figure 14-6. Algorithm depicting the recommended approach for the emergency evaluation and treatment of patients with acute unstable neurologic deficits.

endarterectomy should be advised. This also applies to a non-critical arterial lesion in a patient with crescendo TIAs. We have not, however, performed carotid endarterectomy emergently for stroke in evolution when only a stable, noncritical arterial lesion is identified. We have deferred operation until the neurologic status has stabilized. Patients without significant arterial lesions should continue to receive heparin anticoagulation until their workup is complete and their clinical status optimized.

We do not advocate arteriography or operation in patients with severe fixed neurologic deficits, especially when associated with depressed levels of consciousness. Presumably, cerebral infarction has already occurred in these individuals. Neither do we advocate operations to reestablish flow in a totally occluded internal carotid artery, whether or not there are symptoms of cerebrovascular insufficiency. The superficial temporal artery-to-middle cerebral artery bypass operations have proven beneficial for many patients in this situation.

Finally, the selection of an operative approach to any carotid lesion should be made only if the surgical team can perform such procedures with acceptable morbidity and mortality rates (less than about 3 percent combined), since postoperative neurologic morbidity and mortality vary from surgeon to surgeon and from institution to institution.

REFERENCES

1. Goldstone J, Moore W: Emergency carotid artery surgery in neurologically unstable patients. Arch Surg 111:1284, 1976
2. Mentzer, RM Jr, Finkelmeier BA, Crosby IK, et al: Emergency carotid endarterectomy for fluctuating neurologic deficits. Surgery 89:60, 1981
3. Goldstone J, Effeney DJ: The role of carotid endarterectomy in the treatment of acute neurologic deficits. Prog Cardiovasc Dis 22:415, 1980
4. Goldstone J, Moore WS: A new look at emergency carotid artery operations for the treatment of cerebrovascular insufficiency. Stroke 9:599, 1978
5. Carter AB: Clinical aspects of cerebral infarction, in Vinken JP, Bruyn GS (eds): Handbook of Clinical Neurology: Vascular Disease of the Nervous System, Volume 11. New York, North Holland Publishing Company and American Elsevier Publishing Company, 1972, p 292
6. Ovitt TW, Christenson PC, Fisher HD III, et al: Intravenous angiography using digital video subtraction: X-ray imaging system. AJNR 1:387, 1980
7. Christenson PC, Ovitt TW, Fisher HD III, et al: Intravenous angiography using digital video subtraction: Intravenous cervico-cerebrovascular angiography. AJNR 1:379, 1980
8. Moore WS, Yee JM, Hall AD: Collateral cerebral blood pressure: An index of tolerance to temporary carotid occlusion. Arch Surg 106:520, 1973
9. Thompson, JE, Austin DJ, Patman RD: Carotid endarterectomy for cerebrovascular insufficiency: Long-term results in 592 patients followed up to thirteen years. Ann Surg 172:663, 1970
10. Blaisdell WF, Clauss RH, Galbraith JG, et al: Joint study of extracranial arterial occlusion IV. Review of surgical considerations. JAMA 209:1889, 1969
11. Millikan CH, McDowell FH: Treatment of progressing stroke. Prog Cardiovasc Dis 22:397, 1980
12. Millikan CH: Discussion, in McDowell FH, Brennan RW (eds): Cerebral Vascular Diseases (Transactions of the Eighth Princeton Conference on Cerebral Vascular Disease). New York, Grune and Stratton, Inc., 1973, pp 209
13. Wylie EJ, Hein MF, Adams JE: Intracranial hemorrhage following surgical revascularization for treatment of acute strokes. J Neurosurg 21:212, 1964
14. Bruetman ME, Fields WS, Crawford ES, et al: Cerebral hemorrhage in carotid artery surgery. Arch Neurol 9:458, 1963
15. Gonzalez LL, Lewis CM: Cerebral hemorrhage following successful endarterectomy of the internal carotid artery. Surg Gynecol Obstet 123:773, 1966
16. Fisher CM, in discussion, Meyer JS, Mathew NT, Shimazu K: Clinical management of cerebral ischemia, in McDowell FH, Brennan RW (eds): Cerebral Vascular Disease, Eighth Conference. New York, Grune and Stratton, 1972, p 216
17. Fisher M, Adams RD: Observations on brain embolism with special reference to the mechanism of hemorrhagic infarction. J Neuropsychol Exp Neurol 10:92, 1951
18. Weisberg LA: Computerized tomographic enhancement pattern in cerebral infarction. Arch Neurol 37:21, 1980
19. Weisberg LA: Lacunar infarcts: Clinical and computed tomographic correlations. Arch Neurol 39:37, 1982
20. Sundt TM, Houser OW, Sharbrough FW: Carotid endarterectomy: Results, complications, and monitoring techniques, in Thompson RA, Green JR (eds): Advances in Neurology, vol. 16, New York, Raven, 1977, p 97
21. Sundt TM: Surgical therapy of occlusive vascular diseases of the brain, in Nyhus L (ed): Surgery Annual. New York, Appleton-Century-Crofts, 1974, p 393
22. Plenge KL, Sonntag VKH: Chronic subdural hematoma causing "Transient Ischemic Attacks" in a young woman. Ann Neurol 6:279, 1979

Jesse E. Thompson
C.M. Talkington
Wilson V. Garrett

15

Asymptomatic Carotid Bruit: Course and Surgical Management

It has now been clearly established that in many patients with cerebrovascular insufficiency the responsible atherosclerotic occlusions are in the extracranial vasculature. Since these lesions are in surgically accessible sites, it is technically feasible to increase cerebral blood flow or remove sources of emboli by surgical means. Carotid endarterectomy is highly effective in the treatment of patients with transient cerebral ischemia, since symptoms are relieved in most instances and the incidence of subsequent strokes is markedly reduced.[1,2,3,4]

A controversial area at present concerns the advisability of performing arteriography and operation on patients with asymptomatic carotid bruits. Asymptomatic subclavian bruits, even with a demonstrated subclavian steal syndrome, do not require operative intervention. However, the mid-carotid bruit, which reflects the presence of atherosclerosis at the common carotid bifurcation, is another matter. Seventy-five to 90 percent of such bruits arise from internal carotid plaques, the rest coming from external carotid plaques or other uncommon lesions.[1,5,6] The indications for endarterectomy in patients with asymptomatic carotid bruits, however, have not yet been precisely defined.

Auscultation of the neck for the presence of carotid bruits is an important examination in patients with cerebrovascular insufficiency syndromes. In fact, this should be done in every routine physical examination, especially in patients over the age of 40 and in those with evidence of atherosclerosis elsewhere in the body. Recently developed sophisticated stethoscopes for the heart are inadequate for the head and neck. The standard 3 cm bell stethoscope remains the most satisfactory one for cervical auscultation.

A bruit usually appears when diameter reduction is 50 percent (cross-sectional area reduction 75 percent) or greater, and may actually disappear at

85 to 90 percent diameter stenosis or when the lumen is only 0.5 cm to 1 mm in diameter.[1,7] Rarely, a bruit is present in the absence of any radiographically demonstrable carotid pathology. It has been attributed to a hemodynamic phenomenon of increased carotid flow resulting from total occlusion of the opposite carotid.[8]

Several studies have been done on patients with overt cerebrovascular insufficiency, correlating stenotic lesions demonstrated on arteriograms with carotid bruits heard in the neck.[5,9,10] The degree of correlation is very high when bruits are audible, ranging from 75 to 85 percent. Overall correlation between demonstrable carotid disease and bruits is about 60 percent, since lesions may be present on the arteriogram yet no bruit be audible. These include stenosis of less than 50 percent, ulcerated plaques without stenosis, severe stenosis with a lumen diameter of 1 mm or less, and total occlusions of the internal carotid artery.[3] A carotid bruit when present thus constitutes a significant finding in patients with cerebrovascular insufficiency. The controversy concerns the significance of the bruit in the absence of cerebral symptoms.[11,12]

What are the clinical consequences that have been observed in patients with asymptomatic carotid bruits followed for long periods of time? These may be listed as follows: (1) nothing may happen, (2) transient cerebral ischemic attacks (TIAs) may supervene, (3) frank strokes may occur without intervening episodes of transient ischemia, (4) total occlusion of the artery may occur without symptoms, and (5) total occlusion may occur with production of either transient ischemia or frank stroke. The hazard depends directly upon the lesion giving rise to the bruit and the status of all vessels, both primary and collateral, supplying the brain.

The report of Javid et al.[13] on the natural history of growth of carotid atheromas has important implications with regard to management of carotid bruits. In a study of 86 patients undergoing serial arteriography over a period of 1 to 9 years, they noted no change in size of the atheromas in only 35 (38 percent) of the patients studied but found a significant increase in 51 (62 percent). The increase was greater than 25 percent each year in 32 patients and less than 25 percent each year in 19.

It is thus apparent that the rate at which atherosclerosis progresses is unpredictable in the individual patient. Most common is a moderate rate of progression with a carotid lesion becoming symptomatic over 3 to 4 years. Some lesions progress very slowly or hardly at all, while others may progress rapidly to produce symptoms in a year or two.

It does not appear unreasonable, therefore, to consider the asymptomatic carotid bruit as part of the total picture of cerebrovascular insufficiency rather than an isolated finding on physical examination. The natural history of ischemic thrombotic stroke due to extracranial lesions must begin somewhere.

It may begin as a plaque at the common carotid bifurcation and its first physical manifestation be an asymptomatic bruit. With time, the asymptomatic lesion becomes symptomatic from ulceration and embolization or from impairment of cerebral blood flow. It is to be hoped that the first symptom is a TIA when therapy can be initiated. At times, however, the first symptom is hemiplegia especially if a stenotic carotid undergoes acute total occlusion. This sequence of events is seen repeatedly in retrospective studies of patients with completed strokes.[13,14,15,16] Many other factors enter in to complicate this simplistic scheme: namely, multiple lesions both extracranial and intracranial, anatomic configurations of cerebral collateral pathways, rate of progression of atherosclerosis in the individual patient, hypertension, diabetes, etc., to mention some of the more important ones. The length of time during which these bruits are present is also very important.

A considerable body of data bearing on the asymptomatic carotid bruit is available. These data include our personal experiences and those of others taken from the literature.

ASYMPTOMATIC BRUITS FOLLOWED BUT UNOPERATED UPON

Three series of patients with asymptomatic bruits followed but not operated upon when the bruit was initially detected are available for comparison.[15,17,18] The data are quite consistent in the incidence of ischemic cerebral episodes observed during follow-up from 2 to 16 years. The incidence of transient ischemic attacks thus varies from 11.3 percent to 26.8 percent, while the incidence of strokes, both fatal and nonfatal, varies from 15 percent to 18.6 percent. The incidence of long-term deaths in all series is quite high, averaging almost 40 percent. The majority of these deaths are cardiac in origin although a significant portion result from stroke. It is apparent from these data that the asymptomatic carotid bruit is not a benign lesion if observed for a sufficiently long period of time.

Data are also available on patients with asymptomatic bruits who were followed but not operated upon when the bruit was initially heard but who were studied by noninvasive screening examinations. They are grouped into categories depending upon whether the examination was positive or negative. Kartchner and McRae[14] carried out oculoplethysmography (OPG) while Busuttil et al.[19] performed oculopneumoplethysmography combined with supraorbital Doppler studies. Kartchner and McRae thus reported an incidence of 4.9 percent for TIAs and 11.9 percent for strokes when the OPG was positive, but an incidence of 2.1 percent and 1.9 percent respectively when the OPG was negative. Likewise, Busuttil et al. gave an incidence of 28.9 percent for TIAs and 6.6 percent for strokes when the tests were positive and 7.1 percent and zero when negative. It appears from the data in both series that patients with positive tests, or hemodynamically significant carotid lesions, are at greater risk for subsequent cerebral ischemic episodes, both TIAs and strokes, than are those with negative tests, or who have nonhemodynamically significant lesions.

ASYMPTOMATIC BRUITS OPERATED UPON WITH CAROTID ENDARTERECTOMY

A number of authors have reported short-term results following carotid endarterectomy performed for asymptomatic carotid bruits.[2,15,16,20,21,22,23,24,25,26,27] Operative mortality for these patients is quite low, ranging from zero to 2.4 percent, averaging less than 1 percent. This low mortality is acceptable for this elderly group of atherosclerotic patients whose average age is 65 years.

The incidence of transient neurologic deficits related to operation ranges from zero to 2.9 percent, while that of permanent deficits ranges from zero to 3 percent. It is clear from these reports that operation may be performed in these asymptomatic patients with low mortality and morbidity.

There are several reports on the long-term functional results of carotid endarterectomy for asymptomatic bruits.[2,15,22,23,25] More than 90 percent of the patients subjected to prophylactic endarterectomy remained asymptomatic during follow-up periods ranging up to 16 years. There is a consistent observation that between 2.8 and 4.5 percent of patients developed subsequent TIAs, while an additional 2.9 percent to 4.6 percent developed strokes, either fatal or nonfatal. This incidence of TIAs and strokes is very similar to that found in numerous long-term studies of patients with TIAs subjected to therapeutic endarterectomy, an observation that fits the unified concept enunciated above. The long-term death rate remains high, 30 to 40 percent. In these patients, however, death from stroke is very low, the majority resulting from cardiac disease.

PERSONAL EXPERIENCE

During a 24-year period from 1957 to 1981, we performed 1666 operations on 1323 private patients with the various syndromes of cerebrovascular insufficiency (Table 15-1). Among patients with asymptomatic bruits, two series—an operated group and a non-operated control group—have been followed pari-passu over the years. A total of 270 patients with asymptomatic mid-carotid bruits have been studied. Of these, 132 were subjected to endarterectomy primarily, while 138 were followed but not operated upon when the bruit was first detected. Follow-up extended to 17 years. Results of this long-term follow-up study have previously been reported

Table 15-1
Operative Mortality Following Carotid Endarterectomy
Total Experience = 24 Years

Clinical Category	No. of Patients	No. of Operations	No. of Deaths	Patient Mortality	Procedure Mortality
Frank Stroke	357	433	22	6.2%	5.1%
Transient Ischemia	747	959	11	1.5%	1.1%
Chronic Ischemia	22	28	0	0	0
Asymptomatic Bruit	197	246	0	0	0
Totals	1323	1666	33	2.5%	2%

in detail.[15] There were no operative deaths. Two patients sustained transient neurologic deficits related to operation, which cleared completely, and two additional patients had permanent mild deficits, an incidence of 1.2 percent. Thirty-five patients, or 26.5 percent, had bilateral operations performed in separate stages.

Table 15-2 displays the long-term follow-up data on these two groups of patients. There is a significant difference in the incidence of long-term ischemic episodes in favor of patients operated upon prophylactically as compared with nonoperated controls. The average follow-up period in both groups of patients was 55 months. Among the 138 patients in the nonoperated group, 24 subsequently sustained total internal carotid artery occlusion with disappearance of the bruit. Of these 24, 10 patients developed TIAs and were operated upon, while 10 others sustained frank strokes without an intervening

Table 15-2
Long-term Follow-up Data on Operated and Nonoperated Patients

	Asymptomatic	TIAs	Stroke Nonfatal	Stroke Fatal	Length of follow-up
Operated 132 patients	120 90.9%	6 4.5%	3 2.3%	3 2.3%	6 to 184 months mean—55.1 mos.
Non-operated 138 patients	77 55.8%	37 26.8%	21 15.2%	3 2.2%	To 199 months mean—54.9 mos.
Significance	$p < 0.01$	$p < 0.01$	$p < 0.01$		

episode of transient ischemia. Four patients developed total occlusion without symptoms. Patients treated by prophylactic operation have a more favorable long-term outlook, from the standpoint of subsequent ischemic cerebral episodes, than their nonoperated counterparts. There is a paucity of data in the literature on this matter. The data from our personal experiences represent the only series where operated and nonoperated patients with asymptomatic bruits have been followed simultaneously over the years and their long-term status documented.

During long-term follow-up, 43 of 132 patients in the operated group died (32.6 percent), while 51 of 138 patients in the nonoperated group died (37 percent). Seventy-two percent of the deaths among the operated patients and 48 percent of those in the nonoperated group were due to cardiac disease, thus pointing up the severe and widespread nature of atherosclerosis in these patients with cerebrovascular disease.

Since publication of the data presented above, the series of operated asymptomatic carotid bruits now numbers 246 operations in 197 patients, without operative mortality (Table 15-1). We have continued to follow a number of patients with asymptomatic bruits who were not operated upon when the bruit was first heard. During a 5-year period we have encountered some 90 additional patients. Twenty-two (24.4 percent) have developed TIAs while under observation. Twenty (22.2 percent) have suffered frank strokes of varying severity during this period. These data are in accord with our previously published figures. It appears from our data, and those of others, that certain individuals over the age of 40 with asymptomatic carotid bruits are at definite risk for subsequent ischemic cerebral episodes if allowed to go untreated. Patients treated by prophylactic carotid endarterectomy have a more favorable outlook than the nonoperated group. The problem then is how to identify the patient at risk.

PROTOCOL FOR MANAGEMENT

The questions that arise when one first hears a bruit in an asymptomatic patient are the following: does the bruit denote a significant lesion in the internal carotid artery, and how can one determine its significance without subjecting the patient to the risk of unnecessary arteriography? Several non-invasive screening tests have been developed and still others are under intensive investigation. With perfection of these techniques in the future, it should be possible to assess more accurately both anatomic and functional hemodynamic components of the lesions responsible for bruits, thus making more precise the indications for arteriography, the definitive diagnostic maneuver. Once arteriography has been accomplished, indications for endarterectomy are usually straightforward. Present methods for evaluation of the anatomic components include pulsed and continuous-wave Doppler imaging, B-mode scanning methods, and intravenous digital subtraction angiography (DSA). Techniques assessing the functional hemodynamic components include the OPG-Kartchner, the OPG-Gee and Doppler methods.[28]

One factor that is unpredictable is the rate at which atherosclerosis progresses in the individual patient. The only way that this progression can be determined is by careful follow-up examinations at appropriate intervals by whatever means available: physical examination, non-invasive tests, or invasive arteriograms.

Based on the considerations discussed above, the authors' management of patients with asymptomatic carotid bruit follows three steps: (1) noninvasive screening, (2) cerebral arteriography and (3) carotid endarterectomy.

Noninvasive Screening

Noninvasive screening tests can be applied to all patients. At present, we use principally the OPG-Kartchner and B-mode real-time scanning. The ease and safety of such examinations make possible serial testing at regular intervals to determine if a bruit-producing lesion found initially to be insignificant is indeed progressing toward one of significance, when arteriography may be required.

With the introduction of the intravenous digital subtraction angiographic technique, evaluation of lesions responsible for asymptomatic carotid bruits will in all likelihood become simpler and much more precise, perhaps eliminating invasive arteriography in some cases. We are beginning to use the technique at present and are greatly impressed with the early results.

Cerebral Arteriography

As cerebral arteriography has become increasingly safer with retrograde techniques and local anesthesia, it may be recommended more liberally than previously, but not routinely, in evaluating asymptomatic bruits. The overall general status of each patient should be considered very carefully. Arteriography should not be done if some contraindication to endarterectomy already exists. It is not to be recommended if the bruit is soft and unilateral, if other conditions take priority over study of the bruit such as a painful aneurysm or a gangrenous leg, or if the noninvasive tests are negative. It may be recommended if bruits are bilateral and harsh, in patients with known progressive atherosclerosis elsewhere, prior to other major operations, when noninvasive tests are positive, and when one's best clinical judgement indicates that it is necessary. It should be emphasized that an experienced and skillful arteriographer should be available so that complications remain well under 1 percent.

Carotid Endarterectomy

If the arteriogram shows that the bruit arises from a lesion posing no stroke hazard, such as the external carotid, operation need not be considered. If a significant atherosclerotic stenosis is found in the common or internal carotid, endarterectomy may be recommended. Specific indications include: (1) bilateral stenoses; (2) unilateral stenosis with contralateral occlusion; (3) stenosis in the artery to the dominant hemisphere; (4) known progressive atherosclerosis elsewhere in the peripheral vasculature, especially in younger patients; and (5) contemplated major surgery of another sort, particularly cardiac surgery.

If prophylactic carotid surgery is to be considered, mutiple risk factors such as hypertension, history of myocardial infarction, or congestive heart failure in patients over 65 should not be present.[22] This is emphasized by the high long-term mortality from heart disease during the early years of follow-up[15] and the high operative mortality associated with these factors in patients undergoing carotid endarterectomy.[29] Since no unnecessary technical risks should be taken, an experienced surgical team should be available and appropriate measures for cerebral protection used to avoid neurologic deficits. Some authors recommend selective shunting based on either intra-operative neurologic testing, electroencephalographic monitoring, or mea-

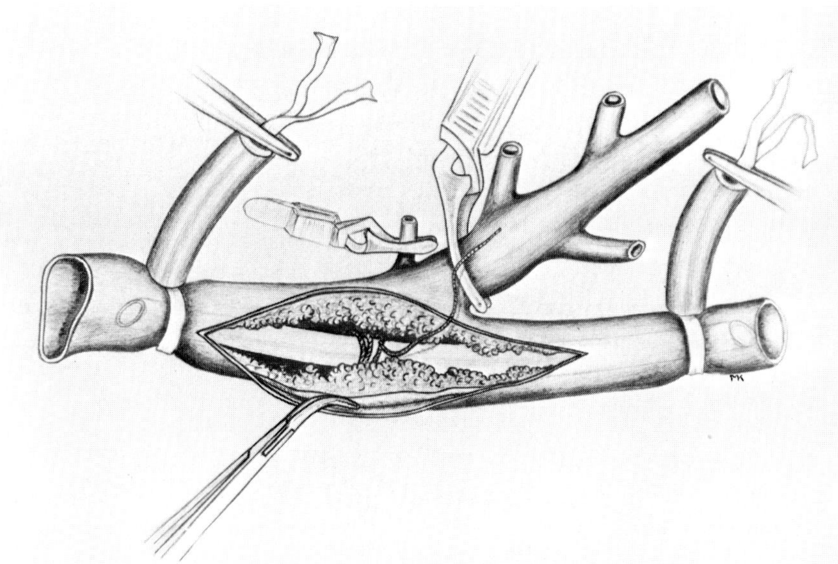

Figure 15-1. Diagram illustrating the technique of carotid endarterectomy in which a temporary inlying shunt is routinely employed with the patient under general anesthesia.

surement of internal carotid artery stump pressure.[4] Our preference is to use general anesthesia and a routine temporary shunt (Fig. 15-1).

Over the years, prophylactic endarterectomy has been recommended for the asymptomatic patient with carotid bruits who is about to undergo a major operation of another sort where a hypotensive episode might well result in a stroke. Two recent reports question the validity of this indication, citing the low degree of correlation between presence of bruits and incidence of postoperative stroke in patients undergoing aortic operations.[11,12] Although at present, with skillful anesthetic management and avoidance of hypotension, the risk of stroke attendant upon most operative procedures in the presence of asymptomatic carotid stenosis is quite low, ischemic accidents do occur.[30] In our own series of 138 patients with asymptomatic bruits not subjected to primary prophylactic endarterectomy, five strokes occurred following femoropopliteal bypass, inguinal herniorrhaphy, lumbar sympathectomy, and transurethral prostatic resection. This is an infrequent but serious problem, and the question is how to identify the patient at risk for stroke without subjecting all patients to carotid arteriography. Recommendations are based largely on opinion rather than on well-documented facts.

Of great concern is stroke complicating coronary artery bypass. In several studies, this figure approximates 2 percent.[31] A number of groups have attempted to reduce the incidence of stroke by prophylactic carotid endarterectomy.[29,31,32,33,34] Three approaches have evolved: carotid endarterectomy prior to, combined with, or subsequent to myocardial revascularization. Feasibility of the combined approach has been documented.[31,32,35] However, Hertzer et al.[31] observed that patients with the combined procedures sustained an operative mortality of 4.3 percent and a stroke rate of 4.3 percent, while those having staged procedures had an operative mortality of 1.7 percent and a stroke rate of 1.5 percent. Recently, Craver et al.[35] in recommending concomitant carotid and coronary artery reconstruction, reported zero mortality, a 2 percent incidence of myocardial infarction, and a 1.3 percent incidence of neurologic deficit related to the combined procedure. From information available in the literature, certain recommendations can be made. In the event of severe simultaneous carotid and cardiac disease, a combined procedure may be necessary.[29] If one system has more severe disease, it takes priority and operations may be staged. Crawford et al.[36] have also demonstrated the feasibility of combined carotid and non-coronary operations in patients with severe carotid disease.

Another approach to the overall problem of whether or not carotid arteriography and operation should be performed prior to other major operations is the application of preoperative noninvasive screening tests to evaluate the hemodynamic significance of carotid bruits. Kartchner and McRae[14] have studied patients with oculoplethysmography (OPG) and carotid phonoangiography (CPA). Among 42 patients with positive OPGs who did not undergo prophylactic endarterectomy, the stroke rate was 17 percent, in contrast to those with negative OPGs in whom the stroke rate was 1 percent.

It appears that a small but significant proportion of patients with asymptomatic bruits are at risk for stroke if subjected to major non-carotid operations. Those patients at greatest risk can be identified by the appropriate use of non-invasive screening tests. Patients with simultaneous carotid and coronary disease are considered to be particularly vulnerable.

REFERENCES

1. Thompson JE, Kartchner MM, Austin DJ, et al: Carotid endarterectomy for cerebrovascular insufficiency (Stroke): Follow-up of 359 cases. Ann Surg 163:751, 1966
2. Moore WS, Boren C, Malone JM, et al: Asymptomatic carotid stenosis. Immediate and long-term results after prophylactic endarterectomy. Am J Surg 138:228, 1979
3. Thompson JE, Patman RD, Talkington CM: Carotid surgery for cerebrovascular insufficiency. Curr Prob in Surg 15: 1978, p 68
4. Thompson JE, Talkington CM: Carotid endarterectomy: Surgical Progress. Ann Surg 184:1, 1976
5. David TE, Humphries AW, Young JR, et al: A correlation of neck bruits and arteriosclerotic carotid arteries. Arch Surg 107:729, 1973
6. Gautier JC, Rosa A, Lhermitte F: Auscultation corotidienne. Correlations chez 200 patients avec 332 angiographies. Rev. Neurol. (Paris) 131:175, 1975
7. Allen N: The significance of vascular murmurs in the head and neck. Geriatrics 20:525, 1965
8. Allen N, Mustian V: Origin and significance of vascular murmurs of the head and neck. Medicine 41:227, 1962
9. Gilroy J, Meyer JS: Auscultation of the neck in occlusive cerebrovascular disease. Circulation 25:300, 1962
10. McDowell F, Rennie L, Ejrup B: Arterial bruit in cerebrovascular disease, in Millikan CH, Siekert RG, Whisnant JP (eds): Cerebral Vascular Diseases. New York, Grune and Stratton, 1966
11. Carney WI Jr, Steward WB, DePinto DJ et al: Carotid bruit as a risk factor in aortoiliac reconstruction. Surgery 81:567, 1977
12. Treiman RL, Foran RF, Cohen L, et al: Carotid bruit. A follow-up report on its significance in patients undergoing an abdominal aortic operation. Arch Surg 114:1138, 1979
13. Javid H, Ostermiller WE, Hengesh JW, et al: Natural history of carotid bifurcation atheroma. Surgery 67:80, 1970
14. Kartchner MM, Mcrae LP: Non-invasive laboratory evaluation, II. The clinical use of oculoplethysmography and carotid phonangiography, in Baker WH (ed): Diagnosis and Treatment of Carotid Artery Disease. Mount Kisco, NY, Futura Publishing Co., 1979, p 62
15. Thompson JE, Patman RD, Talkington CM: Asymptomatic carotid bruit: Long-term outcome of patients having endarterectomy compared with unoperated controls. Ann Surg 188:308, 1978
16. Wylie EJ: Is an asymptomatic carotid stenosis a surgical lesion? in Courbier R, Jausseran JM, Reggi M (eds): Arteriopathies Cerebrales Extracraniennes Asymptomatiques. Lyon, France, Medicale OBERVAL, 1980, p 231:240
17. Cooperman M, Martin EW Jr, Evans WE; Significance of asymptomatic carotid bruits. Arch Surg 113:1339, 1978

18. Dorazio RA, Ezzet F, Nesbitt NJ: Long-term follow-up of asymptomatic carotid bruits. Am J Surg 140:212, 1980
19. Busuttil R, Baker W, Davidson JD, et al: Carotid artery stenosis-hemodynamic significance and clinical course. JAMA 245:1438, 1981
20. Duke LJ, Slaymaker EE, Lamberth WC, et al: Carotid arterial reconstruction: Ten-year experience. Am Surg 45:281, 1979
21. Hertzer NR, Beven EG, Greenstreet RL, et al: Internal carotid back pressure, intraoperative shunting, ulcerated atheroma, and the incidence of stroke during carotid endarterectomy. Surgery 83:306, 1978
22. Javid H, Ostermiller WE, Hegesh JW, et al: Carotid endarterectomy for asymptomatic patients. Arch Surg 102:389, 1971
23. Kanaly PJ, Peyton WD, Cannon JP, et al: The asymptomatic bruit. Am J Surg 134:821, 1977
24. Kremer RM, Ahlquist RE Jr: The prophylactic carotid thromboendarterectomy. Am Surg 45:703, 1979
25. Lefrak EA, Guin GA: Prophylactic carotid artery surgery in patients requiring a second operation. South Med J 67:185, 1974
26. Whitney GW, Kahn EW, Estes JW, et al: Carotid artery surgery without a temporary indwelling shunt. Arch Surg 115:1393, 1980
27. Natali J, Benhamou AC, Kieffer E, et al: Chirurgie des stenoses carotidiennes des patients asymptomatiques apres 70 ans, in Courbier R, Jausseran JW, Reggi M (eds): Arteriopathies Cerebrale Extracraniennes Asymptomatiques, Lyon, France, Medicale OBERVAL, 1980, p 393
28. Barnes RW: Noninvasive evaluation of the carotid bruit. Ann Rev Med 31:201, 1980
29. Ennix CL Jr, Laurie GW, Morris GC Jr, et al: Improved results of carotid endarterectomy in patients with symptomatic coronary disease: An analysis of 1,546 consecutive carotid operations. Stroke 10:122, 1979
30. Kartchner MM, McRae LP: Noninvasive evaluation and management of the "asymptomatic" carotid bruit. Surgery 82:840, 1977
31. Hertzer NR, Loop FD, Taylor PC, et al: Staged and combined surgical approach to simultaneous carotid and coronary vascular disease. Surgery 84:803, 1978
32. Bernhard VM, Johnson WD, Peterson JJ: Carotid artery stenosis: Association with surgery for coronary artery disease. Arch Surg 105:837, 1972
33. Mehigan JT, Buch WS, Pipkin RD, et al: A planned approach to coexistent cerebrovascular disease in coronary artery bypass candidates. Arch Surg 112:1403, 1977
34. Urschel HC, Razzuk MA, Gardner MA: Management of concomitant occlusive disease of the carotid and coronary arteries. J Thor and Cardiovasc Surg 72:829, 1976
35. Craver JM, Murphy DA, Jones EL, et al: Concomitant carotid and coronary artery reconstruction. Ann Surg 195:712, 1982 (in press)
36. Crawford ES, Palamara AE, Kasparian AS: Carotid and noncoronary operations: Simultaneous, staged, delayed. Surgery 87:1, 1980

James J. Schuler
D. Preston Flanigan
Larry R. Williams

16

The Results of Carotid Endarterectomy in Patients with Tandem Carotid Lesions

Endarterectomy of the carotid bifurcation and proximal internal carotid artery is now firmly established as an effective, safe, and durable form of treatment for transient ischemic attacks and resolved strokes in the carotid territory.[1-5] It has been shown that approximately three-fourths of strokes or transient ischemic attacks can reasonably be attributed to either hemodynamically significant stenosis and/or embolic events originating from atherosclerotic plaques at the carotid bifurcation.[6] These lesions are considered surgically accessible, and the beneficial results of operative intervention are well documented.[1-5] However, as many as one-third of patients subjected to complete aortic arch, carotid, and cerebral angiography, can be shown to have both surgically accessible and inaccessible lesions.[6-13] The majority of the surgically inaccessible lesions are located in the area of the carotid siphon.[6-13] The carotid siphon is that segment of the internal carotid artery between its exit from the petrous bone and its division into anterior and middle cerebral arteries. This combination of disease has been termed "tandem" carotid lesions.[14]

Numerous authors have previously suggested that carotid endarterectomy for carotid bifurcation disease may be contraindicated in the presence of concomitant carotid siphon stenosis either because of an increased risk of stroke[15-18] or the potential failure of carotid bifurcation endarterectomy alone to relieve symptoms caused by lesions in tandem.[14,19] The present study was undertaken to assess any differences in stroke rate, mortality, or relief of symptoms in patients with and without such tandem lesions following elective carotid endarterectomy.

METHODS

Between August 1, 1978 and December 31, 1981, 111 patients underwent 126 elective carotid endarterectomies at the University of Illinois Hospital or the West Side Veterans Administration Hospital in Chicago. During January, 1982, the charts, angiograms, and operative notes of these patients were reviewed and the patients were interviewed with specific emphasis on the early or late recurrence of transient ischemic attacks or strokes. Review of the angiograms revealed 26 patients who had undergone 28 carotid endarterectomies in whom intracerebral angiography either was not done or the views obtained were of insufficient quality to assess the presence or absence of disease in the carotid siphon. An additional six patients who had undergone 7 carotid endarterectomies were lost to follow-up. Thus, 91 carotid bifurcation endarterectomies performed in 79 patients were available for analysis.

The percent stenosis involving both the carotid siphon and bifurcation was calculated by measuring the width of the dye column in the diseased portion of the vessel as compared to the width of the dye column in the nearest portion of the artery distal to the stenosis which showed no disease. Both anteroposterior and lateral projections were examined and the projection showing the greatest degree of stenosis was used for calculating the percent stenosis. Stenoses of less than 20 percent were considered normal.

Patients were divided into two groups: Group I (44 patients; 47 endarterectomies) had carotid bifurcation stenosis only; Group II (35 patients; 44 endarterectomies) had carotid siphon stenosis in conjunction with bifurcation stenosis. Follow-up ranged from 1 to 40 months with a mean follow-up of 15.9 months. Differences between groups were determined by chi-square analysis using Yates' correction for continuity. Differences were considered significant at the $p < .05$ level.

All carotid endarterectomies were performed by general surgery residents or fellows in the Division of Peripheral Vascular Surgery and were performed under the direct and constant intraoperative supervision of Dr. Flanigan or Dr. Schuler. All operations were performed under normovolemic, normotensive, normocarbic general anesthesia. Systemic heparin, 5,000 units, was given intravenously prior to clamping the carotid artery. Sodium pentothal, 250 mg, was given as a bolus intravenously approximately 5 minutes before clamping the carotid artery and continued at a rate of 8 milligrams per minute intravenously for the duration of carotid clamping in all patients except those with cardiac contraindications to the use of barbiturates. No shunts were used and all but four arteriotomies were closed without a patch. Intraoperative completion arteriography was not routinely performed. In the latter half of the series, however, real time B-mode intraoperative ultrasonography was performed following closure of the arteriotomy to assess the technical adequacy of the procedure.

RESULTS

Incidence of Carotid Siphon Stenosis

Forty-four of the 91 carotid arterial systems subjected to endarterectomy had carotid siphon stenosis of greater than 20 percent, for an incidence of siphon stenosis in this series of 48 percent. Eighteen of 91 carotid systems (19.8 percent) had carotid siphon stenosis more severe than proximal internal carotid stenosis. No patient had angiographically significant occlusive disease in that segment of the carotid artery proximal to the siphon but distal to the surgically accessible portion of the internal carotid artery.

Patient Characteristics

The demographic data and pertinent patient characteristics are outlined in Table 16-1. The mean age of the patients in Group I was 64.3 years and in Group II 63.8 years. Eighty-six percent of the patients in Group I were males whereas only 71 percent of the patients in Group II were males. Twenty-seven percent of the patients in Group I and 31 percent of the patients in Group II were black. Eighty-two percent of the patients in Group I and 86 percent of the

Table 16-1
Patient Characteristics

	Group I N = 44	Group II N = 35
Mean Age (range)	64.3 (44–81 years)	63.8 (50–75 years)
Male:Female (% male)	38:6 (86%)	25:10 (71%)
Black:White (% black)	12:32 (27%)	11:24 (31%)
Mean Follow-up (range)	16.7 (1–40 months)	15.2 (1–40 months)
Hypertension	$\frac{36}{44}$ 82%	$\frac{30}{35}$ 86%
Required Bilateral Carotid Endarterectomies	$\frac{3}{44}$ 7%	$\frac{9}{35}$ 26%

patients in Group II were hypertensive. None of the above differences was statistically significant.

Only three of the 44 patients (7 percent) in Group I required bilateral carotid endarterectomies, whereas nine of the 35 patients in Group II (26 percent) required bilateral carotid endarterectomies. This difference was statistically significant.

Duration of follow-up in both groups ranged from 1 to 40 months, with an average length of follow-up of 16.7 (±10.7) months in Group I and 15.2 (±12.8) months in Group II. This difference was not statistically significant as assessed by Student's unpaired t-test.

Twenty-five percent of the patients in Group I and 23 percent of the patients in Group II were placed on aspirin or other anti-platelet agents (usually dipyridamole) in the postoperative period on the advice of their referring physician or the medical services. Duration of treatment, dosage, degree of compliance, and efficacy relative to relief of symptoms were all so variable and erratic, however, that meaningful analysis of differences between the groups as regards this particular parameter was impossible.

The indications for operation are detailed in Table 16-2. In Group I the primary indication for carotid endarterectomy was transient ischemic attacks or amaurosis fugax: 66 percent, previous resolved stroke: 19 percent, vertebro-basilar insufficiency: four percent, and asymptomatic lesions: 11 percent. In Group II, the primary indication for operation was transient ischemic attacks or amaurosis fugax: 61 percent, previous resolved stroke: 18 percent, vertebro-basilar insufficiency: two percent, and asymptomatic lesions: 18 percent. None of these differences between groups as regards the primary indication for carotid endarterectomy was statistically significant.

Table 16-2
Operative Indications

	Group I		Group II	
Transient Ischemic Attacks	$\frac{31}{47}$	(66%)	$\frac{27}{44}$	(61%)
Resolved Stroke	$\frac{9}{47}$	(19%)	$\frac{8}{44}$	(18%)
Vertebrobasilar Insufficiency	$\frac{2}{47}$	(4%)	$\frac{1}{44}$	(2%)
Asymptomatic Lesions	$\frac{5}{47}$	(11%)	$\frac{8}{44}$	(18%)

Operative Results

All patients in both groups who were symptomatic preoperatively experienced immediate relief of symptoms postoperatively. The earliest recurrence of symptoms referable to the operated side was at 10 months in a Group I patient and at 12 months in a Group II patient.

The differences in stroke rate, recurrence of symptoms, and mortality between Groups I and II are detailed in Table 16-3. In the 44 Group I patients (no tandem lesions) who underwent 47 endarterectomies, there were no intraoperative strokes and no strokes occurring within 30 days of operation for a zero operative stroke rate. In Group I patients, there were four late strokes (8.7 percent) referable to the cerebral hemisphere on the operated side. These strokes occurred at 2, 3, 6, and 12 months postoperatively and none were fatal. All 4 patients were severely hypertensive and non-compliant on medical management for hypertension. Three of the 4 patients were subjected to repeat arteriography which showed normal endarterectomized carotid bifurcations and no progression of aortic arch or intracerebral small vessel disease. At present, 3 of these 4 patients have had resolution of their strokes and the fourth is bedridden. In Group I patients, there were two late strokes (4.8 percent) referable to the unoperated side. Repeat angiography in both of these hypertensive patients revealed no extracranial or intracranial carotid artery disease which could reasonably account for their strokes.

Three patients (6.5 percent) had late development of symptoms referable to the operated side. One patient had recurrence of mild, vague symptoms of vertebro-basilar insufficiency beginning 25 months postoperatively. Another patient had transient ischemic attacks recur at 10 months postoperatively. Both of these patients refused repeat arteriography. The remaining patient had the recurrence of transient ischemic attacks 3 months postoperatively; repeat angiography revealed a normal endarterectomized segment with no intracerebral small vessel disease and her symptoms resolved spontaneously without specific therapy. One additional patient (2.4 percent) developed late symptoms referable to the unoperated side. Repeat angiography showed enlargement and ulceration of a right-sided carotid bifurcation plaque which had appeared small and smooth in contour on the arteriogram performed prior to the patient's left-sided carotid endarterectomy 27 months earlier. The patient has remained symptom free for 6 months following right carotid endarterectomy. There was one (2.1 percent) operative mortality secondary to myocardial infarction occurring 2 weeks postoperatively. There were no late deaths in the Group I patients.

In Group II (carotid siphon stenosis in conjunction with carotid bifurcation stenosis), there were 35 patients who underwent 44 carotid endarterectomies. In this group, there were two intraoperative strokes (4.5 percent) and three strokes (6.8 percent) at less than 30 days postoperatively for

Table 16-3

	Group I		Group II	
	N	%	N	%
Operative Stroke	0/47	0%	5/44	11.4%
Intraoperative Stroke	0/47	0%	2/44	4.5%
Stroke Within 30 Days of Operation	0/47	0%	3/44	6.8%
Immediate Relief of Symptoms	41*/41	100%	29†/29	100%
Late Stroke Referable to the Operated Side	4/46	8.7%	2/39	5.1%
Late Development of Symptoms Referable to the Operated Side	3/46	6.5%	2/39	5.1%
Late Development of Symptoms Referable to the Unoperated Side	1 ‡/42	2.4%	2 §/28	7.1%
Late Stroke Referable to the Unoperated Side	2 ‡/42	4.8%	0 §/28	0%
Operative Mortality	1/47	2.1%	4/44	9.1%
Late Mortality	0/46	0%	3/40	7.5%

*Excludes 5 carotid bifurcation lesions which were asymptomatic prior to surgery and 1 non-stroke related operative mortality.
†Excludes 8 carotid bifurcation lesions which were asymptomatic prior to surgery, 5 strokes sustained in the operative period, and 2 non-stroke related operative mortalities
‡Excludes 2 patients who underwent staged bilateral carotid endarterectomies 1–3 weeks apart and one operative mortality
§Excludes 6 patients who underwent staged bilateral carotid endarterectomies 1–3 weeks apart and 4 operative mortalities

an operative stroke rate of 11.4 percent. Of the intraoperative strokes, one of these resolved completely in seven days, and the remaining patient went on to die of stroke-related complications 4 weeks postoperatively. Of the strokes occurring at less than 30 days postoperatively one of these patients, having sudden onset of a mild right upper extremity paresis 1 day following left carotid endarterectomy, was re-explored immediately and found to have a thrombosed right internal carotid artery. The thrombus was removed, the right upper extremity paresis resolved in 1 month, and the patient remains symptom free at 33 months follow-up. The second of these 3 patients developed severe hypertension (blood pressure 240/120 mmHg) 2 hours postoperatively, followed by a severe global neurologic deficit and died of stroke-related complications four weeks postoperatively. The third patient developed right hemiplegia ten days following left carotid endarterectomy and died of myocardial infarction 3 weeks postoperatively. Two of the remaining 39 patients (5.1 percent) sustained late strokes referable to the operated side during the follow-up period. One of these patients who was severely hypertensive sustained a fatal stroke 28 months postoperatively. The other patient's stroke (31 months postoperatively) was mild and resolved completely in 2 months. There were no late strokes referable to the unoperated side in Group II patients.

Two of the patients in Group II (5.1 percent) had late recurrence of symptoms referable to the operated side. One of these patients had a single transient ischemic attack 18 months postoperatively, and repeat angiography showed a normal endarterectomized carotid bifurcation with no discernible progression of her carotid siphon disease. She was placed on aspirin, 325 mg b.i.d., and has remained asymptomatic to date (16 months). The remaining Group II patient with recurrence of symptoms referable to the operated side experienced infrequent episodes of right eye amaurosis fugax beginning 2 years after right carotid endarterectomy. Repeat arteriography revealed a normal endarterectomized carotid bifurcation, no discernible progression or ulceration of carotid siphon disease, and what was interpreted as a stenotic and ulcerated lesion of the innominate artery. Innominate artery exploration revealed a completely normal vessel. Postoperatively, the patient was placed on aspirin, 325 mg b.i.d., and has had no recurrence of amaurosis fugax or other focal symptoms to date (14 months). An additional 2 patients (7.1 percent) developed late symptoms referable to the unoperated side. Both patients underwent repeat arteriography which showed enlargement of previously small carotid bifurcation lesions, had successful carotid endarterectomies, and remain asymptomatic. There were four operative mortalities in Group II. Two of these were secondary to myocardial infarction, one secondary to a stroke sustained intraoperatively, and another secondary to a stroke sustained postoperatively. There were three late deaths in Group II. One was secondary to myocardial infarction, one followed a late stroke, and 1 patient died of unknown causes.

Although the Group II patients tended, in general, to fare more poorly than did the patients in Group I in respect to operative stroke rate, operative mortality, and late mortality, none of the above mentioned differences was statistically significant.

Since the major concern regarding tandem lesions has dealt with that group of patients who have a greater degree of siphon stenosis than proximal internal carotid artery stenosis, Group II was subdivided into Group IIa and Group IIb. Group IIa (17 patients undergoing 26 endarterectomies) consisted of those patients with carotid siphon stenosis less severe than proximal internal carotid artery stenosis. Group IIb (18 patients undergoing 18

Table 16-4

	Group IIb		Group I Plus Group IIa	
	N	%	N	%
Operative Stroke	2/18	11.1%	3/73	4.1%
Intraoperative Stroke	1/18	5.6%	1/73	1.4%
Stroke Within 30 Days of Operation Referable to the Operated Side	1/18	5.6%	2/73	2.7%
Immediate Relief of Symptoms	12*/12	100%	58†/58	100%
Late Stroke Referable to the Operated Side	1/17	5.9%	5/68	7.4%
Late Development of Symptoms Referable to the Operated Side	1/17	5.9%	4/68	5.9%
Late Development of Symptoms Referable to the Unoperated Side	2/17	11.8%	1‡/53	1.9%
Late Stroke Referable to the Unoperated Side	0/17	0%	2‡/53	3.8%
Operative Mortality	1/18	5.6%	4/73	5.5%
Late Mortality	1/17	5.9%	2/69	2.9%

*Excludes 4 carotid bifurcation lesions which were asymptomatic prior to surgery plus 2 operative strokes

†Excludes 9 carotid bifurcation lesions which were asymptomatic prior to surgery, 3 operative strokes, 2 non-stroke related operative mortalities and 1 death 6 weeks postoperatively of unknown causes

‡Excludes the 8 patients who underwent staged bilateral carotid endarterectomies 1–3 weeks apart and 4 operative mortalities

endarterectomies) consisted of those patients with carotid siphon stenosis greater than proximal internal carotid stenosis. The results in Group IIb were then compared to the results of the combined Group I and Group IIa patients and are outlined in Table 16-4. In this subgroup of 18 patients (Group IIb), there was one intraoperative stroke (5.6 percent), and one patient (5.6 percent) had a stroke referable to the operated side within 30 days of operation. In this subgroup of patients with siphon disease more severe than bifurcation disease, there was one operative mortality (5.6 percent). Of the remaining 17 patients, one (5.9 percent) sustained a late stroke referable to the operated side, and one patient (5.9 percent) developed late recurrence of symptoms referable to the operated side. Two patients in Group IIb (11.8 percent) went on to develop focal symptoms referable to the unoperated side whereas only one of the patients in the combined Group I and Group IIa (1.9 percent) went on to develop symptoms referable to the unoperated side. There was one late death (5.9 percent) in Group IIb. These differences between Group IIb and the combination of Group I and Group IIa patients were not statistically significant.

DISCUSSION

An examination of Tables 16-1 and 16-2 reveals that the two groups were evenly matched as regards age, sex and racial distribution, duration of follow-up, incidence of hypertension, and primary indication for operation. An examination of Tables 16-3 and 16-4 reveals that there was no significant difference between the groups as regards operative stroke rate, late stroke rate, operative mortality, or late mortality. The 35 Group II patients in this series, however, had a higher incidence of bilateral extracranial carotid disease severe enough to require operation than did the Group I patients. This difference was the only discernible difference between the two groups in regard to the parameters analyzed. This difference may be indicative of a generally more extensive or widespread distribution of atherosclerotic occlusive disease in the Group II patients.

The difference in operative stroke rate approaches but does not reach statistical significance. It is possible, but speculative, that a larger experience or a more prolonged period of follow-up would show a significant difference between the groups as regards this end point since the Group I patients likewise remain at risk. It is more pertinent, however, to compare the results of carotid endarterectomy in patients with tandem lesions, as observed in this study, with the natural history of untreated tandem lesions. Several studies[20–25] have shown that 30-35 percent of untreated patients who experience transient ischemic attacks will develop frank strokes during a 5 year follow-up period with the majority of these strokes occurring during the first 1-2 years of follow-up. The combined operative and late stroke rate in Group II (14.3 percent) observed during a follow-up period extending to 40 months is less than the stroke rate which would be expected based on previously reported natural history studies.[20–25] Since an accurate definition of the natural history of patients with tandem carotid lesions does not presently exist, the need for a prospective randomized study employing carotid endarterectomy, medical management, and no treatment is obvious.

The 14.3 percent incidence of total strokes in the Group II patients is identical to the 14.3 percent incidence of total strokes derived by Thompson's[26] application of a more meaningful analysis of the total stroke rate in the aspirin-treated group of patients reported in the Canadian Cooperative study.[27] The 14.3 percent incidence of total strokes in Group II of the present study is also quite similar to the 12.5 percent incidence of total strokes in the aspirin-treated group of patients reported in the American aspirin trial.[28] Neither of the above studies, however, defines the incidence of carotid siphon disease in the aspirin-treated group. Thus, meaningful comparisons between the results of carotid endarterectomy in patients with tandem lesions derived from the present study and the results of medical management derived from the Canadian and American studies are impossible. This again emphasizes the need to include carotid endarterectomy as a treatment modality in any future studies comparing efficacy of various forms of treatment in patients with transient ischemic attacks.

One of the concerns expressed in the literature is that carotid bifurcation endarterectomy in the presence of carotid siphon stenosis would fail to relieve symptoms.[14,19] In the present study, all symptomatic patients in both Groups I and II experienced immediate relief of symptoms regardless of the primary indication for surgery. The earliest recurrence of symptoms referable to the operated side was at 10 months in a Group I patient and at 12 months in a Group II patient. This indicates that the vast majority of symptomatic patients with tandem lesions have their symptoms secondary to either hemodynamic and/or embolic events originating in the carotid bifurcation and not the carotid siphon. Since patients with carotid tandem lesions are uniformly relieved of symptoms by carotid bifurcation endarterectomy and are at no greater operative or late risk than patients with only carotid bifurcation lesions, it would at present appear unwise to deprive a patient with tandem lesions of the proven benefits of carotid endarterectomy because of the theoretical possibility of continued symptoms originating from the carotid siphon.

Based on the observations made in the present study, the following conclusions can be drawn: (1) Approximately half of all patients with symptoms of cerebrovascular disease have tandem lesions, and approximately 20 percent of the total group have a greater degree of carotid siphon stenosis than proximal internal carotid stenosis. (2) Patients with tandem lesions do not have a statistically significantly higher rate of operative stroke, operative mortality, or late mortality as compared to patients without tandem lesions. (3) Patients with tandem lesions subjected to carotid endarterectomy have a stroke rate that is less than the stroke rate that would be anticipated if no therapy were rendered based on the natural history of untreated patients. (4) All symptomatic patients in both groups experienced immediate relief of symptoms thus indicating that even in patients with tandem lesions the vast majority of symptoms originate in the carotid bifurcation.

REFERENCES

1. Thompson JE, Talkington CM: Carotid endarterectomy. Ann Surg 184:1, 1976
2. Callow AD: An overview of the stroke problem in the carotid territory. Am J Surg 140:181, 1980
3. West H, Burton R, Roon AJ, et al: Comparative risk of operation and expectant management for carotid artery disease. Stroke 10:117, 1979
4. Blaisdell FW, Clauss RH, Galbraith JG, et al: Joint study of extracranial arterial occlusion: IV—A review of surgical considerations. JAMA 209:1889, 1969
5. DeWeese JA, Rob CG, Satran R, et al: Results of carotid endarterectomies for transient ischemic attack—five years later. Ann Surg 178:258, 1973
6. Hass WK, Fields WS, North RR, et al: Joint study of extracranial arterial occlusion. II—Arteriography, techniques, sites, and complications. JAMA 203:159, 1968
7. Bauer RB, Sheehan S, Wechsler N, et al: Arteriographic study of sites, incidence, and treatment of arteriosclerotic cerebrovascular lesions. Neurology (Minneap) 12:698, 1962
8. Luessenhop AJ: Occlusive disease of the carotid artery: Observations on the prognosis and surgical treatment. J Neurosurg 16:705, 1959
9. Fieschi C, Bozzao L: Transient embolic occlusion of the middle cerebral and internal carotid arteries in cerebral apoplexy. J Neurol Neurosurgery Psychiatry 32:236, 1969
10. Bostrom K, Hassler O: Radiological study of arterial calcification. Neurology (Minneap) 15:1168, 1965
11. Ratinov G: Extradural intracranial portion of carotid artery. A clinicopathologic study. Arch Neurol 10:66, 1964
12. Fisher CM, Gore I, Okabe N, et al: Atherosclerosis of the carotid and vertebral arteries—extracranial and intracranial. J Neuropath Exp Neurol 24:455, 1965
13. Blaisdell WF, Hall AD, Thomas AN, et al: Cerebrovascular occlusive disease. Experience with panarteriography in 300 consecutive cases. Calif Med 103:321, 1965
14. Wylie EJ, Ehrenfeld WK: Extracranial Occlusive Cerebrovascular Disease: Diagnosis and Management. Philadelphia, W.B. Saunders, 1970, p 126
15. Hugenholtz H, Elgie RG: Carotid thromboendarterectomy: A reappraisal: Criteria for patient selection. J Neurosurg 53:776, 1980
16. Day AL, Rhoton AL, Quisling RG: Resolving siphon stenosis following endarterectomy. Stroke 11:278, 1980
17. Sundt TM, Sandok BA, Whisnant JP: Carotid endarterectomy. Complications and preoperative assessment of risk. Mayo Cl Proc 50:301, 1975
18. Bauer RB, Meyer JS, Fields WS, et al: Joint study of extracranial arterial occlusion. III—Progress of controlled study of long-term survival in patients with and without operation. JAMA 208:509, 1969

19. Fields WS: Selection of stroke patients for arterial reconstructive surgery. Am J Surg 125:527, 1973
20. Goldner JC, Whisnant JP, Taylor WF: Long-term prognosis of transient cerebral ischemic attacks. Stroke 2:160, 1971
21. Millikan CH: Reassessment of anticoagulant therapy in various types of occlusive cerebrovascular disease. Stroke 2:201, 1971
22. Acheson J, Hutchinson EC: The natural history of 'focal cerebral vascular disease'. Quart J Med 40:15, 1971
23. Toole JF, Janeway R, Choi K, et al: Transient ischemic attacks due to atherosclerosis. A prospective study of 160 patients. Arch Neurol 32:5, 1975
24. Millikan CH, McDowell FH: Treatment of transient ischemic attacks. Stroke 9:299, 1978
25. Thomson JE, Patman RD, Talkington CM: Carotid surgery for cerebrovascular insufficiency. Curr Prob Surg 15:1, 1978
26. Thompson JE: Letter to the Editor. N Eng J Med 299: 954, 1978
27. Barnett HJM, Sackett DL, Taylor DW, et al: A randomized trial of aspirin and sulfinpyrazone in threatened stroke. N Eng J Med 299:53, 1978
28. Fields WS, Lemak NA, Frankowski RF, et al: Controlled trial of aspirin in cerebral ischemia. Stroke 8:301, 1977

Charles S. O'Mara

17

Surgical Significance of the External Carotid Artery

The importance of the internal carotid artery and its intracranial branches in maintaining satisfactory cerebral perfusion is readily apparent. As a result of this importance, endarterectomy of the internal carotid artery has become a standard operative technique for treatment of atheromatous plaques of the proximal part of the artery. The external carotid artery and its branches can also contribute significantly to cerebral blood flow, especially when other extracranial arteries are diseased. The potential role of external carotid artery revascularization in treating cerebral ischemia, however, has received relatively little attention.

Internal carotid endarterectomy is an effective method of treatment of lesions that are ulcerative or stenotic. Cerebral and retinal ischemic symptoms occasionally occur, however, in the presence of total occlusion of the ipsilateral internal carotid artery. When internal carotid occlusion coexists with contralateral internal carotid stenosis, endarterectomy of the contralateral carotid artery often alleviates symptoms.[1,2] When no significant compromise of the opposite internal carotid exists, the choice of therapy for symptomatic internal carotid artery occlusion is more difficult.

Results of thromboendarterectomy of the totally occluded internal carotid artery have been discouraging, and this procedure is infrequently performed today.[3] Use of antiplatelet agents such as aspirin and dipyridamole has been advocated, and these drugs may have a role in managing nonoperatively certain patients with cerebral ischemia. Nevertheless, the precise indications for and the long-term results of these agents are unsettled issues.[4] Studies have documented the technical feasibility of microvascular anastomosis of the distal superficial temporal artery and the middle cerebral artery in treating symptomatic internal carotid occlusion. This operation can be performed with relatively low morbidity and mortality when done by experienced microvascular surgeons.[5] The therapeutic value of extracranial-intracranial (EC-IC) bypass, however, is still unproven, and its indications remain controversial.[6,7]

When a patient is symptomatic from internal carotid artery occlusion and has ipsilateral external carotid artery stenosis or common carotid occlusion, revascularization of the external carotid artery represents yet another therapeutic alternative. Wetzel and associates[8] were among the first to draw attention to the clinicopathologic significance of the external carotid artery in 1964, when they reported ten patients with symptoms of cerebrovascular insufficiency secondary to external carotid stenosis. In 1967, Jackson[9] emphasized the potential role of external carotid artery revascularization by reporting 5 patients with cerebral ischemia treated successfully by external carotid endarterectomy. Two years later, in a clinical evaluation of 3 patients, Ehrenfeld and Lord[10] cited the importance of external carotid collateral pathways as mediators of retinal ischemia. Studies have subsequently documented the beneficial effect of external carotid revascularization in properly selected patients.[11-16] The purpose of this chapter is to consider the rationale behind external carotid revascularization, as well as its indications, operative techniques, and results.

EXTERNAL CAROTID COLLATERAL PATHWAYS

Extensive anatomic and arteriographic evidence documents the existence of numerous potential collateral pathways between the external carotid artery and the intracranial circulation.[17-24] Five of the 8 branches of the external carotid communicate with the blood supply of the ipsilateral retina and cerebral hemisphere. These branches include the superficial temporal, internal maxillary, occipital, facial, and posterior auricular arteries. The external carotid collateral pathways are shown in Figure 17-1.

The most abundant external carotid collaterals to the brain and retina course around the orbit to connect with the ophthalmic artery. The ophthalmic artery, a branch of the intracranial internal carotid, enters the orbit through the optic canal within the dural sheath of the optic nerve. Several branches of the ophthalmic artery supply the contents of the orbit. Among these branches is the central artery, which nourishes the retina as an end artery. Six branches of the ophthalmic artery pass beyond the orbit. These branches include the dorsal nasal artery to the face; the supraorbital and supratrochlear arteries to the forehead; the lacrimal artery to the eyelid, cheek, and temporal region; and the anterior and posterior ethmoidal arteries to the nasal cavity. Each of these branches communicates freely with branches of the external carotid artery.

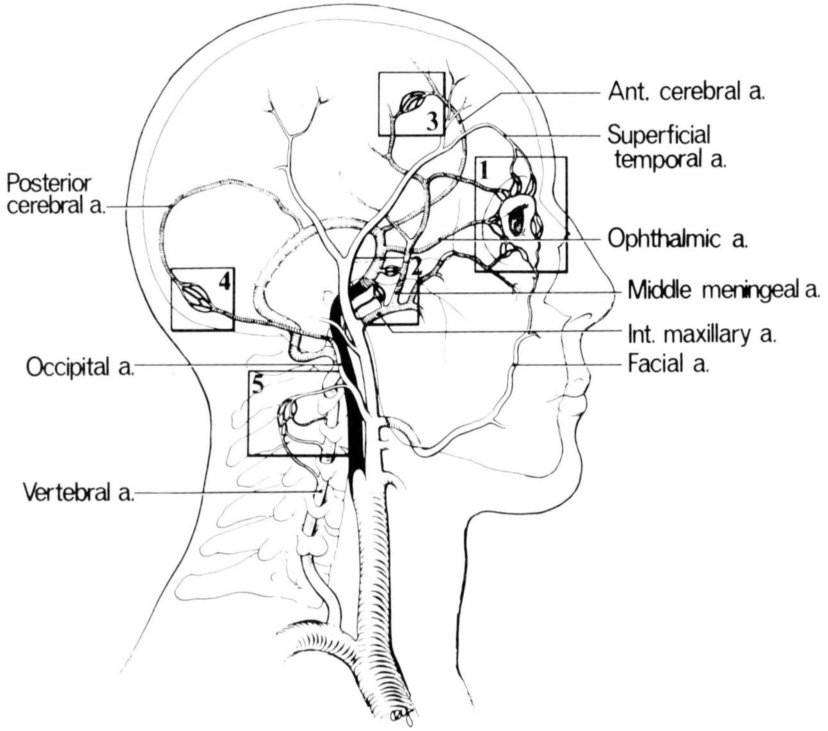

Figure 17-1. Numerous collateral pathways exist between the external carotid artery and the intracranial arteries. The superficial temporal, facial, and internal maxillary branches of the external carotid participate in rich periorbital anastomoses with numerous branches of the ophthalmic artery (Box 1). The posterior auricular and internal maxillary arteries communicate with small branches of the petrous and cavernous portions of the internal carotid artery (Box 2). The middle meningeal and occipital arteries connect by way of leptomeningeal arteries with the anterior and posterior cerebral arteries, respectively (Boxes 3 and 4). The occipital artery also communicates with muscular branches of the vertebral artery (Box 5).

The dorsal nasal artery connects with both the lateral nasal and the angular branches of the facial artery. The supraorbital and supratrochlear branches of the ophthalmic artery communicate with the frontal branch of the superficial temporal artery. The lacrimal artery anastomoses with the middle meningeal branch of the internal maxillary artery. The lacrimal artery also connects with the zygomatico-orbital branch of the superficial temporal artery by way of zygomatico-facial and zygomatico-temporal anastomoses. The anterior and posterior ethmoidal branches of the ophthalmic artery communicate with the sphenopalatine artery, which is a branch of the internal maxillary artery. Periorbital collaterals which fill the ophthalmic artery in retrograde fashion and which allow reconstitution of the intracranial internal carotid artery can be documented arteriographically in about three-fourths of patients with ipsilateral occlusion of the cervical portion of the internal carotid artery.[18]

In addition to collaterals to the ophthalmic artery, other potentially important communications exist between external carotid branches and intracranial arteries. The carotico-tympanic branch of the internal carotid artery arises within the petrous portion of the temporal bone. This vessel communicates with the external carotid by way of both the stylomastoid branch of the posterior auricular artery and the anterior tympanic branch of the internal maxillary artery. The meningohypophyseal trunk and the artery to the inferior cavernous sinus, both branches of the cavernous portion of the internal carotid, anastomose with branches of the middle meningeal artery. The carotico-tympanic, meningohypophyseal, and cavernous branches of the internal carotid are small and usually difficult to demonstrate arteriographically. Their potential significance as collateral channels after occlusion of the cervical internal carotid artery is implied when the petrous and cavernous portions of the internal carotid are reconstituted by them on delayed arteriographic exposures.[25]

Branches of the external carotid artery occasionally communicate with the anterior or posterior cerebral circulation. The middle meningeal branch of the internal maxillary artery connects with cortical leptomeningeal branches of the anterior cerebral artery. The occipital artery likewise communicates with cortical leptomeningeal branches of the posterior cerebral artery. In addition, the descending portion of the deep branch of the occipital artery connects with muscular branches of the vertebral artery, which then reach the posterior cerebral circulation by way of the basilar artery. Although this occipital-vertebral anastomosis can be documented in less than 1 percent of consecutive cerebral arteriograms, it is more commonly demonstrated when diffuse extracranial occlusive disease exists.[26]

PATHOLOGIC CONSIDERATIONS

Atherosclerosis is the primary pathologic process in the vast majority of patients with extracranial cerebrovascular disease. The most common site of extracranial obstructive lesions responsible for cerebrovascular insufficiency is the carotid bifurcation. Atheromatous plaque at the bifurcation usually extends for only 1 or 2 cm in the proximal internal carotid artery and then abruptly merges into normal intima. Plaque in the internal carotid may progressively enlarge, narrow the lumen of the vessel, and produce hemodynamic alterations. In addition, the plaque may undergo degenerative changes, ulcerate, and become the nidus for formation of platelet aggregates and thrombi which, along with atheromatous debris from the plaque itself, may dislodge and embolize to the brain or retina.

Progressive growth of the plaque may result in gradual narrowing and ultimate total occlusion of the internal carotid artery, whereas hemorrhage into a plaque may cause sudden thrombosis. Following closure of the internal carotid origin by either of these mechanisms, clot propagates distally in the vessel to the site of a major branch, usually the ophthalmic artery, which reconstitutes the distal internal carotid artery by retrograde flow and usually prevents further thrombus propagation. In the proximal internal carotid, a patent remnant or "stump" is a common finding following occlusion of the vessel.

As illustrated in Figure 17-2, the atheromatous process of the carotid

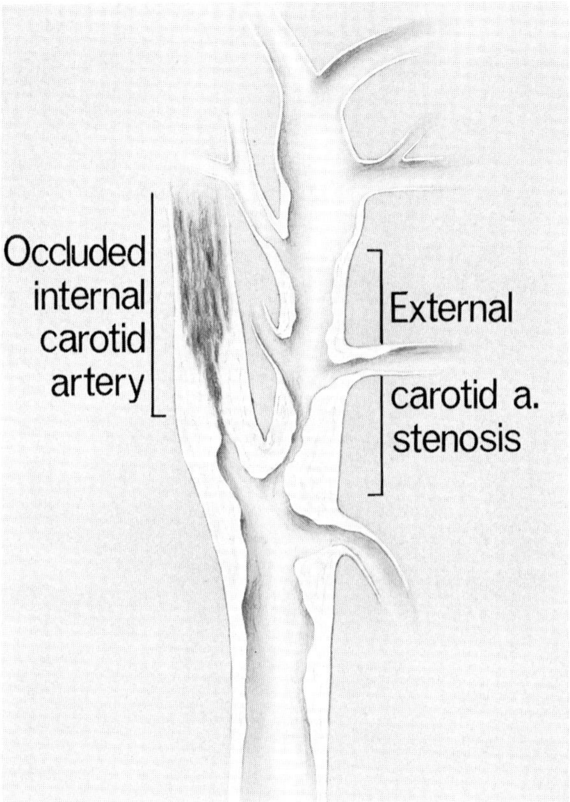

Figure 17-2. This drawing depicts typical pathologic characteristics of the carotid bifurcation in patients with symptomatic internal carotid occlusion. A patent remnant of the occluded internal carotid exists at its origin. Coexisting irregular atheromatous plaque in the external carotid artery narrows the origin of the vessel, extends relatively far distally, and is associated with mild poststenotic dilatation. The flow surface of the common carotid artery is also irregular.

bifurcation usually involves the external carotid as well as the internal carotid artery.[27] Plaque in the external carotid varies considerably in extent, but it is often longer than the corresponding plaque in the internal carotid artery. Poststenotic dilatation may be present. External carotid plaque often has a gradual transition into normal intima in contrast to the usual abrupt juncture of plaque with nondiseased distal intima in the internal carotid. In most other respects, the atheromatous process is similar in the two vessels. External carotid plaque may narrow the lumen and produce a hemodynamically significant pressure gradient. As with the internal carotid artery, plaque in the external carotid may ulcerate and become a source of emboli, which can migrate to the brain or retina through external carotid collateral pathways.[28,29] When the internal carotid has previously become occluded, progressive plaque formation or sudden hemorrhage into an external carotid plaque may result in closure of the external carotid orifice. Complete occlusion of the origin of both the internal and the external carotid arteries causes thrombosis of the common carotid. Like other arteries with multiple muscular branches, proximal occlusion of the external carotid seldom results in distal propagation of thrombus. Instead, vessel patency is maintained by retrograde flow from external carotid branches. In this situation, patency of the external carotid artery can usually be documented on delayed arteriographic views. When common carotid thrombosis is caused by progressive narrowing of the vessel proximal to its bifurcation, retrograde blood flow in the external carotid and its branches may maintain antegrade flow in the internal carotid artery. Such continued patency of the internal carotid is important surgically because it affords the possibility of direct internal carotid revascularization by bypass techniques.

INDICATIONS FOR OPERATION

When the internal carotid artery is totally occluded, the external carotid and its branches can provide up to 30 percent of the blood flow to the ipsilateral cerebral hemisphere and retina through collateral circuits.[17] As previously described, however, the origin of the external carotid artery is often involved in the same atherosclerotic process which has caused internal carotid occlusion. Such external carotid artery stenosis may prevent recruitment of external carotid collateral pathways when the internal carotid is occluded. The resultant hemodynamic alterations may produce generalized symptoms of diffuse cerebral ischemia such as ataxia, dizziness, vertigo, and syncope. In the presence of arteriographically documented external carotid stenosis and coexisting bilateral internal carotid occlusion, such nonlateralizing cerebrovascular symptoms are an indication for repair of the external carotid narrowing to augment cerebral blood flow through external carotid collateral channels. This indication for external carotid revascularization is exemplified in the following patient summary.

Example 1

A 55-year-old woman presented with a six-month history of vertigo and ataxia. Arteriography documented bilateral internal carotid occlusion and severe stenosis of the left external carotid artery (Fig. 17-3). The right external carotid was not compromised, but both vertebral arteries were narrowed at their origins. In the presence of diffuse cerebral ischemic symptoms combined with arteriographic evidence of bilateral internal carotid occlusion and left external carotid stenosis, left

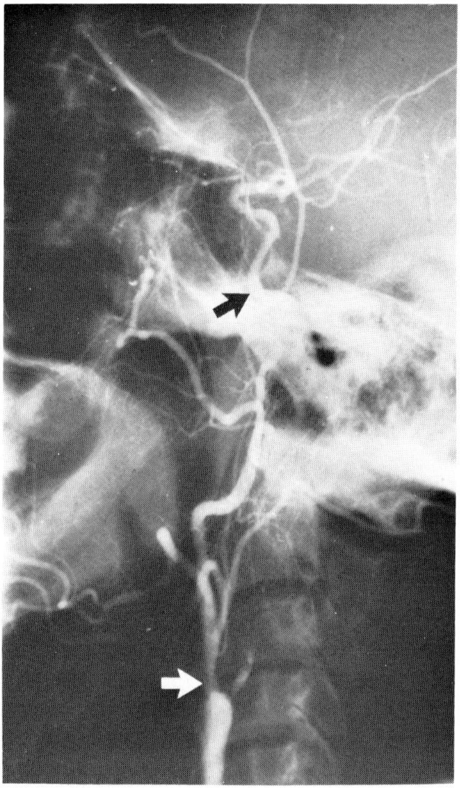

Figure 17-3. Selective left carotid arteriogram from Example 1 shows internal carotid occlusion and stenosis of the external carotid origin (white arrow). A long irregular remnant of the proximal occluded internal carotid artery persists. Notice reconstitution of the distal internal carotid artery (dark arrow) by way of the ophthalmic artery and the small branches of the petrous and cavernous portions of the artery.

external carotid endarterectomy was performed. Subsequent superficial temporal-middle cerebral artery anastomosis had initially been considered, but alleviation of symptoms by external carotid endarterectomy alone rendered any additional operation unnecessary.

Symptoms of diffuse cerebral ischemia may be associated with total occlusion of both the common and internal carotid arteries. In this situation, bypass grafting to the patent external carotid artery offers the possibility of increased cerebral blood flow through external carotid collaterals with resultant alleviation of cerebrovascular symptoms. Examples of this indication for external carotid revascularization are given below in the section on operative techniques of external carotid bypass.

Like atheromatous lesions of the internal carotid artery, external carotid plaques may degenerate and develop ulcers. Platelet aggregates, small blood clots, and atheromatous debris can dislodge from these ulcers and embolize distally. When the internal carotid is occluded, such emboli can be transmitted through external carotid collateral channels to either the retina or cerebral hemisphere. These emboli result in amaurosis fugax or transient episodes of focal cerebral ischemia such as hemiparesis, hemidysesthesia, and dysphasia. Emboli may also originate either at the site of irregular plaques in the common carotid artery or within the occluded remnant of the internal carotid artery where blood flow is turbulent and additional atheromatous ulcers may exist. These emboli, like those developing within the external carotid artery, can also migrate through external carotid collaterals to either the retina or the brain.

When transient cerebral or retinal ischemia occurs in the presence of ipsilateral internal carotid occlusion, the arteriogram should be examined carefully for a potential source of emboli which can migrate through external collaterals. If an embolic nidus such as an irregular plaque of the external or common carotid artery or a large internal carotid remnant exists, repair of the embolic source should be considered. If success is to be expected, the contralateral carotid bifurcation should be free of significant disease and not represent a potential source from which the emboli might have originated. Moreover, arteriographic documentation of the existence of collateral channels from external carotid branches to the involved eye or cerebral hemisphere optimizes the chance of successful operation[30] (Fig. 17-4). However, in the presence of severe stenosis of the proximal external carotid artery and resultant markedly diminished flow through its branches, collateral circuits may be difficult to document even with optimal arteriographic techniques.

Example 2

A 60-year-old man suffered a right hemispheric stroke and had a residual mild left hemiparesis. One month later, he developed right amaurosis fugax which occurred

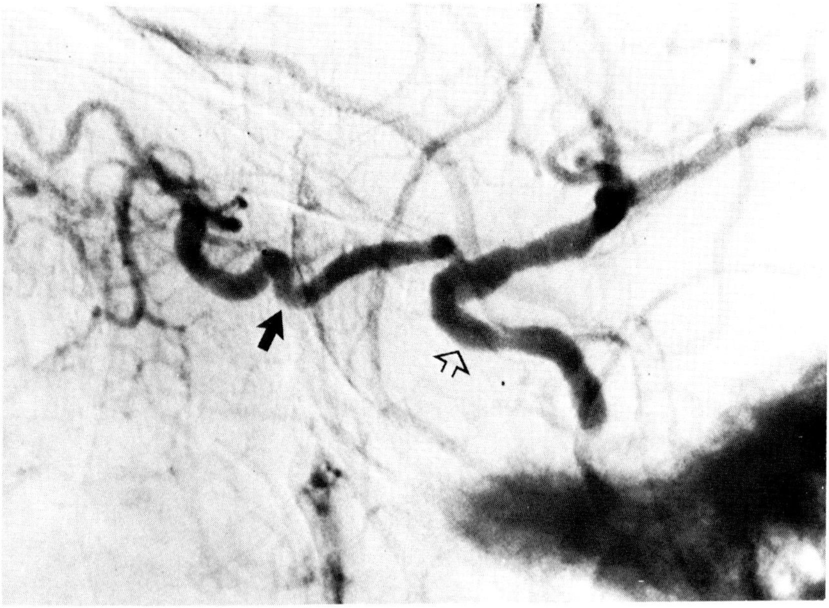

Figure 17-4. This carotid arteriogram documents reconstitution of the carotid siphon (open arrow) by retrograde flow in a large ophthalmic artery (solid arrow) from periorbital external carotid collaterals.

once every other day. Carotid arteriography three months later documented complete occlusion of the right internal carotid artery and severe stenosis of the common carotid just proximal to the bifurcation (Fig. 17-5). The left internal carotid artery was mildly stenotic with collateral filling of the right cerebral hemisphere from the left vertebral and left carotid arteries. The right ophthalmic artery was supplied by collateral branches of the right external carotid artery. The patient underwent endarterectomy of the right common and external carotid arteries. He has had no amaurosis fugax during an 18 month follow-up period.

Example 3

This 55-year-old woman had bilateral harsh midcervical bruits. Oculoplethysmography documented bilateral severe eye pulse delay. Carotid arteriography showed 95 percent stenosis of the left internal and the left external carotid arteries (Fig. 17-6A) and 75 percent stenosis of the right internal carotid artery. She was scheduled to return for left carotid endarterectomy, but prior to readmission she sustained a left hemispheric stroke with right hemiparesis. She gradually improved during the following 2 months and had no significant residual neurologic deficit. She then began to have transient right arm numbness. Repeat carotid arteriography documented the presence of the proximal remnant of an occluded left internal carotid, persistent left external carotid stenosis (Fig. 17-6B), and slight worsening of the right internal carotid stenosis. Right carotid endarterectomy was performed. Five days postoperatively she

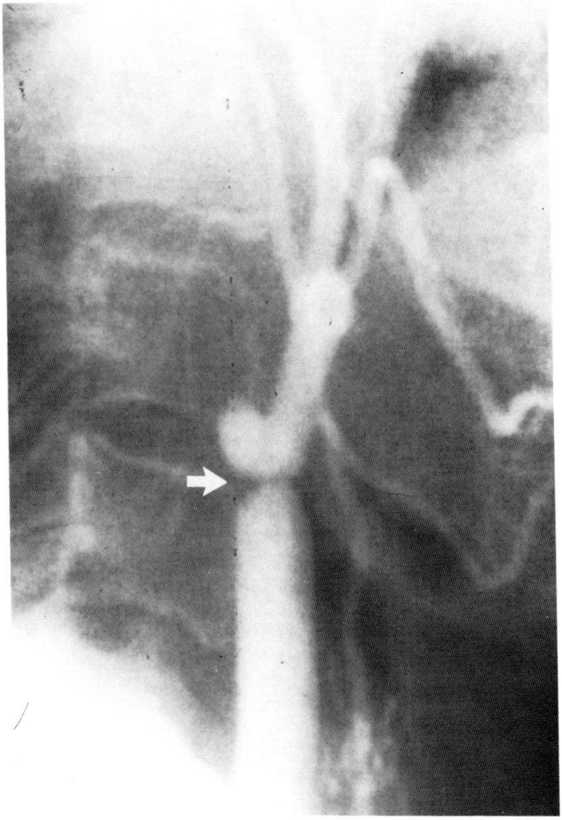

Figure 17-5. Right carotid arteriogram from Example 2 documents internal carotid occlusion and severe stenosis of the common carotid just proximal to the bifurcation (arrow).

experienced recurrent right arm numbness. Because of suspected embolization through left external carotid artery collateral pathways, the patient underwent left external carotid endarterectomy. She experienced no subsequent neurologic problems.

OPERATIVE TECHNIQUE

External Carotid Endarterectomy

External carotid endarterectomy is a suitable technique for cerebral revascularization when internal carotid occlusion is associated with a common carotid artery which provides satisfactory inflow to a stenotic

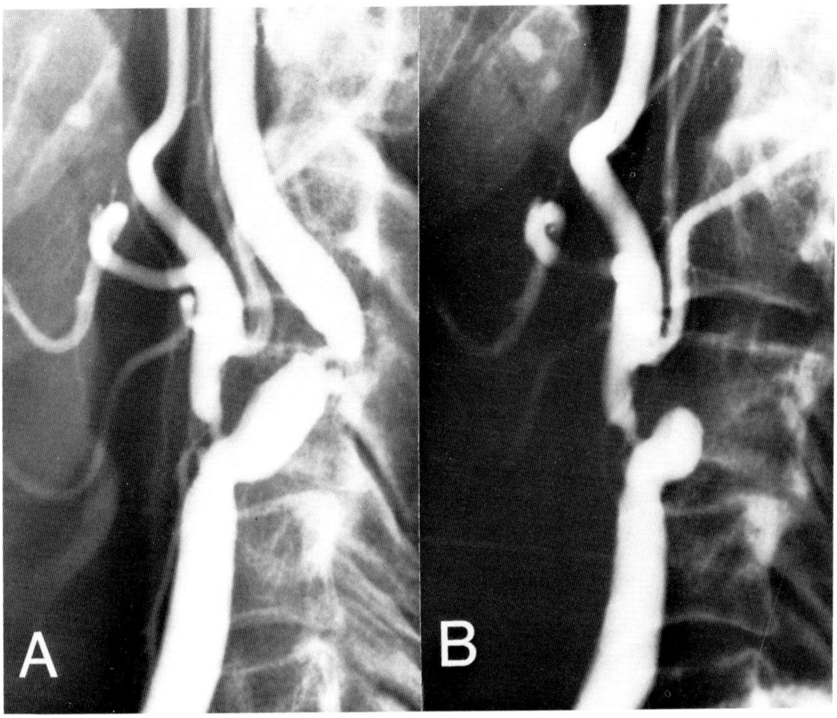

Figure 17-6. Left carotid arteriogram of Example 3 shows severe stenosis of both the internal and the external carotid arteries (A). Repeat arteriography 2 months later demonstrates occlusion of the internal carotid artery (B). Both the external carotid plaque and the internal carotid stump were potential causes of post-occlusive hemispheric transient ischemic attacks in this patient.

external carotid artery. The essential steps of the operation have been described previously[14,31] and are shown in Figure 17-7. Operative exposure is similar to that of standard carotid endarterectomy. The extent of exposure of the external carotid artery, however, is determined by the extent of atherosclerotic involvement of the artery. Atheromatous plaque often extends beyond the initial branches of the external carotid, in which case extensive exposure of the external carotid and its distal branches is necessary. This dissection sometimes requires division of the posterior belly of the digastric muscle and gentle elevation of the hypoglossal nerve.

After administration of systemic heparin, the external carotid artery and its branches are doubly encircled with soft silastic loops for distal control. A vascular clamp is applied for control of the common carotid artery. A longitudinal arteriotomy is begun on the distal common carotid and extended

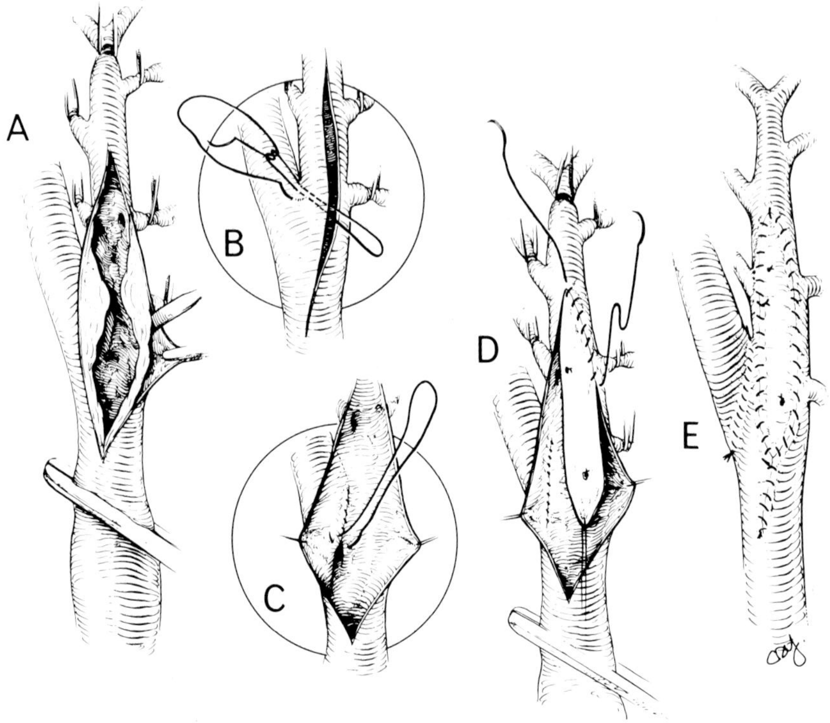

Figure 17-7. Important features of the operative technique for external carotid endarterectomy are shown. A longitudinal arteriotomy is begun in the common carotid artery and extended beyond the distal limit of atheromatous plaque in the external carotid (A). The plaque is removed in a standard endarterectomy plane. After removal of the plaque, the internal carotid orifice is obliterated using a continuous suture which is placed from within the common carotid but which has its knots tied outside the vessel (B and C). Because of the small size of the external carotid artery, vein patch angioplasty closure of the external carotid portion of the arteriotomy is often necessary (D and E). Notice that the internal carotid orifice has been obliterated to avoid creation of a cul-de-sac.

onto the external carotid artery to a point beyond the distal limit of the plaque. The appropriate cleavage plane for endarterectomy is established. The plaque is transected proximally in the common carotid artery, and the distal portion of the plaque is separated smoothly from the external carotid artery. As with internal carotid endarterectomy, special care is taken to be certain that there is no distal intimal flap which will cause postoperative occlusion. If a distal intimal shelf is present, the arteriotomy should be extended distally to a point beyond the plaque. If this is done, intimal tacking sutures should seldom be necessary. The plaque is extracted by eversion from the origin of the occluded internal carotid artery. The remnant of occluded internal carotid artery is obliterated either with a continuous suture technique from within the common carotid artery or by transecting the proximal internal carotid and oversewing each end.

An indwelling shunt from the common carotid artery to the distal external carotid may be necessary in selected situations. We have not routinely used an intraluminal shunt with this procedure, however, because of the small size of the distal external carotid artery and also because of the usually severe external carotid stenosis in association with internal carotid occlusion.

Patch angioplasty closure of the arteriotomy is rarely necessary for internal carotid endarterectomy: however, a patch is often needed for external carotid endarterectomy because of the small diameter of the endarterectomized external carotid artery. Autogenous vein is preferred for use as a patch. The vein patch is carried down only to the origin of the external carotid artery. The remaining portion of the arteriotomy on the common carotid, which is of adequate diameter, can be closed without a patch. An alternative technique involves use of an endarterectomized segment of the occluded internal carotid artery for either patch or flap angioplasty closure of the arteriotomy[9] (Fig. 17-8). Following completion of arteriotomy closure, flow is restored initially to the superior thyroid artery and then to the more important distal branches of the external carotid. The reconstruction can be easily monitored in the postoperative period by palpation or Doppler flow detection of the facial or superficial temporal artery.

External Carotid Bypass

When both the internal and common carotid arteries are occluded, the external carotid artery almost invariably is reconstituted by retrograde flow in its initial branches. In this circumstance, revascularization of the external carotid artery can be performed by bypass grafting from a remote source to the proximal external carotid artery.[32,33] The choice of source for the bypass depends upon clinical and angiographic findings. Bypass to the external carotid artery can be performed from the ipsilateral subclavian artery, from the contralateral carotid artery, and from the ascending aorta. Description of these techniques will be given in the following case summaries.

Subclavian-External Carotid Bypass

Example 4

A 45-year-old man had sustained three previous right hemispheric strokes with residual mild left hemiparesis. He also had rest pain and ischemic ulceration of the

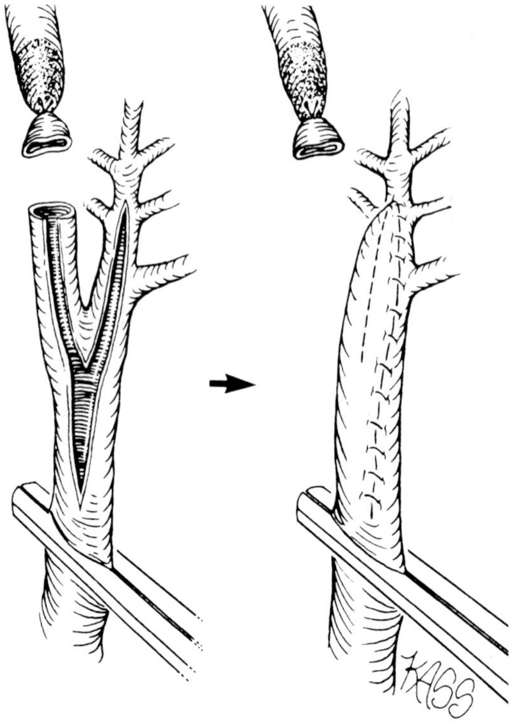

Figure 17-8. An alternative technique is to use an endarterectomized segment of occluded internal carotid artery for flap angioplasty closure of the carotid arteriotomy (From O'Mara CS, et al: External Carotid Endarterectomy. In Bergan JJ, Yao JST, (eds): Operative Techniques in Vascular Surgery. New York, Grune and Stratton, 1980. Reproduced by permission of Grune and Stratton, Inc.)

right great toe. Arch aortography disclosed complete occlusion of both common carotid arteries (Fig. 17-9A). Delayed views showed that the right external carotid artery was reconstituted at its origin, but the left carotid system was not seen. Each vertebral artery was severely stenotic at its origin. Revascularization of the right external carotid artery was felt warranted to increase the safety of aortic reconstruction and to minimize the risk of subsequent stroke. The right carotid bifurcation was exposed through an oblique right neck incision. The external carotid artery was patent beyond the superior thyroid branch. The right subclavian artery was exposed through a separate right supraclavicular incision. A 6 mm Dacron graft was anastomosed end-to-side to the subclavian artery. The proximal external carotid artery was transected and the initial portion of the artery was endarterectomized. The graft was passed posterior to the sternocleidomastoid muscle and was anastomosed end-to-end in spatulated fashion to the external carotid artery (Fig. 17-9B).

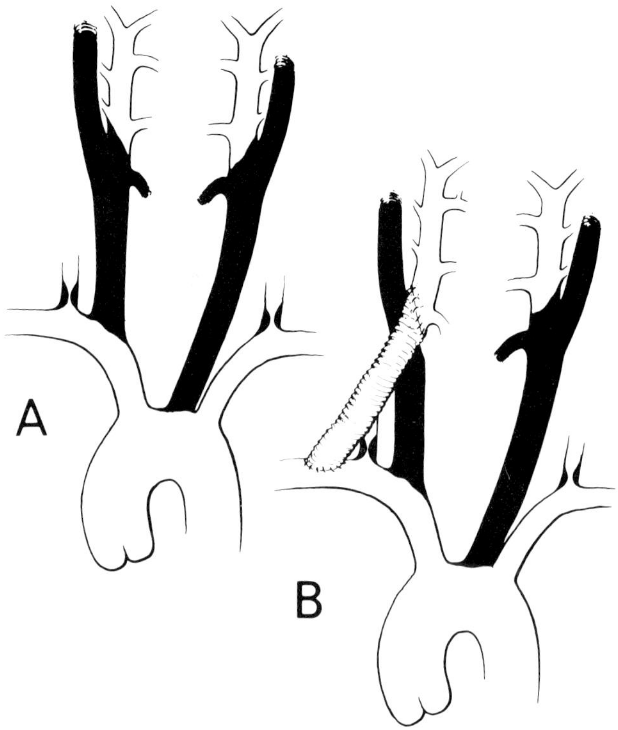

Figure 17-9. Drawing depicts preoperative arteriographic documentation in Example 4 of bilateral common and internal carotid occlusions and bilateral proximal vertebral stenoses. Both external carotid arteries were patent (A). Revascularization of the right external carotid artery was accomplished by bypass from the subclavian artery (B).

Contralateral Carotid-External Carotid Bypass

Example 5

This 76-year-old man had experienced transient episodes of lightheadedness and syncope with increasing frequency during the previous 2 years. Arch aortography documented complete occlusion of the left common carotid, right internal carotid, and both vertebral arteries. There was also severe stenosis of the right external carotid artery with reconstitution of the right vertebral artery by way of a large collateral from the occipital artery (Fig. 17-10A). Revascularization was performed to alleviate symptoms of diffuse cerebral ischemia. Each carotid bifurcation was exposed through bilateral oblique neck incisions. Right external carotid endarterectomy was performed as described above. The proximal left external carotid artery was transected and its

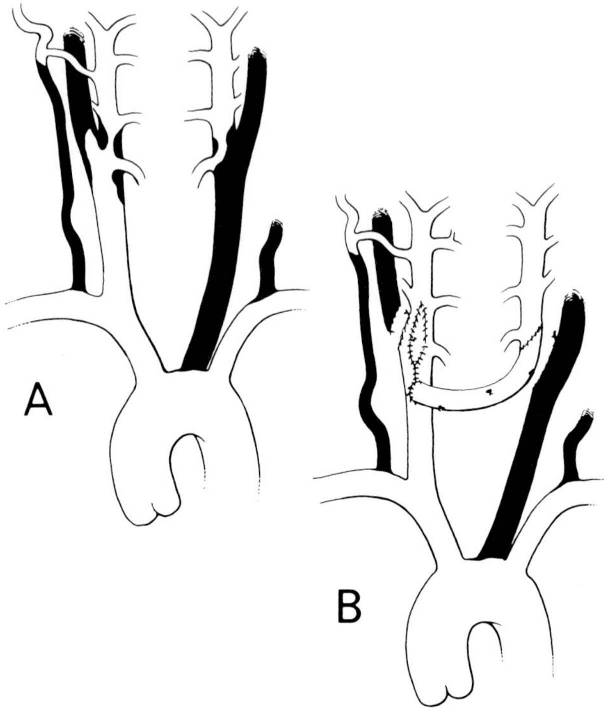

Figure 17-10. Arteriography documented extensive extracranial occlusive lesions in Example 5 (A). Note the severe stenosis at the origin of the right external carotid artery, which was the principal source of blood flow to the brain by way of large occipital-vertebral artery collateral. To improve total cerebral perfusion, this patient underwent right external carotid endarterectomy combined with right common-to-left external carotid bypass (B).

initial segment was endarterectomized. End-to-end anastomosis between left external carotid artery and saphenous vein graft was performed. The graft was passed beneath the platysma muscle across the neck and was anastomosed end-to-side to the common carotid artery (Fig. 17-10B). An intraluminal shunt from the right common carotid to the right external carotid artery was used during performance of the right external carotid endarterectomy and during creation of the anastomosis between saphenous vein graft and common carotid artery. Cerebral ischemic symptoms were relieved and the patient has remained well during 1 year of follow-up.

Aortic Arch-External Carotid Bypass

Example 6

A 57-year-old woman presented with a two month history of intermittent transient episodes of lightheadedness, syncope, dysphasia, and right hand numbness.

She also experienced left forearm claudication upon moderate left upper extremity exertion. Systolic blood pressure was 40 mm Hg less in the left arm than in the right arm. Arch aortography documented bilateral common and internal carotid occlusions with reconstitution of both external carotid arteries. There was 70 percent stenosis of the proximal left subclavian artery and 50 percent stenosis of the proximal right subclavian artery. Both vertebral arteries were moderately stenotic at their origin (Fig. 17-11A). Revascularization was warranted to alleviate symptoms of cerebral and left upper extremity ischemia. The distribution of stenotic and occlusive lesions precluded a simple extraanatomic bypass outside the chest cavity. Therefore, the ascending aorta was exposed through a median sternotomy incision. The right carotid bifurcation was dissected using a right neck incision, and the left subclavian artery was exposed through a left infraclavicular incision. Controlled hypotension was pharmacologically induced while the ascending aorta was clamped tangentially. A longitudinal aortotomy was used for end-to-side anastomosis of the body of a bifurcated Dacron graft to the ascending aortic arch. One limb of the graft was tunnelled to the right neck incision where it was anastomosed end-to-end to the transected proximal external carotid artery. The other limb of the graft was passed across the apex of the left pleural cavity and through the first intercostal space to the left infraclavicular

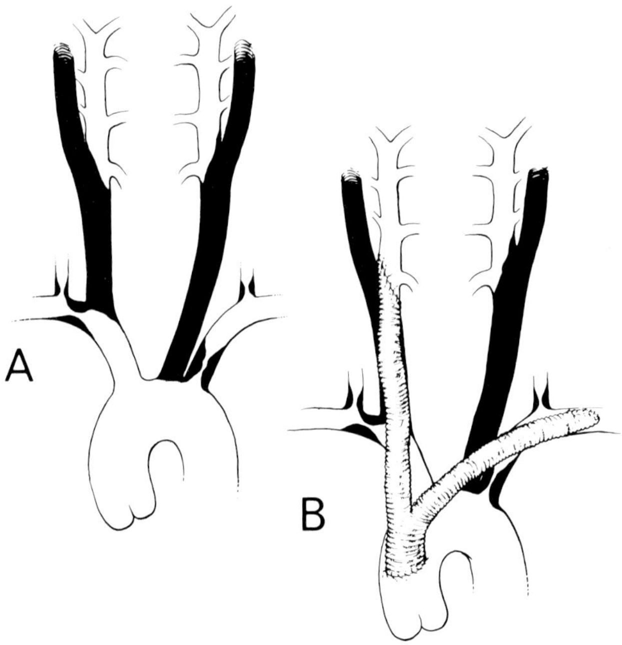

Figure 17-11. The patient in Example 6 also had diffuse extracranial occlusive disease as depicted in (A). Cerebral and left upper extremity revascularization was accomplished by median sternotomy and placement of a prosthetic graft from the ascending aortic arch to the right external carotid artery and to the left subclavian artery (B).

incision. This limb of the graft was anastomosed end-to-side to the subclavian artery (Fig. 17-11B). Cerebral and left arm ischemic symptoms were relieved, and the patient has been well for the past 3 years.

DISCUSSION

Transient ischemic attacks secondary to atheromatous internal carotid plaque often cease after the stenotic lesion progresses to complete occlusion. Ischemic events in the ipsilateral eye or cerebral hemisphere, however, sometimes persist or recur.[34,35] Fields and Lemak[36] reported an 8 percent incidence of new strokes involving the ipsilateral cerebral hemisphere in 359 patients with unilateral internal carotid occlusion during a mean follow-up period of 44 months. The incidence of delayed transient ischemic attacks in the territory of the occluded internal carotid may be as high as 35 percent.[37] A consideration of the pathogenesis of post-occlusive cerebroretinal ischemia is useful in planning management.

Post-occlusive ischemic episodes are occasionally best explained on a hemodynamic basis.[5,38] Decreased cerebral perfusion results from alterations in blood flow through precarious anastomotic channels when cardiac output is diminished secondary to cardiac rhythm disturbances or when systemic blood pressure is decreased by either postural changes or abnormal autoregulatory responses. Decreased cerebral blood flow results in symptoms of diffuse cerebral ischemia. These hemodynamic alterations usually occur only in the presence of widespread extracranial occlusive disease, such as bilateral internal carotid occlusion combined with external carotid stenosis or occlusion of both the common and internal carotid arteries. In these circumstances, revascularization of the external carotid artery is recommended to augment external carotid collateral blood flow and to increase total cerebral perfusion.

Amaurosis fugax and symptoms of focal cerebral ischemia usually result from emboli rather than from altered hemodynamics. Lesions in either the contralateral internal carotid artery or the posterior cerebral circulation are rarely the source of emboli which course through intracranial anastomotic channels to lodge in a more remote territory of the brain. This indirect route is usually difficult to substantiate and seems inconsistent with the absence of the ischemic episodes on the nonoccluded side in most patients.[34,37] Several reports have suggested that ischemic events after internal carotid occlusion in some patients result from fragmentation and embolization of thrombotic material dislodged from the soft distal tail of the intracranial portion of the artery.[39,40] Nevertheless, evidence to support this mechanism has been lacking in other studies.[30,34,41]

Finally, emboli may arise from the ipsilateral carotid system and pass through extracranial carotid collateral channels to the retina or cerebral hemisphere.[28,42] The precise site of origin of emboli may be either irregular atheroma in the common carotid or external carotid arteries or the proximal remnant or stump of the occluded internal carotid artery. All of 9 patients with hemispheric or retinal ischemia after occlusion of the appropriate internal carotid artery in the study of Barnett and associates[41] had arteriographic evidence of an internal carotid stump. The internal carotid remnants in these patients varied in length from 2 to 25 mm and averaged 10 mm. In six of seven operated patients, lesions were pathologically consistent with an active process of thrombus formation adherent to ulcerative atheromatous lesions in the stump. In two patients, the carotid stump was the apparent sole source of emboli formation, whereas in the remaining 7 patients irregularity of the common or external carotid arteries represented an alternative source. Turbulent blood flow in the stump was considered an important mechanism for thrombogenesis with subsequent embolization through anastomotic channels.

Among 23 patients with internal carotid occlusion followed up to 60 months after arteriography and reported by Bogousslavsky and co-workers,[37] eight had delayed transient ischemic attacks in the territory of the occluded internal carotid artery. Each of these 8 patients had atheromatous stenosis of the ipsilateral external/common carotid artery or an ulcerated stump of the occluded internal carotid artery. All eight showed good collateral supply from the ipsilateral external carotid artery. In the remaining 15 patients without delayed transient ischemic attacks, only three had a potential source for emboli formation combined with angiographic evidence of external carotid collateral flow to the cerebral circulation. These studies provide circumstantial evidence that the presence of atheromatous stenosis of the external or common carotid artery on the side of an occluded internal carotid, or the presence of an irregular stump of the occluded internal carotid artery, is an important factor in further occurrence of cerebroretinal ischemic events.

Communications between external carotid branches and the intracranial circulation must be substantial if one is to accept the theory that emboli originating proximally can be transmitted to the brain or retina by way of external carotid collateral pathways and if one is to expect total cerebral blood flow to be improved significantly by revascularization of the external carotid artery. As mentioned previously, the existence of potential communications between the external carotid artery and the cerebral circulation has been fully documented by anatomic and arteriographic studies. The clinical relevance of these potential communications, however, is best indicated by their functional significance.

Physiologic documentation of communications from the external carotid artery to the ophthalmic artery is provided by Doppler-derived periorbital flow detection techniques.[43,44] The functional significance of the external carotid collateral pathways is also suggested by intraoperative pressure measurements obtained in the study of Machleder and Barker.[45] Among 8 patients undergoing standard carotid endarterectomy, internal carotid back pressure increased by an average of 21 percent (mean rise of 11 mm Hg) when ipsilateral external carotid blood flow was restored as compared to when the artery was clamped. These measurements documented that flow through the external carotid artery can significantly augment internal carotid back pressure. It is logical to assume that the contribution of the external carotid artery is even greater in patients with chronic internal carotid occlusion when external carotid collaterals have had sufficient time to develop fully.

The study of Zarins et al.[16] provided additional objective information to confirm the functional significance of external carotid collateral blood flow. They reported ten patients undergoing external carotid revascularization for cerebral ischemia associated with internal carotid occlusion and external carotid stenosis. Cerebral blood flow was measured with ^{133}Xe in 6 patients preoperatively and in five postoperatively. Four of the 6 patients had diminished mean blood flow on the affected side, while three had decreased flow on the contralateral side. Regional cerebral blood flow abnormalities were present in each of the 6 patients. All patients had significant postoperative increase in mean blood flow on the treated side, and four had contralateral improvement. All had improvement in regional cerebral blood flow. These objective measurements not only confirm the importance of external carotid collateral pathways in maintaining cerebral perfusion when the internal carotid artery is occluded, but they also document improvement in cerebral blood flow after external carotid revascularization. In their study, symptomatic improvement was achieved in all but 1 patient, who was subsequently relieved of symptoms by EC-IC bypass.

Other clinical studies have also documented relief of cerebral and retinal ischemic symptoms after external carotid revascularization in patients with internal carotid occlusion and therefore have provided additional support for the functional significance of external carotid collateral flow. Diethrich and co-workers[13] described 10 patients with cerebrovascular insufficiency secondary to combined internal carotid occlusion and external carotid stenosis. Each was treated with external carotid endarterectomy. Nine patients available for follow-up were asymptomatic up to 5 years after operation. In the series of Clayson and Edwards,[11] 8 patients with internal carotid occlusion underwent revascularization of only the external carotid by either endarterectomy or bypass. All had significant or complete relief of symptoms. Karmody and associates[15] reported 9 patients who underwent external carotid endarterectomy for treatment of ischemic hemispheric dysfunction secondary to internal carotid occlusion and external carotid stenosis. Of 8 patients available for follow-up ranging from 6 months to three and one-half years, none had neurologic symptoms. Jacques and associates[46] documented improvement in cognitive testing after external carotid endarterectomy. The safety of external carotid revascularization is exemplified by the fact that no operative strokes occurred in any of these series.

Recurrent cerebral ischemia after internal carotid occlusion is frequently presumed to result from intermittent hemodynamic alterations that can be improved by EC-IC bypass.[38,47] Post-occlusive ischemia, however, is often secondary to an embolic mechanism.[28,30,34] A surgical procedure designed to augment cerebral blood flow by direct anastomosis will have questionable benefit when the procedure utilizes branches of an external carotid artery with proximal disease which may be either the source of continued embolization or the cause of restricted inflow to the bypass. Therefore, external carotid endarterectomy may be necessary prior to EC-IC bypass. However, among 9 patients who had external carotid endarterectomy performed to increase inflow for anticipated EC-IC bypass in the study of Moran and associates,[48] two became asymptomatic and did not require subsequent intracranial anastomosis. In 3 patients reported by Kamody and others,[15] external carotid endarterectomy was done solely to provide satisfactory inflow to the superficial temporal artery for subsequent intracranial anastomosis. Nevertheless, each of the 3 patients was relieved of cerebral ischemic symptoms and EC-IC bypass was not required. Such occurrence reemphasizes the importance of extracranial collateral channels. Moreover, successful application of EC-IC bypass requires in each patient a consideration of the mechanism of cerebral ischemia and careful evaluation of the role of the external carotid artery and its collateral pathways in restoring satisfactory cerebral perfusion.

SUMMARY

The presence of cerebral or retinal ischemia after atherosclerotic occlusion of the internal carotid artery should indicate the possibility of coexisting pathology of the external carotid artery. Important collateral channels exist between the external carotid artery and the cerebral circulation. Revascularization of the external carotid not only can prevent embolization by way of external carotid collaterals to the cerebral hemisphere or retina but also can allow augmentation of collateral circuits which improve total cerebral blood flow. In properly selected patients, alleviation of diffuse or focal ischemic symptoms can be expected from external carotid artery revascularization performed either by external carotid endarterectomy or by bypass to the external carotid artery. Consideration of external carotid revascularization is important during investigation prior to EC-IC bypass both to avoid facilitating intracranial embolization and to obviate unnecessary operation in patients who may receive a sufficient increase in cerebral blood flow from external carotid revascularization alone.

REFERENCES

1. Riles TS, Imparato AM, Kopelman I: Carotid artery stenosis with contralateral internal carotid occlusion: Long-term results in fifty-four patients. Surgery 87:363, 1980
2. Thompson JE, Talkington CM: Carotid endarterectomy. Ann Surg 184:1, 1976
3. Thompson JE, Austin DJ, Patman RD: Endarterectomy of the totally occluded carotid artery for stroke. Results of 100 operations. Arch Surg 95:791, 1967
4. Carson SN, Demling RH, Esquivel CO: Aspirin failure in symptomatic atherosclerotic carotid artery disease. Surgery 90:1084, 1981
5. Chater N: Patient selection and results of extra- to intracranial anastomosis in selected cases of cerebrovascular disease. Clin Neurosurg 23:287, 1976
6. Samson DS, Boone S: Extracranial-intracranial (EC-IC) arterial bypass: Past performance and current concepts. Neurosurg 3:79, 1978
7. Whisnant JP: Extracranial-intracranial arterial bypass. Neurology (Minneap) 28:209, 1978
8. Wetzel N, Tunchbay E, Kaupp HA, et al: Stenotic lesions of external carotid artery. Arch Surg 88:842, 1964
9. Jackson BB: The external carotid as a brain collateral. Am J Surg 113:375, 1967
10. Ehrenfeld WK, Lord RSA: Transient monocular blindness through collateral pathways. Surgery 65:911, 1969
11. Clayson KR, Edwards WH: Importance of the external carotid artery in extracranial cerebrovascular occlusive disease. South Med J 70:904, 1977
12. Connolly JE, Steimer EA: Endarterectomy of the external carotid artery. Arch Surg 106:799, 1973
13. Diethrich EB, Liddicoat JE, McCutchen JJ, et al: Surgical significance of the external carotid artery in the treatment of cerebrovascular insufficiency. J Cardiovasc Surg 9:213, 1968
14. Hertzer NR: External carotid endarterectomy. Surg Gynecol Obst 153:186, 1981
15. Karmody AM, Shah DM, Monaco VJ, et al: On surgicial reconstruction of the external carotid artery. Am J Surg 136:176, 1978
16. Zarins CK, DelBeccaro EJ, Johns L, et al: Increased cerebral blood flow after external carotid artery revascularization. Surgery 89:730, 1981
17. Fields WS, Bruetman ME, Weibel J: Collateral circulation of the brain. Monogr Surg Sci 2:183, 1965
18. Gado M, Marshall J.: Clinico-radiological study of collateral circulation after internal carotid and middle cerebral occlusion. J Neurol Neurosurg Psychiatry 34:163, 1971
19. Lasjaunias P, Vignaud J, Hasso AM: Maxillary artery blood supply to the orbit: Normal and pathological aspects. Neuroradiol 9:87, 1975
20. Marx F: An arteriographic demonstration of collaterals between internal and external carotid arteries. Acta Radiol 31:155, 1949
21. Mount LA, Taveras JM: Arteriographic demonstration of the collateral circulation of the cerebral hemisphere. Arch Neurol Psychiat (Chic) 78:235, 1957
22. Richter H: Collaterals between the external carotid artery and the vertebral artery in cases of thrombosis of the internal carotid artery. Acta Radiol (Stockh) 40:108, 1953
23. Taveras JM, Mount LA, Friedenberg RM: Angiographic demonstration of external-internal carotid anastomosis through the ophthalmic artery. Radiology 63:525, 1964
24. Vignaud J, Hasso AN, Lausjaunias P, et al: Orbital vascular anatomy and embryology. Radiology 111:617, 1974
25. Margolis MT, Newton TH: Collateral pathways between the cavernous portion of the internal carotid and external carotid arteries. Radiology 93:834, 1969
26. Schecter MM: The occipital-vertebral anastomosis. J Neurosurg 21:758, 1964
27. Martin MJ, Whisnant JP, Sayre GP: Occlusive vascular disease in extracranial circulation. Arch Neurol 3:530, 1960

28. Countee RW, Vijayanathan T: Intracranial embolization via external carotid artery: Report of a case with angiographic documentation. Stroke 11: 465, 1980
29. Lord RSA: Monocular transient ischemic attacks and the external carotid artery. Med J Aust 1:742, 1973
30. Countee RW, Vijayanathan T: External carotid artery in internal carotid artery occlusion. Angiographic, therapeutic, and prognostic considerations. Stroke 10:450, 1979
31. O'Mara CS, Yao JST, Bergan JJ: External carotid endarterectomy, in Bergan JJ, Yao JST (eds): Operative Techniques in Vascular Surgery. New York, Grune and Stratton, 1980, pp 71–80
32. Berguer R, Bauer RB: Subclavian artery to external carotid artery bypass graft. Arch Surg 111:893, 1976
33. Palma EC: Revascularizacion cerebral anastomotica mediante la carotida externa, en la obliteracion de carotida interna. Angiologia 25:277, 1973
34. Barnett HJM: Delayed cerebral ischemic episodes distal to occlusion of major cerebral arteries. Neurology (Minneap) 28:769, 1978
35. McDowell FH, Potes J, Groch J: The natural history of internal carotid and vertebro-basilar artery occlusions. Neurology (Minneap) 11:153, 1961
36. Fields WS, Lemak NS: Joint study of extracranial arterial occlusion. X. Internal carotid artery occlusion. JAMA 235:2734, 1976
37. Bogousslavsky J, Regli F, Hungerbuhler J, et al: Transient ischemic attacks and external carotid artery. A retrospective study of 23 patients with an occlusion of the internal carotid artery. Stroke 12:627, 1981
38. Austin G, Loffin D, Hayward W: Physiologic factors in selection of patients for superficial temporal artery-to-middle cerebral artery anastomosis. Surgery 75:861, 1974
39. Einsiedel-Lechtape H: Secondary emboli: A frequent sequela of complete extracranial internal carotid artery occlusion. Neuroradiol 16:96, 1978
40. Finklestein S, Kleinman GM, Cuneo R, et al: Delayed stroke following carotid occlusion. Neurology 30:84, 1980
41. Barnett HJM, Peerless SJ, Kaufman JCE: "Stump" of internal carotid artery. A source for further cerebral embolic ischemia. Stroke 9:448, 1978
42. Burnbaum MD, Selhorst JB, Harbison JW, et al: Amaurosis fugax from disease of the external carotid artery. Arch Neurol 34:532, 1977
43. Machleder HI: Evaluation of patients with cerebrovascular disease using the Doppler ophthalmic test. Angiology 24:374, 1973
44. Muller HR: The diagnosis of internal carotid artery occlusion by directional Doppler sonography of the opthalmic artery. Neurology 22:816, 1972
45. Machleder HI, Barker WF: External carotid artery shunting during carotid endarterectomy. Evidence of feasibility. Arch Surg 108:785, 1974
46. Jacques S, Garner JT, Tager R, et al: Improved cognition after external carotid endarterectomy. Surg Neurol 10:223, 1978
47. Heilbrun MP, Reichman OH, Anderson RE, et al: Regional cerebral blood flow studies following superficial temporal-middle cerebral artery anastomosis. J Neurosurg 43:706, 1975
48. Moran JM, Reichman OH, Baker WH: Staged intracranial and extracranial revascularization. Arch Surg 112:1424, 1977

J.M. Cormier
J-B. Ricco

18

Carotid Graft for Cerebrovascular Insufficiency

Although early attempts at carotid artery surgery by Carrea et al.[1] and Eastcott, Pickering and Rob[2] were by direct anastomosis of the resected carotid artery, thromboendarterectomy as introduced by DeBakey[3] has become the standard surgical procedure in patients who suffer from cerebral ischemia. Regardless of whether or not an indwelling shunt is used,[4-12] the most serious complication of the procedure is cerebral embolization during surgery. Emboli may develop from debris at the thromboendarterectomy site, at the suture line, or from incomplete endarterectomy. In an effort to minimize this complication, we have used a vein bypass graft from the common carotid artery to the internal carotid artery, with distal ligation of the internal carotid artery to exclude the diseased segment from the circulation. Currently, 285 patients have undergone this procedure. The present report summarizes our surgical approach and results in 321 procedures performed in these 285 patients.

PATIENT POPULATION

Between January, 1979 and December, 1981, 321 carotid grafts were done for atherosclerotic disease in 285 patients. Takayasu's disease and complex supra-aortic trunk revascularizations were excluded from this study. The patient age ranged from 40 years to 84 years. Table 18-1 shows the age distribution in these patients. The indications for surgery were transient ischemic attacks in 91 patients, reversible neurologic deficit (RIND) in 27 patients, and non-reversible neurologic deficit but stable stroke in 18 patients. One hundred nine patients were asymptomatic, and 76 had vertebro-basilar or contralateral hemispheric symptoms (Table 18-2).

Table 18-1
Carotid Grafts—Age Distribution of Patients (N = 285)

Age	Number of Patients	%
50	9	3
50–59	49	17
60–69	128	45
70–79	92	33
80	7	2

Prior to surgery, all patients underwent extracranial carotid Doppler examination and B-mode ultrasound scan of the carotid arteries. In addition, the collateral circulation of the carotid and vertebral arteries was studied by Doppler recording, as described previously.[13] All patients underwent arteriography using a bilateral retrograde brachial injection and a direct left carotid injection. Biplane extracranial and intracranial views were obtained.

OPERATIVE TECHNIQUE

No indwelling shunts or stump pressure measurements were used in the study. Also, there was no attempt to monitor the EEG changes in these patients. An arterial line was used routinely to monitor the blood pressure immediately before, during, and after the operation.

Under general anesthesia, the patient was placed in the supine position, with the shoulders elevated on a folded sheet and with the head turned away from the side of operation. A vertical neck incision along the anterior border of the sternocleidomastoid muscle was used all cases. Retraction of this

Table 18-2
Indications For Carotid Graft (N = 321)

Symptomatology	Number of Patients	%
Transient Ischemic Attack	91	28
Reversible Ischemic Neurologic Deficit	27	9
Stable Stroke	18	6
Vertebro-Basilar or Contralateral Hemispheric Symptoms	76	23
Asymptomatic	109	34

muscle laterally allowed ample exposure of the carotid artery. The common facial vein was ligated and divided, permitting exposure of the underlying carotid sheath.

The carotid sheath was then entered and the common carotid, internal carotid, and external carotid arteries were dissected free. In order to obtain satisfactory length of the internal carotid artery, the hypoglossal nerve was carefully dissected out. Sometimes, the digastric muscle had to be transected for additional exposure. Once dissection of the carotid arteries was completed, attention was turned to harvesting the saphenous vein from the groin. This was done by placing a vertical incision in the groin, with removal of the vein in the usual manner.

After systemic administration of 5000 units of heparin, the common carotid artery was clamped and a longitudinal arteriotomy done on the anterior lateral aspect at a point beyond the extent of atherosclerotic disease (Fig. 18-1). The proximal anastomosis was done between the vein graft and the common carotid artery in end-to-side fashion, using a 6-0 prolene suture in continuous fashion. Before completion of this anastomosis, the end of the vein graft was ligated.

Once the anastomosis was completed, the inferior clamp was removed from the common carotid artery, allowing blood to flush through the

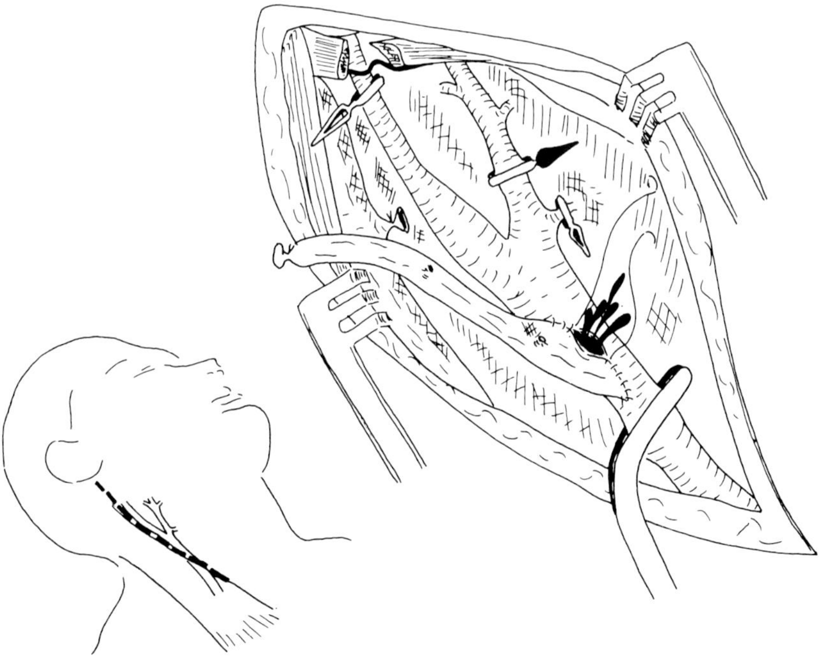

Figure 18-1. Carotid graft proximal anastomosis

anastomosis to the vein graft. Thereafter, the superior clamp was removed and flow through the internal and external carotid arteries thus temporarily reestablished. At this time, the vein graft was filled with blood and perfused at systemic pressure. This maneuver determined the correct length of the graft and straightened it to avoid any twisting.

After the exact length of the graft was determined, the common, external, and distal internal carotid arteries were again clamped to prepare for the distal anastomosis. The internal carotid artery was opened longitudinally above the stenosis on two-thirds of its circumference. The distal anastomosis was done between the vein graft and the internal carotid artery as an end-to-side anastomosis using 7-0 running prolene suture. Once the anastomosis was done, the internal carotid artery was transected completely below the anastomosis (Fig. 18-2).

If the vein graft contained a valve, air bubbles might be trapped by the valve. In order to flush these bubbles from the graft, the clamp at the proximal end-to-side anastomosis was first released (Fig. 18-2A); therefore, blood could flow through the open end of the distal internal carotid artery. If the vein contained no valve, the flush was done in retrograde fashion by releasing the internal carotid clamp (Fig. 18-2B). Once flushing was completed, the transected stump (proximal and distal) was closed using a running 6-0 prolene suture.

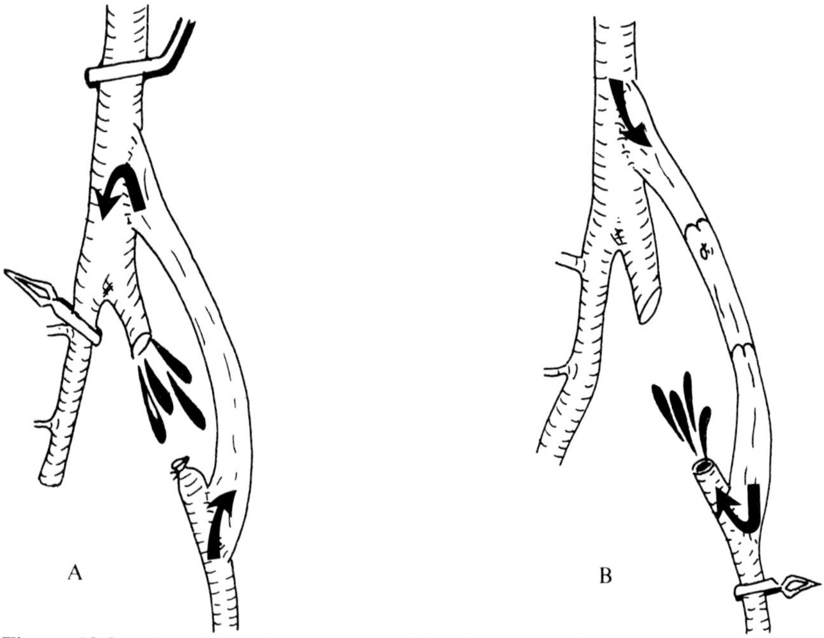

A B

Figure 18-2. Carotid graft technique of flush (A) valvulated saphenous vein (B) avalvulated saphenous vein

Several technical maneuvers of the bypass operative technique require special emphasis. First, the end-to-side anastomosis of the internal carotid artery must be done before transection of the artery to prevent any twisting or error in length. Transection of the internal carotid artery transforms the end-to-side anastomosis to a somewhat end-to-end anastomosis. Second, a thromboendarterectomy of the common carotid stump may be done if there is severe disease process involving the external carotid artery. This is done by an incision made in the common carotid and external carotid artery junction, with the endarterectomy performed in usual manner from inside the artery.

RESULTS

All patients who awoke from surgery with a neurologic deficit were considered as immediate complications, whereas those who developed a neurologic deficit during the postoperative period (30 days) were listed as late complications. Immediate neurological complications were noted in 5 patients. All five deficits were transient and reversed completely within 24 hours. Table 18-3 summarizes the neurological complications in these patients. A seizure and transient ischemic attack occurred in 2 patients who had transient ischemic attacks as their presenting symptoms. Of 3 patients with preoperative, non-reversible neurologic deficit (stable stroke), one had a seizure, and two had their preoperative neurologic status worsened after surgery (Table 18-4).

The occurrence of these five immediate postoperative neurologic complications was analyzed in relation to the existence of a contralateral carotid stenosis or occlusion (Table 18-5). Of 246 patients with unilateral carotid stenosis, only two had complications (0.8 percent). No immediate permanent neurologic deficit occurred in the 75 patients who had either a complete occlusion or a significant stenosis of the contralateral carotid artery at the time of surgery, although three of these (4 percent) demonstrated transient deficits.

Three patients suffered delayed neurological complications. All of these had a normal neurologic status immediately after surgery. One patient had a stroke during a hypertensive crisis and died from a bleeding stress ulcer 12 days postoperatively. Another had a brain stem infarction and died on the sixth postoperative day. A third patient had an acute thrombosis of the vein graft, with a reversible neurologic deficit occurring during the first 24 hours postoperatively.

Mortality within 30 days postoperatively for the entire group was 0.6 percent (2 patients), and was related to delayed stroke. Among the survivors, there was no permanent neurologic deficit and, for the entire series, the incidence of temporary neurologic deficit was 1.8 percent (6 patients).

Table 18-3
Early Postoperative Results of Carotid Bypass Without a Shunt In 321 Procedures

Preoperative Neurological Status	No. of Operations	Immediate Neurologic Postoperative Complications		Delayed Neurologic Postoperative Complications		Hospital Mortality
		Temporary	Permanent	Temporary	Permanent	
Asymptomatic	109	0	0	0	0	0
Symptomatic	212	5	0	1	2	2*

*Overall hospital mortality = .6%

Table 18-4
Immediate Postoperative Neurologic Complications in Carotid Bypass Without a Shunt in 321 Procedures

Preoperative Neurological Status	No. of Operations	Seizure	Transient Ischemic Attack	Reversible Neurologic Deficit
TIA	91	1	1	0
Reversible Neurologic Deficit (RIND)	27	0	0	0
Non-Reversible Neurologic Deficit (stable stroke)	18	1	0	2

DISCUSSION

The use of saphenous vein bypass grafts for carotid artery stenosis was first reported by Javid et al. in 1955,[14] but the procedure retained little interest after the introduction of thromboendarterectomy. Other bypasses, such as the subclavian-carotid bypass, right brachiocephalic trunk-carotid bypass or carotid-carotid bypass have been described as surgical treatment for extra-cranial carotid artery disease. Although we reported earlier on the use of bypass grafting in carotid artery disease from irradiation, Takayasu's disease, or aneurysm,[15] there has not yet been a large series on the use of direct vein bypass grafting from the common carotid to the internal carotid artery in patients with atherosclerotic disease. The present report represents an extensive experience in the use of vein bypass grafting for atherosclerotic carotid artery disease. In this series, the mortality rate of 0.6 percent and the 1.6 percent incidence of reversible neurologic deficit compare favorably with other reports using the thromboendarterectomy technique, with or without a shunt.[4-12] Carotid vein bypass may be a safe alternative procedure for surgical treatment of cerebral ischemia.

Carotid bypass vein grafting offers several advantages over thrombo-endarterectomy. In many instances, the main technical problem of carotid endarterectomy is the distal plane of the plaque. Sometimes, the plane ends smoothly, and the entire plaque is removed easily. Not infrequently, the plaque is continuous with the cephalad portion of the internal carotid artery and must be transected abruptly. This creates a steep edge of the plaque that must be sutured to prevent flap formation. The presence of such residual plaque may

Table 18-5
Carotid Bypass
Immediate Postoperative Neurologic Complications
Correlation With Contralateral Carotid Disease in 321 Procedures

Preoperative Arteriographic Findings	No. of Operations	Seizures	Transient Ischemic Attack	Reversible Neurologic Deficit
Unilateral Carotid Stenosis	246	1	0	1
Bilateral Carotid Stenosis	55	1	1	0
Contralateral Carotid Occlusion	20	0	0	1

cause re-stenosis, or it may serve as the site for distal embolization. Although patch angioplasty as advocated by some surgeons may avoid re-stenosis, the imperfect size of the patch may lead to dilatation, causing turbulence. The latter may also play a role in distal embolization. Finally, the endarterectomy site may serve as a focus for platelet aggregation, and platelet emboli may account for neurological problems after surgery. The bypass graft with distal ligation of the artery described here excludes the atheromatous plaque from the circulation. In doing so, the source of embolization is completely eliminated. The technique is particularly suited for patients with atherosclerotic plaques or stenosis associated with kinking or looping. The use of the vein bypass corrects the stenosis and kinking simultaneously. In addition, the carotid vein bypass graft is ideal in trauma, spontaneous dissecting aneurysm, or aneurysm of the carotid artery.

No attempt was made to use an indwelling shunt or to record stump pressure in the present series. EEG monitoring was also not employed. We doubt that these two manuevers advocated by many authors are essential in carotid artery surgery. As demonstrated in the present report, only 5 patients (1.6 percent) had immediate neurological deficits, and all recovered 5 days later. The result is comparable to those series in which shunt or EEG monitoring were used.[8,16,17] The incidence of postoperative neurologic deficit, however, appears to be higher in patients with contralateral carotid artery occlusion (5 percent) or stenosis (4 percent). As noted in previous reports, the presence of a neurological deficit prior to surgery influences significantly the outcome of surgery. Of 18 patients with preoperative, non-reversible neurological deficit (stable stroke), three developed postoperative neurological complications (17 percent). One of these three patients had a seizure and the other two had transient aggravation of the pre-existing neurologic deficit. The seizure may be explained on the basis of an embolic event or cerebral edema during carotid clamping. It is possible that a zone of ischemic brain tissue persists after a stroke, and such a zone may be supplied by highly resistant collateral vessels. Thus, during cross-clamping, a drop in perfusion pressure to this critical region may cause worsening of neurologic symptoms.[16] Perhaps the use of a shunt in patients with neurologic deficit may reduce the morbidity in these patients.

There are minor drawbacks in the bypass technique. The dissection of the internal carotid artery needs to be more extensive than that for a thrombo-endarterectomy, the total clamping time is appreciably longer, and the vein must be harvested in the groin. As a result, the total operating time using carotid bypass is longer than for carotid endarterectomy.

Long-term follow-up is not yet available. At 3 years, however, we have yet to observe dilatation or fibrosis of the vein graft, as has been reported in renal or femoral bypass grafts. The bypass graft technique described in this report offers a safe alternative in the treatment of atheromatous lesions of the carotid artery. Although it may be premature to recommend this technique as a routine procedure, we feel that bypass grafting is particularly suited for stenotic lesions with kinking or looping of the internal carotid artery, post-irradiation damage of the internal carotid artery, and possibly, in re-do surgery for recurrent stenosis after a thromboendarterectomy.

REFERENCES

1. Carrea R, Molius M, Murphy G: Surgical management of spontaneous thrombosis of the internal carotid artery in the neck: Carotid-carotideal anastmosis, report of a case. Acta Neurol Lat Am 1:71, 1955
2. Eastcott HHG, Pickering GW, Rob C: Reconstruction of the internal carotid artery in a patient with intermittent attacks of hemiplegia. Lancet 2:994, 1954
3. DeBakey ME, Crawford ES, Cooley DA, et al: Cerebral arterial insufficiency: One to 11 year results following arterial reconstruction operation. Ann Surg 161:921, 1965
4. Thompson JE, Austin DJ, Patman RD: Carotid endarterectomy for cerebrovascular insufficiency: Long-term results in 592 patients followed up to 13 years. Ann Surg 172:633, 1970
5. Giannotta SL, Dicks RE, Kindt GW: Carotid endarterectomy technical improvements. Neurosurg 7:309, 1980
6. Ojemann RG, Crowell RM, Roberson GH, et al: Surgical treatment of extracranial carotid occlusive disease. Clin Neurosurg 22:214, 1975
7. Sundt TM, Sandok BA, Whisnant JP: Carotid endarterectomy: Complications and pre-operative assessment of risk. Mayo Clin Proc 50:301, 1975
8. Sundt TM, Sharbrough FW, Piepgras DG, et al: Correlation of cerebral blood flow and encephalographic changes during carotid endarterectomy with results of surgery and hemodynamics of cerebral ischemia. Mayo Clin Proc 56:533, 1981
9. Baker WM, Dorner DB, Barnes RW: Carotid endarterectomy: Is an indwelling shunt necessary? Surgery 82:321, 1977

10. Whitney DG, Kahn EM, Estes JW, et al: Carotid surgery without a temporary indwelling shunt: 1917 consecutive procedures. Arch Surg 115:1393, 1980
11. Ott DA, Cooley DA, Chapa L, et al: Carotid endarterectomy without temporary intraluminal shunt: Study of 390 consecutive operations. Ann Surg 191:708, 1980
12. Bland JE, Lazar ML: Carotid endarterectomy without a shunt. Neurosurg 8:153, 1981
13. Franchesi C: Exploration Doppler des voies de suppleance des arteres cervico-cerebrales. J Maladie vasculaires (Paris), vol. 6. p 89, 1981
14. Javid H: Current status of carotid surgery. Contemp Surg 16:13, 1980
15. Cormier JM, Lagneau P, Janneau D: Cent trois revascularisations de la carotide interne par greffe veineuse. J Chir (Paris), 115:7, 1978
16. Rosenthal D, Stanton PE, Lamis PA: Carotid endarterectomy. The unreliability of intraoperative monitoring in patients having had stroke or reversible ischemic neurologic deficit. Arch Surg 116:1569, 1981
17. Chiappa KM, Burke SR, Young RR: Results of electroencephalographic monitoring during 367 carotid endarterectomies. Stroke 10:381, 1979

PART VI

Specialized Management During Carotid Surgery

Thoralf M. Sundt, Jr.
Frank W. Sharbrough
David G. Piepgras

19

The Significance of Cerebral Blood Flow Measurements during Carotid Endarterectomy

We analyzed 1352 consecutive carotid endarterectomies for carotid artery ulcerative-stenosis, which were categorized into 4 groups according to preoperative risk factors and monitored with intraoperative cerebral blood flow (CBF) measurements and electroencephalograms (EEGs) and postoperative EEGs and retinal artery pressure (RAP) measurements. Overall mortality was 1.2 percent, major morbidity 1 percent, minor morbidity 1 percent, and transient neurological dysfunction 2 percent. However, these statistics varied from a minor morbidity of 1 percent and transient neurological dysfunction of 1 percent in the lowest risk group (grade 1) to a 5 percent mortality, 2.5 percent major morbidity, 2 percent minor morbidity, and 3.5 percent transient neurological dysfunction in the highest risk group (grade 4). CBF and EEG changes correlated closely with preoperative neurological function, intraoperative complications, and postoperative hyperperfusion syndromes. The critical flow (CBF required to maintain normal EEG) approximated 30 percent (15 ml/100g/min) of normal CBF (50 ml/100g/min), but shunts were usually placed if flow fell below 18 to 20 ml/100g/min during occlusion for endarterectomy. Baseline and occlusion CBF values were significantly lower in the highest risk group in comparison to similar measurements in the lowest risk group. Occlusion flows below 10 ml/100g/min were recorded in 4 percent of grade 1 patients, 9 percent of grade 2 patients, 11 percent of grade 3 patients, and 20 percent of grade 4 patients. Intraoperative embolization and postoperative hyperperfusion syndromes in which CBF increased to over 200 percent the baseline flow were the most common neurological complications; the former was the leading cause for ischemic infarction and the latter the apparent cause for transient seizures, migraine variants, and intracerebral hemorrhages. Myocardial infarction was the primary cause of death and occurred exclusively in patients with known coronary artery disease. This study supports a hemodynamic component for ischemic events when cerebral autoregulation is paralyzed but a microembolic cause when it is preserved. The two theories or mechanisms for the production of ischemia are not mutually exclusive and were often found together in the grade 4 group in which embolization into regions of marginal ischemia was frequently observed and in which, because of marginal collateral flow, were the cause of a progressing deficit.

Over the past decade elective carotid endarterectomies at the Mayo Clinic have routinely had intraoperative electroencephalographic (EEG) and cerebral blood flow (CBF) monitoring and pre- and post-operative EEG and retinal artery pressure (RAP) measurements. These collected data, stored in a computer along with pertinent aspects of each patient's record, have provided information concerning normal and marginal CBF, which has contributed to our understanding of the pathophysiology of cerebral ischemia. Furthermore, this data has made feasible a detailed analysis of results and, more importantly, complications of carotid endarterectomy. Many of the latter are generally recognized. They include the following: intraoperative embolization, inadequate cerebral protection during the period of carotid occlusion at surgery, and postoperative occlusion at the site of endarterectomy.[1,2,3,4,5] Others related to postoperative unilateral cerebral hyperperfusion have not been described, or if described, have not been attributed to that phenomenon.[6,7] In order to place in perspective the changes in CBF from surgery and the complications of the operation, it is necessary to review the entire series. The indications for surgery and long-term follow-up data will not be considered here,[8,9] nor will we broach the controversial subject of the role of thromboendarterectomy in acute occlusions.[10]

METHODS

This report includes all patients operated on for carotid stenosis by our neurovascular surgical services between January 1, 1972 and January 1, 1982. Patients were operated on by one of two staff surgeons or by a chief resident with one of those staff surgeons acting as the first assistant. All patients had detailed pre- and postoperative neurological examinations and RAPs and most, including all with a complication, had a postoperative EEG.

Preoperative Risk Factors

A correlation has been noted between certain preoperative risk factors and complications.[11,12] The following represent the major, but by no means the only, considerations in determining the patient's surgical risk: (1) medical risk factors—the presence of symptomatic coronary artery disease (angina pectoris) or a myocardial infarction within 6 months prior to the date of surgery, severe hypertension (blood pressure greater than 180/110), chronic obstructive pulmonary disease, physiological age of more than 70 years, and severe obesity; (2) neurological risk factors—a progressing neurological deficit, a deficit less than 24 hours old prior to surgery, frequent daily transient ischemic attacks, or symptoms of generalized (in contrast to focal) cerebral ischemia; and (3) angiographically determined risks—coexisting stenosis of the internal carotid artery in the siphon area, extensive involvement of the vessel to be operated on with the plaque extending more than 3 cm distally in the internal carotid artery or 5 cm proximally in the common carotid artery, bifurcation of the carotid artery at the level of the second cervical vertebra in conjunction with a short or thick neck, occlusion of the opposite internal carotid artery, evidence of a soft thrombus extending from the ulcerative lesion or small vessel occlusions from multiple emboli, and a slowed intracranial circulation time on angiography. The degree of stenosis per se was not considered a risk factor.

Classification of Cases

On the basis of the foregoing general risk factors, it is possible to create a system for grading a patient's potential risk for surgery.[11] Although a given patient does not always fit neatly into a particular grouping, this system does provide a framework for comparative purposes. The patients were graded as follows: grade 1—neurologically stable (no neurological risk factors) with no major medical or angiographically determined risks, with unilateral or bilateral ulcerative-stenotic diseases; grade 2—neurologically stable with no major medical risks but with significant angiographically determined risks; grade 3—neurologically stable with major medical risks with or without significant angiographically determined risks; grade 4—major neurological risks with or without associated major medical or angiographically determined risks; angiograms in this group frequently showed both a slowed flow and multiple small vessel occlusions.

Preoperative Evaluation

All patients had detailed medical, neurological, and neuro-ophthalmological evaluation prior to surgery. Preoperative EEGs were performed in the operating room prior to the induction of anesthesia.

Intraoperative Monitoring

Anesthesia

The anesthetic technique used has been reported previously.[13] The depth of anesthesia is carefully controlled in order to have a sensitive EEG tracing and the arterial carbon dioxide tension ($PaCO_2$) held constant in order to have comparable conditions for the comparison of CBF measurements. With subjects grouped according to anesthetic agent used and grade level, the mean $PaCO_2$ and mean MABP values for the baseline, occlusion, shunt, and post-occlusion determinations were nearly identical with groups (see tables). Furthermore, the mean baseline $PaCO_2$ values were the same for each anesthetic group (overall mean $= 40 \pm 4.9$), whereas the mean baseline MABP determination was significantly higher ($p < .001$) in the halothane group than in the ethrane group (111 ± 16 vs. 103 ± 14). There were too few patients operated under other anesthetic agents to consider them in the analysis of CBF measurements.

Cerebral Blood Flow Measurements

Regional cerebral blood flow measurements were determined from clearance curves obtained from the extracranial detection of intra-arterially injected Xenon-133.[14] The technique for this has been described in detail previously.[15,16] All instruments for recording counts were located in an adjacent monitoring room (Fig. 19-1). No cumbersome equipment was present in the operating suite. The indicator was injected through a No. 27 needle into the common carotid artery with the external carotid artery temporarily occluded. Each injectate contains 200 to 300 μCi of xenon-133 diluted to 0.2 to 0.3 ml total volume with physiological saline. Customarily, three measurements are obtained: one prior to occlusion, one during occlusion, and one after restoration of flow. If a shunt is employed, a fourth measurement and sometimes a fifth is performed with the shunt in place.

Electroencephalographic Technique

A continuous 16-channel EEG tracing is initiated prior to induction of anesthesia and terminated with extubation.[13] An experienced technician interprets the EEG intraoperatively, but all tracings are formally read by Dr. Sharbrough after the operation.

Operative Technique

A saphenous vein patch graft is used routinely except in cases with particularly large vessels. A shunt is always placed when both the EEG and CBF indicate cerebral ischemia during the period of occlusion and frequently is placed if the CBF is marginal even if the EEG remains unchanged. This latter indication for shunting is particularly important in patients with a preoperative infarction and an abnormal EEG because changes in the EEG are more difficult to identify and there appears to be a lower tolerance for ischemia in these individuals.[13] A shunt is never placed until the normal wall of the vessel is visualized beyond the limits of the plaque. If a temporal pulse is

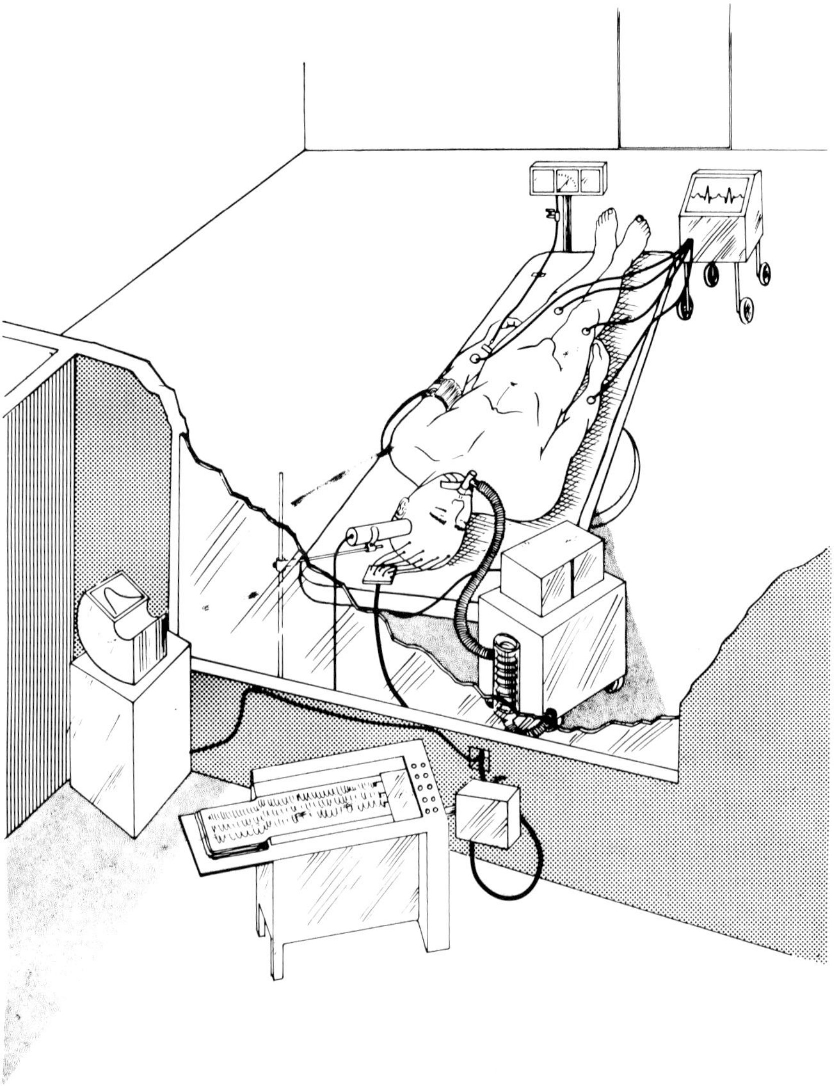

Figure 19-1. Equipment for monitoring carotid endarterectomies is maintained in room adjacent to operating theater and does not interfere with anesthesia or surgical teams.

not present after flow has been restored, the origin of the external carotid artery is temporarily occluded and the shelf of elevated plaque or intima at the distal limit of the resection excised through a separate short arteriotomy in that vessel. Routinely 4,000 to 5,000 units of heparin are given prior to occlusion of the vessels. This heparin is not reversed.

Postoperative Monitoring

All patients have a detailed neurological examination when they awaken from anesthesia. They remain in the intensive care unit for 24 hours during which time postoperative retinal artery pressure measurements are obtained. All patients, elective and non-elective, have postoperative RAPs; these have been proven to be highly accurate for the identification of occlusion or severely stenotic lesions.[17] Most patients have postoperative EEGs, which usually are completed on the 6th or 7th postoperative day. Some patients are discharged within that period, however, prior to having a postoperative EEG.

Categorization of Complications

We defined morbidity as any deficit not present prior to the operation. A minor morbidity was considered any deficit—e.g. a slight visual field defect—that did not interfere with normal daily living or employment present at the time of hospital discharge or follow-up examination. A patient with a new postoperative EEG abnormality and a normal neurological examination was considered to have a minor morbidity on the basis of an infarction in a silent area of the brain. Major morbidity did interfere with normal daily living and employment.

Categorization of Results

Complications were divided into those that occurred during the operation and those that followed surgery. In the latter grouping, complications were subdivided into medical (generally cardiac) and neurological types.

Data Analysis

Information from the preoperative grading of the patient, intraoperative monitoring, postoperative studies, and ultimate clinical results was recorded on a standard form and the information from that form stored in a computer. The data retrieved were analyzed using standard techniques, and those data have served as the basis for this report.

CASES ILLUSTRATIVE OF LOW AND HIGH PERFUSION SYNDROMES

Case 1

This 65-year-old diabetic male with a 95 percent stenosis of the right internal carotid artery underwent carotid endarterectomy on July 13, 1974, because of a progressive, non-stepwise, deterioration in neurological function in the left lower extremity. Proximal function was retained in that extremity, but the foot was essentially paralyzed and the patient was unable to walk without assistance. Dexterity in the left hand was decreased, and the family reported problems with cerebration. Blow flows at surgery were as follows: baseline, 20 ml/100g/min; occlusion, 15 ml/100g/min; shunt, 50 ml/100g/min; and postocclusion, 78 ml/100g/min. The EEG remained abnormal and unchanged except for transient worsening with occlusion. Following surgery there was a dramatic increase in the RAPs on the right (40/10 pre-op, 90/40 post-op), and he gradually regained near normal neurological function, retaining only weakness in dorsiflexion of the foot when last evaluated by his referring neurologist.

Comment

This case characterizes some of those patients classified as grade 4 candidates for surgery and typifies the "slow stroke" syndrome. The normal preoperative computerized tomogram and functional recovery following surgery suggests the low CBF of 20 ml/100g/min was adequate for the maintenance of neuronal viability but inadequate for normal function.

Case 2

This 74-year-old mildly hypertensive male on anticoagulant therapy was referred for neurological evaluation on April 20, 1980, because of a progression in the frequency and severity of daily posturally related events of near syncope with visual blurring. There was no history of focal TIAs but mental function had deteriorated. Cardiac function was monitored and found to be normal during these attacks. The episodes were not changed by intravenous heparin therapy. RAPs sitting were 42/20 bilaterally. Angiography revealed bilateral 99 percent stenotic (less than 1 mm residual lumen) carotid lesions. Blood flows during left carotid endarterectomy were as follows: baseline, 19 ml/100g/min; occlusion, 15 ml/100g/min; shunt, 26 ml/100g/min; and postocclusion, 64 ml/100g/min. Neurological function following surgery was normal, but the patient complained of severe ipsilateral headache, which was more severe supine. His blood pressure was 160/90, no different from preoperative measurements. Flame-shaped hemorrhages were noted on ophthalmoscopic examination, and the RAPs had more than doubled on the side of operation. Five days after the operation, the patient had a massive intracerebral hemorrhage and died.

Comment

This case characterizes another subgroup of the grade 4 category and typifies the "generalized cerebral ischemia" or "orthostatic cerebral ischemia" syndrome. The intracerebral hemorrhage following surgery was probably the result of a paralysis of the cerebral autoregulatory control mechanisms. We believe CBF continued to increase following the operation and was the cause of the unilateral headaches.

RESULTS

Morbidity-Mortality

Table 19-1 summarizes the morbidity-mortality of the series according to risk classification for surgery. The causes for both transient and permanent neurological deficits are considered further below but will be briefly summarized here. There were 19 cases with transient neurological dysfunction who had, compared to preoperative testing, both normal or unchanged neurological examinations at hospital discharge. The causes for these transient deficits were as follows: postoperative ICA occlusion, four; embolic TIAs, three; migraine variants, five; transient seizure activity, six; and intraoperative embolization, one. Twelve patients sustained a major ischemic stroke; the causes were as follows: postoperative ICA occlusion, one; positional occlusion of vessel during surgery, one; intraoperative embolization, seven; failure to place shunt, one; and myocardial infarction with hypotension, two (one opposite to side of surgery). Fourteen patients retained a minor new deficit; the causes were as follows: intraoperative embolization, two; postoperative embolization, four; postoperative ICA occlusion, two; seizures with residual deficit, three; small intracerebral hemorrhage, one; and migraine variant, two. There were five fatal intracerebral hemorrhages; one occurred during the operation and four following surgery.

Intraoperative CBF Measurements

Mean baseline, occlusion, shunt (when used), and postocclusion (flow following completion of endarterectomy) blood flows are summarized in

Table 19-1
Results of Carotid Endarterectomy*
January 1 1972-January 1, 1982

		Neurologic Function				Morality		
Grade of Risk	Procedures	Normal, unchanged, or improved†		New Deficit Major	New Deficit Minor	From intracerebral hemorrhage	From myocardial infarction	From other complications
1	472	468	(4)	0	4	0	0	0
2	282	278	(4)	2	2	0	0	0
3	357	342	(4)	5	3	0	6	1
4	241	222	(7)	5	5	5	2	2
Total	1,352	1,310	(19)	12	14	5	8	3

*Overall, mortality was 1.2%, major morbidity was 1%, and minor morbidity was 1%.
†Numbers in parentheses are patients with transient neurologic dysfunction (transient ischemic attacks, seizures, migraine variants)

Table 19-2 according to the anesthetic agent used (halothane and ethrane only, other agents not included) and the grade of the patient. The precise degree of stenosis is difficult to determine from only one plane on an angiogram, and the relative effect from this stenosis on CBF is a function of its length and available collateral flow to the ipsilateral hemisphere. Thus, this table does not include the degree of stenosis. Virtually all of the grade 4 group, however, had greater than a 90 percent stenosis. There were 25 grade 4 cases with a baseline CBF below 25 ml/100g/min. Generally, a shunt was used if the occlusion flow fell below 18 to 20 ml/100g/min. The distribution of occlusion flows with halothane and ethrane anesthesia is summarized in Table 19-3. Occlusion flows below 10 ml/100g/min for all anesthetic agents, however, were recorded in 15 grade 1, 20 grade 2, 35 grade 3, and 35 grade 4 patients.

Intraoperative EEGs and Complications

Intraoperative EEGs were recorded in all cases. A focal change with occlusion occurred in 361 cases and in 359 of these, the EEG reverted to baseline with placement of a shunt. The relative change in the EEG from ischemia paralleled the severity of CBF reduction below the critical flow. Typical EEG changes are illustrated in Figure 19-2. In one case with diffuse proximal atherosclerosis, the EEG suddenly worsened after the shunt had been in place and in one case, also with severe proximal disease, there was a dramatic worsening with placement of the shunt. It was concluded that embolization through the shunt explained both of these events. A focal transient change occurred in 141 cases not associated with the time of carotid occlusion for endarterectomy. In 131 cases this was minor, transient, and related to changes in the depth of anesthesia in patients with a minor preexisting abnormality. It was persistent, however, in 11 cases and in each of these, the patient awoke from anesthesia with a new neurological deficit. This was transient in one and permanent in 10 cases. Intraoperative embolization was assumed to be the cause for nine of these events (one from contralateral vessel) and positional occlusion of a high grade stenosis for one. One was related to a massive intracerebral hemorrhage, which in turn occurred from a major increase in CBF in a patient who had a coexisting, autopsy-proven sagittal sinus thrombosis. Retrospectively, this was identified on the preoperative angiograms.

Postoperative Neurologic Complications

A postoperative ICA occlusion, identified by a reduction in the RAP and subsequent angiography, occurred in eight cases. These were the only cases in the entire series with low postoperative RAPs or reduced oculoplethysmographic (OPGs) readings. Six of these cases occurred in endarterectomies without patch grafting. Five remained patent following reoperation with

Table 19-2
Cerebral Blood Flow According to Anesthetic Used and Grade of Risk
(Mean ± SD)

Halothane

Time of measurement	Grade 1 n	Grade 1 $\bar{x}$ ± SD	Grade 2 n	Grade 2 $\bar{x}$ ± SD	Grade 3 n	Grade 3 $\bar{x}$ ± SD	Grade 4 n	Grade 4 $\bar{x}$ ± SD
Baseline	149	63 ± 26	85	59 ± 27	135	52 ± 21	80	48 ± 20
Occlusion	149	35 ± 18	85	31 ± 18	137	27 ± 15	78	24 ± 14*
Shunt	40	45 ± 15	40	53 ± 18	62	44 ± 17	46	41 ± 12
Postocclusion	150	70 ± 27†	86	69 ± 25†	137	62 ± 23†	82	61 ± 21†

Ethrane

Time of measurement	Grade 1 n	Grade 1 $\bar{x}$ ± SD	Grade 2 n	Grade 2 $\bar{x}$ ± SD	Grade 3 n	Grade 3 $\bar{x}$ ± SD	Grade 4 n	Grade 4 $\bar{x}$ ± SD
Baseline	278	49 ± 18	168	45 ± 20	180	42 ± 18	127	38 ± 21
Occlusion	276	27 ± 12	167	24 ± 14	176	21 ± 11	127	18 ± 11*
Shunt	97	38 ± 14	86	36 ± 12	97	36 ± 12	78	36 ± 15
Postocclusion	280	51 ± 18	170	51 ± 20†	187	49 ± 19†	133	51 ± 22†

*Two-sample t test applied to differences between grade 1 and grade 4 values at occlusion was significant at $p < 0.001$.
†Paired t test applied to differences between baseline and postocclusion values was significant at $p < 0.001$.

Table 19-3
Cerebral Blood Flow Versus Electroencephalogram From Carotid Occlusion

	Number of patients with change in electroencephalogram from occlusion		Number of patients without change in electroencephalogram from occlusion	
Flow*	Halothane	Ethrane	Halothane	Ethrane
0–4	6	27	0	0
5–9	18	73	1	0
10–14	46	84	6	36
15–19	41	64	19	73
20–24	7	8	41	101
25–29	0	0	54	101
≥30	0	0	222	253
Total	118	256	343	564

*In ml/100 g per minute

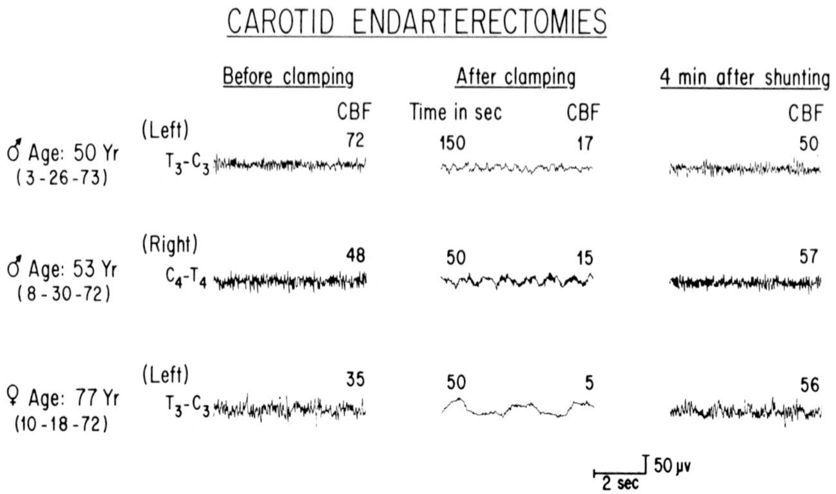

Figure 19-2. Changes in the EEG mirror the severity of CBF reduction during carotid occlusion. The more severe the change in the EEG, the longer it takes to return to normal.

grafting. The two occlusions in patched vessels occurred in patients with evidence of hypercoagulability status (proven disseminated intravascular coagulopathy in one and vitamin K induced in the other); both of these remained patent following reoperation with postoperative anticoagulant therapy. The one patient in whom we could not restore flow developed a major infarction from this cause, and two others retained a minor deficit related to the period of occlusion. Five left the hospital with normal function, however, after an average period of hospitalization (four had had brief single posturally related TIAs from the occlusion, and one had been asymptomatic).

Microemboli were the apparent cause of typical TIAs in three cases and minor infarcts in four. These patients were treated with anticoagulants or anti-platelet agents.

Atypical TIAs with migrainous components occurred in seven cases. These usually developed 5 to 7 days following surgery, occurred in the morning before breakfast, were associated with unilateral headache, evolved over a period of several minutes rather than suddenly as in a typical TIA, and were not accompanied by an elevation in blood pressure. One of these patients, after five daily morning events, sustained a quadrantic homonymous field defect. The mean baseline CBF in this group was 43.2 ± 16 and post-endarterectomy was 83.2 ± 39.8 ml/100g/min. Postoperative angiograms in these patients were normal. Two of these patients retained a minor fixed deficit.

Transient focal seizure activity occurred in 11 cases, ten of which were considered grade 4 candidates for surgery. The seizures resolved in all cases, and no patients developed a chronic seizure focus. Seizures usually developed between the fifth and seventh postoperative day and were not related to elevations in blood pressure. The mean baseline CBF in this group was 37.3 ± 13.4 ml/100g/min, and the mean postocclusion flow was 85.5 ± 31.8 ml/100g/min. All patients had a major increase in the RAP measurements. Two patients, treated with heparin, developed intracerebral hemorrhages (fatal in one, minor fixed deficit in one), three retained a minor new fixed deficit, and six recovered entirely with no deficit. There were no major ischemic infarctions in this group. Angiograms were normal.

Intracerebral hemorrhages occurred postoperatively in five cases and were fatal in four. The mean baseline CBF was 29.6 ± 20 ml/100/min, and the mean postocclusion CBF was 76.8 ± 18.5 ml/100g/min. Two of these patients, relatively early in our experience and before we recognized the possible relevancy of seizures to reactive hyperemia, were on heparin at the time of the hemorrhage. Two other patients were on aspirin because they were operated during a clinical trial period when we had used this drug routinely. This complication usually developed 5 to 7 days after surgery and was not associated with a significant change in blood pressure.

Postoperative Non-Neurologic Complications

There were thirteen myocardial infarctions (one in a patient who had undergone simultaneous coronary bypass grafting); eight were fatal, and two led to major neurological complications. One patient died from a mesenteric artery thrombosis. One patient developed phlegmasia cerulea dolens which led to amputation of a lower extremity. There were two minor wound infections.

DISCUSSION

EEG-Neurological Function

The EEG has proved to be a sensitive monitor of neurological function.[12,13] We have never had a patient emerge from anesthesia with a new deficit not predicted by the EEG. Pre- and post-operative EEGs have correlated closely with positive neurological findings and, although patients with TIAs have often had normal tracings, no patients have had a prolonged or fixed neurological deficit without an associated EEG abnormality. The converse has not been true as focal EEG changes in so-called silent areas—e.g. frontal and temporal—have been seen commonly in preoperative EEGs in patients (usually grade 4) with no recorded fixed neurological deficit.

EEG-CBF Correlation

The EEG has corresponded well with changes in the CBF, and reductions in flow with carotid occlusion below the critical range for that anesthetic agent invariably created changes in the EEG, the severity of which were proportional to the degree of ischemia. There was some variability from case to case in the critical flow (defined as the CBF required to sustain a normal EEG). Patients with pre-existing EEG abnormalities were more vulnerable to reductions in CBF than those who had a normal EEG. Patients operated under ethrane anesthesia appeared to have a lower critical flow than patients operated under halothane. Occlusion flows below 10 ml/100g/min always produced rapid changes in the EEG in both groups, however, and flows below 15 usually caused EEG changes. Furthermore, in that patients with occlusion flows below 18 ml/100g/min were shunted routinely, it is probable that many of the patients with flows between 10 and 18 ml/100g/min who did not have immediate EEG changes would have developed abnormalities in the EEG had the ischemia been permitted to persist. Thus it seems safe to conclude that critical flow approximates 15 ml/100g/min. This concept of critical flow is of such importance that it is necessary to comment about the accuracy of the CBF measurements.

These measurements are uniquely free of artifacts related to Compton scatter and "look through" as the radioactive indicator is delivered to the area predestined for ischemia, and only after the indicator has arrived in that area is the parent vessel occluded.[18] This is in contrast to other clinical studies in which the true severity of the ischemia is not measured because of impaired delivery of indicator into the region of reduced flow and the non-spatial characteristics of these types of measurements.[19,20]

Although there were modest but significant increases in CBF following endarterectomy in all four groups, the major increases were achieved in the grade 4 patients where CBF was brought to normal levels. These were static measurements, which were altered by the vasodilating anesthetic agents (halothane > ethrane). They do indicate the probability, however, that the brain's autoregulatory reserve was restored from the operation. As previously reported, lesions creating less than a 90 percent stenosis have not usually been hemodynamically significant.[14]

The very significantly lowered occlusion flows in the grade 4 group reflected the precarious collateral flow available in those patients. This finding supports a hemodynamic component for symptomatology in this group.

Ischemic Tolerance of Neural Tissue

The ischemic tolerance of neural tissue is proportional to the severity of flow reduction and the period of the ischemia.[21] At zero flow, as with cardiac arrest, this approximates 4 minutes. At 15 ml/100g/min, laboratory studies suggest a tolerance of 1 hour under barbiturate anesthesia. The shape of the curve between two points is undetermined, but we have been very cautious and assumed on the basis of laboratory studies and the severity of the EEG changes that ischemia below 10 ml/100g/min is tolerated only for a matter of minutes before there is infarction.[22]

Analysis of Results

Clearly the best results, in terms of frequency of complications, were achieved in those patients considered to be in the low risk category. As in illustrative Case 1, however, dramatic improvements were often achieved in patients considered neurologically unstable. It is necessary to balance the risks of surgery against those of not operating and to remember that virtually all of the grade 4 group had continued to have a progression in their symptomatology while on anticoagulants or anti-platelet agents.

Analysis of Complications

Intraoperative

There were 12 major and 14 minor new fixed neurological deficits in the series; seven of the former and three of the latter occurred from intraoperative embolization (one contralateral to the side of surgery in a patient with bilateral disease) or positional occlusion of a high grade stenosis. As shunts were used whenever doubt existed regarding the adequacy of cerebral perfusion, no infarctions were attributed to inadequate cerebral protection during the period of occlusion. There were, however, 33 cases (2 percent) with occlusion flows below 5, 92 cases (7 percent) with occlusion flows between 5 and 9, and 172 cases (13 percent) with occlusion flows between 10 and 14 ml/100g/min. Therefore, depending on the occlusion time required for endarterectomy, the complication rate from not using a shunt would probably have been between 9 percent and 22 percent in this series. The occlusion flows were significantly lower and the need for shunting significantly higher in the poorer risk patients. Some surgeons believe the risk of using a shunt exceeds the protection derived from its use,[23,24] while others recommend that patients be monitored or routinely shunted.[1,2,3] Differences in patient populations, case selection, and presence or absence of active participation by neurologists in the pre- and post-operative neurological evaluation and analysis of the case material make comparisons among reported series quite difficult. It seems apparent, however, that "the sicker the patient, the more likely a shunt will be required."

Postoperative

In contrast to intraoperative complications of hypoperfusion from a major vessel occlusion, postoperative neurological complications were most commonly related to hyperperfusion. These were encountered in grade 4 patients with a high grade carotid stenosis in whom there had been the following: (1) a very major increase in CBF (over 100 percent and very significantly different from mean values in the series) following completion of the endarterectomy (suggesting paralysis of cerebral autoregulatory mechanisms) and (2) a marked rise in the RAP (indicating a major increase in the profusion pressure). We believe our data support the contention that cerebral hyperperfusion can result in a form of unilateral hypertensive encephalopathy with the following: intracerebral hemorrhages (especially if anticoagulated), seizures, and migraine variants (possibly as an exaggerated or uncontrolled vasoconstrictive response to hyperperfusion). Prior to the development of this triad of complications, these patients frequently complained of unilateral headache. All but one of the patients with an intracerebral hemorrhage were on anticoagulants or anti-platelet agents at the time of the bleed. Anticoagulants are contraindicated in patients who develop seizures postoperatively.

Postoperative internal carotid artery occlusion was quite uncommon and usually occurred in vessels not patched at surgery. Prompt attention averted a major deficit in all except one case. This complication was unrelated to the grade of the patient.

Postoperative embolization producing typical TIAs or infarction was relatively uncommon, possibly as a result of our policy of not reversing heparin administered intraoperatively in order to protect the endarterectomized surface during the first few hours when it is most thrombogenic.[25] This same policy may have predisposed our cases to seizures by creating petechial hemorrhages which subsequently developed into a seizure focus and may explain the infrequent reports in the literature of this complication.[11,26]

Postoperative non-neurological complications were those one might expect in patients with diffuse atherosclerosis. The occurrence of myocardial infarction declined later in the series, possibly due to the extensive use of propranalol pre- and post-operatively in the grade 3 group.

Hemodynamics of Cerebral Ischemia

It was not our purpose in this report to discuss the symptoms of carotid artery atherosclerosis or the indications for surgery.[5] The availability of this CBF-EEG data and corresponding clinical symptomatology, however, has given us the opportunity to make some observations regarding the hemodynamic character of ischemic events in the anterior circulation and to correlate them with classic pathological studies.

There are recognized differences in the patterns of atherosclerosis in the anterior and posterior circulations.[27,28,29,30] In contrast to the vertebral and basilar arteries, where plaques are diffusely distributed and seldom ulcerate to produce embolic complications, plaques in the carotid arteries are frequently localized to the carotid bifurcation, and ulceration with secondary embolization is common. Superimposed thrombosis is the primary cause for occlusion of the basilar and vertebral arteries, but middle cerebral artery occlusion usually is embolic in origin.[28,30]

Although Fisher and his colleagues were among the first to call attention to the fact that secondary embolization from the carotid artery was a potential source of middle cerebral artery occlusion and infarction,[31] these workers reported that often infarction in the territory of the middle cerebral artery occurred with no major intracranial vessel occlusion and postulated a hemodynamic basis secondary to a proximal internal carotid artery occlusion.[27] These careful studies were later corroborated by other investigators. It was not necessary for a clot to propagate distally in the internal carotid artery to produce infarction.[30]

Microembolism as a cause for TIAs and some cerebral infarctions seems well established, but it has recently been challenged in two eloquent studies as a uniform explanation for all such events.[32,33] This has essentially revived the concept of a hemodynamic source for some ischemic events (i.e., alterations in effective perfusion pressure across the stenosis or distal to a point of occlusion).[34,35] The results of this study support the observations and contentions of those workers.[32,33] It seems clear that in those patients with occlusion flows below the critical levels, cerebral infarction would have occurred before the propagation of a clot from the site of occlusion. The posturally related nature of TIAs in patients with postoperative occlusions and the relief of these symptoms with restoration of flow are suggestive, but not conclusive evidence that, at least in this small group of patients, the TIAs were related to hemodynamic changes. More substantial support for this position is derived from that large subgroup of grade 4 candidates who had baseline CBF values between 20 and 25 ml. Clearly this flow (40 percent of normal awake CBF) is marginal.[36] The reactive hyperemia or "luxury perfusion" observed with the restoration of a normal perfusion pressure confirms that cerebral autoregulation was severely impaired, thus rendering the brain incapable of controlling its own flow and making it passively dependent on the perfusion pressure.[35,37,38]

Effects of Endarterectomy

It is important to note that our measurements were of cerebral blood flow—not flow through the artery—and were performed under static controlled conditions. Even in cases in which there was not a major change in

CBF, Boysen and co-workers, using electromagnetic arterial flow probes along with simultaneous CBF measurements, found an increase in arterial flow and the contribution to total CBF from the vessel operated if a high grade stenosis was present.[39]

The cerebral hemispheric arterial circulation can be divided into two general types of arteries: (1) the conducting vessels consisting of the internal carotid artery and its major trunks which then divide into a network of interlacing and anastomosing smaller branches on the brain's surface and (2) the penetrating or nutrient arterioles which arise on the surface of the brain from the conducting vessels and enter the brain parenchyma.[40] In normal man, there is only a 10 to 15 percent drop in perfusion pressure between the origin of the internal carotid artery and the penetrating vessels.[41] The conducting vessels can be regarded as a pressure equalization reservoir modulated by the sympathetic nervous system.[42,43] True cerebral autoregulation probably resides in the penetrating arterioles which apparently are modulated by an intrinsic nervous system taking origin in the brain stem.[44,45,46,47] Those arterioles must be supplied with an adequate perfusion pressure to function normally. The normalization of RAPs following endarterectomy indicates the restoration of a normal perfusion pressure in the conducting vessels. This increase in the distal perfusion pressure permits the parenchymal arterioles to return to a more normal tone—from one of maximal dilatation—and thus the brain's autoregulatory ability is restored.

The microembolic[48,49] and hemodynamic theories[33] for TIAs and infarcts are not mutually exclusive. Areas of brain functioning on a marginal flow of 40 to 50 percent of normal are particularly vulnerable to the effects of emboli. Furthermore, plaques with a severe degree of stenosis and which, therefore, represent a significant hemodynamic lesion, are more likely to develop deep ulcer craters than plaques of lesser severity.

Thus, endarterectomy in a patient with a high grade stenosis and ulceration does the following: (1) removes a source of emboli,[48] (2) restores a normal distal perfusion pressure and the capability for normal autoregulation, (3) increases flow through the artery and—depending on collateral flow—increases CBF, and (4) prevents progression of the stenosis to occlusion.

We do not believe patients with the so-called "mini-ulcer" should be operated but rather treated conservatively. We have noted that not infrequently in plaques removed at surgery, for a high grade stenosis or deep ulcer crater, there will be proximal small pits covered with endothelium that probably represented at one time minor ulcerations. Carotid stenosis is not the only cause for TIAs[50,51] and one should be very cautious about recommending surgery on the basis of a presumed ulcer crater. Conversely, not all strokes from carotid stenosis or occlusion are preceded by a TIA[50], and, therefore, asymptomatic patients with a tight stenosis and reduced RAPs may be candidates for surgery.[48,52,53]

REFERENCES

1. Thompson JE: Complications of carotid endarterectomy and their prevention. World J Surg 3:155, 1979
2. Hertzer NR, Beven EG, Greenstreet RL, et al: Internal carotid back pressure, intraoperative shunting, ulcerated atheromata, and the incidence of stroke during carotid endarterectomy. Surgery 83:306, 1978
3. Hays RJ, Levinson SA, Wylie EG: Intraoperative measurements of carotid back pressure as a guide to operative management of carotid endarterectomy. Surgery 72:953, 1972
4. Thompson JE, Garrett WV: Peripheral-arterial surgery. New Engl J Med 302:491, 1980
5. Ojemann RG: The surgical treatment of cerebrovascular disease. N Engl J Med 274:440, 1966
6. Wylie EJ, Hein MF, Adams JE: Intracranial hemorrhage following surgical revascularization for treatment of acute stroke. J Neurosurg 21:212, 1964
7. Bruetman ME, Fields WS, Crawford ES, et al: Cerebral hemorrhage in carotid artery surgery. Arch Neurol 9:458, 1963
8. DeWeese JA, Rob CG, Satran R, et al. Results of carotid endarterectomies for transient ischemic attacks—five years later. Ann Surg 178:258, 1973
9. Blaisdell WF, Clauss RH, Galbraith JG, et al: Joint study of extracranial arterial occlusion. IV, A review of surgical consideration. JAMA 209:1889, 1969
10. Hunter JA, Julian OC, Dye WS, et al: Emergency operation for acute cerebral ischemia due to carotid artery obstruction: Review of 26 cases. Ann Surg 162:901, 1965
11. Sundt TM Jr, Sandok BA, Whisnant JP: Carotid endarterectomy: complications and preoperative assessment of risk. Mayo Clin Proc 50:301, 1975
12. Phillips MR, Johnson WC, Scott RM, et al: Carotid endarterectomy in the presence of contralateral carotid occlusion. Arch Surg 114:1232, 1979
13. Sharbrough FW, Messick JM, Sundt TM Jr: Correlation of continuous electroencephalograms with cerebral blood flow measurements during carotid endarterectomy. Stroke 4:674, 1973
14. Sundt TM Jr, Sharbrough FW, Anderson RE, et al: Cerebral blood flow measurements and electroencephalograms during endarterectomy. J Neurosurg 41:310, 1974
15. Waltz AG, Wanek AR, Anderson RE: Comparison of analytic methods for calculation of cerebral blood flow after intracarotid injection of ^{133}Xe. J Nucl Med 13:66, 1972
16. Anderson RE, Sundt TM Jr: An automated cerebral blood flow analyzer: Concise communication. J Nucl Med 18:728, 1977
17. Kobayashi S, Hollenhorst RW, Sundt TM Jr: Retinal arterial pressure before and after surgery for carotid artery stenosis. Stroke 2:569, 1971
18. Hanson EJ Jr, Anderson RE, Sundt TM Jr: Comparison of ^{85}Krypton and ^{133}Xenon cerebral blood flow measurements before, during, and following focal, incomplete ischemia in the squirrel monkey. Circ Res 22:220, 1975
19. Fieschi C, Agnoli A, Battistini N, et al: Derangement of regional cerebral blood flow and of its regulatory mechanisms in acute cerebrovascular lesions. Neurology (Minneap) 18:1166, 1968
20. Paulson OB: Regional cerebral blood flow in apoplexy due to occlusion of the middle cerebral artery. Neurology (Minneap) 20:63, 1970
21. Sundt TM Jr, Michenfelder JD: Focal transient cerebral ischemia in squirrel monkey: Effect on brain ATP and lactate levels with electrocorticographic and pathologic correlation. Circ Res 30:702, 1972
22. Astrup J, Symon L, Branston NM, et al: Cortical evoked potential and extracellular K^+ and H^+ at critical levels of brain ischemia. Stroke 8:51, 1977
23. Baker WH, Dorner DB, Barnes RW: Carotid endarterectomy: Is an indwelling shunt necessary? Surgery 82:321, 1977

24. Whitney DG, Kahn EM, Estes JW, et al: Carotid artery surgery without a temporary indwelling shunt. 1,917 consecutive procedures. Arch Surg 115:1393, 1980
25. Dirrenberger RA, Sundt TM Jr: Carotid endarterectomy. Temporal profile of the healing process and effects of anticoagulation therapy. J Neurosurg 48:201, 1978
26. Wilkinson JT, Adams HP, Wright CB: Convulsions after carotid endarterectomy. JAMA, 244:1827, 1980
27. Fisher, CM, Gore I, Okabe N, et al: Atherosclerosis of the carotid and vertebral arteries—extracranial and intracranial. J Neuropathol Exp Neurol 24:455, 1965
28. Castaigne P, Lhermitte F, Gautier JC, et al: Arterial occlusions in the vertebro-basilar system: A study of 44 patients with post-mortem data. Brain 96:133, 1973
29. Fisher CM: Occlusion of the vertebral arteries causing transient basilar symptoms. Arch Neurol 22:13, 1970
30. Lhermitte F, Gautier JC, Derouesne C, et al: Ischemic accidents in the middle cerebral artery territory. Arch Neurol 19:248, 1968
31. Fisher CM: Occlusion of the internal carotid artery. Arch Neurol Psychiat 69:346, 1951
32. Caplan LR, Sergay S: Positional cerebral ischaemia. J Neurol Neurosurg Psychiat 39:385, 1976
33. Pessin MS, Hinton RC, Davis KR, et al: Mechanisms of acute carotid stroke. Ann Neurol 6:245, 1979
34. Meyer JS, Denny-Brown D: The cerebral collateral circulation. Neurology (Minneap) 7:447, 1957
35. Waltz AG: Effect of blood pressure on blood flow in ischemic and in non-ischemic cerebral cortex. Neurology (Minneap) 18:613, 1968
36. Kety SS, Schmidt CF: The nitrous oxide method for the quantitative determination of cerebral blood flow in man: Theory, procedure and normal values. J Clin Invest 27:476, 1948
37. Lassen NA: Control of cerebral circulation in health and disease. Brief reviews. Circ Res 34:749, 1974
38. Lassen NA: The luxury-perfusion syndrome and its possible relation to acute metabolic acidosis localized within the brain. Lancet 2:1113, 1966
39. Boysen G: Cerebral hemodynamics in carotid surgery. Acta Neurol Scand (Suppl) 41:310, 1973
40. Saunders RL, Bell MA: X-ray microscopy and histochemistry of the human cerebral blood vessels. J Neurosurg 35:128, 1971
41. Bakay L, Sweet WH: Cervical and intracranial intra-arterial pressures with and without vascular occlusion. Surg Gynecol Obstet 95:67, 1952
42. Symon LA: A comparative study of middle cerebral pressure in dogs and macaques. J Physiol (Lond) 191:449, 1967
43. Harper AM, Deshmukh VD, Rowan JO, et al: The influence of sympathetic nervous activity on cerebral blood flow. Arch Neurol 27:1, 1972
44. Langfitt TW, Kassell NF: Cerebral vasodilatation produced by brainstem stimulation: Neurogenic control vs. autoregulation. Am J Physiol 215:90, 1968
45. Bates D, Weinshilboum RM, Campbell RJ, et al: The effect of lesions in the locus coeruleus on the physiological responses of the cerebral blood vessels in cats. Brain Res 136:431, 1977
46. Shalit NM, Reinmuth OM, Shimojyo S, et al: Carbon dioxide and cerebral circulatory control: III. The effects of brainstem lesions. Arch Neurol 17:342, 1967
47. Raichle ME, Hartman BK, Eichling JO, et al: Central noradrenergic regulation of cerebral blood flow and vascular permeability. Proc Nat Acad Sci 72:3726, 1975
48. Siekert RG, Whisnant JP, Millikan CH: Surgical and anticoagulant therapy of occlusive cerebral vascular disease. Ann Intern Med 48:637, 1963
49. Whisnant JP, Millikan CH, Sayre GP, et al: Effect of anticoagulants on experimental cerebral infarction. Circulation 20:56, 1959

50. Pessin MS, Duncan GW, Mohr JP, et al: Clinical and angiographic features of carotid transient ischemic attacks. N Engl J Med 296:358, 1977
51. Mohr JP, Caplan LR, Melski JW, et al: The Harvard cooperative stroke registry: A prospective registry. Neurology 28:754, 1978
52. Javid H: Development of carotid plaque. Am J Surg 138:224, 1979
53. Moore WS, Boren C, Malone JM, et al: Asymptomatic carotid stenosis: Immediate and long-term results after prophylactic endarterectomy. Am J Surg 138:228, 1979

Hushang Javid

20

Intraluminal Shunting during Carotid Endarterectomy

Since the advent of carotid surgery for atheromatous disease in 1954,[1] much knowledge and experience has been accumulated. At the present time, the effectiveness of this mode of management in the amelioration of symptoms and prevention of stroke has been generally accepted. Diagnostic methods have been developed for a safe and non-invasive technique of screening and monitoring the progression of atheromatous lesions. Indications for surgery and technical maneuvers necessary for carotid endarterectomy have been standardized. The results of surgery have gradually improved to an acceptable level and are measured by the rate of postoperative mortality and stroke. The safety of carotid surgery depends upon proper case selection, well-administered anesthesia, meticulous surgical technique, and protection of the brain during the mandatory carotid cross-clamping. In spite of the general agreement in the above stated principles, three schools of thought have developed regarding the need and methods of cerebral protection. The majority believes in selective shunting based on the need which is determined by various methods of monitoring employed to measure the adequacy of collateral supply. A second group of surgeons believe vehemently that carotid cross-clamping is safe and methods designed to preserve the adequacy of cerebral perfusion are never needed. To assert their point of view, they compare their rate of morbidity and mortality with those who believe differently. As members of the third group, those at our center have employed routine intraluminal shunting during the past 20 years. Our policy has been based on the assumption that collateral supply is inadequate in certain individuals requiring carotid cross-clamping and that intraluminal shunting is the safest and most effective means of maintaining the regional cerebral perfusion at the preclamping level. Based on our own past experience, the routine use of intraluminal shunting eliminates the need for time-consuming, cumbersome, and often inaccurate methods of determining the adequacy of collateral supply. Shunting also eliminates the need for haste, thus permitting meticulous endarterectomy and debridement of the vessel wall. The catheter in the internal carotid artery does not interfere with exposure of the distal end of the atheromatous plaque and, in fact, facilitates the repair of the arterial incision and prevents stricture caused by a faulty suture line. It is our contention that the proper use of an intraluminal catheter and appropriate use of the clamps will protect the brain, will not cause injury to the arterial wall, and is totally free of complications. A review of the literature and our own experience confirms our belief that shunting reverses ischemic changes as detected by electroencephalogram and regional cerebral blood flow determinations. The usefulness of shunting in the surgical management of internal carotid aneurysms, kinked carotid artery, carotid body tumor, and concomitant carotid endarterectomy with carotid subclavian bypass graft will also be described.

The goal of carotid surgery is the elimination of hemispheric or nonhemispheric cerebral symptoms and the prevention of stroke. The results of surgery should be judged by the rate of mortality, incidence of stroke, and incidence of minor cerebral damage. Mortality has mainly been the result of myocardial infarction. Liberal use of coronary angiography during the preoperative evaluation in the future will identify patients in need of coronary bypass graft prior to carotid endarterectomy. Stroke rate can, and should be, reduced by proper case selection, careful dissection of the carotid artery to avoid embolization, a thorough endarterectomy, and maintenance of adequate cerebral perfusion during the period of cross-clamping. The success of these measures is determined by the incidence of postoperative neurologic deficit. Stroke represents a major insult to the brain tissue. It is quite possible, however, that minor injuries due to limited ischemia occur but go undetected because of inadequate pre- and post-operative neurologic evaluation which should include both intellectual and psychological assessments. A parallel example in the recent past when ischemic arrest in cardiac surgery was considered safe should be recalled. The irreversible damage caused by even a brief period of ischemia went undetected in the early postoperative stage. Late evaluation of the patients, however, detected evidence of myocardial fibrosis. The object of this presentation is to summarize the information available regarding methods designed to determine the adequacy of collateral circulation during a carotid cross-clamping and to demonstrate the efficacy, ease, and the superiority of routine intraluminal shunting.

COLLATERAL CIRCULATION

The principal extracranial sources of collateral circulation, in the presence of internal carotid artery occlusion, are communications between the ophthalmic artery and the branches of both the ipsilateral and contralateral external carotid arteries. The most important intracranial cross-circulation is that of the circle of Willis. Ordinarily, there is little flow crossing from one side to the other or between the posterior and anterior circulation. In the presence of either basilar or internal carotid artery occlusion, however, the posterior communicating arteries may become extremely important conduits for collateral blood flow. Anomalies of the circle of Willis occur frequently, and the prediction of its patency and adequacy is clinically impossible. Whether cerebral ischemia and infarction will occur following carotid artery cross-clamping will depend, to a great extent, on the patency of the circle of Willis and the extracranial collateral channels. The need to determine the adequacy of collateral supply prompted the development of various methods including the ones discussed below.

Angiographic Evaluation

With the techniques available, visualization and quantification of the collateral supply to the brain have been inadequate. Complete patency of the Circle of Willis has been estimated at 50 percent of patients studied, based on angiographic and necropsy examinations.

Test Clamping

Preparation of patients for carotid artery ligation, by intermittent compression of the carotid artery, was practiced and abandoned years ago. During the early phase of the development of carotid artery surgery, test clamping in unanesthetized patients was attempted to evaluate the tolerance to cross-clamping during surgery. The hypothesis that tolerance to a 3 minute period of clamping is predictive of adequacy of collateral flow proved to be false. Bland and associates[2] reported 11 patients in their series who tolerated 3 minutes of trial occlusion under local anesthesia but developed neurologic deficits following a longer period of operative carotid artery cross-clamping. Kwaan and associates[3] recently reported that 24 out of 125 consecutive patients undergoing carotid endarterectomy under local anesthesia lost consciousness immediately following carotid artery cross-clamping. These patients regained consciousness after the employment of intraluminal shunting. It was also pointed out in this paper that stump pressure measurements were an unreliable guide. In 8 patients who lost consciousness during carotid cross-clamping, stump pressures were above 50 mm Hg.

Stump Pressure Measurement

Michal and associates,[4] in 1966, advocated measurement of the internal carotid back pressure during trial clamping of the common and external carotid arteries as an indicator of collateral blood supply. Moore and Hall,[5] in 1969, reported their experience in the measurement of the internal carotid back pressure in a series of 40 patients undergoing carotid endarterectomy under local anesthesia. They found a critical lower value of 25 mm Hg carotid stump pressure. Pressures below this level were associated with a substantial postoperative neurologic deficit. Hays, Levinson, and Wylie,[6] on the other hand, suggested that a stump pressure of 50 mm Hg was the critical level needed to provide adequate collateral blood flow during an average period of 20 minutes of carotid clamping. Fifteen of the 73 operations in which the internal carotid back pressure was less than 50 mm Hg were performed without an internal shunt with a 53 percent incidence of stroke (8 of 15 cases). Carotid occlusion time varied from 15 to 22 minutes in these 15 patients. In a similar group of 21 operations in which intraluminal shunting was employed, the incidence of stroke was 5 percent, occurring in 1 patient out of 21 operations. The deficit was temporary, and the authors thought that the incident was not related to the operative ischemia. This patient was the only one in the series who had a neurologic deficit of recent origin at the time of the operation. The deficit increased postoperatively and was attributed to revascularization of a small cerebral infarct. There were 224 operations performed without a shunt in patients with internal carotid back pressure greater than 50 mm Hg, and 9 patients in this group developed postoperative neurologic deficits, an incidence of 4 percent.

Hertzer and associates,[7] who also designated a back pressure of 50 mm Hg as the critical level for shunt insertion, reported their experience in a series of 260 operations involving 253 patients. Back pressure of less than 50 mm Hg was found in 100 patients, and shunts were used in this group. Another 55 operations were done using temporary shunts despite back pressure of greater than 50 mm Hg, for various reasons, including contralateral carotid stenosis or occlusion, past history of previous stroke, and combined carotid endarterectomy and myocardial revascularization. A total of 105 operations were completed without shunts; 30 of these patients had back pressure of less than 50 mm Hg. The incidence of permanent stroke in the shunted group of 155 operations was 1.3 percent, as compared to 2.8 percent in the nonshunted group of 105 operations. (Considering the fact that shunting was done in patients with contralateral lesions and a history of previous stroke, as well as in patients with internal carotid back pressure below 50 mm Hg [6.9

percent.]) Boysen,[8] in a scholarly study, showed that a stump pressure below 50 mm Hg was accompanied by a critical reduction of regional cerebral blood flow and also by EEG changes suggestive of significant brain ischemia. Thompson and Talkington[9] noted that the incidence of patients with internal carotid back pressure below 50 mm Hg varied considerably (from 25-70 percent) in various series, indicating the unreliability of this method.

Electroencephalographic Monitoring

Electroencephalographic monitoring during a test occlusion of the carotid artery was advocated by Harris and co-workers[10] who performed carotid endarterectomy under local anesthesia. They suggested that general anesthesia would render EEG changes less sensitive to alterations in cerebral perfusion. Baker and associates[11] employed continuous EEG monitoring during 213 carotid endarterectomies in 157 patients. General anesthesia was used in all of these patients. Electroencephalographic abnormalities, associated with ischemia, occurred in 31 operations. Four patients with internal carotid back pressures of 75-100 mm Hg developed EEG abnormalities. These changes disappeared following insertion of an intraluminal shunt. A comprehensive study by Sundt and associates,[12] analyzing 1145 consecutive carotid endarterectomies, reported significant alterations of EEG and/or cerebral perfusion to justify the use of intraluminal shunt in 511 cases. They concluded that when the regional cerebral blood flow fell below 18-20 ml/100g/min after carotid cross-clamping, shunting was necessary and, in fact, the use of the shunt restored the flow to the pre-clamping level.

Regional Cerebral Blood Flow Measurement

Boysen,[8] using the intra-arterial injection of ^{133}Xenon, found that hemispheric regional cerebral blood flow was reduced during cross-clamping from a mean of 51 to 30 ml/100g/min, a mean reduction of 41 percent. In 19 of the 60 endarterectomies, regional cerebral blood flow was so severely reduced as to necessitate the use of a shunt (Table 20-1). In approximately half of the patients requiring shunts, the contralateral angiogram appeared normal. Of the patients studied, 32 percent had electroencephalographic changes that corresponded with reduction of regional cerebral blood flow values below 25 ml/100g/min. Twenty percent of the patients evaluated had flattening of the electroencephalogram. All of these patients had regional cerebral blood flow values below 20 ml/100g/min. Boysen[8] thus concluded that one-third of the patients requiring carotid surgery deserved intraluminal shunting. In a similar study, Rowed and Vilaghy[13] reached the conclusion that when mean ipsilateral hemispheric regional cerebral blood flow exceeds 20 ml/100g/min, an intraluninal shunt is not necessary. In 37 percent of their patients, however,

Table 20-1
Hemodynamic data in patients with Javid shunts inserted during carotid endarterectomy

	Mean Systemic arterial Blood pressure	Range	Mean $PaCO_2$	Range	Mean rCBF	Range	Number
Before endarterectomy	108	87–136	43.6	28–74	40.6	24–76	14
During test clamping	118	101–140	43.8	28–74	22.6	12–39	16
With shunt in situ	127	92–170	43.7	27–61	41.4	25–60	16

(From Boysen G: Studies in cerebral circulation. Am Coll Surg Bull June, 1973.)

test clamping of the carotid artery reduced the regional cerebral blood flow below this critical level. In these patients, intraoperative shunting was capable of restoring the flow to a preocclusion level.

Other non-invasive methods, such as oculopneumoplethysmography or supraorbital Doppler flow measurements have similarly isolated a certain percentage of patients who have collateral supply which is insufficient to permit safe cross-clamping of the carotid artery.

The challenge remains for those who advocate the use of non-shunting technique. They must demonstrate that flattening of the electroencephalogram, ischemia of the brain tissue determined by rCPF measurements, and the state of unconsciousness are harmless and should be totally ignored.

BRAIN PROTECTION

Considerable attention has been given to the need for protection of brain tissue during carotid artery surgery. Methods employed include general anesthesia, induced hypertension, hypercarbia, hypocarbia, and the use of a temporary intraluminal shunt. General anesthesia not only provides a quiet operative field but also decreases the metabolic demands of the brain tissue. Halothane, barbiturates, and nitrous oxide are credited with reducing cerebral metabolic oxygen consumption.

Induced Hypertension

The concept that cerebral blood flow increases by induced systemic hypertension has been questioned by many investigators.[14,15] Fog,[16] in 1934, showed that vasopressor drugs have no direct effect on cerebral blood flow. He described vasoconstriction of cerebral arterioles during induced hypertension, and vasodilatation as a response to hypotension, thus presenting the phenonenon of cerebral autoregulation. Boysen[8] found also a minimal effect of induced hypertension on regional cerebral blood flow in patients with poor collateral circulation and concluded that induced hypertension was not recommended as a precautionary measure during carotid endarterectomy. The ill effects of induced hypertension in elderly individuals far outweigh the potential benefit.

Hypercarbia

On theoretical grounds, it seems logical that the addition of hypercarbia and induced hypertension to general anesthesia should provide optimal brain protection. Unfortunately, the benefits of induced hypertension are quite limited, and the beneficial effect of increased CO_2 has been questioned. In the presence of local cerebral ischemia, hypercarbia may produce an intracerebral steal. A general cerebral vasodilatation increases the blood flow to the normal brain and decreases flow to the ischemic portion of the brain, the so-called, "reversed Robin Hood phenomenon."[17,18] Recent experimental studies suggest that with increased $PaCO_2$, a higher cerebral perfusion is needed to maintain normal cerebral metabolism. According to Boysen,[8] hypocapnea does not prevent marked changes in the EEG at low regional cerebral blood flow values.

To conclude, it seems that general anesthesia protects the brain during carotid artery cross-clamping by reducing the oxygen demand of cerebral tissue. Induced hypertension and alteration of $PaCO_2$ do not seem to be protective of brain tissue. Most surgeons dealing with carotid artery surgery have unanimously agreed that intraluminal shunting does reverse the deleterious effects of carotid clamping.[11,19] It results in prompt recovery from a comatose state in patients operated on under local anesthesia, reversing EEG abnormalities, and the regional cerebral blood flow returns to preocclusive levels. According to various authors, from 1/3 to 2/3 of patients require some sort of protective measure during carotid artery surgery. The objections raised in the literature to the use of the intraluminal shunt include difficulty in insertion, the potential for embolization, intimal damage, and difficulty of exposure, particularly in lesions extending high in the internal carotid artery.[20,21,22]

During the last quarter of a century, 2753 carotid endarterectomies were performed (Table 20-2) for a variety of conditions. During the first few years, the majority of patients were operated under local anesthesia. Intraluminal shunt was employed occasionally. During the last twenty years,[23] however, routine use of general anesthesia and intraluminal shunting was instituted, and the rate of postoperative neurologic deficits was drastically reduced. During this 20-year period, over 2300 internal carotid endarterectomies have been performed. There have been only 12 instances where insertion of the

Table 20-2
Results of carotid endarterectomy, performed from December, 1955 to December, 1981

Clinical category	Number of patients	Number of operations	Neurologic deficits Transient	Permanent	Mortality
Transient ischemic attacks	1295	1776	17 (.9%)	13 (.7%)	16 (.9%)
Asymptomatic	280	340	5 (1.4%)	2 (.5%)	—
Prior stroke	400	462	7 (1.5%)	10 (2.2%)	12 (2.5%)
Emergency procedures	126	126	8 (6.3%)	11 (8.7%)	12 (9.5%)
Total	2098	2704	37 (1.3%)	36 (0.75%)	40 (1.4%)

shunt was not possible, due to proximal or distal extension of the atheromatous disease. In only 4 patients, the internal carotid artery was too small to permit the introduction of the distal end of the polyvinyl tube. On rare occasions, it was necessary to remove the distal extension of the atheromatous tongue prior to the insertion of the distal end of the intraluminal shunt. All patients were systemically heparinized. There have been no instances of intraluminal thrombosis, intimal tear, or dissection. It should be emphasized, however, that there is need for gentle manipulation of the carotid bifurcation, adequate exposure, a generous longitudinal carotid incision, meticulous and gentle insertion of the distal end of the flexible olive-tip catheter, adequate filling of the tube to remove air bubbles by retrograde carotid blood flow, adequate inspection of the proximal end of the incision to make certain that there is no debris present within the lumen, and finally, gentle insertion of the proximal end after filling the intraluminal pouch with blood to again prevent introduction of air bubbles into the system. The Javid ring clamps have been designed to fit the proximal and distal ends of the tube appropriately; the distal clamp is placed underneath the carotid bifurcation, providing better exposure of the operative site for endarterectomy. Early in our experience, blood flow measurements proved to our satisfaction that the flow through the shunt is adequate and significantly higher than the preocclusive internal carotid flow. This flow is dependent on the pressure gradient between the systemic and stump back pressure.[24] When the shunt is in place and functioning, the need for haste is eliminated, and the surgeon can meticulously remove the entire atheromatous plaque, which includes the plaque within the lumen of the external carotid artery, as well as the portion extending above the normal intima in the internal carotid artery. Removal of the tongue-like extension of the atheroma is most important in the prevention of recurrent stenosis following carotid endarterectomy. Routine use of the shunt increases the experience of the operator, and it is rare for the insertion time to extend beyond 2 minutes. The exposure of the atheroma is excellent since the flexible

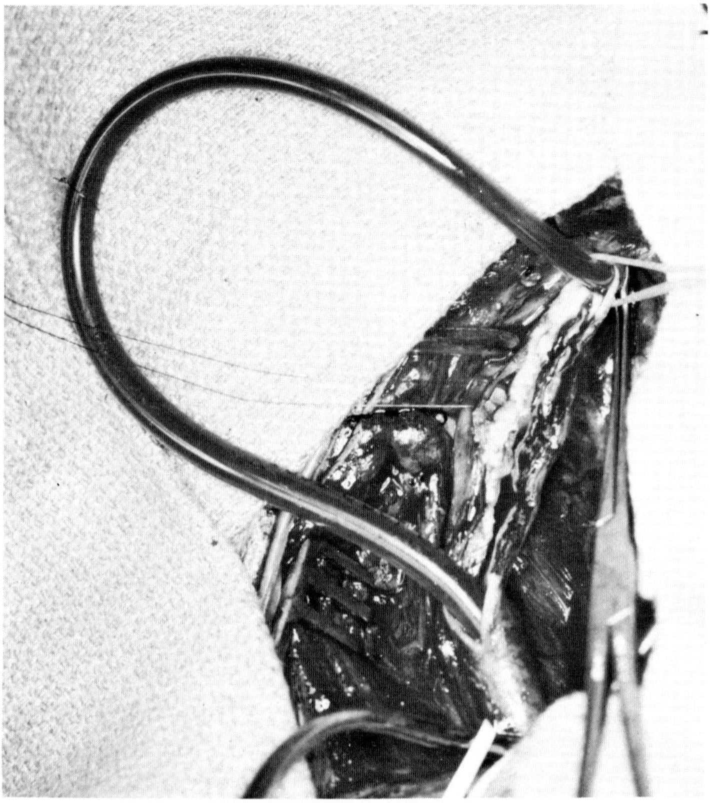

Figure 20-1. Atheroma can be retracted without kinking to accomplish a careful and meticulous endarterectomy.

tube is looped outside of the artery and can be retracted without kinking to accomplish a careful and meticulous endarterectomy (Fig. 20-1). The intima should be routinely inspected to make certain that the distal end is firmly adherent to the outer layers. Better exposure and careful removal of the atheroma have eliminated the need for tacking sutures to the distal intima and the use of patch angioplasty. The presence of the tube within the artery facilitates suturing and avoids constriction by faulty suture technique.

RESULTS

Table 20-2 shows a review of our experience during the last quarter of a century. The rate of stroke following surgery has gradually been reduced by better case selection and further refinement of surgical technique. Fields and

Lemak[25] in 1976, reporting the experience of a joint study of extracranial arterial occlusion, concluded that the centers with the best surgical results appeared to use operative shunts. Thompson,[9] in a review of the literature, came to the same conclusion and indicated that the rate of pemanent deficit in centers using no shunt was higher. The rate of stroke following surgery is significantly greater in patients with contralateral carotid occlusion. This is particularly true in centers where shunt is not used. Baker, Dorner, and Barnes[26] reported an 8.8 percent incidence of neurologic deficit following carotid endarterectomy in patients with contralateral carotid occlusion, as compared to a 2 percent incidence in patients whose contralateral internal carotid artery was patent. On the other hand, using routine intraluminal shunting in 23 patients with contralateral occlusion, Patterson[27] reported no postoperative mortality or morbidity. Thompson[9] reported 123 carotid endarterectomies in patients with contralateral occlusion, with 1 neurologic deficit, an incidence of 0.8 percent. In our series,[28] we had a similar experience. Using routine intraluminal shunting in 94 patients with contralateral carotid occlusion, we had 1 instance of immediate postoperative neurologic deficit, for an incidence of 1 percent. From the foregoing review, it becomes evident that the maintenance of cerebral perfusion by an intraluminal shunt can drastically reduce the incidence of postoperative stroke.

As mentioned previously, stroke represents a major, easily detectable neurologic deficit. Minor ischemic damage may seriously alter the function of vulnerable portions of the brain but remain undetected. Ammon's horn, the Sommer sector and the endfolium of the hippocampus are most vulnerable to anoxia[29]; unless the intellectual, emotional and personality changes of patients are routinely assessed pre- and post-operatively, an estimate cannot be made of the degree of insult imposed by cross-clamping of the carotid artery for 20-30 minutes. A review of the literature[30] indicates that centers reporting an increase in average IQ and perceptual organization intelligence scores following carotid endarterectomy employed routine intraluminal shunting. Haynes and associates[31] compared 17 endarterectomy patients with 9 control patients and concluded that following carotid artery surgery, there was an increase in perceptual organization IQ; a decrease in time to complete a perceptual motor task; and a significant reduction in suspicion, confusion, and other personality symptoms generally associated with senility. In our institution, 31 patients with transient ischemic attacks were extensively evaluated before and 3 months after carotid endarterectomy.[32] The intellectual and psychological parameters were compared with 15 control patients with vascular disease, undergoing other types of surgical procedures. There were statistically significant improvements in memory and learning capabilities in the group that had carotid endarterectomy, as compared to the control series. It is hoped that in the future, other studies in centers where shunting is not used routinely can be evaluated, so that comparisons between various groups can be made.

The use of a shunt is also helpful in other carotid lesions, such as aneurysm, kinked carotid artery, carotid body tumor or in performing carotid-subclavian bypass. Five patients with acquired aneurysms of the internal carotid artery and 3 individuals with traumatic aneurysms were surgically treated with the use of an intraluminal shunt without an incidence of postoperative stroke. Aneurysms in the midportion of the cervical segment of the internal carotid artery (Fig. 20-2) are particularly suitable for intraluminal shunting. Carotid bifurcation and the aneurysmal segment of the internal carotid artery are exposed through a longitudinal neck incision (Fig. 20-3). The distal end of the tube is advanced to an area beyond the aneurysm and secured in place with the ring clamp (Fig. 20-4). Excision and primary repair of the aneurysm was accomplished in 6 patients, while in 2 individuals a graft interposition was necessary to bridge the defect. In situations requiring graft implantation, the distal end of the tube was threaded through the graft prior to insertion of the tube within the internal carotid artery, in order to permit end-to-end anastomosis between the graft and the host artery above the aneurysm high in the neck. The entire operation can be accomplished with only a brief period of carotid artery cross-clamping.

Shunting is also important in the surgical management of the kinked

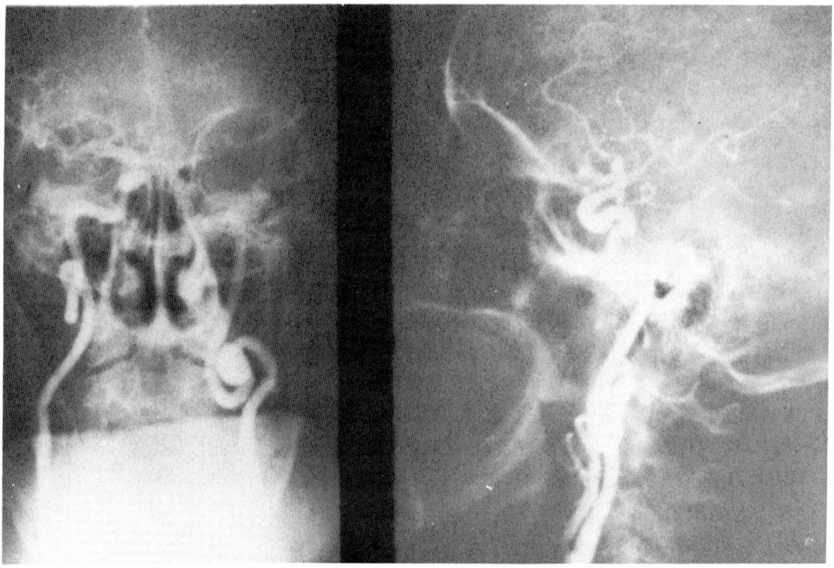

Figure 20-2. Aneurysms in the midportion of the cervical segment of the internal carotid artery are particularly suitable for intraluminal shunting.

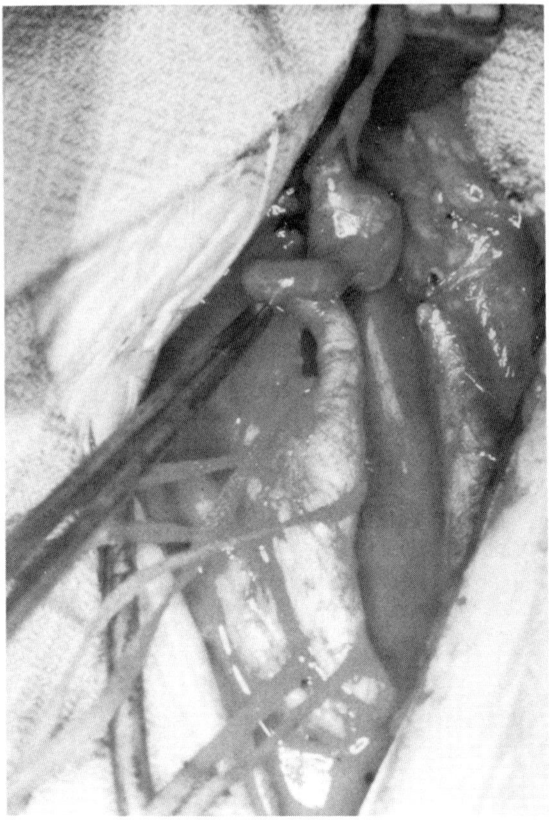

Figure 20-3. Carotid bifurcation and the aneurysmal segment of the internal carotid artery are exposed through a longitudinal neck incision.

internal carotid artery since, in the majority of patients with kinked internal carotid arteries, obstruction of the channel occurs intermittently with changes of neck position, and the collateral arterial supply may not be fully developed. In our experience,[33] reimplantation of the origin of the internal carotid artery to a more proximal level is the procedure of choice (Fig. 20-5).

Carotid body tumor is a vascular lesion that is often intimately attached to the carotid bifurcation, thus making the surgical procedure most difficult. External carotid artery branches are often embedded within the substance of the tumor, providing the vascularity of the lesion. Total removal of large tumors and preservation of the internal carotid artery flow is often most difficult. Shunting renders the tumor avascular and facilitates excision of the tumor without excessive blood loss. This technique was employed in 11 of 27

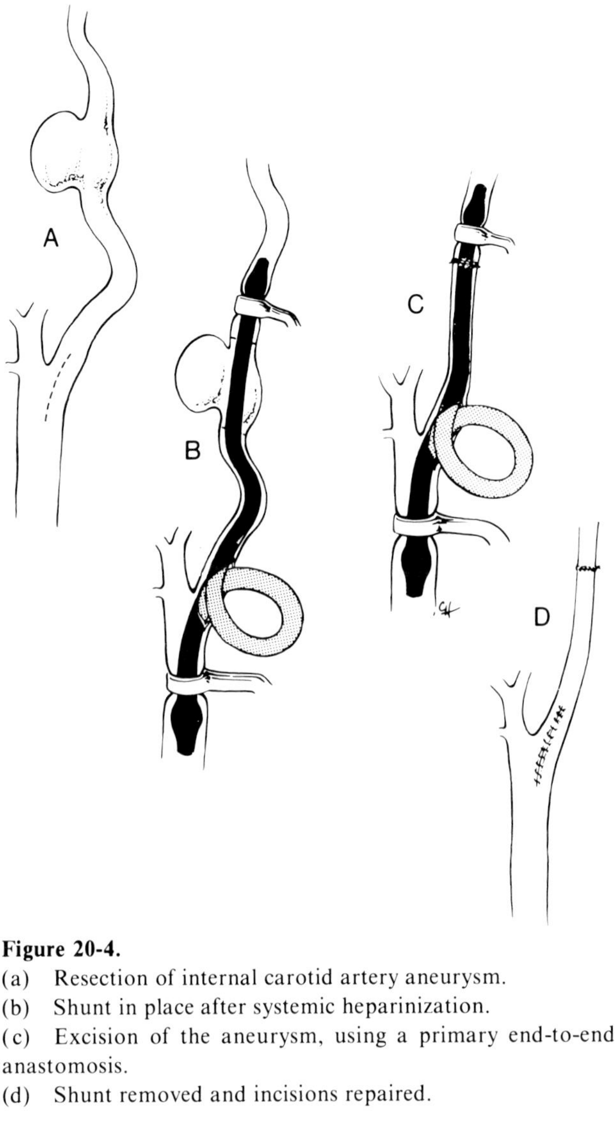

Figure 20-4.
(a) Resection of internal carotid artery aneurysm.
(b) Shunt in place after systemic heparinization.
(c) Excision of the aneurysm, using a primary end-to-end anastomosis.
(d) Shunt removed and incisions repaired.

patients in our series. In each instance, the carotid flow was preserved, and no neurologic deficit resulted. The shunt is inserted through an incision in the common carotid artery, below the tumor (Fig. 20-6). The distal end is introduced into the internal carotid artery and is passed to a level above the tumor, where it is secured in place with the Javid clamp. Thus, separation of the avascular tumor from the artery becomes simple. Often it is necessary to

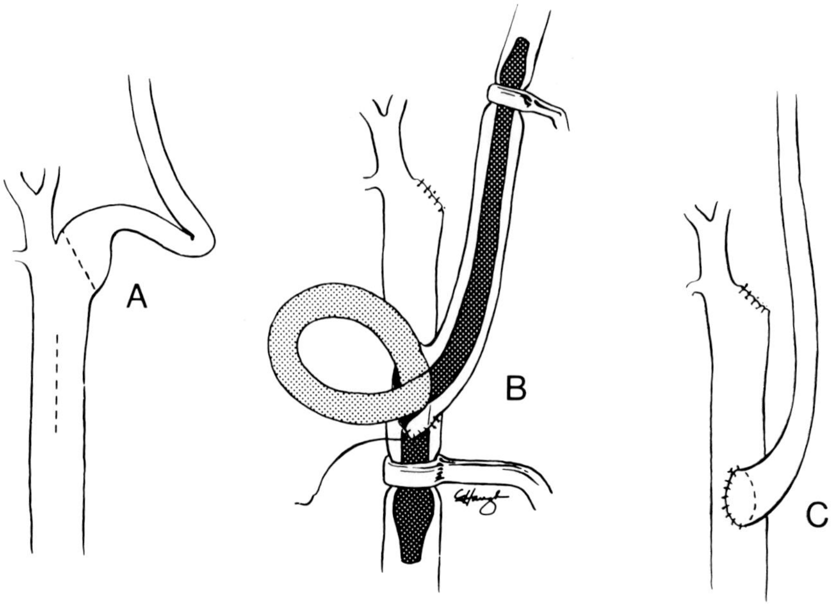

Figure 20-5. Reimplantation of the internal carotid artery using an intraluminal shunt.

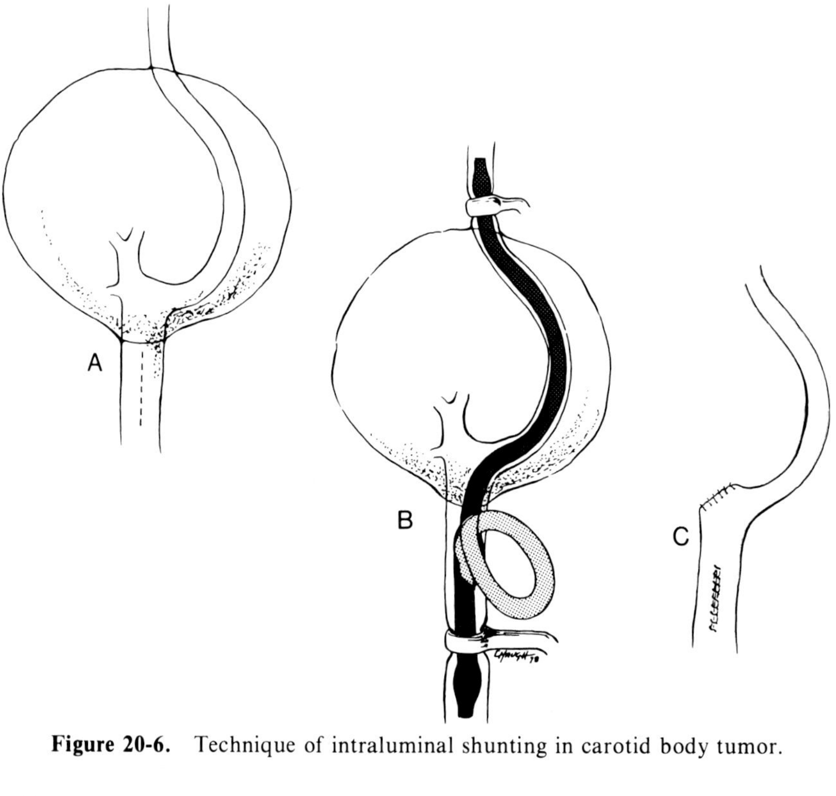

Figure 20-6. Technique of intraluminal shunting in carotid body tumor.

sacrifice the external carotid artery. In 1 patient, it was necessary to use a segment of long saphenous vein graft to replace the portion that was encircled by a densely adherent and vascular tumor.

Carotid endarterectomy and ipsilateral carotid-subclavian bypass often require a lengthy period of carotid clamping which, in turn, increases the risk of postoperative stroke. The technique described in Figure 20-7 attempts to maintain cerebral blood flow during the surgical procedure. Through 2 separate incisions, the carotid bifurcation and the subclavian artery are exposed. An 8 mm Gore-Tex graft is first anastomosed to the subclavian

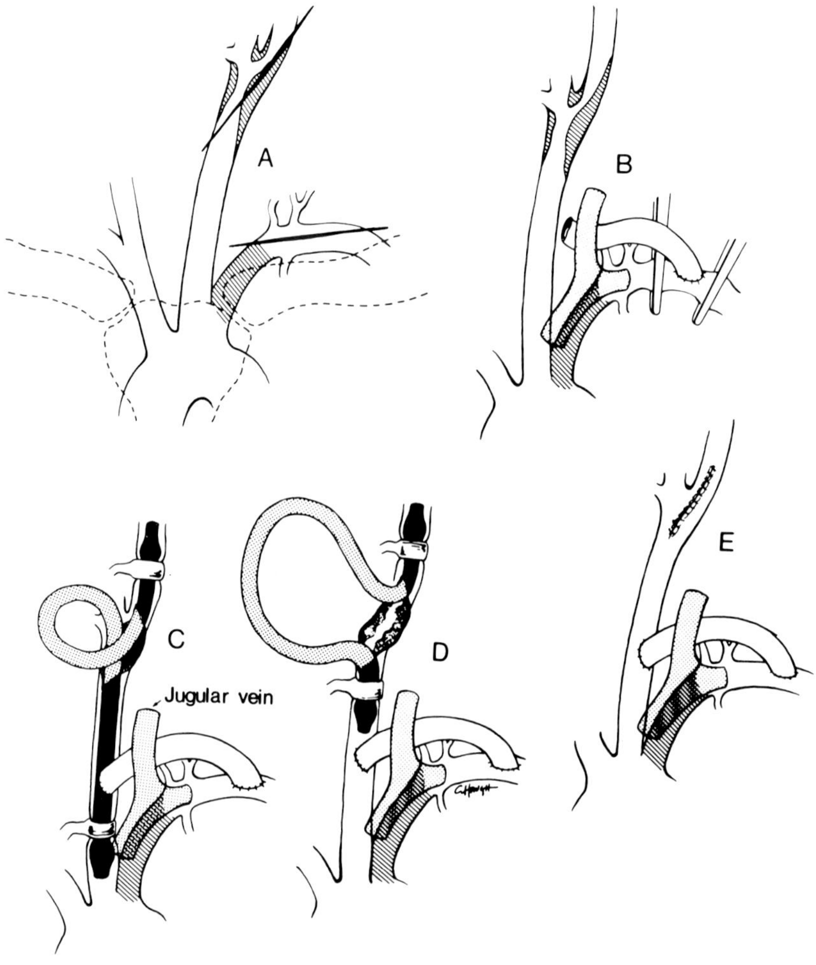

Figure 20-7. Concomitant carotid endarterectomy and carotid-subclavian bypass graft.

artery after systemic heparinization by using an end-to-side technique. Internal carotid shunting is then established. The proximal end of the tube is passed downward to an area just above the clavicle and is secured in place. A longitudinal incision is then made on the lateral wall of the common carotid artery, above the lower clamp. The graft is passed behind the jugular vein and is anastomosed to the common carotid artery with an end-to-side technique. The proximal end of the tube is then pulled upward to a level above the anastomosis and is secured in place again. Thus, carotid-subclavian bypass flow is accomplished. Carotid endarterectomy is then completed in the usual fashion, and the operation is completed.

REFERENCES

1. Eastcott HHG, Pickering GW, Rob CG: Reconstruction of the internal carotid artery. Lancet 2:994, 1954
2. Bland JE, Lazar ML: Carotid endarterectomy without shunt. Neurosurgery 8:153, 1981
3. Kwaan JM, Peterson GJ, Connolly JE: Stump pressure an unreliable guide for shunting during carotid endarterectomy. Archives of Surgery 115:1083, September, 1980
4. Michal VV, Hejhal L, Firt P: Zeitweilige shunts in der vaskularen chirurgie. Thorax-chirurgie 14:35, 1966
5. Moore WS, Hall AD: Carotid artery back pressure. Arch Surg 99:702, 1969
6. Hays RJ, Levinson SA, Wylie EJ: Intraoperative measurement of carotid back pressure as a guide to operative management for carotid endarterectomy. Surgery 72:953, 1972
7. Hertzer NR, Beven EG, Greenstreet RL, et al: Internal carotid back pressure, intraoperative shunting, ulcerated atheroma and the incidence of stroke during carotid endarterectomy. Surgery 83:306, 1978
8. Boysen G: Cerebral hemodynamics in carotid surgery. Acta Neurol Scand 49(suppl 52):1, 1973
9. Thompson JE, Talkington CM: Surgical progress in carotid endarterectomy. Ann Surg 184:1, 1976
10. Harris EJ, Brown WH, Pavy RN, et al: Continuous electroencephalographic monitoring during carotid artery endarterectomy. Surgery 62:441, 1967
11. Baker JD, Gluecklich B, Watson CW, et al: An evaluation of electroencephalographic monitoring for carotid study. Surgery 78:787, 1975
12. Sundt TM, Sharbrough FW, Piepgras DG, et al: Correlation of cerebral blood flow and electroencephalographic changes during carotid endarterectomy. Mayo Clinical Proceedings 56:533, 1981
13. Rowed DW, Vilaghy MI: Intraoperative regional cerebral blood flow during carotid endarterectomy. Le Journal Canadien des Sciences Neurologique 8:235, 1981
14. Waltz AG: Effect of blood pressure on blood flow in ischemic and non-ischemic cerebral cortex: The phenomena of autoregulation and luxury perfusion. Neurology 18:613, 1968
15. Bloodwell RD, Hallman GL, Keats AS, et al: Carotid endarterectomy without a shunt: Results using hypercarbia general anesthesia to prevent cerebral ischemia. Arch Surg 96:644, 1968
16. Fog M: Om Piaarteriernes Vasomotoriske Reaktioner. Thesis Copenhagen, Munksgaard, 1934.
17. Youmans JR, Kindt GW: Efficacy of carbon dioxide in the treatment of cerebral ischemia. Surg Forum 19:425, 1968

18. Brawley BW, Strandness DE, Kelly WA: The physiologic response to therapy in experimental cerebral ischemia. Arch Neurol 17:180, 1967
19. Callow AD, Matsumoto G, Baker D, et al: Protection of the high-risk carotid endarterectomy patient by continuous electroencephalography. J Cardiovasc Surg 19:55, 1978
20. Piepgras DG, Sundt TM: Clinical and laboratory experience with heparin impregnated silicone shunts for carotid endarterectomy. Ann Surg 184:637, 1976
21. Moore WS, Yee JM, Hall AD: Collateral cerebral blood pressure: An index of tolerance to temporary carotid occlusion. Arch Surg 106:520, 1973
22. Smith LL, Jacobson JG, Hinshaw DB: Correlation of neurological complications and pressure measurements during carotid endarterectomy. Surg Gyn & Obstet 143:233, 1976
23. Julian OC, Dye WS, Javid H, et al: Cardiovascular Surgery. Chicago, YearBook Medical Publishers, Inc., 1962
24. Chung FF, Chen RZ, Chien S, et al: Bypass blood flow during carotid endarterectomy. Anesthesiology 55:305, 1981
25. Fields WS, Lemak NA: Joint study of extracranial arterial occlusion and internal carotid artery occlusion. JAMA 235:2734, 1976
26. Baker WH, Dorner DB, Barnes RW: Carotid endarterectomy: Is an indwelling shunt necessary? Surgery 82:321, 1977
27. Patterson RH: Risk of carotid surgery with occlusion of contralateral carotid artery. Arch Neurol 30:188, 1974
28. Meng RL, Javid H, et al: Internal carotid artery occlusion: Risk of evaluation and surgical management. Conn Med J 42:441, 1978
29. Brierly JB: Cerebral hypoxia. In Greenfield's Neuropathology, Third Edition, Blackwood, W, Corsellis, JAN, editors. London, Edward Arnold Publishers, 1976
30. King GD, Gideon DA, Haynes CD, et al: Intellectual and personality changes associated with carotid endarterectomy. J Clin Psychol 33:215, 1977
31. Haynes CD, Gideon DA, King GD, et al: The improvement of cognition and personality after carotid endarterectomy. Surg 80:699, 1976
32. Kelly MP, Garron DC, Javid H: Carotid artery disease, carotid endarterectomy and behavior. Archives of Neurology volume 37, December, 1980
33. Najafi H, Javid H, Dye WS, et al: Kinked internal carotid artery. Arch Surg 89:134, 1964

Allan D. Callow
Thomas F. O'Donnell, Jr.

21

EEG Monitoring in Cerebrovascular Surgery

The Artery of Sleep was the label applied to the vessel palpable at the neck by the ancient Greek physicians. The word carotid appears to be derived from *karos* meaning heavy sleep and from *karoun,* to stupefy. Pressure on this artery was believed to result in unconsciousness and even death. The statuary, originally from the Parthenon and by an unknown sculptor of about the middle of the 5th century B.C., and now one of the Elgin marbles in the British Museum, depicts a centaur striving to render a Greek citizen unconscious by compressing his carotid artery (Fig. 21-1) (Written communication, The British Museum). A first stroke in the carotid territory is associated with a mortality of 20 percent, a two year recurrence rate of approximately 60 percent, and a 60 percent mortality at five years. Fifty percent of individuals suffering an acute stroke in the carotid artery territory ultimately die of stroke. The incidence rate for stroke escalates rapidly with advancing age from 3.5/100,000 persons under 35 years to more than 1800/100,000 persons 85 years of age or older.[1] Cerebral thrombotic infarction incidence rates more than double for every 10 year age increment from 45 years onward. Nearly 75 percent of patients with a completed stroke had a history of transient ischemic attacks and when internal carotid territory ischemia resulted in a completed stroke, prior transient ischemic attacks almost invariably involved the same arterial territory.[2,3] The incidence of stroke in patients with transient ischemic attacks is more than ten times that in a randomly selected series of persons of the same age and sex.[4] The transient ischemic attack must therefore be recognized as a warning of potential catastrophe. In 1976, the economic impact of stroke in the United States in terms of total cost to society was 7.36 billion dollars of which 3.26 billion were direct expenditures.[5]

Present day knowledge suggests that the transient ischemic attack may be the consequence of ulceration and embolization of an atheromatous plaque—

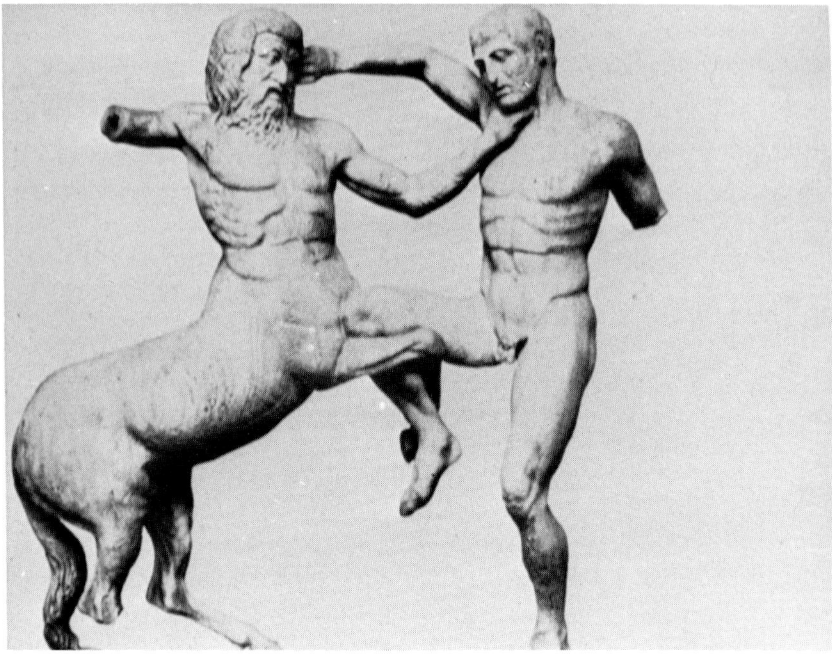

Figure 21-1. Courtesy of the Trustees of the British Museum.

the embolic theory[6] or as a consequence of reduction in flow secondary to an area of narrowing at the origin of or within the course of the internal carotid artery or vessels of the intracranial distribution—the stenotic theory.[7] These two theories are not mutally exclusive for areas of the brain which function on a marginal flow—50 percent of normal or less—are particularly vulnerable to the effects of emboli, and severely stenotic plaques, on the other hand, are more likely to form deep ulcerative craters and give rise to emboli than plaques of lesser hemodynamic severity. In the presence of high grade stenosis and ulceration and subject to variations in the severity of disease and the rate of maturation and degeneration of the atherosclerotic plaque, carotid endarterectomy removes the source of potential emboli, increases cerebral blood flow and perfusion pressure distal to the endarterectomy site, and prevents progression of the stenosis and ulceration to thrombosis and occlusion. In a sense, all carotid endarterectomies are prophylactic operations aimed at the prevention of an irreversible neurologic deficit, or in occasional instances, the extension of an already existing deficit.

Published series have repeatedly demonstrated that operative mortality and morbidity vary with the severity of the disease in the carotid artery and with the number and severity of risk factors in a given patient.[8,9] Based on clinical findings, Thompson and his associates have identified 4 categories for the classification of patients: (1) frank stroke, (2) transient cerebral ischemia, (3) chronic cerebral ischemia, and (4) the asymptomatic carotid bruit.[10,11] Noting a correlation between identifiable preoperative risk factors and complications of operation, Sundt and his associates have classified patients by the following: (1) medical risk factors, (2) neurologic risk factors, and (3) angiographically determined risk.[12] The major risk factors included the presence of symptomatic coronary artery disease or a myocardial infarction within the prior 6 months, severe hypertension, chronic obstructive pulmonary disease, a progressing or stable neurologic deficit or an unstable neurologic state characterized by frequent transient ischemic attacks, and multiple or extensive lesions within the carotid system as determined angiographically. This category also included occlusion of the opposite internal carotid, evidence of soft thrombus within the carotid artery under consideration and a high bifurcation of the carotid. Curiously, the degree of stenosis was not included as a risk factor. With these factors the following grades were evolved: (1) neurologically stable with no major medical or angiographically defined risks, (2) neurologically stable with no major medical risks but significant angiographically determined risks, (3) neurologically stable with major medical risks with or without significant angiographically determined risks, and (4) major neurologic risks with or without associated major medical or angiographically determined risks. Operative results varied according to risk factors. On the basis of intraoperative cerebral blood flow measurements determined from Xenon-133 clearance curves[13,14,15] and continuous electroencephalographic monitoring, the baseline and occlusion cerebral blood flow values were significantly lower in the highest risk group in comparison with those in the lowest risk group.[16] Failure to categorize patients makes comparison between results reported in published series difficult if not impossible. The patient with the least disease in the arterial system irrespective of other preoperative risk factors, and especially the patient operated for the asymptomatic bruit and who may need the operation least, will have the lowest risk of cerebral hypoxia during endarterectomy. The patient with extensive occlusive disease and with reduced or marginal cerebral blood flow has a greater probability of requiring a temporary intraluminal shunt during endarterectomy because of inadequate collateral supply.

Measures to determine the adequacy of collateral circulation include clinical assessment of the level of consciousness in the awake patient operated under local and regional anesthesia, or, when the patient is under general anesthesia, measurement with oculoplethysmographic readings of the back or carotid stump pressure and continuous monitoring with a multiple lead electroencephalogram. Induced hypertension or hypercarbia have been largely abandoned as ineffective and, in the case of hypertension, is contraindicated because of the unnecessary and hazardous burden imposed upon the myocardium of the patient with coexisting coronary artery disease.

Cerebral hypoxia may be avoided by the use of a temporary inlying shunt used either routinely in all cases or selectively. The inlying shunt permits the use of general anesthesia, maintains normal regional cerebral blood flow, eliminates the need for any type of monitoring system, and avoids a sense of haste. Its disadvantages include the possibility of embolization or injury to the arterial wall particularly at the distal end of the arteriotomy where satisfactory visualization may be difficult. These limitations may be avoided in most patients because, except in the highest risk group, the majority of patients do not require a shunt.[17]

Selective intraluminal shunting may be utilized based upon changes in the level of consciousness while the operation is proceeding under regional or local anesthesia; the adequacy of the critical carotid "stump" pressure usually taken at 50 mm Hg but with a lower level accepted by others; changes in the oculoplethysmographic findings during cross-clamping; or as preferred by us and some others, changes in the electroencephalogram with the patient under general anesthesia. As customarily performed, the stump pressure measurement is a single determination providing no monitoring during cross-clamping to detect possible changes in association with changes in level of anesthesia or cardiac function. Some confusion exists as to what is the adequate minimum back pressure, and pressure certainly must not be equated with flow. In a series of 125 awake patients operated under local anesthesia, Connolly found that 24 lost consciousness within 1 minute of cross-clamping with stump pressures ranging from 55 to 85 mm Hg. Eight patients (33 percent) had stump pressures above 50 mm Hg. In our series of 289 consecutive carotid endarterectomies performed in 204 patients and utilizing continuous electroencephalographic monitoring, EEG evidence of ischemia developed in 6 percent of the total series despite a stump pressure of greater than 50 mm Hg. The degree of disparity and its incidence between stump pressure and the EEG tracings varied according to the clinical category. In all cases where a temporary shunt was used, it was done on the basis of EEG criteria alone and regardless of the stump pressure. For patients operated for an asymptomatic bruit, 11 percent displayed ischemic changes on the EEG and required a temporary shunt. For patients operated with a classical carotid transient ischemic attack, 15 percent required a shunt, and for patients in the third and fourth categories, namely a history of a carotid territory stroke with recovery or with vertebral-basilar insufficiency symptoms superimposed upon carotid artery stenosis, 24 percent required a shunt (Figs. 21-2 and 21-3).[18] Twenty-eight operations (10 percent of the total series) required shunts with stump pressures less than 50 mm Hg, and 17 operations required shunts with stump pressures greater than 50 mm Hg (6 percent). Twenty-one operations or 7 percent of the series revealed a stump pressure of less than 50 mm Hg but did not require a shunt because of the continuation of a normal encephalographic tracing. In this group, there was a zero incidence of

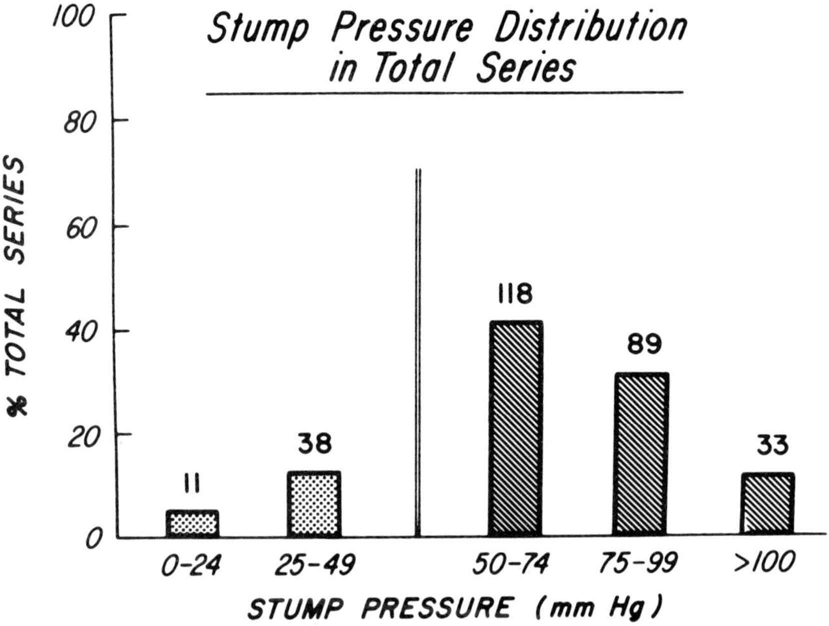

Figure 21-2. Reprinted with permission from AD Callow: The Leriche Memorial Lecture. Fact or fancy: A twenty year personal perspective in the detection and management of carotid occlusive disease.

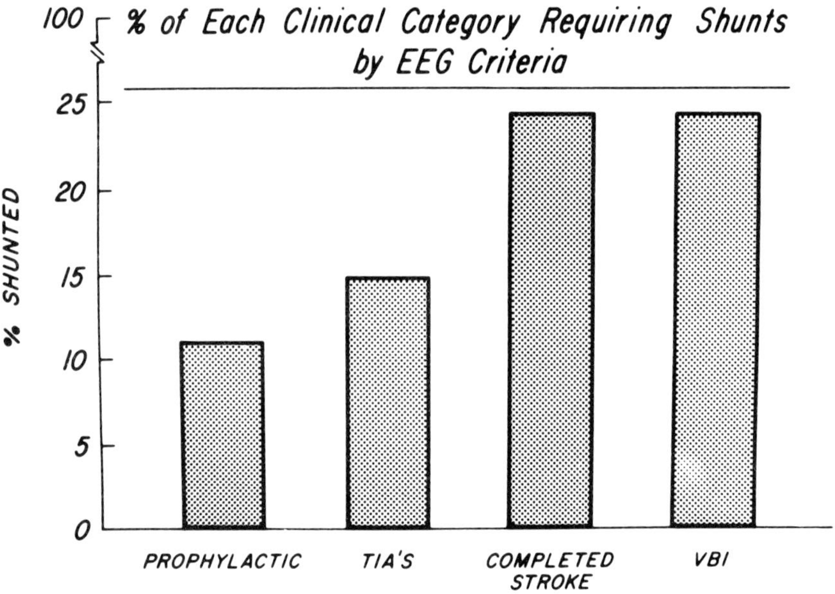

Figure 21-3. Reprinted with permission from AD Callow: The Leriche Memorial Lecture. Fact or fancy: A twenty year personal perspective on the detection and management of carotid occlusive disease.

neurologic deficit indicating the safety of EEG monitoring in patients with a low stump pressure. Finally, in those individuals operated with vertebral basilar insufficiency symptoms superimposed upon carotid artery stenosis and in whom one could assume that the available collateral circulation might be deficient, 77 percent of those patients requiring an intraoperative shunt had a carotid stump pressure of greater than 50 mm Hg.[19,20,21]

Archie and Feldtman have assumed that somewhere between 20 to 35 percent of patients operated without the use of an internal shunt have some degree of cerebral ischemia during the clamp period. The insensitivity of the neurologic deficit as an endpoint and the short clamp times with prompt reperfusion may explain the infrequency with which a temporary or permanent neurologic deficit is found.[22] Boysen et al.[23] have demonstrated that regional cerebral blood flow studies with radionuclide Xenon (Xe 133) indicate that flows of less than 18 ml/100g/min, which occur in approximately 20 to 25 percent of patients who undergo carotid endarterectomy, are associated with ischemic EEG changes and neurologic deficits.[23] Normal regional cerebral blood flow[24,25] is 50 to 55 ml/100g/min in patients with complete arterial hemoglobin oxygen saturation and a normal hematocrit reading. Since the autoregulatory lower limit of the cerebral perfusion pressure in humans is 50 to 55 mm Hg,[26] perfusion pressures below 18 mm Hg should correlate with flows below 18 ml/100g/min. Thus, a pressure of 18 mm Hg may be the cutoff point for safe perfusion pressure in humans with a normal cerebral vascular bed. Archie further reasons that if there is a brain region with a higher than normal minimum resistance or inability to autoregulate to a minimum cerebrovascular resistance, for example, a zone around a previous infarction or individuals with lowered collateral circulation such as a history of a previous stroke or vertebral-basilar insufficiency symptoms as well, as in the cases cited above, the lower limit of a safe perfusion pressure may be higher locally than 18 mm Hg. The results of Archie's study indicate that patients who undergo a carotid endarterectomy with general anesthesia have a mean ipsilateral collateral cerebral perfusion pressure of 29 mm Hg with a wide and skewed standard deviation. Twenty-five percent of these patients had a cerebral perfusion pressure less than 18 mm Hg and might therefore be considered the high risk group. The carotid back pressure alone identified only two-thirds of this group: "clearly patients with carotid back pressures as high as 40 to 45 mm Hg but high jugular venous pressures may have a perfusion pressure less than 18 mm Hg and, thereby, be at risk for cerebral ischemic injury."[22] The authors point out that measurements of the cerebral perfusion pressure, the carotid back pressure minus the jugular venous pressure, provide a more accurate estimate of collateral flow and are independent of patient position and anesthetic effect. This is particularly important if the carotid back pressure is in the lower 50 percent of the normal distribution because it is in this subgroup that a high or low venous pressure can lead to an erroneous identification of patients at risk.

METHOD

Twenty gold electrodes to the scalp and two ear electrodes are applied with collodion according to the 10–20 International Montage of Electrode Placement (Fig. 21-4).[27] A 16 channel Grass EEG machine is employed and a baseline trace obtained prior to induction and following the induction of the anesthetic level. The EEG is recorded continuously, ending only with extubation and in some individuals repeated in the recovery room or 4 to 5 days after operation. A careful log is kept of all medications administered preoperatively and throughout the anesthesia a variety of anesthetic agents are used, including halothane, ethrane, nitrous oxide, and furane. And in high risk patients, because of coexisting coronary artery disease, a narcotic technique utilizing Fentanyl, morphine, oxygen, and nitrous oxide are used. An arterial line is placed to permit continuous direct arterial pressure monitoring and intermittent arterial carbon dioxide tension, oxygen tension, and pH determinations. The electrocardiogram and the arterial pressures are

E.E.G. MONITORING FOR CAROTID ENDARTERECTOMY
INTERNATIONAL (20) ELECTRODE PLACEMENT

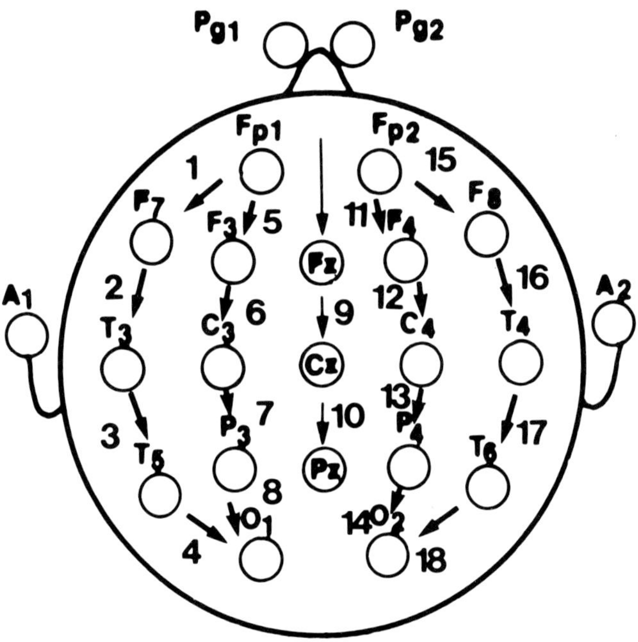

Figure 21-4. International montage—20 leads. Reprinted with permission from R Spehlmann: EEG Primer. Amsterdam, Elsevier/North-Holland Biomedical Press, 1981, p 472.

monitored continuously by an oscilloscopic display. In a few high risk patients, Swan Ganz catheters are placed for more precise monitoring.

Although on first glance, EEGs may appear to be very difficult to interpret and indeed under some instances they are, the changes of underperfusion of the brain and hypoxia are usually so obvious when seen by the individual who is familiar with the normal tracing as to be recognizable even though the individual is not a trained electroencephalographer. The variations in electrical activity were given Greek letters and then assigned in the order of their discovery, which explains the illogical sequence of the standard nomenclature. The frequencies are divided into four major bands. The 8-13 cycle per second band, the most striking rhythm of the normal EEG, was discovered first and labeled the alpha rhythm. Beta, theta, and delta frequencies are designations of frequency and carry no connotations as to localization or other parameters. The beta band is in excess of 13 cycles per second and is depressed or even absent in progressive to severe hypoxia. The theta band has a frequency of 4 to 7 cycles per second and delta, sometimes referred to as slow wave activity, is under 4 cycles per second (Fig. 21-5) [27] (Fig. 21-6).[28] Although the electroencephalographic record varies widely from one person to another and brain activity in the same subject changes from one second to the next, an individual's EEG, as a whole, remains remarkably constant over the mainspan of adult life.

In almost all patients with adequate cerebral perfusion during operation, a basic symmetric pattern consisting of sustained rhythmic activity of 10 to 14 Hertz ranging between 25 and 100 microvolts is obtained.[29]

Anoxia causes a progressive increase in amplitude and frequency, eventually followed by decreased amplitude and electrical silence.[30] As anoxia proceeds, delta frequency becomes the dominant rhythm. Slowing of the EEG occurs when the cerebral metabolic rate for oxygen has decreased by about 30 percent. It rapidly deteriorates with slowing first in the theta range, then in the delta range, and finally decreases in amplitude and becomes flat. The appearance of delta activity on the EEG coincides with a decrease of approximately 65 to 70 percent in the cerebral metabolic rate for oxygen. That

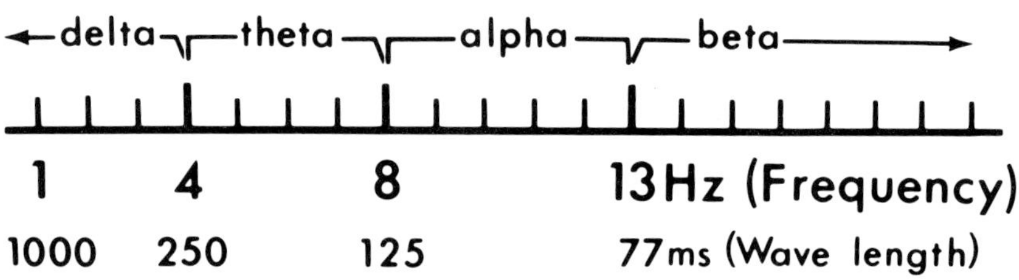

Figure 21-5. Diagrammatic representation of common EEG bands. See Fig. 21-6 for comparison of wave forms. Reprinted with permission from R Spehlmann: EEG Primer. Amsterdam, Elsevier/North-Holland Biomedical Press, 1981, p 472.

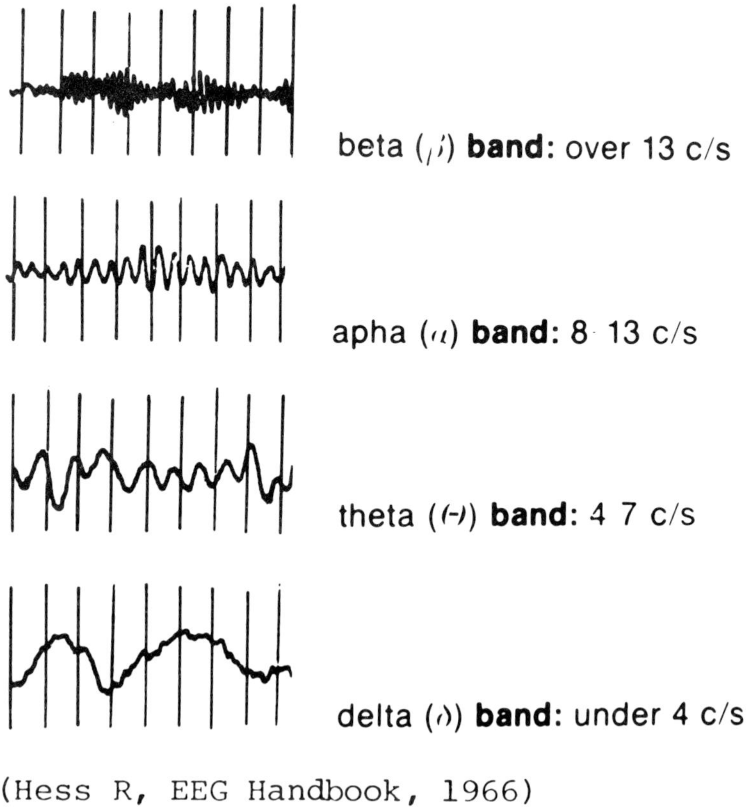

Figure 21-6. Reprinted with permission from R Hess: EEG Handbook. (Sandoz Monographs) EEG Laboratory of University Hospital, Zurich, Sandoz 1966, p 148.

oxygen pressure alone is not responsible for EEG changes has been shown during insulin-induced hypoglycemia[31] where the EEG changes parallel those of anoxia. Anesthesia produces depression of both consciousness and the cerebral metabolic rate. Focal changes, usually consisting of reduction of the normal background activity associated with variable amounts of irregular slowing, may be noted as evidence of hypoperfusion. In such cases, a shunt is used, and the focal changes usually resolve within a few seconds of opening the shunt, or where reduction in flow is more marked and collateral circulation limited, within 7 to 8 minutes (Fig. 21-7). In these instances, which involve the faster background frequencies, the beta component is replaced by a lower amplitude slow wave activity—the delta component. In the patient with advanced ischemia, the residual EEG activity is usually reduced to a very low voltage, irregular slow activity, and absence of the faster background components (Fig. 21-8). As the depth of anesthesia increases, the electroencephalogram becomes dominated by slow waves of 2 to 6 Hertz with some

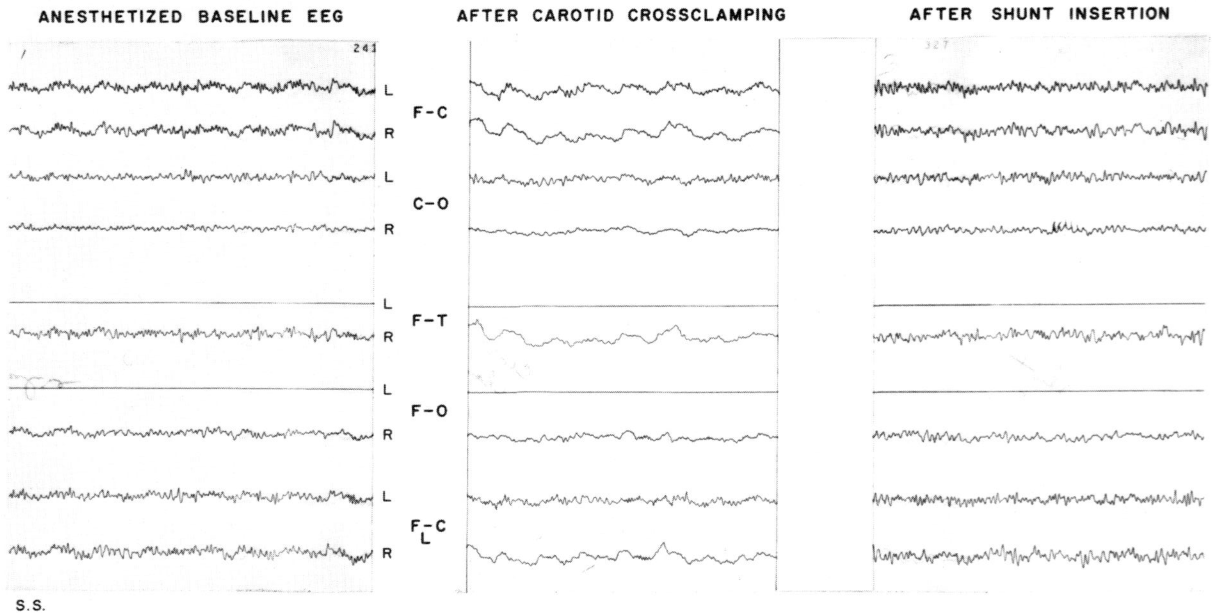

Figure 21-7. Ten lead electroencephalograph tracing showing the anesthetized baseline (left panel); the loss of fast wave and appearance of slow wave activity in the right hemisphere following right carotid cross-clamping (center panel), and prompt return of beta and disappearance of delta activity upon restoration of flow following a temporary intraluminal shunt insertion. The top five tracings are from the left hemisphere, the bottom five in each panel from the right hemisphere. Two electrodes in each panel are not functioning.

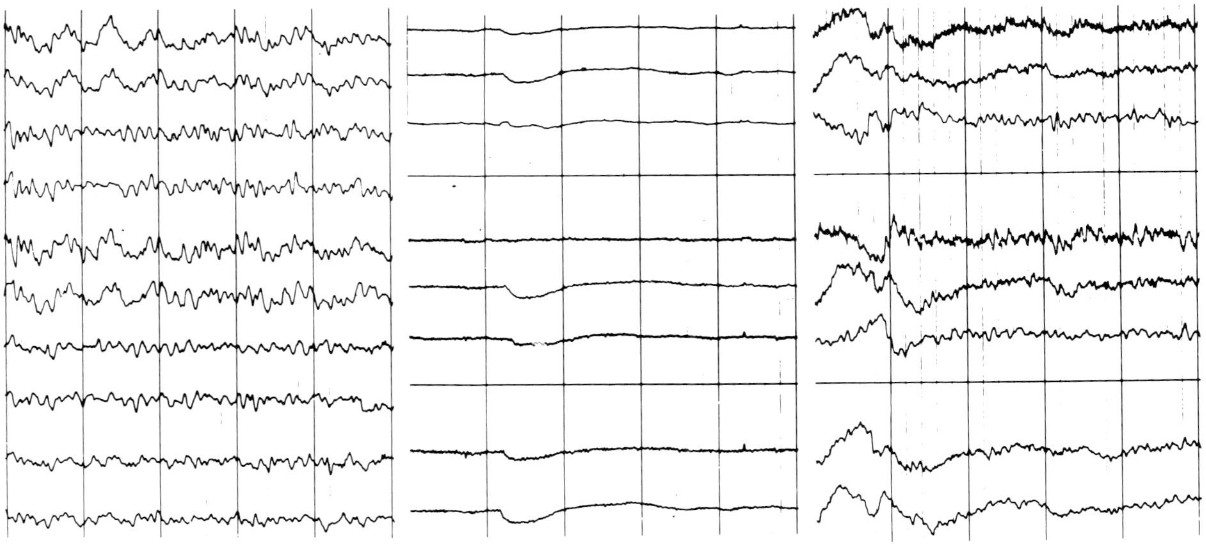

Figure 21-8. Ten lead electroencephalograph tracing showing anesthetized baseline in the left panel, severe loss of electrical activity in the central panel following cross-clamping of the left common carotid artery, and somewhat delayed return of electrical activity (8 minutes) after insertion of the shunt in the right panel. The top five in each panel are from the left, the bottom five from the right hemisphere. Two leads in the central and right panel are non-functioning. This individual's total cerebral supply was from 50 percent stenotic and ulcerated left internal carotid artery. The right internal and both vertebral arteries were occluded. The more severe the deprivation of blood flow, the more marked is the suppression of electrical activity and the longer the delay in restoration of normal electrical activity after restoration of flow.

loss of the faster components. This is a generalized change making recognition of focal abnormalities more difficult. Furthermore, the $PaCO_2$ must also be carefully controlled as EEG fluctuations have been reported with changes in the arterial tension of this gas.[32] Contralateral focal EEG changes not associated with occlusion of the ipsilateral carotid probably indicate significant contralateral vascular disease. Transient or permanent ipsilateral EEG changes occurring during surgery or after closure of the arteriotomy may indicate thromboembolism from or thrombosis within the endarterectomy site. Because of the importance of an adequate endarterectomy at the distal end of the arteriotomy, it is our custom not only to complete this portion of the endarterectomy prior to inserting a shunt when the EEG dictates its need, but to do so routinely for the need of a shunt may not be immediately apparent after carotid cross-clamping.

The electroencephalogram provides close correlation between cerebral perfusion and electric activity[19,24,25,32]; provides continuous surveillance of cerebral flow; avoids reliance on a single stump pressure measurement; avoids a sense of haste; and provides adequate protection for all patients irrespective of undetected variations in collateral flow, depth of anesthesia, and transient

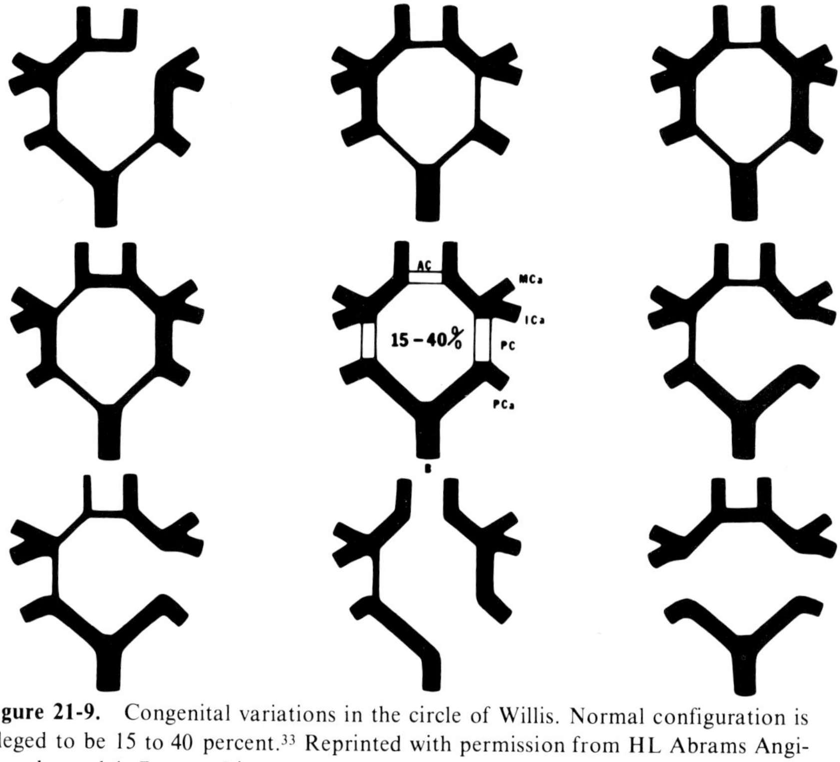

Figure 21-9. Congenital variations in the circle of Willis. Normal configuration is alleged to be 15 to 40 percent.[33] Reprinted with permission from HL Abrams Angiography, vol 1. Boston, Little Brown, 1961–62.

or permanent cardiac malfunction under anesthesia. Its disadvantages, which seem trivial to us, are added expense and time.

For those surgeons who do not utilize any type of monitoring or shunting or even measurement of the carotid back pressure, their speed of operation and the abundant collateral circulation help to avoid neurologic complications. For others, however, and particularly when dealing with patients in a high risk category in whom the collateral circulation may be marginal, too great reliance upon the circle of Willis can be hazardous. Various studies have revealed that not over 40 percent of individuals and as few as 15 percent in another series have a so-called normal configuration. Congenital anomalies include lack of communication through the circle of Willis via posterior communicating arteries, between the posterior and anterior circulations, or between one hemisphere and the other. Anomalies of lesser flow significance are numerous (Fig. 21-9).[33]

"To maintain that a shunt is never necessary puts one in an indefensible position—indefensible philosophically and scientifically."[34] Carotid endarterectomy is conceptually simple and technically easy to accomplish, but devastating complications may follow as a consequence of seemingly trivial surgical derelictions. It is not an operation for the beginner or the occasional vascular surgeon. In the words of Willman, "Although it is attractive to consider oneself as being numbered among the twelve minute endarterectomists, most surgeons will, in the companionship of their conscience, choose the security of measuring, shunting and monitoring."[35]

REFERENCES

1. The National Survey of Stroke. Weinfeld FD, Ed. American Heart Association Monograph No. 75. Stroke 12(2); Mar/Apr, 1981. Robins M, Baum HM, Chap 4. Incidence, pp I-45
2. McDowell F: Report of the New Orleans (1970) meeting concerning the epidemiology of cerebrovascular disease. Stroke 2:101, 1971
3. Lyons C: Progress report of the joint study of extracranial arterial occlusion, in Siekert RG, Whisnant JP (eds): Cerebral Vascular Diseases. New York, Grune and Stratton, 1965, p 221
4. Fields WS: Selection of patients with ischemic cerebrovascular disease for arterial surgery. World J Surg 3:147, 1979
5. Adelman SM: Economic impact, in Weinfeld FD (ed): The National Survey of Stroke, chap 6. American Heart Association Monograph No. 75. Stroke 12(2); Mar/Apr, 1981, p I-69
6. Gomensoro JB, Maslenikov V, Azambuja N, et al: Joint study of extracranial arterial occlusion. VIII. Clinical-radiographic correlation of carotid bifurcation lesions in 177 patients with transient cerebral ischemic attacks. JAMA 224:985, 1973
7. Yates PO, Hutchinson EC: Cerebral infarction: The role of stenosis of the extracranial cerebral arteries. Medical Research Council Special Report Series No. 300, London, Her Majesty's Stationery Office, 1961
8. Wylie EJ, Hein MF, Adams JE: Intracranial hemorrhage following surgical revascularization for treatment of acute strokes. J Neurosurg 21:212, 1964

9. Riles TS, Imparato AM, Mintzer R, et al: Comparison of results of bilateral and unilateral carotid endarterectomy five years after surgery. Surgery 91:258, 1982
10. Thompson JE, Patman RD, Talkington CM: Carotid surgery for cerebrovascular insufficiency. Curr Probl Surg 15 No. 12:1, 1978
11. Thompson JE: Complications of carotid endarterectomy and their prevention. World J Surg 3:155, 1979
12. Sundt TM Jr, Sandok BA, Whisnant JP: Carotid endarterectomy: complications and preoperative assessment of risk. Mayo Clin Proc 50:301, 1975
13. Sundt TM Jr, Sharbrough FW, Anderson RE, et al: Cerebral blood flow measurements and electroencephalograms during carotid endarterectomy. J Neurosurg 41:310, 1974
14. Waltz AG, Wanek AR, Anderson RE: Comparison of analytic methods for calculation of cerebral blood flow after intracarotid injection of ^{133}Xe. J Nucl Med 13:66, 1972
15. Anderson RE, Sundt TM Jr: An automated cerebral blood flow analyzer: concise communication. J Nucl Med 18:728, 1977
16. Sundt TM, Sharbrough FW, Piepgras DG, et al: Correlation of cerebral blood flow and electroencephalographic changes during carotid endarterectomy with results of surgery and hemodynamics of cerebral ischemia. Mayo Clin Proc 56:533, 1981
17. Kwaan JHM, Peterson GJ, Connolly JE: Stump pressure. An unreliable guide for shunting during carotid endarterectomy. Arch Surg 115:1083, 1980
18. Callow AD: The Leriche Memorial Lecture. Fact or fancy: A twenty year personal perspective on the detection and management of carotid occlusive disease. J Cardiovas Surg 21:641 1980.
19. Kelly JJ, Callow AD, O'Donnell TF, et al: Failure of carotid stump pressures. Its incidence as a predictor for a temporary shunt during carotid endarterectomy. Arch Surg 114:1361, 1979
20. Matsumoto GH, Baker JD, Watson CW, et al: EEG surveillance as a means of extending operability in high risk carotid endarterectomy. Stroke 7:554, 1976
21. Baker JD, Gluecklich B, Watson W, et al: An evaluation of electroencephalographic monitoring for carotid surgery. Surgery 78:787, 1975
22. Archie JP, Feldtman RW: Determinants of cerebral perfusion pressure during carotid endarterectomy. Arch Surg 117:319, 1982
23. Boysen G, Engell HC, Pistolese GR, et al: On the critical lower level of cerebral blood flow in man with particular reference to carotid surgery. Circulation 49:1023, 1974
24. Boysen G, Ladegaard-Pedersen HJ, Engell HC: Cerebral blood flow studies during carotid surgery, in Brock M, Fieschi C, Ingvar DH, et al (eds.): Cerebral Blood Flow. New York, Springer-Verlag, Inc, 1969, p 155
25. Boysen G, Engell HC, Henriksen H: The effect of induced hypertension on internal carotid artery pressure and regional blood flow during temporary carotid clamping for endarterectomy. Neurology 22:1133, 1972
26. Fieschi C, Angoli A, Battistina N, et al: Derangement of regional cerebral blood flow and its regulatory mechanisms in acute cerebrovascular lesions. Neurology 18:1166, 1968
27. Spehlmann R: EEG Primer. Amsterdam, Elsevier/North-Holland Biomedical Press, 1981, p 472
28. Hess R: EEG Handbook. (Sandoz Monographs) EEG Laboratory of University Hospital, Zurich, Sandoz Ltd, (Publ) 1966, p 148
29. Westmoreland BF: Normal and benign EEG patterns. Am J of EEG Tech 22:3, 1982
30. Constant S: Understanding hypoxia and its effects on the EEG recordings. Am J of EEG Tech 22:33, 1982
31. Handbook of EEG and Clinical Neurophysiology. Amsterdam, Elsevier Scientific Publishing Co, vol. 7B-29, 54:14A-6,7

32. Sharbrough FW, Messick JM, Sundt TM: Correlation of continuous electroencephalograms with cerebral blood flow measurements during carotid endarterectomy. Stroke 4:674, 1973
33. Abrams HL: Angiography, vol. 1. Boston, Little Brown, 1961 p 62
34. Thompson JE: Discussion. Arch Surg 115:1398, 1980
35. William VL: Editorial Comment. Arch Surg 115:942, 1980

D. Preston Flanigan
Bernard Sigel
James J. Schuler

22

Intraoperative Ultrasonic Carotid Artery Imaging

Stroke, as a result of carotid endarterectomy, is usually reported at less than five percent in most series.[1] There is a growing realization that most strokes resulting from carotid endarterectomy are not due to transient cerebral hypoperfusion during carotid clamping but, rather, are due to technical errors made at the time of surgery. These errors are mainly responsible for intraoperative strokes or strokes occurring in the early postoperative period. As a result, many surgeons are now deemphasizing intraoperative protection of cerebral perfusion and are emphasizing the importance of meticulous operative technique. Technical errors at surgery may result from excessive manipulation of the carotid artery during dissection or shunt placement resulting in intraoperative embolization and stroke. Errors also may result from inadequate attention to the details of the endarterectomy itself such that defects including arterial strictures, intimal flaps, or intraluminal thrombi occur. These latter complications may result in either intraoperative or early postoperative strokes. Reduction in the incidence of such errors would most likely reduce the incidence of strokes associated with carotid endarterectomy.

The suggestion that technical errors may be responsible for most operative strokes is not new. In 1967, Blaisdell, in an attempt to decrease the neurologic sequelae of carotid endarterectomy, studied 100 elective procedures which were evaluated by completion intraoperative carotid arteriography as a means of detecting defects created at operation.[2] In Blaisdell's series, 26 percent of the procedures were found to be unsatisfactory because of defects shown arteriographically. The importance of completion intraoperative arteriography following carotid surgery has been emphasized more recently by others.[3-5]

Intraoperative cerebral arteriography is not without risk. Permanent stroke has been reported as a result of technical problems with intraoperative carotid arteriography.[4,5] Andersen, in analyzing the Walter Reed Army Medical Center experience with carotid endarterectomy in which completion carotid arteriography was routine, indicated that the risk of complications from the arteriogram outweighed its benefit for routine application and suggested that it be applied only in selected situations.[4] In addition to neurologic sequelae, the general hazards of arteriography must be considered. These hazards include radiation exposure to both the patient and surgeon and allergic reactions, which at times may be life threatening. A completely safe, yet accurate, technique of intraoperatively evaluating the technical results of carotid endarterectomy which could be applied in a routine fashion should be useful in decreasing the neurologic sequelae occasionally associated with the procedure. To this purpose, we have explored the use of intraoperative, real-time, high resolution, B-mode, ultrasonic imaging.

INTRAOPERATIVE ULTRASOUND

The use of intraoperative ultrasound is not new. Several reports in the early 1960s considered its use in the detection of common duct stones, breast tumors, and renal calculi.[6–9] With the recent advances in ultrasound, resulting in high resolution, real-time, B-mode imaging, and the development of small parts scanners, the application of the technique to intraoperative arterial imaging seemed promising.

Ultrasound Technique

Our technique utilizes a High Stoy real-time, B-mode instrument having a resolution of 1 mm. Either a 7.5 MHz or 10 MHz probe may be used. The probe is hand held and the cord from the gas sterilized transducer is handed off the operative field for attachment to the main ultrasound unit. The operative wound is filled with warm saline for acoustic coupling. Scan angles are limited only by the confines of the wound, and transverse and multiple longitudinal scan planes can usually be obtained. Real-time images are visualized on a black and white television monitor and may also be recorded on video tape or Polaroid® prints for subsequent review.

Early Evaluation

Preliminary evaluation was made in the canine laboratory to assess the accuracy of the ultrasound technique. Arteries 5 mm-10 mm in external diameter were surgically entered and defects were created. The defects consisted of strictures, thrombi, subintimal hematomas, and intimal flaps. Intimal flap size varied from 1 mm-5 mm. All cases of stricture, thrombi, and subintimal hematomas were correctly identified by ultrasound (Figs. 22-1-

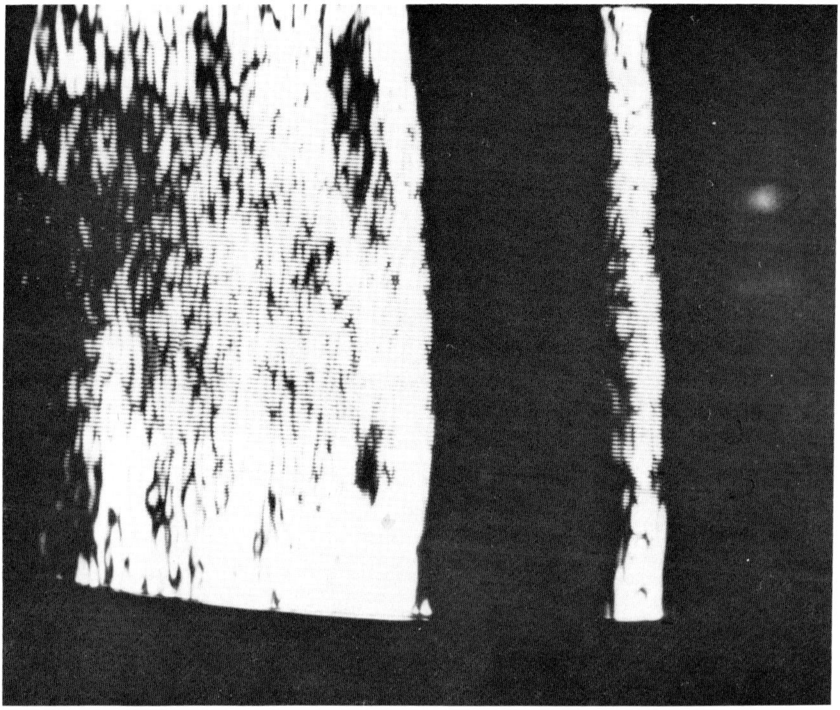

Figure 22-1. Normal arterial ultrasonogram (canine aorta).

22-5). Intimal flaps measuring 1 mm were detected 68 percent of the time, and all flaps 2 mm or greater in size were identified. Correlation between ultrasonically measured flap size and actual flap size was very good ($r = .84$, $p < 0.001$) (Table 22-1). There were no false positive examinations.[10]

Since we were evaluating ultrasound as a potential replacement for intraoperative arteriography, an experiment was designed to compare the two techniques. Intimal defects, 2 mm and 5 mm intimal flaps, thrombi, and strictures were created in canine aortas (approximately 1 cm diameter) and evaluated by ultrasound and both portable and serial bi-plane arteriography. The accuracy and sensitivity of ultrasound was higher than both types of arteriography for 2 mm and 5 mm flaps and thrombi. Both types of arteriography were more sensitive than ultrasound in detecting intimal defects. All three techniques were equally accurate in detecting arterial strictures (Table 22-2).[11] Based on these experimental results, intraoperative ultrasound appeared to be at least as accurate if not more accurate than arteriography and, thus, warranted clinical evaluation.

The accuracy of ultrasound in comparison to operative arteriography was evaluated clinically in 48 patients having lower extremity arterial bypass

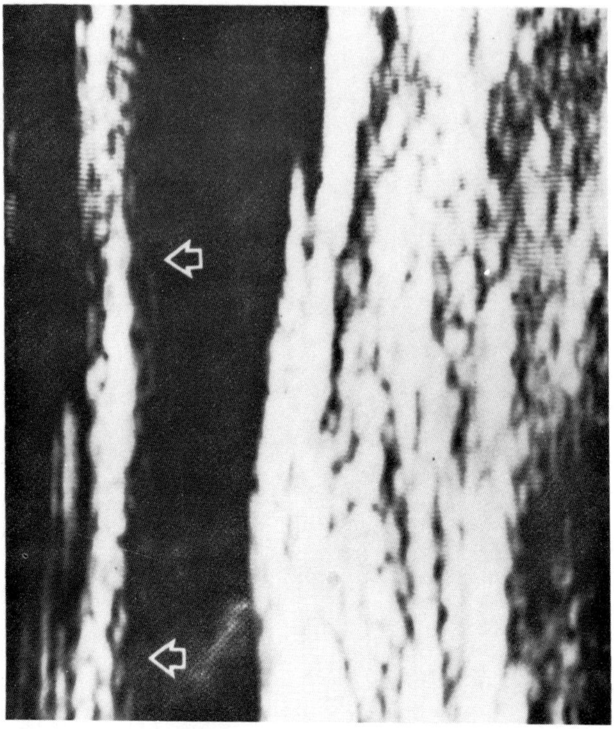

Figure 22-2. Ultrasonogram showing an arterial stricture (canine aorta).

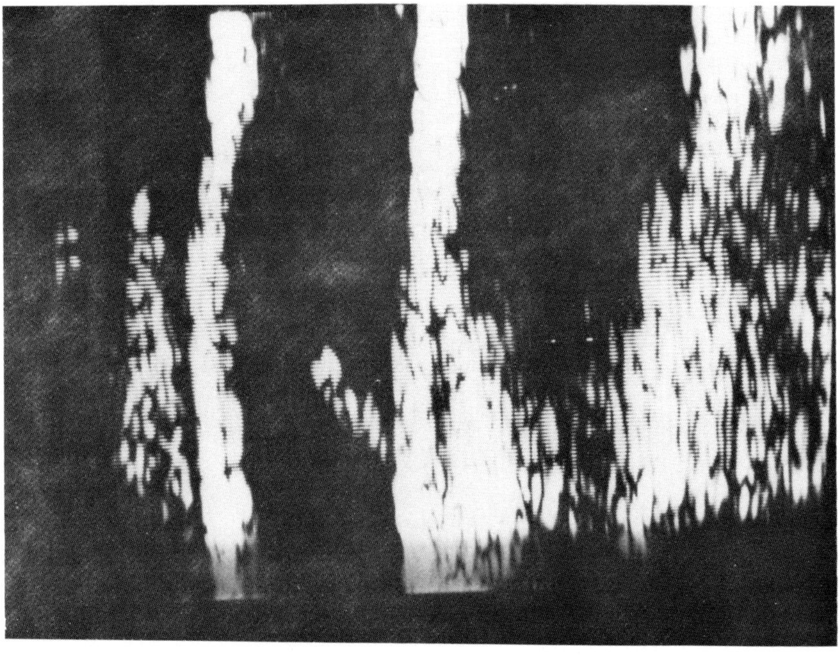

Figure 22-3. Ultrasonogram showing a 5 mm intimal flap (canine aorta).

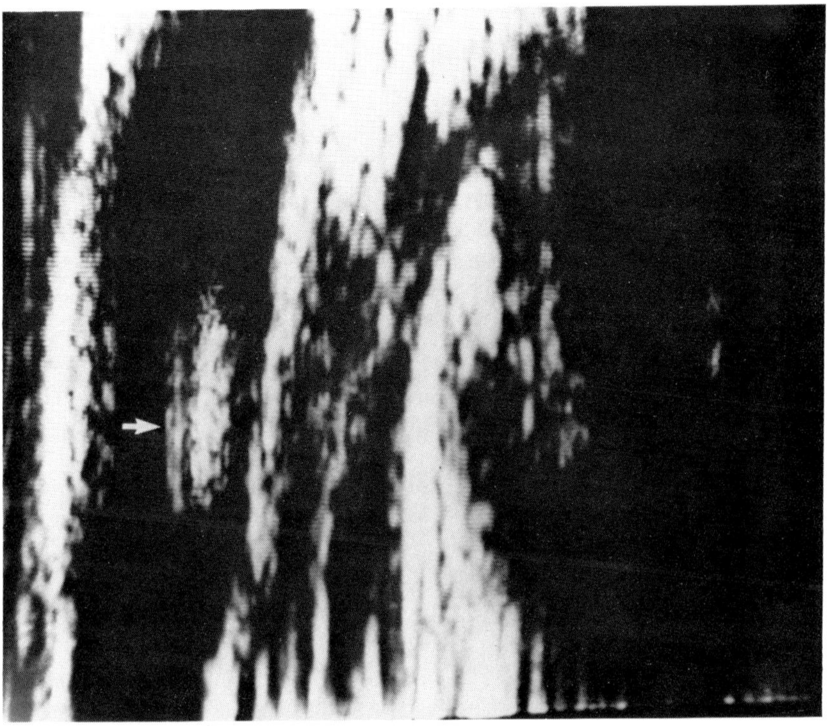

Figure 22-4. Ultrasonogram showing intraluminal thrombus (canine aorta).

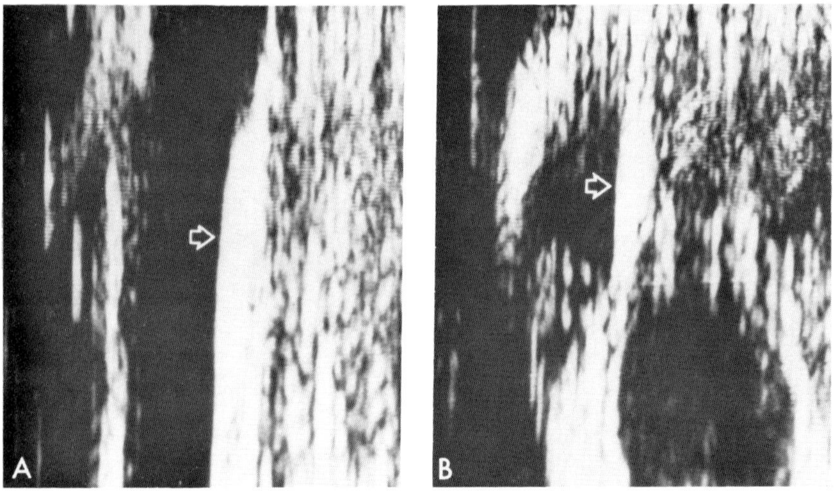

Figure 22-5. Ultrasonogram showing subintimal hematoma (A) longitudinal scan (B) transverse scan (canine aorta).

Table 22-1
Ultrasonic Detection of Intimal Flaps

Ultrasound Result	Normal Artery	Flap Size (mm) 1	2	3	4	5
True Positive	0	17	25	25	25	25
False Negative	0	8	0	0	0	0
True Negative	20	0	0	0	0	0
False Positive	0	0	0	0	0	0
Total	20	25	25	25	25	25

procedures.[12] The standards for comparison in these patients were the presence or absence of postoperative graft complications or the findings within the arteries upon reexploration in these vessels found to have significant defects by either ultrasound or arteriography. Any patient having a postoperative graft complication was considered as having a correctable defect which should have been detected by the diagnostic techniques. Table 22-3 shows the results of this analysis. The accuracies for ultrasound and arteriography were 96 percent and 85 percent respectively.

COMPLETION CAROTID ULTRASONOGRAPHY

Our total experience to date includes 48 carotid endarterectomies which have been evaluated by intraoperative ultrasound. In 13 patients (27 percent),

Table 22-2
Comparison of Ultrasound to Portable and Serial Biplane Arteriography

	Portable Arteriography			Serial Arteriography		
Defects	Sens.	Spec.	Acc.	Sens.	Spec.	Acc.
2 mm Flaps	21	99	59	54	97	75
5 mm Flaps	24	100	61	48	100	73
Intimal Defects	24	99	60	27	99	62
Thrombi	37	100	67	70	100	84
Strictures	52	94	73	62	96	79

	Ultrasonography		
Defects	Sens.	Spec.	Acc.
2 mm Flaps	92	99	95
5 mm Flaps	92	100	96
Intimal Defects	7	94	49
Thrombi	100	100	100
Strictures	76	96	85

Table 22-3
Clinical Evaluation of Ultrasound vs. Arteriography

Test Result	Ultrasound	Arteriography
False Positive	33%	67%
False Negative	0	3%
Sensitivity	100%	75%
Specificity	95%	86%
Accuracy	96%	85%

defects were detected (Table 22-4). In all patients, the defect was an intimal flap (2 mm-7 mm). Eight flaps were in the common carotid artery, three flaps were in the external carotid artery, and only two flaps were in the internal carotid artery. Flaps in 11 patients were considered not to be of clinical significance. In 2 patients, flaps were considered significant, and this led to reopening of the carotid arteriotomies and successful correction of the defects. One repaired flap was 5 mm in size and was located at the distal end point of the plaque resection (Fig. 22-6). The other repaired flap measured 7 mm in size and was located in the common carotid artery (Fig. 22-7) (Table 22-5). Both patients having their defects corrected and the 11 patients having defects judged not to require repair had uneventful postoperative courses. The 35 patients with normal intraoperative ultrasonograms also did well except for 1 patient who awoke from anesthesia with a monoparesis which lasted two weeks (Table 22-4). Oculopneumoplethysmographic recordings in the post-operative period in this patient indicated lack of hemodynamically significant stenosis or occlusion in the operated artery. It was felt that this transient stroke was secondary to intraoperative embolization; however, this cannot be known with certainty.

DISCUSSION

Although this represents an early clinical experience with only 48 patients, there were, nevertheless, defects found in 27 percent of the arteries examined. This is extremely similar to the larger series reported by Blaisdell

Table 22-4
Results of Operative Carotid Ultrasound

Defects	Number (%)	Subsequent Repair	Stroke
Yes	13 (27)	2	0
No	35 (73)	0	1
Total	48 (100)	2	1

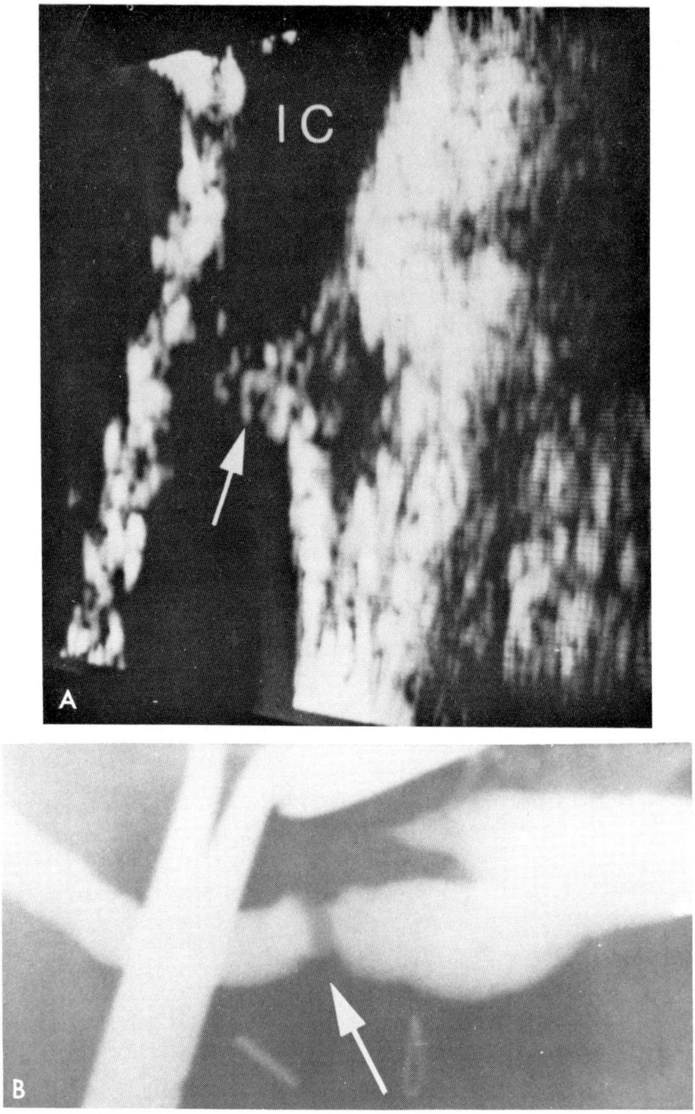

Figure 22-6. (A) Ultrasonogram showing a 5 mm flap in the internal carotid artery (B) an arteriogram done in this patient also demonstrated the defect.

using intraoperative arteriography.[2] Since the clinical experience with intraoperative ultrasound is yet small, its value must be assumed based on the previously determined value of intraoperative arteriography and the fact that we have demonstrated a superior accuracy for the ultrasound technique. As applied to carotid surgery, the demonstration of the efficacy of intraoperative ultrasound is especially difficult because of the low stroke rate now associated

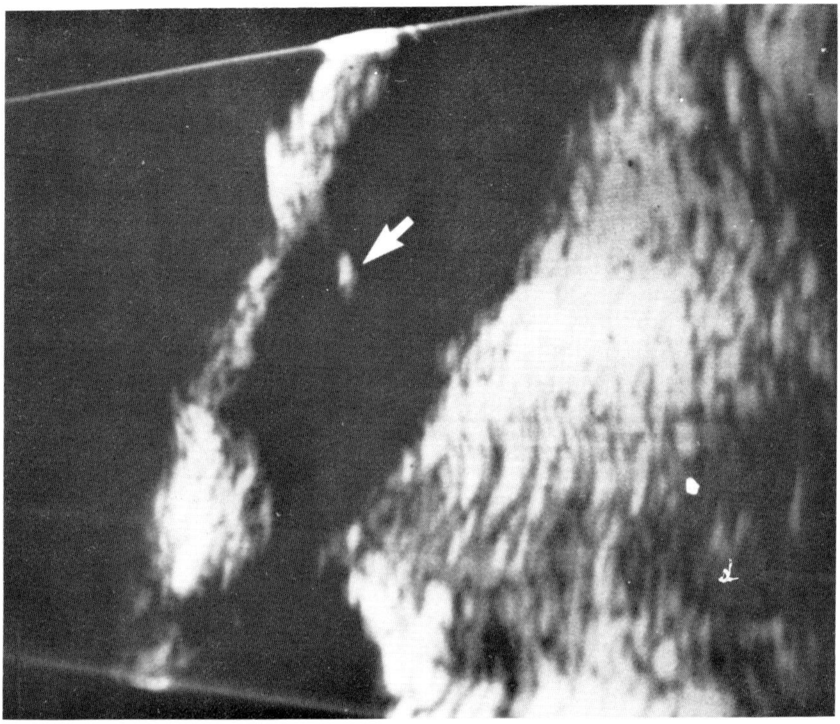

Figure 22-7. Ultrasonogram demonstrating a 7 mm intimal flap in the common carotid artery following carotid endarterectomy.

with the surgical procedure. Because of the demonstrated high accuracy of the technique, we could not justify not revising defects that were felt to be of significant risk to the patient. The decision regarding the importance of a defect is very subjective and involves not only the type and size of the defect but its location as well. In the current series, no patient with an unrevised defect developed a stroke. This suggests that the current technology regarding

Table 22-5
Defects Found at Operative Carotid Ultrasonography

Defect	Number	Location
2 mm Flap	8	Common Carotid (5), External Carotid (2), Internal Carotid (1)
3 mm Flap	2	Common Carotid, External Carotid
4 mm Flap	1	Common Carotid
5 mm Flap	1	Internal Carotid*
7 mm Flap	1	Common Carotid*

*Subsequently repaired

image resolution is reasonably good since even defects having no clinical significance were well visualized.

There is a need, however, for further refinement in the ultrasound equipment. Progress toward smaller probes and lateral apertures for scanning is essential to improve imaging capabilities. Also, development of affordable equipment dedicated to operative use would be beneficial.

There were no complications in this experience that could be related to ultrasound. The safety of the ultrasound technique plus better accuracy when compared to arteriography make ultrasound a superior method for detecting defects at vascular operative sites. The better precision of ultrasound is probably due to the real-time feature allowing dynamic imaging and the ability to scan in multiple projections. As demonstrated by our canine study,[11] ultrasound is not as accurate as arteriography in detecting shallow intimal defects, but this shortcoming is of questionable significance since areas of denuded intima are necessitated by carotid endarterectomy and, in the absence of flaps, are probably of no clinical significance.

There are two other shortcomings of intraoperative ultrasound that deserve mention. One is the need for the surgeon to learn a new technique and the problems associated with the always attendant "learning curve." The other is the inability of the ultrasound to image beyond the confines of the operative wound. When imaging outside the area of the wound is required, arteriography is currently the better choice.

REFERENCES

1. Thompson JE, Talkington CM: Carotid endarterectomy. Ann Surg 184:1, 1976
2. Blaisdell FW, Lim R Jr, Hall AD: Technical result of carotid endarterectomy: Arteriographic assessment. Am J Surg 114:239, 1967
3. Rosental JJ, Gasper MR, Movius HJ: Intraoperative arteriography and carotid thromboendarterectomy. Arch Surg 106:806, 1973
4. Andersen CA, Collins GJ JR, Rich NM: Routine operative arteriography during carotid endarterectomy: A reassessment. Surgery 83:67, 1978
5. Collins GJ Jr, Rich NM, Andersen CA, et al: Stroke associated with carotid endarterectomy. Am J Surg 135:221, 1978
6. Schlegel JU, Diggdon P, Cuellar J: The use of ultrasound for localizing renal calculi. J Urol 86:367, 1961
7. Hayashi S, Wagai T, Miyazawa R, et al: Ultrasonic diagnosis of breast tumor and cholelithiasis. West J Surg 70:34, 1962
8. Knight RP, Newell JA: Operative use of ultrasonics in cholelithiasis. Lancet 1:1023, 1963
9. Eiseman B, Greenlaw RH, Gallagher JQ: Localization of common duct stones by ultrasound. Arch Surg 91:195, 1965
10. Coelho JCU, Sigel B, Flanigan DP, et al: Detection of arterial defects by real-time ultrasound scanning during vascular surgery: An experimental study. J Surg Res 30:535, 1981
11. Coelho JCU, Sigel B, Flanigan DP, et al: An experimental evaluation of arteriography and imaging ultrasonography in detecting arterial defects at operation. J Surg Res 32:130, 1982
12. Sigel B, Coelho JCU, Flanigan DP, et al: Detection of vascular defects during operation by imaging ultrasound. Annals of Surgery (in press)

Steven R. Larson Max R. Gaspar
Herbert J. Movius John J. Rosental
Donald D. Bell Guy G. Lemire

23

Intraoperative Arteriography in Cerebrovascular Surgery

Most vascular surgeons seem to subscribe to the tenet that completion arteriography is necessary after reconstructive arterial operations in the lower extremities, but few have adopted the same doctrine for carotid thrombo-endarterectomy. In 1967, Blaisdell and his co-authors reported 100 patients in whom routine arteriography was performed in the operating room after carotid endarterectomy.[1] In 26 cases, there were significant defects which necessitated revision of the endarterectomized carotid vessels. Following Blaisdell's report and his challenge to perform routine completion arteriography, we developed a simple method which provides a minimum loss of operating time.[2]

TECHNIQUE

The patient's chest and head are placed on a plywood tunnel which will accept an x-ray cassette. The anesthesiologist is positioned to the side opposite the one to be operated upon (Fig. 23-1). The surgeons place themselves about the head of the patient in a comfortable position for the operation (Fig. 23-2). After completion of the endarterectomy, the x-ray technician is called to the operating room as closure of the arteriotomy is commenced. Following closure of the arteriotomy in the carotid artery, the occluding vessel loops are removed. A 10 cc syringe with attached tubing and needle are brought to the operating table and filled with saline solution. All bubbles of air are carefully flushed from the tubing, and the needle is introduced into the common carotid artery proximal to the arteriotomy. When a vertical incision is used, a scalp

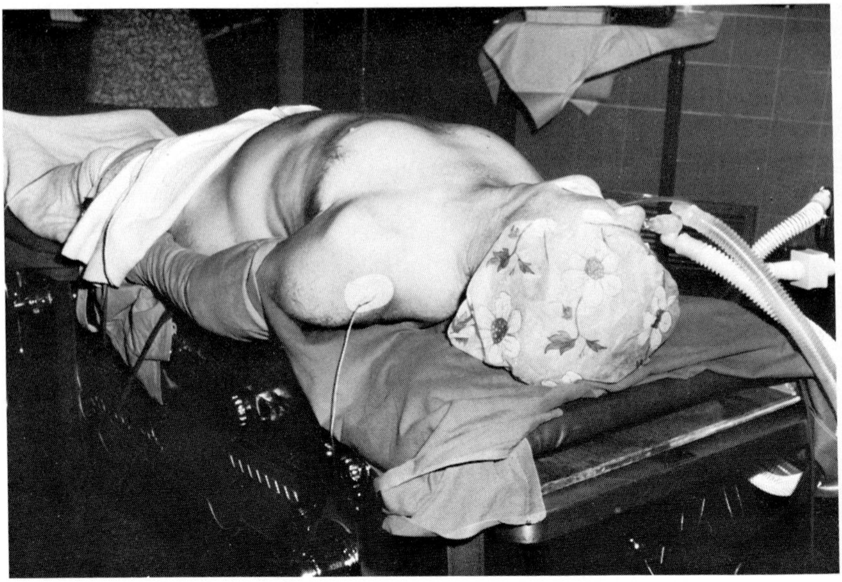

Figure 23-1. Patient in position on a wooden tunnel which will accept an x-ray cassette. Anesthesiologist positioned to the side opposite to the one being operated upon.

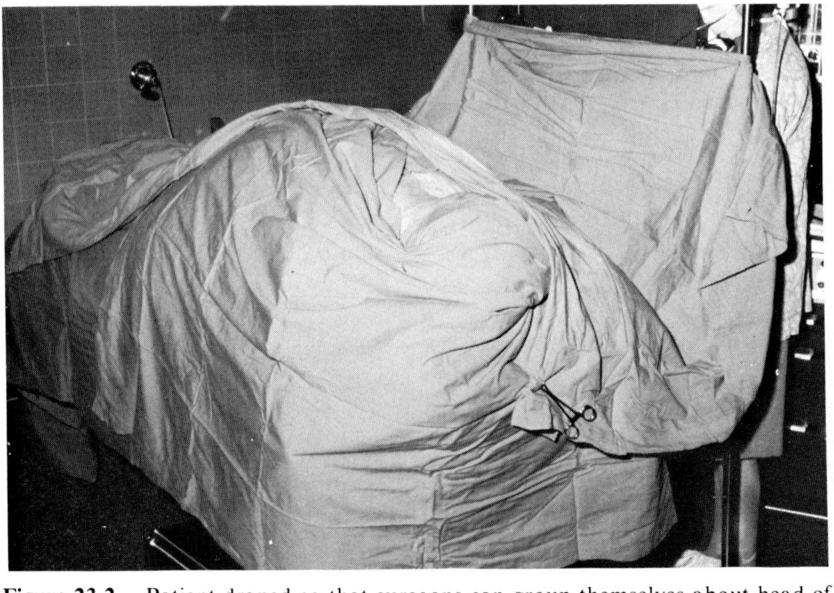

Figure 23-2. Patient draped so that surgeons can group themselves about head of patient with easy access to carotid artery. Anesthesiologist positioned to side of patient.

vein needle can be placed directly into the artery, with one or both wings positioned so as to hold the needle in place. When a transverse or skinline incision is used, a 1-1/2 in. needle is introduced through the skin and into the artery (Fig. 23-3). The tubing is clamped to a surrounding drape to secure it from being dislodged. A temporary Vitallium clip left on the superior thyroid artery provides orientation and a means of measuring the distance of potential defects from the clip.

A portable frame with a lead shield adjusted to the height of the physician is draped with a sterile sheet and rolled in front of the surgeon for protection from the x-rays (Fig. 23-4). An 11 × 14 in. x-ray cassette is placed into the tunnel under the head and neck of the patient so as to obtain an intracranial arteriogram, as well as a cervical carotid arteriogram. A battery operated portable x-ray machine is rolled into position and centered over the incision. A syringe containing 10 cc of Conray 60 is attached to the hub of the connecting tubing, and the occluding clamp is removed. Again, precautions are taken to be certain there is no air in the syringe or tubing. The x-ray technician is alerted to start his rotor and to be alert for the signal to take the x-ray. The entire bolus of contrast material is injected as rapidly as possible. The command to trigger the x-ray machine is given as the plunger of the syringe passes the 5 cc mark. A tendency to stop the injection after giving the

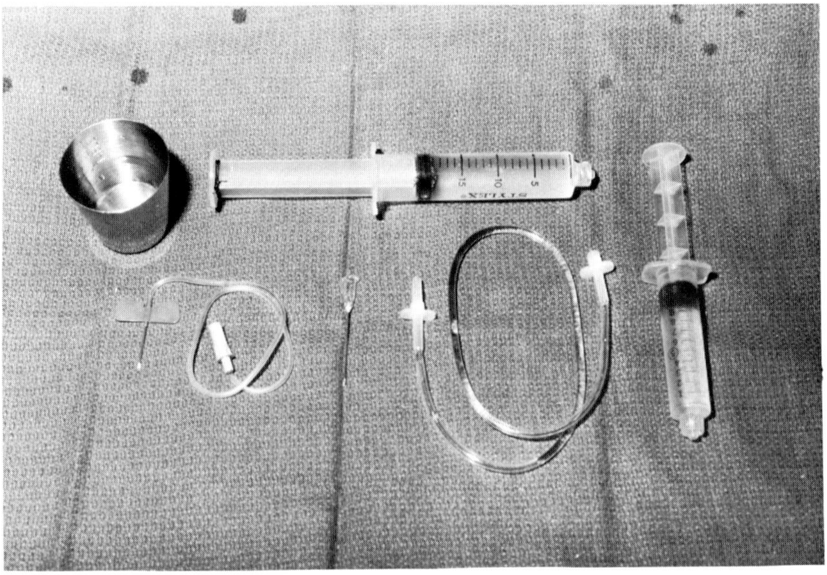

Figure 23-3. Apparatus needed for intraoperative arteriogram. A 20 cc syringe contains saline solution. A 10 cc syringe contains Conray-60. A 21-gauge needle and connector tubing is used when a transverse incision is made. A 21-gauge butterfly needle is used when a vertical incision is made.

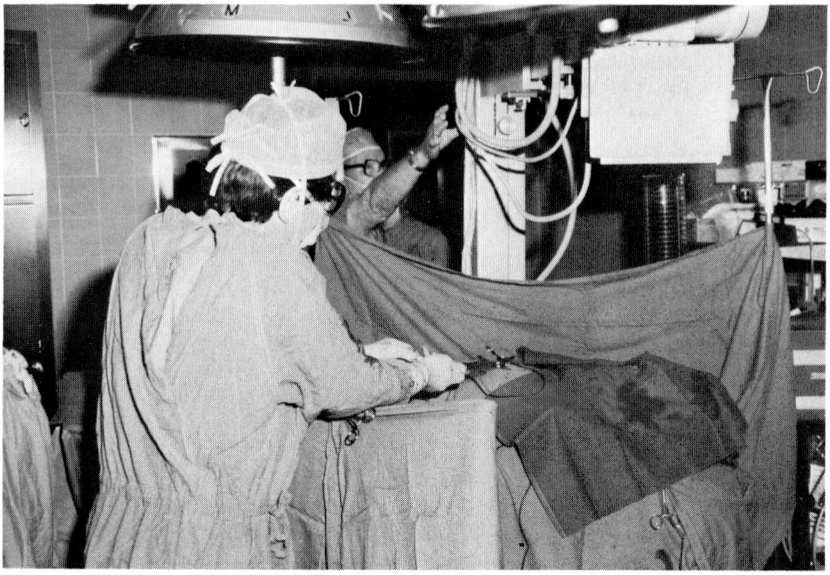

Figure 23-4. Surgeon standing in front of a portable lead shielded frame while injecting dye into carotid artery as portable x-ray unit is used.

signal must be overcome. The usual x-ray factors are 80 to 90 kilovolts at two-fifths of a second.

The tubing and needle are flushed with saline solution, but the needle is not removed until the film has been returned and studied. The entire procedure usually takes between 5 to 10 minutes if only one film is necessary.

PREVIOUS REPORTS

In previous publications, we documented the results of performing routine completion arteriograms in 356 cases of carotid thromboendarterectomy.[2,3] In those studies, 8.07 percent of the endarterectomies as shown by completion arteriography were unsatisfactory. These were divided between the external carotid artery (3.9 percent), the internal carotid artery (3.37 percent), and the common carotid artery (0.8 percent).

MATERIAL AND RESULTS

Four hundred fifty seven consecutive carotid endarterectomies with routine completion arteriograms have been performed since the previous reports. In 420 cases, the endarterectomy as shown by the completion arteriogram was considered satisfactory at the surgical site by the operating surgeon (Fig. 23-5). In 37 cases (8.09 percent), a defect was noted in either the common carotid, external carotid, or internal carotid arteries. There was a

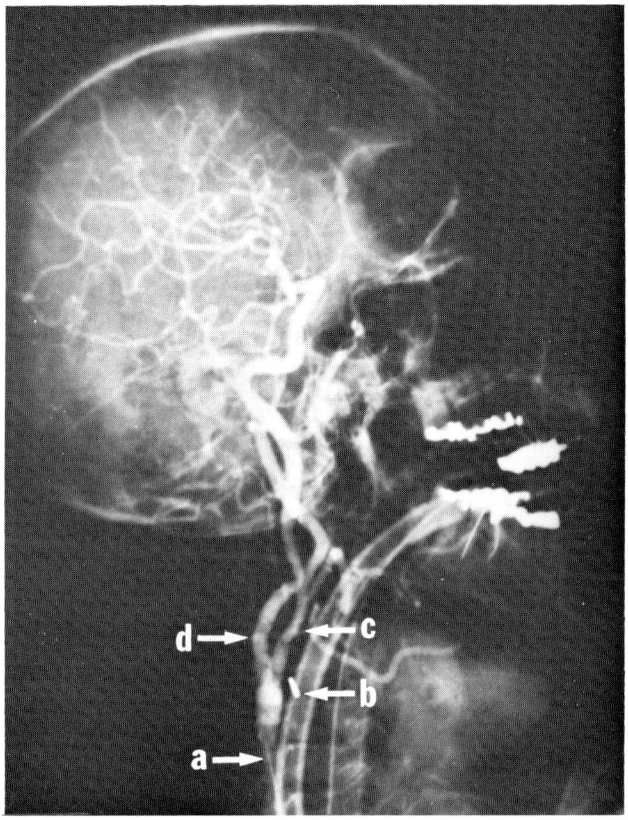

Figure 23-5. Satisfactory completion arteriogram. Common, external, and internal carotid arteries are patent. Intracerebral angiogram shows patent vessels. Anterior cerebral artery does not fill (a common finding). (A) Needle in common carotid artery (B) Clip on superior thyroid artery (C) External carotid artery (D) Internal carotid artery.

suspected intraluminal defect in the internal carotid artery in 18 (3.93 percent), in the external carotid artery in 14 (3.06 percent), and in the common carotid artery in 5 (1.09 percent) of the cases. Necessary revisions were made, and another arteriogram obtained. More than one revision was necessary in 3 cases.

ARTERIOGRAPHIC FINDINGS

The surgical result was considered inadequate if the arteriogram showed complete occlusion or more than 30 percent stenosis of any of the three vessels, evidence of fresh thrombus, remaining atheromatous plaques, or faintly visible transverse defects interpreted as intimal flaps. These strict criteria have been adhered to as closely as possible, although subject to interpretation by the operating surgeon. Later interpretation by a radiologist has tended to agree with the surgeon's opinion made at the time of the operation.

COMMON CAROTID DEFECTS

Care is taken to extend the arteriotomy in the common carotid artery as far proximalward as necessary to remove the thick atherosclerotic plaque. Usually a thin area is reached without extending the arteriotomy more than 4 to 5 cm below the carotid bifurcation. The plaque is usually cut sharply with angled Iris scissors, although bites of a sharp pituitary rongeur will also accomplish a smooth ending of the plaque. Only five common carotid defects were recognized, and two of these were revised. The other three were not considered to be significant enough to require revision. In one of the two, which were revised, there was a thick shelf and a moderate amount of fresh thrombus. In the other, there was fresh thrombus only (Fig. 23-6).

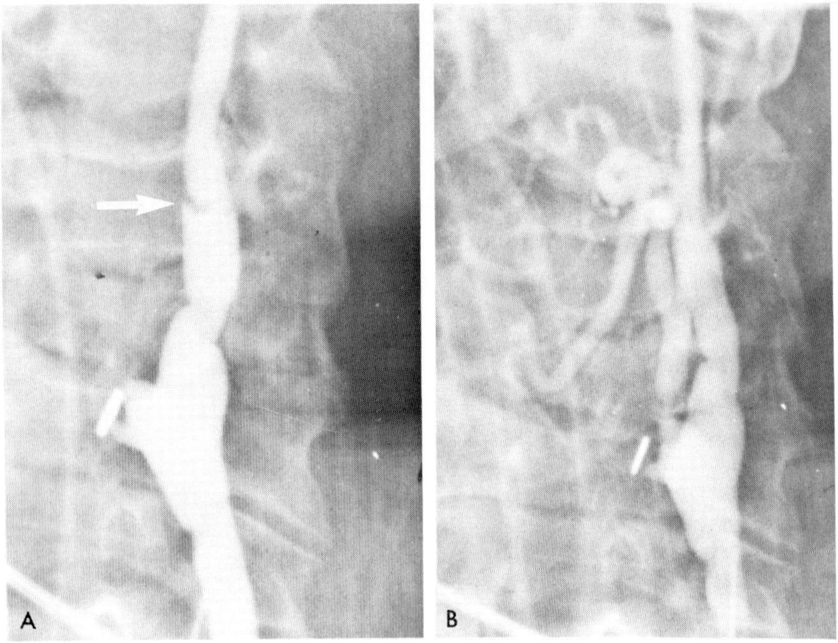

Figure 23-6. (A) Completion arteriogram showing fresh clot in common carotid artery.
(B) Arteriogram after clot has been removed.

Early in our experience, one patient had a stroke 5 days after leaving the hospital because of a fresh thrombus which developed at the site of a ragged edge of a thick plaque in the common carotid artery. Another patient developed a thin web-like obstruction at the proximal end of the endarterectomy 5 months after operation. In the present series, none of the patients who had common carotid defects suffered any postoperative complications.

EXTERNAL CAROTID DEFECTS

Allegedly, up to 30 percent of the blood supply to the cerebral hemisphere can be delivered through the external carotid artery.[4] Indeed, Connolly and Stemmer have advocated external carotid endarterectomy in certain circumstances when the ipsilateral internal carotid artery is occluded and in all conventional carotid endarterectomies.[5] In addition, a patent external carotid would be necessary if extracranial-intracranial bypass surgery would be needed in the future. Other authors have noted the importance of the external carotid artery.[6,7,8,9]

We have included external carotid endarterectomy as a routine part of our carotid operations. The bifurcation plaque is divided between the internal and external carotid orifices so that each segment can be handled separately. The plaque in the external carotid artery is gently separated from the arterial wall using spatulas or small curved hemostats. The plaque usually ends at the origin of either the lingual artery or the external maxillary artery. Usually it can be extracted much like a dentist extracts a tooth, leaving a smooth inner wall. A pituitary rongeur can be used to nibble out remaining bits of intima. Thus, the terminal end of the endarterectomy in the external carotid artery is done blindly.

If the completion arteriogram shows an inadequately endarterectomized external carotid artery, the revision is accomplished by occluding the external carotid at its origin, opening it with a small transverse or vertical incision, and removing whatever plaque or intimal shreds are left (Fig. 23-7).

We have not been able to significantly improve our results of endarterectomy in the external carotid artery. There were defects in 3.93 percent of the first 356 cases and in 3.06 percent of the most recent 457 cases. The terminal end of the plaque extraction is not accomplished under direct vision, nor is the remaining intima tacked down with sutures. Therefore, our results may be at an irreducible minimum. Completion arteriography would seem to be essential if the surgeon considers external carotid endarterectomy important.

INTERNAL CAROTID DEFECTS

Our technique, in which we routinely extend the incision in the internal carotid artery to the end of the plaque, and routinely use a shunt, allows us to

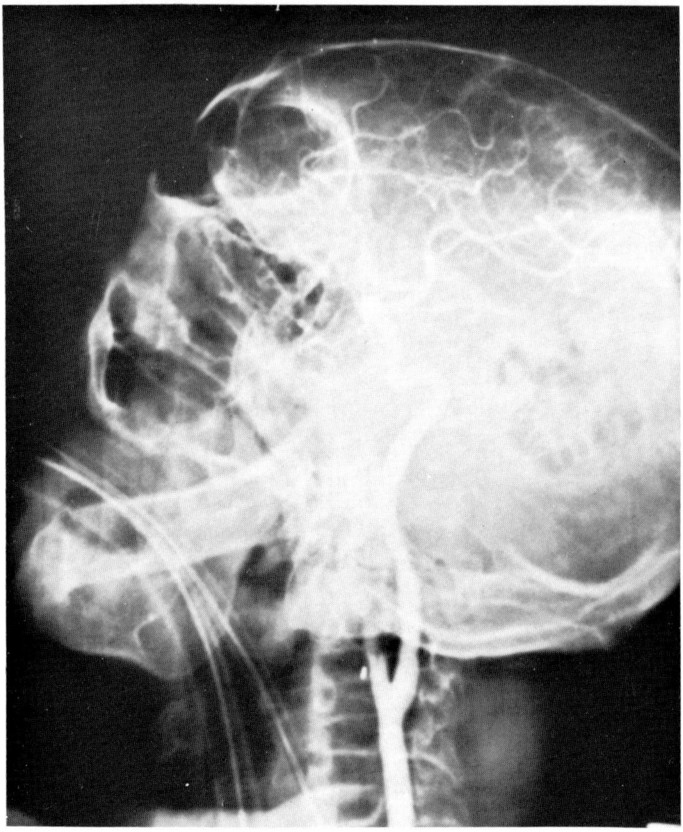

Figure 23-7. Completion arteriogram showing occlusion of external carotid artery by incompletely removed plaque. Common carotid and internal carotid arteries patent.

precisely remove the terminal end of the internal carotid plaque under direct vision. We rarely employ tacking sutures to the distal intima, and we rarely use a patch.

In the last 457 cases, we have had to revise the internal carotid artery about as often as we reported in the earlier series.[2,3] This implies either that we have not improved our technique or have been more critical of the completion arteriograms. There were one complete occlusion, ten stenoses greater than 30 percent, and five intimal flaps or remaining plaques (Fig. 23-8). There were also 3 cases in which there was fresh thrombus in the internal carotid artery. When these defects were found, the common carotid artery was occluded, and the suture line was opened. In the usual case, a small piece of atheroma or intima, or a small clot had to be removed. The shunt was reinserted, and the

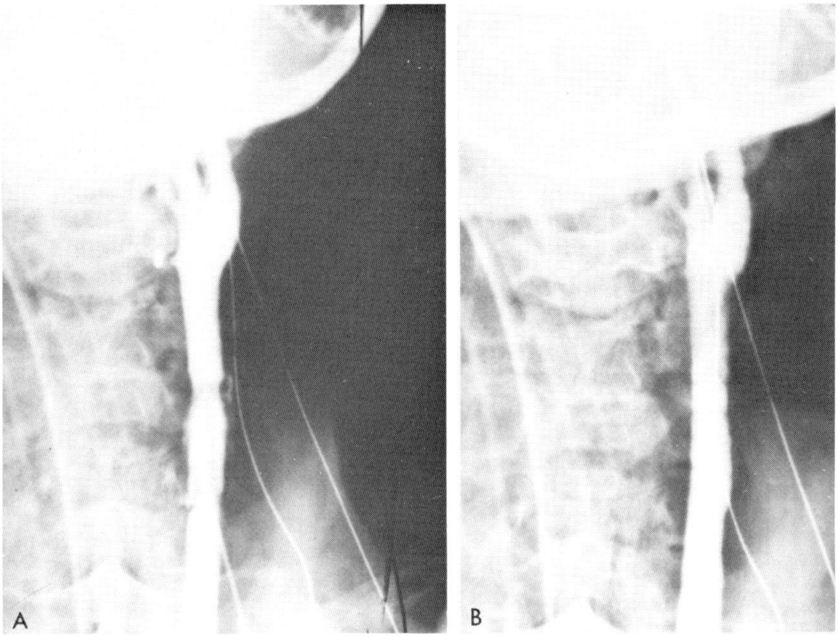

Figure 23-8. (A) Completion arteriogram showing intimal flap in internal carotid artery (arrow). External carotid artery is occluded.
(B) Arteriogram showing removal of internal carotid intimal flap. External carotid occlusion was corrected but origin of vessel was narrowed.

arteriotomy was closed again. The occlusion time was usually less than 6 minutes. In four instances a patch angioplasty was performed (Fig. 23-9). In one case, two small defects were seen which appeared to be bubbles of air. A second angiogram showed these to be gone. The patient had no postoperative complications. In only two instances did exploration of the angiographic defect fail to reveal any pathology.

In the most recent 457 cases, four of the 18 patients requiring internal carotid artery revision had postoperative problems. There was one death, 1 patient with a reversible ischemic neurological deficit, 1 patient with permanent hemiplegia, and 1 patient who had a hypertensive crisis on the third postoperative day with resultant intracerebral hemorrhage. This patient recovered completely.

Without question, the internal carotid artery must be cleared of obstructions and debris before being found acceptable. After revising the endarterectomy, another arteriogram was made in all cases. It was necessary to revise the internal carotid artery more than once in two cases. Both of these patients recovered without problems.

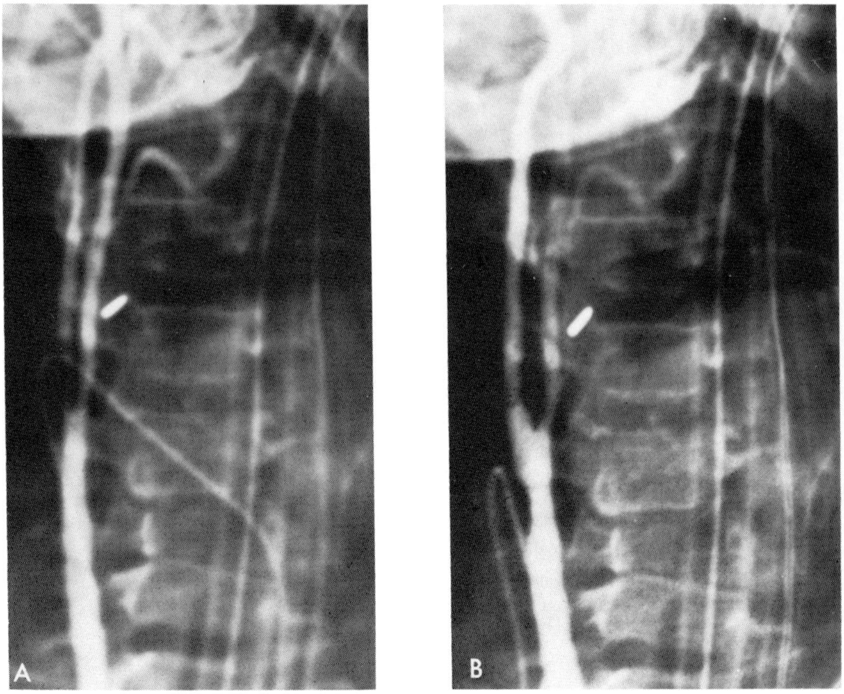

Figure 23-9. (A) Completion arteriogram showing stenosis of internal carotid artery. Grossly, this appeared to be a satisfactory result, and a pulse was present in the internal carotid artery distally. On the basis of the arteriogram, it was realized that suturing of the arteriotomy caused stenosis.
(B) Completion arteriogram after application of a vein patch graft.

COMMENT

Surgeons have expressed the opinion that completion arteriography after carotid endarterectomy is cumbersome and time-consuming and that the films often are of inadequate quality. We solved these problems by obtaining the help of a senior radiology technologist (R. W. Biddle, R.T.) to oversee the equipment and supervise the taking and development of the x-rays. The key to success is having an experienced radiology technologist present in the surgery suite at all times during elective operations, available for cholangiography, orthopedic procedures, and intraoperative angiography. He is called to the operating room as closure of the carotid arteriotomy is begun. The x-ray films are developed in the surgery suite using an automatic film processor. Two and one-half minutes are necessary for development of the film. In most cases, the quality of the films has been excellent with only one injection, but occasionally inadequate films have been obtained, particularly if an experienced technician is not available, such as sometimes happens late in the day or during emergency operations. In such circumstances, a preliminary scout film may save time by providing the proper technique on the first film.

The films have been reviewed by a radiologist working at his leisure. There has been concurrence with the surgeon's interpretation in all but four of the last 457 cases (99 percent agreement). In two instances, the radiologist read the defect in the internal carotid artery as being more severe than that read by the surgeon. One of these had been revised, and the other had not. Both patients had uncomplicated postoperative courses. In another patient, the radiologist overlooked a fresh thrombus which was removed by the surgeon. The other instance of disagreement involved the external carotid artery.

Some have expressed concern that contrast material injected into the brain is harmful. Conray 60 does not pass the intact blood brain barrier and in our experience has not caused complications. The quantity of dye used is small, and the risk/benefit ratio, in our opinion, lies in favor of angiography.

Intracerebral angiography has been a spin-off of our procedure. During one period, 50 intraoperative intracerebral angiograms were reviewed by a radiologist (Vincent Esposito, M.D.). No intracerebral defects were noted. Nevertheless, an occasional problem has been noted by the surgeon studying the films in the operating room. On occasion, these have helped explain postoperative neurological deficits (Fig. 23-10). In the last 457 cases, intracerebral defects were recognized in 11 (2.4 percent) cases. Two deaths occurred in these cases, and one postoperative neurological deficit (9.09 percent) was noted. Therefore, three (27.27 percent) of the 11 patients in whom an intracranial defect was identified had a severe postoperative complication.

In the past, we have not routinely obtained selective carotid studies with intracranial views because of the increased risk to the patient. Angiography has become increasingly safer, however, and although the yield may be low (2.4 percent), the high percentage of complications associated with these findings (27.27 percent) suggests we should be more aggressive in our use of selective angiography to identify signs of intracerebral atherosclerosis.

Those surgeons who do not use routine completion arteriography must depend upon their conviction that they have performed a perfect operation, or perhaps they depend upon feeling a pulse in the internal carotid artery, a finding known to be misleading. Their knowledge that completion arteriography in femoral-popliteal reconstructive operations often shows correctable defects should suggest that defects might also occur after carotid thromboendarterectomy. The fact that revision was necessary in 26 percent of Blaisdell's cases, and in 8 percent of our cases, also offers evidence that completion arteriography should be routine after carotid endarterectomy. Completion arteriography is a form of quality control that, in our opinion, subtly encourages one to do a better endarterectomy. It is also a good teaching modality.

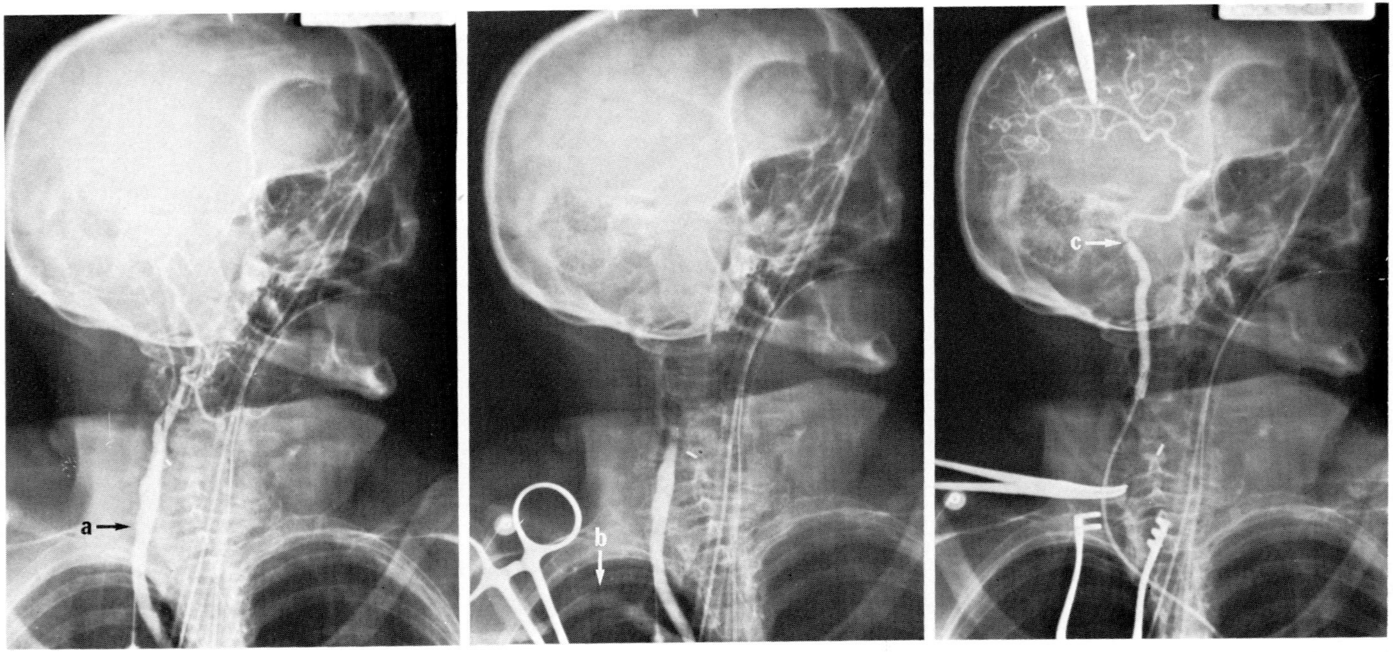

Figure 23-10. (A) Completion arteriogram showing no flow in the internal carotid artery above the level of the mandible in spite of a good pulse. There is unusual filling of the common carotid artery below the site of needle insertion (a).
(B) A second arteriogram with the external carotid artery occluded by a vessel loop showing blockage of the internal carotid artery and retrograde flow filling the common carotid and subclavian arteries (b) indicating high resistance to flow.
(C) Arteriogram made with a feeding tube in the internal carotid artery showing severe stenosis of the intracranial carotid artery (c). A retrospective review of the preoperative angiogram was suggestive of the high internal carotid stenosis.

CONCLUSION

Excellent arteriograms can be obtained after carotid endarterectomy in any operating room with minimum confusion and by adding only 5 to 10 minutes to the operating time. Correctable defects in the common carotid, external carotid, or internal carotid arteries will probably be found in eight percent or more of cases. Therefore, we recommend that completion arteriography become a routine after carotid thromboendarterectomy.

REFERENCES

1. Blaisdell FW, Lim R Jr, Hall AD: Technical results of carotid endarterectomy: Arteriographic assessment. Am J Surg 114:239, 1967
2. Rosental JJ, Gaspar MR, Movius HJ: Intraoperative arteriography in carotid thromboendarterectomy. Archives of Surg 106:806, 1973
3. Gaspar MR, Movius HJ, Rosental JJ: Routine intraoperative arteriography in carotid artery surgery. J Cardiovas Surg, Special Issue: 477, 1974
4. Fields WS, Breutman ME, Weibel J: Collateral circulation of the brain. Monogr Surg Sci 2:183, 1965
5. Connolly JE, Stemmer EA: Endarterectomy of the external carotid artery. Arch Surg 106:799, 1973
6. Clayson KR, Edwards WH: Importance of the external carotid artery in extracranial cerebrovascular occlusive disease. South Med J 70:904, 1977
7. Diethrich EB, Liddicoat JE, McCutcheon JJ, et al: Surgical significance of the external carotid artery in the treatment of cerebrovascular insufficiency. J Cardiovasc Surg 15:213, 1968
8. Jacques S, Garner JT, Tager R, et al: Improved cognition after external carotid endarterectomy. Surg Neurol 10:223, 1978
9. Lord RSA: Monocular transient ischemic attacks and the external carotid artery. Med J Aust 1:742, 1973

PART VII

Special Problems in Cerebrovascular Insufficiency

William C. Krupski
David J. Effeney
William K. Ehrenfeld

24

Fibromuscular Dysplasia, Aneurysms, and Spontaneous Dissection of the Carotid Artery

This chapter discusses fibromuscular disease of the internal carotid artery as well as the uncommon disorders of spontaneous dissection and aneurysm formation of this vessel. It is our purpose to review our own experience and that of others in the management of these diseases and to present appropriate management plans.

FIBROMUSCULAR DISEASE

Fibromuscular dysplasia (FMD) was first described by Leadbetter and Burkland in 1938.[1] Subsequently in 1958, McCormack et al.[2] described four categories of obstructive renal artery disease and called one of them "fibromuscular hyperplasia." Until 1964, when Palubinskas and Ripley[3] described fibromuscular disease of the internal carotid artery, it was thought to be a disease confined to the renal arteries. It is now known that many of the medium-sized arteries are affected,[4] and an increasing number of reports implicate fibromuscular disease as a cause of symptoms of cerebrovascular insufficiency.[5,6,7,8,9,10,11,12] Fibromuscular dysplasia involves the carotid and vertebral arteries as well as the intracranial arteries and is associated with intracranial aneurysms.[12,13]

Pathology and Pathogenesis

Stanley and his co-workers have described four histologic types of fibromuscular dysplasia.[14] These are intimal fibroplasia, medial hyperplasia, medial fibroplasia, and perimedial dysplasia. The most common form is medial fibroplasia. Fibromuscular dysplasia affects segments of long arteries with few primary branches. There is a female predominance that has caused speculation about the role of estrogens and other female hormones in its pathogenesis; however, there is no evidence to incriminate oral contraceptives or postmenopausal estrogen therapy as causative agents, and the role of hormones may be a facilatative one. The observations made pathologically have led to a concept of pathogenesis: stresses act on a segment of artery that is somewhat longer than normal and that has a relatively poor blood supply derived from vasa vasorum. Medial damage progresses to one or another of the histologic types of dysplasia depending on the particular artery involved, the level of medial injury, and the repair mechanisms (all of which may be modified by the hormonal environment).[14,15]

Clinical Findings

The clinical findings of the patients operated on at the University of California, San Francisco, up to December 1979, have been reported previously.[6,16,17] Since that time, 15 new patients have been evaluated and operated on for symptomatic FMD. Patients have ranged in age from 27 to 86 years of age (mean 58). Tables 24-1 and 24-2 summarize the major symptoms and physical findings in this group of patients.

Fibromuscular dysplasia disease is responsible for a wide variety of symptoms. The proportion of patients with this disease who develop symptoms, however, remains unknown. Once symptoms have developed, there is a disturbingly high incidence of completed stroke in this relatively

Table 24-1
Fibromuscular Disease Internal Carotid
(101 Patients)

Symptoms at Presentation	
Transient Ischemic Attacks	41.4%
Non-Localizing Neurologic	31 %
Bruits Heard by Patient	23 %
Amaurosis Fugax	23 %
Completed Strokes	22 %
Asymptomatic Bruits	8 %
Prolonged Ischemic Attack	2 %
Other	6 %

Table 24-2
Fibromuscular Disease Internal Carotid (101 Patients)

Findings at Presentation	
Carotid Bruit	77%
Hypertension	33%
Neurologic Deficits	9%
ECG Abnormalities	17%

young group of people, and a significant number of patients were left with residual neurologic deficits at the time of presentation. The recent report by Kelly and Morris[8] reviewing the personal experience of Dr. Morris in 25 operated patients revealed that 4 patients had presented with a stroke—a figure almost identical to our own. They, likewise, confirmed the predominance of localizing symptoms such as TIAs and amaurosis fugax over nonlocalizing neurologic complaints. This clinical presentation lends strong support to a thromboembolic cause for symptoms. The true cause of symptom production in this disorder, however, remains unknown.

Angiographic Findings

Fibromuscular dysplasia disease usually occurs in internal carotid arteries that are longer than normal.[13,16] In our series, the bifurcation of the carotid is frequently at the C-4/5 disc level or below. When the bifurcation is placed high, the internal carotid is coiled or kinked. The disease spares the proximal and distal portions of the vessel. It affects the middle and distal thirds of the vessel, with lesions most commonly seen at the level of C 1-3 vertebral bodies. The disease is usually bilateral, although one side may be more advanced than the other. Three types of appearances—classical string of beads, tubular, or localized[13,17,18]—are generally recognized, while the presence of a carotid dissection should prompt examination of the other vessels for fibromuscular dysplasia.[16,17] About a fifth of the patients have associated atherosclerosis of the carotid bifurcation (Figs. 24-1 and 24-2).

Surgical Methods

Surgical methods have been described previously.[6,9,16,18] First described by Morris et al., the technique of graduated intraluminal dilatation has been used almost exclusively since 1970. The internal carotid is mobilized to the level of the styloid process and, if required, the carotid sinus nerve is divided. A soft rubber sling is placed around the proximal internal carotid and is used to straighten the vessel during dilatation. A short longitudinal arteriotomy is

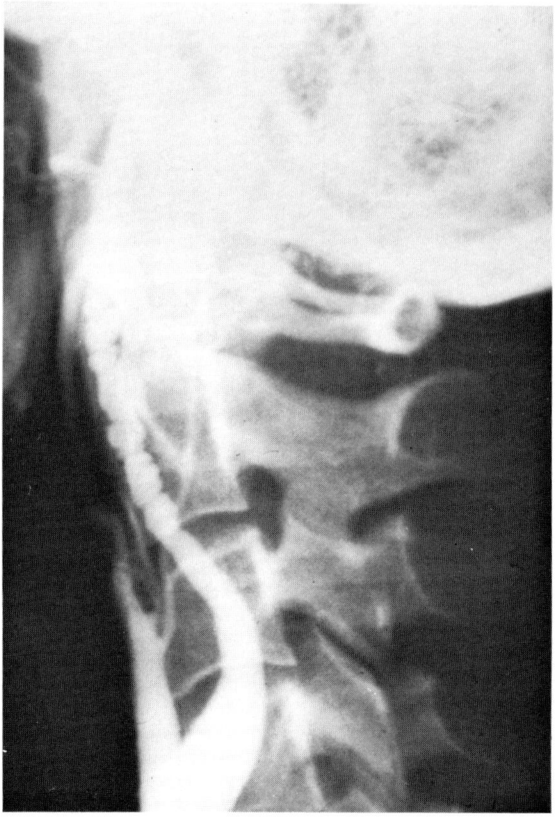

Figure 24-1. Angiogram showing the classical appearance of carotid FMD. Note the low bifurcation, resulting in an artery that is relatively longer than normal, and the proximal and distal artery free of disease, with the maximum disease opposite the C1-2 bodies and disc. This is the clinical "string of beads" pattern.

made in the carotid bulb, and the vessel is progressively dilated, beginning with a 1.5 mm or 2 mm Bakes dilator. The dilator is passed upwards until resistance is felt. Gentle pressure is applied, and the advance of the instrument is accompanied by loss of this resistance. Subsequent passage of 3, 3.5, and 4 mm dilators is usually accomplished with less resistance being encountered. If the vessels are unusually small, a maximal 3.5 mm dilator is used. The artery is allowed to back bleed vigorously for a few seconds to flush out debris and clot, and the arteriotomy is closed with continuous suture. Occasionally, standard techniques of resection and end-to-end anastomosis or vein grafting have been used to treat patients with accessible carotid fibromuscular dysplasia, (Fig.

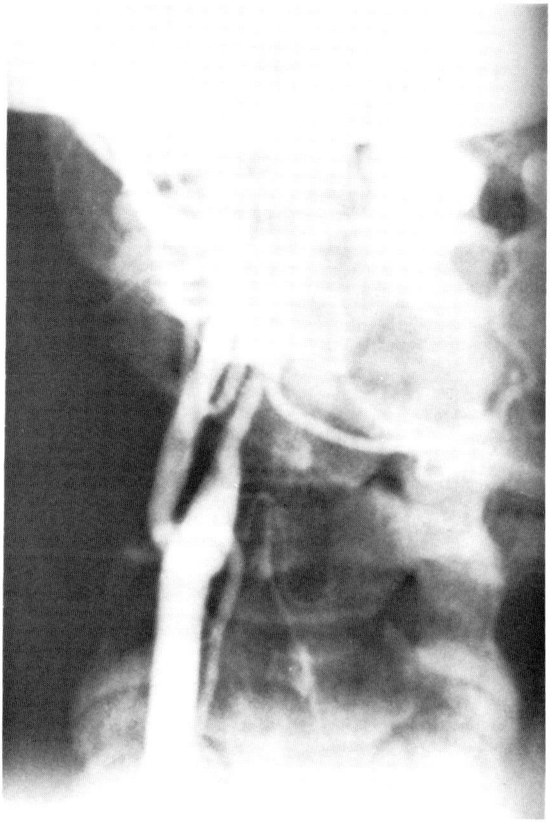

Figure 24-2. Angiogram showing the tubular pattern of FMD.

24-3).[19] Since 1970, 2 patients have required resection of redundant carotid artery combined with intraluminal dilatation. Approximately 18 percent of our patients required endarterectomy at the time of dilatation, while in about 5 percent of cases, endarterectomy was performed on a contralateral carotid, minimally affected by fibromuscular dysplasia.

Results of Therapy

Our results and those of others[6,8,16,17] support the conclusion that the treatment of symptomatic fibromuscular dysplasia is safe. In 150 operations, there have been no deaths, while 3 patients have suffered strokes in the early postoperative period. Nine patients have had transient neurologic deficits (TIA) or amaurosis fugax. The patients have been followed from 1 to 17 years. Two patients have had strokes in this time, 1 due to an embolus

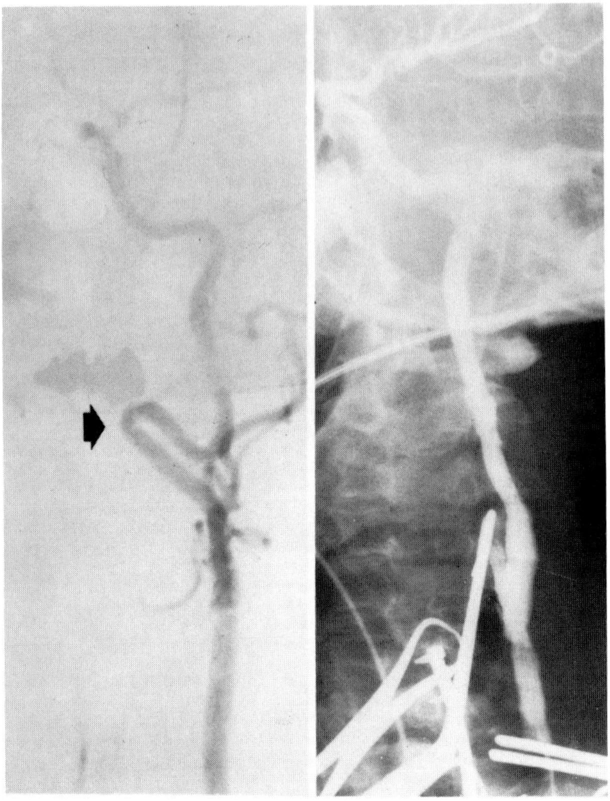

Figure 24-3. Preoperative arteriogram showing a pronounced kink in a very redundant internal carotid affected by FMD. The intraoperative view demonstrates the completed resection with end-to-end anastomosis.

to the right middle cerebral artery. The cause of the other stroke is unknown. Two patients have had subarachnoid hemorrhages from intracranial aneurysms, while 3 patients have had recurrence of generalized neurologic symptoms and represent a poor patient selection.

The immediate patency of the reconstruction has been confirmed in all patients by arteriograms, and patients have been studied serially for up to 5 years. These studies confirm the durability of intraluminal dilatation in fibromuscular dysplastic disease, and in only one patient was a previously dilated artery found to be occluded. One patient has required a redilatation 1 year after the first procedure for a persistent band and three episodes of transient ischemia. The non-neurologic complications of surgical management of symptomatic fibromuscular dysplasia are those associated with carotid endarterectomy and occur with about the same frequency. There is one potential intraoperative complication peculiar to dilatation, and that is the risk of arterial perforation (Fig. 24-4). This complication has occurred once, reinforcing the need for straightening the artery and gentle passage of the dilator.

Discussion

Fibromuscular dysplasia disease remains an enigma. Its incidence is not known, although reports range from 2.5 to 6.8 percent[12,15] in all patients undergoing carotid arteriography. This is a disease primarily of women, and its natural history remains unclear. Many patients remain asymptomatic, while in others the first symptom of fibromuscular dysplasia may be a stroke.

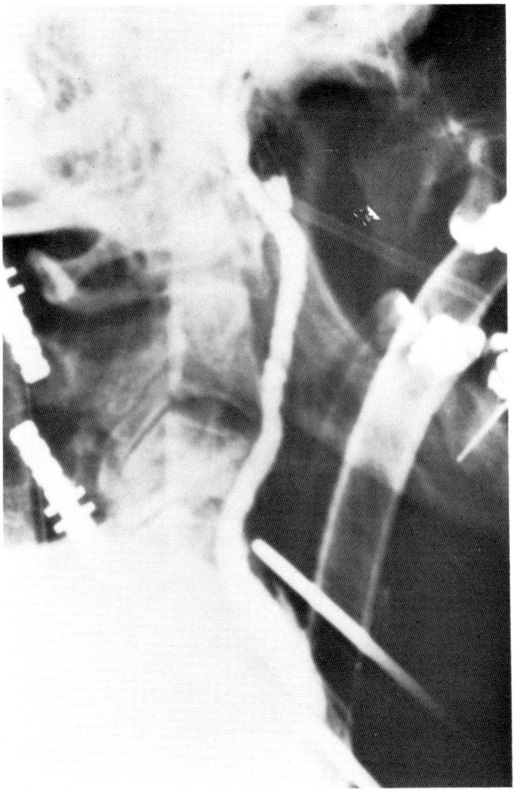

Figure 24-4. Intraoperative arteriogram showing perforation of the internal carotid very high in the neck at the site of a curve in the vessel's course. This reinforces the need for meticulous straightening of the artery prior to passage of the dilator.

The initial clinical and radiological assessment should be complete. Careful history and detailed physical examination are mandatory. The radiologic assessment requires views to look for aneurysms intracranially and an arch injection to document vertebral artery disease as well as the standard views of the extracranial carotids. We routinely perform a midstream aortogram to visualize the renal and external iliac arteries prior to catheter removal.

No data are available to confirm or deny efficacy of any form of medical therapy for fibromuscular dysplasia. We use aspirin prophylactically and recommend surgery for those with symptomatic disease. The results have been gratifying in terms of symptom relief, prevention of stroke, and durability of the repair. Great care must be exercised in patient selection and operative technique. Since no control data on the natural history of this disease are known, prophylactic surgery in asymptomatic patients is not recommended.

SPONTANEOUS DISSECTION OF THE CAROTID ARTERY

Anderson and Schechter first described a case of spontaneous dissection of the internal carotid artery in 1959.[20] Subsequently, 72 cases have been reported in the literature.[21-26] Increased recognition of spontaneous non-traumatic dissection of the carotid artery in recent years suggests that this entity may be more common than was previously appreciated. Furthermore, it is clear that many cases resolve spontaneously, raising speculation that the true incidence may have been largely underestimated in the past.

Pathology and Pathogenesis

The cause of spontaneous dissection of the internal carotid artery remains uncertain. In 1976, we reported our experience with a group of 19 patients thought to have this disorder. Five new patients have been evaluated since that time. Ten patients underwent operative neck exploration, and a portion or all of the dissected arterial segment was removed in 4 patients. In each of these, the characteristic double lumen was demonstrated with the outer lumen filled with thrombus. Although at least one report[27] has implicated cystic medial necrosis as an etiologic factor in the development of carotid dissection, this was not present in our specimens. Atherosclerosis was notably absent. Microscopic findings were similar in all specimens: smooth muscle cells were decreased in number and widely separated; elastic tissue was decreased with degeneration of the internal elastic membrane; mucoid substance was deposited throughout all layers of the vessel wall. The dissection occurred in the outer layer of the media (Figs. 24-5, 24-6, 24-7).

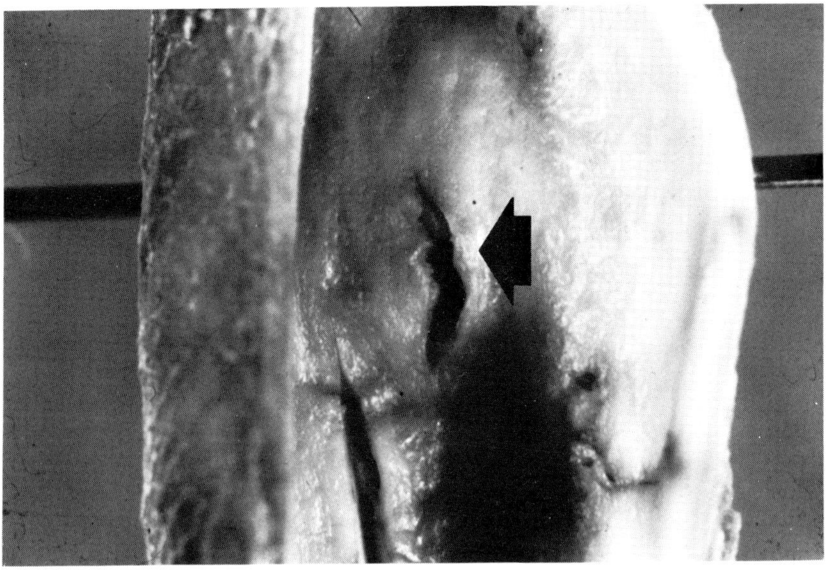

Figure 24-5. Photograph of a resected internal carotid dissection showing the slit-like proximal opening.

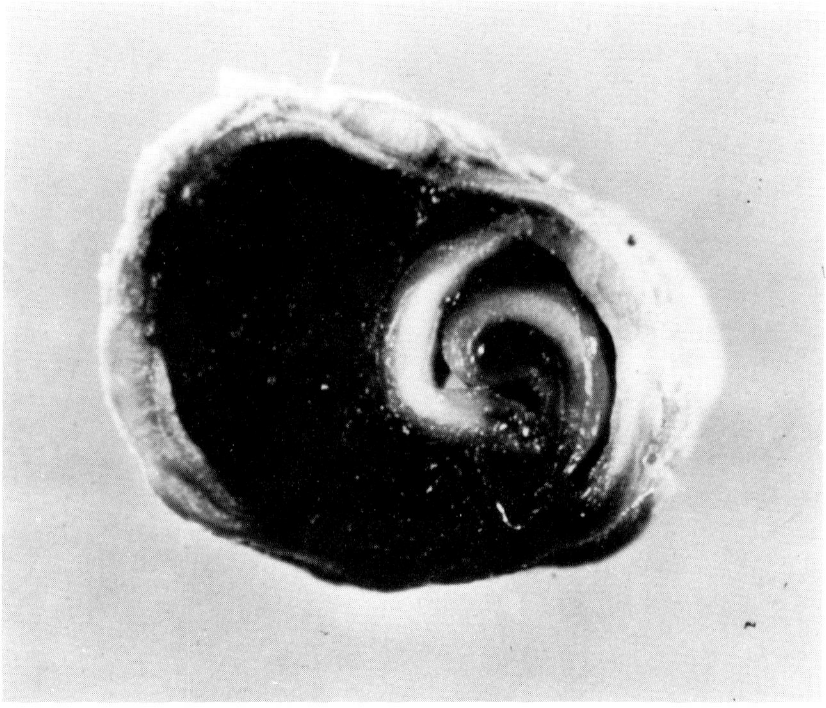

Figure 24-6. Cross-section of a resected internal carotid dissection with the "jelly roll" appearance. Note the dissection plane in the media with compromise of the true lumen due to the infolding of the inner media and intima.

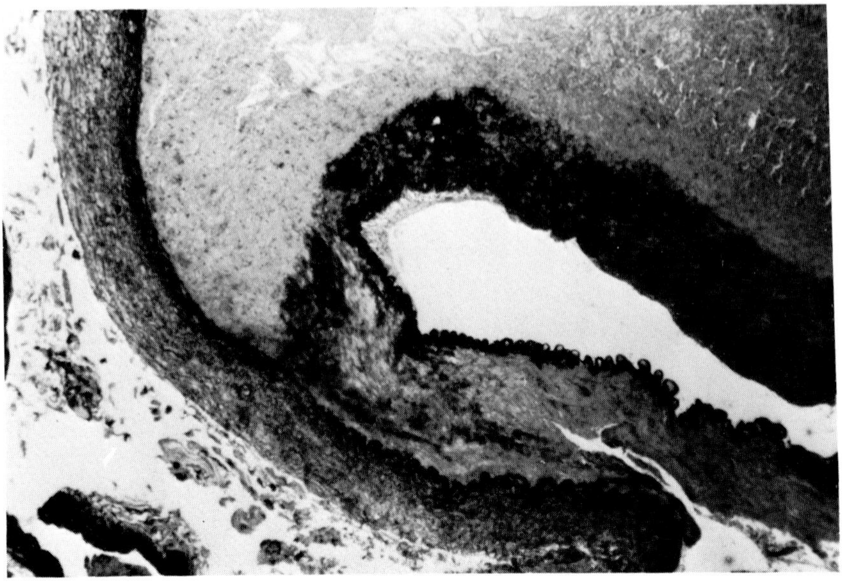

Figure 24-7. Low power view of carotid dissection demonstrating the dissection plane in the outer media and the false lumen filled with unorganized thrombus.

While none of the resected specimens revealed fibromuscular dysplasia (FMD), arteriograms in 3 patients showed irregularities consistent with fibromuscular dysplasia in the contralateral internal carotid artery. Five additional patients without evidence of fibromuscular dysplasia had a uniform cylindrical dilatation of the contralateral internal carotid artery, suggesting some form of generalized arterial ectasia.

Clinical Findings

The twenty-four patients who have presented with spontaneous dissection of the carotid arteries at the University of California during the past 16 years are comprised of 11 women and 13 men, aged 11 to 66 years (mean 50). The clinical presentation of these twenty-four patients is summarized in Table 24-3.

Transient or permanent neurologic deficits are the most common presenting symptoms in these patients. Seven patients in our series had continued transient ischemic attacks after the initial episode, presumably caused by embolization or intermittently decreased cerebral perfusion. Ipsilateral headache, tinnitus and neck pain, and tenderness adjacent to the angle of the mandible were additional symptoms noted in some patients. Although hypertension has been mentioned as an etiologic factor by some authors,[28] this was present in only 5 (21 percent) of our patients. No patient

Table 24-3
Spontaneous Dissection Internal Carotid
(24 Patients)

Symptoms at Presentation	No. Pts.	%
Completed Stroke	8	33
Transient Ischemic Attacks	13	53
Amaurosis Fugax	5	21
Headache	4	20
Neck Pain	3	12
Tinnitus	2	8

gave a history of recent or past cervical trauma or unusual movement preceding the onset of symptoms.

Angiographic Findings

The radiologic appearance of carotid artery dissection depends on the site and extent of the lesion. In our patients, the dissection was limited to the internal carotid artery in 22 patients. In 2 patients, dissection started in the common carotid artery close to the carotid bifurcation and extended into both the internal and external carotid arteries.

Of the 22 lesions confined to the internal carotid artery, 3 groups emerged. In the first pattern of disease (12 patients), narrowing began approximately 2.5 cm distal to the carotid bifurcation. A long tapered reduction in caliber with a resulting wavelike pattern was observed along the cervical course of the vessel until it entered the petrous canal where the artery regained its normal caliber. Lucent filling defects were occasionally seen as well as a delay in passage of contrast (Fig. 24-8). The subtraction technique in the processing of films was often valuable in visualizing the narrow lumen in the zone of dissection—one of the causes of the carotid "string sign."[37]

In the second pattern of disease (7 patients), the dissection was more limited. In these patients, the narrowing began more distally in the internal carotid artery and did not extend to the petrous canal. The narrowed segment was of variable length, and distal to this short segment the vessel regained its normal caliber.

Ultimate occlusion of the internal carotid artery is the third pattern of disease (3 patients). The tapered narrowing again begins beyond the carotid bifurcation ending in a pointed total occlusion at or near the petrous canal.

Associated radiographic abnormalities were noted in 9 patients. As noted previously, 3 patients had contralateral fibromuscular dysplasia. Three others had embolic occlusions of the ipsilateral middle cerebral artery. Two patients had carotid artery aneurysms: it was uncertain whether these were pre-existent

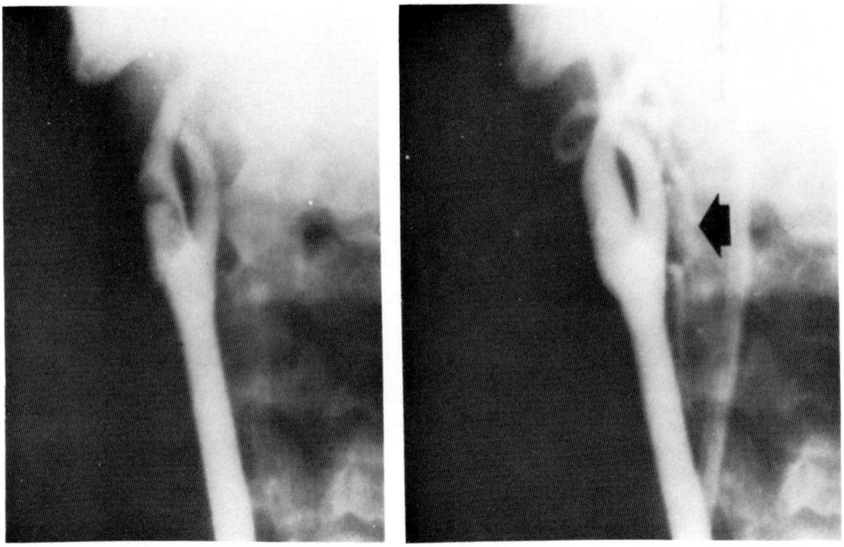

Figure 24-8. Two views of an internal carotid bulb demonstrating the need for multiview technique. The intraluminal defect of a dissection is shown clearly in the left panel, while only a faint outline of the lesion is seen in the right.

or false aneurysms resulting from the dissections (Fig. 24-9). Only 1 patient had an indication of atherosclerosis, namely atheromatous stenosis in the contralateral internal carotid artery.

Surgical Methods

Early in our experience, we believed that some form of surgical management was desirable for all patients with internal carotid artery dissection. A total of 10 patients underwent operation. Three had segmental resection and interposition grafting using saphenous vein. One had graduated intraluminal dilation. Removal of mural thrombus using a balloon catheter was attempted in 2 patients. Two patients with satisfactory carotid back pressure (65 mm Hg) had internal carotid artery ligation and 3 patients with low or marginal stump pressure underwent exploration alone, leaving the patent dissected artery undisturbed.

Results of Therapy

When our patients are combined with those of Fischer,[27] a total of 14 patients underwent attempts at operative repair. In these 14 patients, postoperative angiography is available in ten. There have been eight documented failures of arterial repair and only two documented successes.

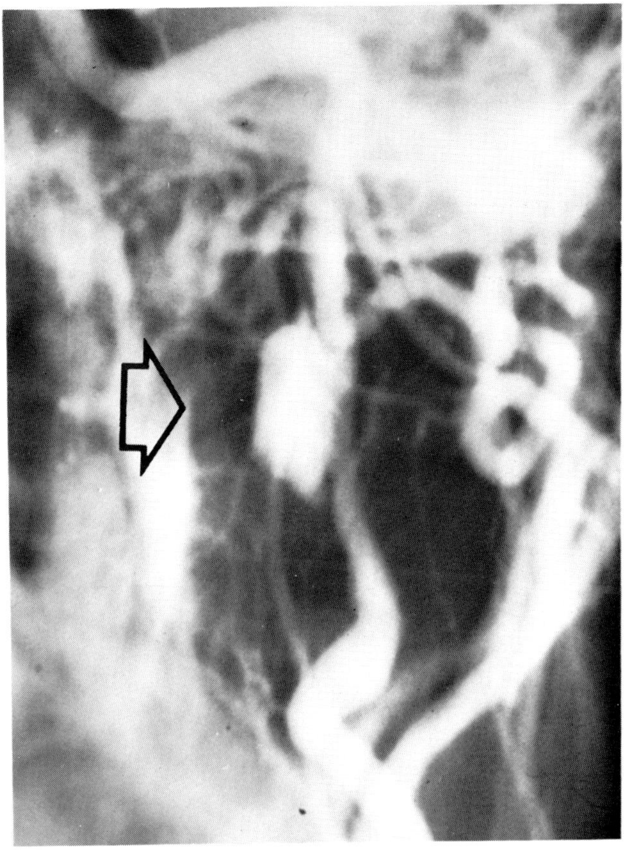

Figure 24-9. Angiogram showing a false aneurysm due to dissection high in the neck. Note the collar stud appearance of the false aneurysm, the narrowed true lumen of the internal carotid, and the dissection continuing above the aneurysm.

In marked contrast to this dismal record is the apparent good prognosis in patients treated expectantly. Fourteen patients in our series had no attempt at arterial reconstruction, and none suffered further neurologic symptoms. A second arteriogram has been obtained in eight of these patients from 2 to 16 months after the original study. One of the eight arteries progressed to total occlusion, but the remaining 7 patients were noted to have patent carotid arteries with essentially near-normal caliber (Fig. 24-10).

Discussion

While there was no consistent etiologic factor associated with our series, it is probable that fibromuscular dysplasia, trauma, and cystic medial necrosis

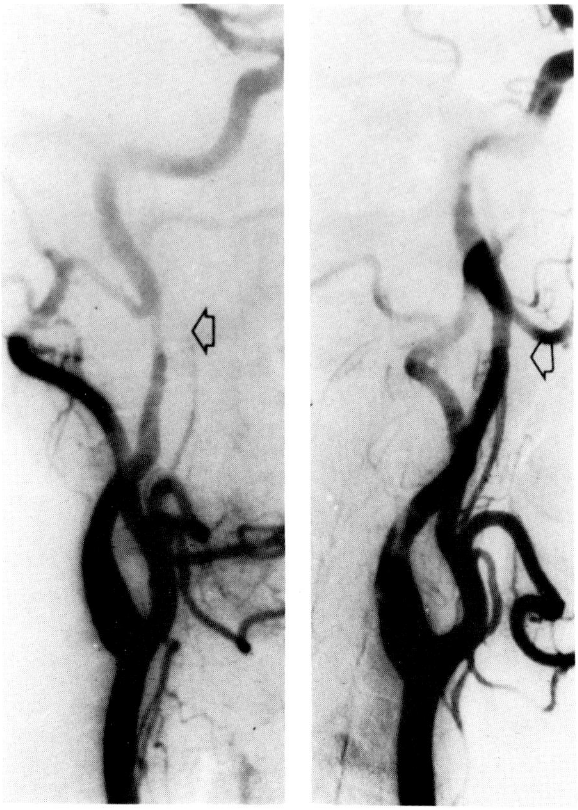

Figure 24-10. The left panel shows the appearance of a dissection at the time of presentation 2 days after onset of a RIND. Note the tapered appearance of the internal carotid artery limited by the base of the skull. The right panel shows the same patient two weeks later. Note the expansion of the distal artery to a more normal caliber.

play a role in some patients with spontaneous dissection of the carotid artery. While it has been our observation that a generalized vascular ectasia is present in many of these patients, no specific microscopic structural abnormality has yet been discovered. Serologic tests for collagen vascular disease were not routinely performed on our patients, but none have had late development of vasculitis.

In view of the good results obtained in patients treated expectantly, we recommend observation and anticoagulation for most patients with spontaneous dissection of the internal carotid artery. Gee[28] has recently suggested that use of occular pneumoplethysmography provides useful prognostic information. He used serial OPG-Gee measurements in 4 patients with spontaneous carotid dissection to demonstrate spontaneous restoration of functional patency. Repeat angiography confirmed patency previously indicated by the noninvasive tests in all four patients.

Gee and others[28,31-32] have advocated anticoagulation in patients with carotid dissection. This would seem advantageous in hastening the repair process as well as decreasing the chance of subsequent embolization from clotted blood present in the wall of the artery exposed to the arterial lumen at the site of the rent or present as mural thrombus within the true lumen. Anticoagulation is contraindicated if the patient has suffered a completed stroke or if a false aneurysm has developed in the cleavage plane between the media and adventitia.

Need for long-term anticoagulation is controversial. One report[31] described an implantable infusion device used for continous administration of heparin over a 5-month period. If such lengthy treatment is desired, use of oral anticoagulants would seem much easier and equally effective. In Gee's series, ocular pressures generally returned to near-normal in 7 weeks. Thus, a more limited treatment period appears indicated.

Surgical intervention should be reserved for those patients who have recurrent transient ischemic attacks despite adequate anticoagulation. If adequate collateral blood supply to the ipsilateral cerebral hemisphere is evident and if the distal end of the involved internal carotid artery is surgically inaccessible, simple ligation of the involved proximal internal carotid artery is appropriate. Our own experience suggests that a carotid stump pressure in excess of 65-70 mm Hg indicates adequate collateral blood flow.[38] This determination can be made preoperatively with reasonable accuracy by ocular pneumoplethysmography performed during digital occlusion of the common carotid artery. If the dissection is relatively short and its endpoint is surgically accessible, resection and graft replacement is indicated in this small group of patients. Instrumental graduated dilation or thrombectomy by withdrawal of a balloon catheter is hazardous and should not be employed.

CAROTID ARTERY ANEURYSMS

Aneurysms of the carotid artery are relatively rare and may occur along the course of the artery in its cervical position, petrous portion, or intracranial extension. While there are many publications in the neurosurgical literature dealing with intracranial aneurysms, little has been written about cervical carotid aneurysms. While rupture and hemorrhage are uncommon modes of presentation, these complications do occur.[39-42] Neurologic sequelae due to embolism or thrombosis are often seen.[43-46] Because of their relative rarity, however, it is impossible to define the true incidence of these aneurysms or to determine whether they are increasing in frequency.

Pathology and Pathogenesis

The most frequent causes of extracranial carotid artery aneurysms are atherosclerosis, previous carotid surgery, and trauma.[47,48] This represents a change in etiology, since prior to World War II, syphilis was by far the most common cause.[49] In the nineteenth century, children were often seen with profuse oropharyngeal bleeding due to erosive aneurysms of the internal carotid artery during streptococcal epidemics.[50] Infectious aneurysms in the pharynx were occasionally incised under the assumption that bulging of the tonsillar area represented a peritonsillar abscess. Other rare causes of carotid aneurysm include cystic medial necrosis,[51] Marfan's syndrome,[52] idiopathic medial arteriopathy,[53] fibromuscular dysplasia, and bacterial and fungal infection.[54]

In the past 20 years, we have treated eighteen patients with nineteen carotid aneurysms at the University of California, San Francisco. Three aneurysms were thought to be congenital. One occurred in an eleven-year-old boy (Fig. 24-11). A 21-year-old Latin American woman had bilateral aneurysms. There appeared to be some degree of acute inflammation in all three specimens, but there was no evidence of systemic vasculitis. Because of their similar appearance to the "berry" type of intracranial aneurysm, and the absence of pathologic changes characteristic of other entities, a congenital defect of the media is postulated.[55]

Six patients had extracranial carotid artery aneurysms caused by atherosclerosis. There were 5 men and 1 woman, ranging in age from 54 to 71 years (mean 65). Aneurysms began at the carotid bifurcation and measured from 2 to 7 cm in diameter. Only one extended to the bony canal and was deemed surgically unresectable. Pathologic examinations of resected specimens revealed typical atherosclerotic changes with focal necrosis and variable amounts of necrotic debris.

Eight patients had false aneurysms of the internal carotid after carotid endarterectomy. Four cases were originally reported in 1972.[56] Six men and two women aged 50-72 (mean 62) presented with false aneurysms from 2 weeks to 8 years after their original operations. Infection played a role in 5 cases. Cultures were positive for staphlococcus aureus in 2 cases, streptococcus viridans in 1 case, and pseudomonas in 2 cases. Pseudoaneurysms occurred in 3 patients who had undergone carotid endarterectomy with saphenous vein patch grafting. Increased incidence of false aneurysm formation after infection and after patch grafting (especially when Dacron is used) has been reported by others.[47,57]

One of our patients had a mycotic common carotid aneurysm. The patient, a 59-year-old man, developed staphlococal septicemia from a pulmonary abscess. Subsequently, a 5 × 6 cm aneurysm of the common carotid artery beginning 4 cm from the aortic arch and extending to the carotid

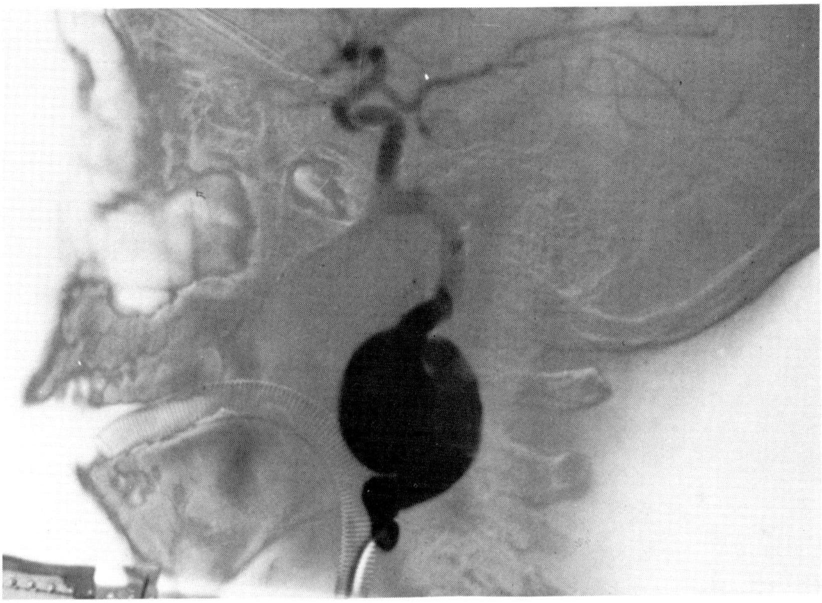

Figure 24-11. Angiogram showing a congenital carotid aneurysm in an 11-year-old child

bifurcation presented as a mass at the base of the neck. Cultures of the arterial wall were positive for staphlococcus aureus.

Although trauma did not cause any carotid aneurysms in our series, this is another major etiology.[58] Penetrating injuries may lead to pseudoaneurysm formation secondary to disruption of the continuity of the arterial wall and periarterial hematoma formation. In a review of World War II injuries, Elkin and Shumacker reported 13 such cases, as well as the more common traumatic arteriovenous fistula (48 cases).[59] Blunt cervical trauma may result in thrombosis of the vessel or false aneurysm formation.[60] Hyperextension and rotation of the neck can cause compression of the internal carotid artery on the transverse process of the atlas, resulting in intimal fracture and thrombosis or disruption of the wall and aneurysm formation. Mandibular fracture, percutaneous needle puncture, and ingested foreign bodies have also been associated with development of pseudoaneurysms.[60-62]

Clinical Findings

The most frequent presenting symptom (summarized in Table 24-4) in our patients was neck or pharyngeal mass. Shipley[63] emphasized that aneurysms of the internal carotid present in the pharynx, whereas those of the

Table 24-4
Carotid Artery Aneurysms (18 Patients)

Symptoms at Presentation	No. Pts.	%
Neck or pharyngeal mass	16	90
Pain	10	60
Transient Ischemic Attack	5	3
Hemorrhage	3	20
Dysplagia	2	11
Hoarseness	2	11

common carotid present in the neck. While this was true in our patients with atherosclerotic aneurysms, most patients with pseudoaneurysms after carotid endarterectomy had pulsatile neck masses, presumably because of surgical disruption of normal tissue planes and extension of the arteriotomy onto the common carotid artery. Two patients with pharyngeal masses complained of dysphagia.

Pain was a complaint in 60 percent of our patients. Most commonly, pain was dull and aching in nature and located at the angle of the mandible over the aneurysm. Fay[64] demonstrated in 1932 that irritation of the wall of the carotid artery produced ipsilateral pain in the head, neck, and face.[64] Thus, these patients may complain of pain because of aneurysmal expansion or impingement on the facial or trigeminal nerves—depending on the size and location of the aneurysm.

Five patients had transient ischemic attacks prior to repair of their aneurysms. Two of these patients had atherosclerotic aneurysms, and three had pseudoaneurysms after carotid endarterectomy. It was felt that embolization of thrombotic material emanating from the aneurysmal wall explained these symptoms, although one patient had significant luminal narrowing combined with a 90 percent stenosis of the contralateral internal carotid artery. This patient may have had flow-related phenomena.

Hoarseness due to vagal nerve compression was present in 2 patients. Other peripheral neurologic sequelae that have been reported include the following: palsy of the 5th, 6th, 7th, 9th, 11th, and 12th cranial nerves and Horner's syndrome.[48]

Spontaneous hemorrhage did not occur in atherosclerotic aneurysms but was a problem in 3 patients who presented with pseudoaneurysms. Intermittent bleeding episodes in the postoperative period heralded major hemorrhage. All these patients had an infectious etiology of their pseudoaneurysms with draining wounds or cellulitis overlying their neck incisions.

Hypertension was present in the vast majority of our patients. Four of the 6 patients with atherosclerotic aneurysms had blood pressure greater than 140/90 mm Hg even while taking antihypertensive medication. In the patients with pseudoaneurysms, hypertension was present in 50 percent and severe postendarterectomy hypertension had occurred in half of these. Rhodes reviewed 23 extracranial carotid artery aneurysms in 19 patients and reported that severe arterial hypertension was a constant finding in all 12 patients who had atherosclerotic aneurysms.[45]

Angiographic Findings

Angiography was diagnostic in all patients. Morphologically, two types of extracranial aneurysms were observed: saccular and fusiform. All atherosclerotic aneurysms were fusiform, beginning at the carotid bifurcation. The smallest aneurysm seen measured 2 cm so that differentiation from the normal dilation of the carotid bulb was not difficult in our patients, although this problem has been reported[65] (Fig. 24-12).

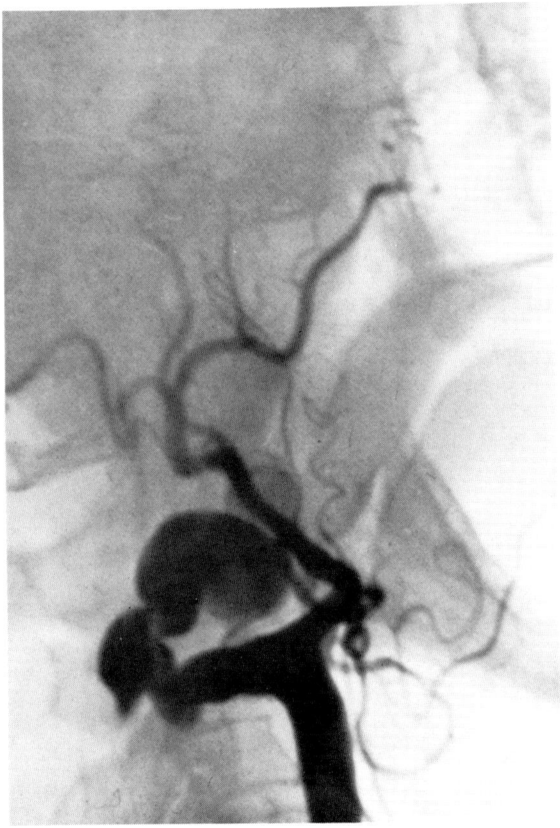

Figure 24-12. Angiogram showing a fusiform atherosclerotic aneurysm of the internal carotid artery.

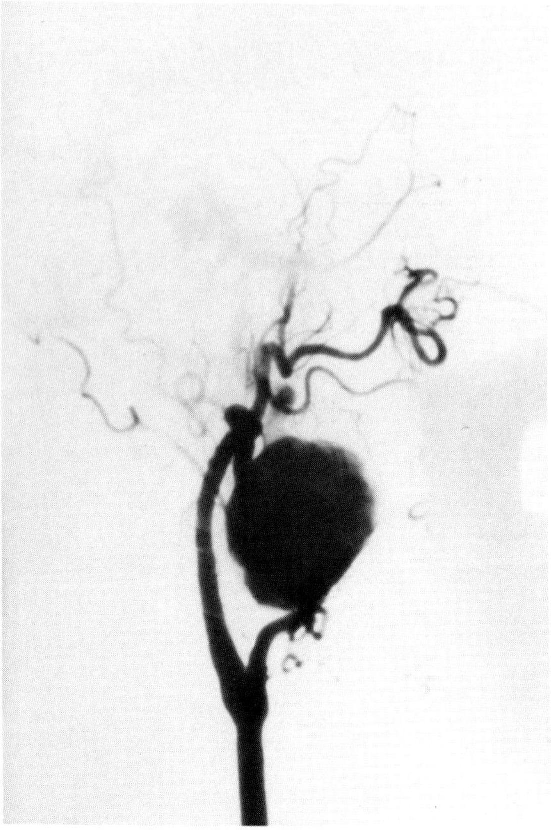

Figure 24-13. Angiogram showing a false aneurysm following a carotid endarterectomy. Note the small tract from the upper end of the arteriotomy leading into the expanded sac lower in the neck.

The three congenital aneurysms were saccular and began just distal to the carotid bifurcation. The mycotic common carotid aneurysm was fusiform and quite extensive.

In patients with false aneurysms of the internal carotid artery after carotid artery endarterectomy, differentiation between saccular and fusiform was more difficult. These aneurysms often assumed bizarre shapes depending on their location and their containment by contiguous structures (Fig. 24-13). None of our patients had B-mode ultrasound scans. Ultrasonography would be expected to demonstrate the aneurysms.

Surgical Methods and Results of Therapy

The first carotid ligation for hemorrhage following traumatic laceration was performed in 1552 by Ambroise Pare. Aphasia and left hemiparesis occurred postoperatively. In 1805, Astley Cooper performed the first carotid ligation for aneurysm. His patient developed hemiplegia and died soon thereafter. Several years later Cooper[66] successfully treated an extracranial carotid artery aneurysm by proximal and distal ligation of the internal carotid artery, and this remained the procedure of choice until Matas introduced endoaneurysmorrhaphy. In 1926, Winslow reported a 71 percent mortality with conservative therapy compared with 30 percent mortality for carotid ligation.[1]

Four of our patients have required carotid ligation because aneurysms extended to the base of the skull. Three patients had carotid stump pressures greater than 65 mm Hg, and none of these had postoperative neurologic sequelae. One patient with a carotid false aneurysm infected with pseudomonas had a low stump pressure but underwent carotid artery ligation because of massive hemorrhage. She suffered postoperative aphasia and hemiparesis and died on the 20th postoperative day. Another patient with a large atherosclerotic aneurysm had neck exploration but neither resection (because of extension of aneurysm to the carotid foramen) nor carotid ligation (because of low stump pressure) was performed. This patient suffered no complications from his aneurysm to the time of his death 5 years later.

Resection of the aneurysm with restoration of blood flow is the procedure of choice for symptomatic carotid artery aneurysms. We advocate the use of autogenous tissue in carotid artery reconstruction. This is mandatory in repairing false aneurysms where infection is suspected. Of the thirteen patients who had arterial reconstruction, the following techniques were employed: patch grafting with saphenous vein (5); resection with primary anastomosis (2); interposition grafting using saphenous vein (3) or iliac artery (2); and anastomosis between external and distal internal carotid artery (2). Temporary intraluminal shunts were used when the stump pressure was below 50 mm Hg. Two patients in this group had central neurologic deficits postoperatively. Each had an excellent recovery. The vagus and hypoglossal nerves were injured in 3 patients with large aneurysms. Infection rate was difficult to determine in the false aneurysm patients, many of whom had infectious causes of their aneurysms. There were no infections in patients with atherosclerotic aneurysms.

Discussion

Diagnosis of carotid artery aneurysms can be confusing. The most frequently encountered lesion that must be distinguished from a carotid artery aneurysm is a tortuous or kinked carotid artery.[67] Differentiation can be accomplished on physical examination by noting whether pulsation occurs parallel to the long axis of the vessel (carotid kink) or at right angles to the artery (carotid aneurysm). In soft tissue x-rays of the neck, calcification can occasionally be seen in the walls of aneurysms but not in tortuous arteries.

Other masses easily confused with carotid artery aneurysm include carotid body tumors, lymph nodes, and branchial cleft cysts.

Improved techniques of ultrasonic scanning make this the method of choice for the noninvasive diagnosis of carotid artery aneurysms. Angiography established the diagnosis in all our patients and provided essential information regarding resectability and assessment of intracranial circulation. Computerized digital intravenous angiography will certainly have a place among diagnostic procedures and may entirely replace standard arteriography in certain patients.

Decisions regarding surgical therapy of asymptomatic atherosclerotic aneurysms are complicated by a lack of knowledge of their natural history. Clearly, our experience as well as that of others supports the view that these lesions may cause serious symptoms. When possible, symptomatic aneurysms should be resected with restoration of cerebral blood flow. Wrapping and endoaneurysmorrhaphy have been largely abandoned. If distal control cannot be accomplished, carotid artery ligation may be done safely if carotid stump pressure exceeds 65-70 mm Hg taken in conjunction with usual ward pressures. Preoperative estimation of stump pressure can be obtained using ocular pneumoplethysmography.

Pseudoaneurysm after carotid endarterectomy is unusual but results in significant morbidity. Because of a propensity to cause embolism and hemorrhage, all neck false aneurysms should be repaired. In the majority of cases, false aneurysms occur in a surgically accessible location and can be treated with resection and patch angioplasty or interposition grafting. Autogenous tissue must be used in such repairs because of the danger of infection. Gratifying results can be expected with a carefully selected operative approach to this unusual lesion.

REFERENCES

1. Leadbetter WF, Burkland CE: Hypertension in unilateral renal disease. J Urol 39:611, 1938
2. McCormack LJ, Hazard JB, Poutasse EF: Obstructive lesions of the renal artery associated with remedial hypertension. Am J Pathol 34:582, 1958
3. Palubinskas AJ, Ripley HR: Fibromuscular hyperplasia in extrarenal arteries. Radiology 82:451, 1964
4. Nunn DB: Fibromuscular hyperplasia of the internal carotid artery. Am Surg 40:309, 1974
5. Connett MC, Lansche JM: Fibromuscular hyperplasia of internal carotid artery. Report of a case. Ann Surg 162:59, 1965
6. Ehrenfeld WK, Wylie EJ: Fibromuscular dysplasia of the internal carotid artery. Surgical management. Arch Surg 109:676, 1974
7. Harrington OB, Crosby VG, Nicholas L: Fibromuscular hyperplasia of the internal carotid artery. Ann Thorac Surg 9:516, 1971
8. Kelly TF, Morris GC: Arterial fibromuscular disease. Am J Surg 143:232, 1982
9. Morris GC Jr, Lechter A, DeBakey ME: Surgical treatment of fibromuscular disease of the carotid arteries. Arch Surg 96:636, 1968

10. Patman RD, Thompson JE, Talkington CM, et al: Natural history of fibromuscular dysplasia of the carotid artery. Stroke 2:135, 1980
11. Perry MO: Fibromuscular dysplasia. Surg Gynecol Obstet 139:97, 1974
12. Stanley JC, Fry WJ, Seeger JF, et al: Extracranial internal carotid and vertebral artery fibrodysplasia. Arch Surg 109:215, 1974
13. Osborn AG, Anderson RE: Angiographic spectrum of cervical and intracranial fibromuscular dysplasia. Stroke 8:617, 1977
14. Stanley JC, Gewertz BL, Bove EL, et al: Arterial fibrodysplasia: Histopathologic character and current etiologic concepts. Arch Surg 110:561, 1975
15. Effeney DJ, Ehrenfeld WK, Stoney RJ, et al: Fibromuscular dysplasia of the internal carotid artery. World J Surg 3:179, 1979
16. Effeney DJ, Ehrenfeld WK, Stoney RJ, et al: Why operate on carotid fibromuscular dysplasia? Arch Surg 115:1261, 1980
17. Houser OW, Baker HL: Fibrovascular dysplasia and other uncommon diseases of the cervical carotid artery: Angiographic aspects. Am J Roentgenol 104:201, 1978
18. Palubinskas AJ, Perloff D, Newton TH: Fibromuscular hyperplasia: An arterial dysplasia of increasing clinical importance. Am J Roentgenol 98:907, 1966
19. Ehrenfeld WK, Stoney RJ, Wylie EJ: Fibromuscular hyperplasia of the internal carotid artery. Arch Surg 95:284, 1967
20. Anderson R, Schechter M: A case of spontaneous dissecting aneurysm of the internal carotid artery. J Neurol Neurosurg Psychiatry 22:195, 1959
21. Brice JG, Crompton MR: Spontaneous dissecting aneurysms of the cervical internal carotid artery. Br Med J 2:790, 1964
22. Bostrom K, Liliequist B: Primary dissecting aneurysm of the extracranial part of the internal carotid and vertebral arteries. Neurology 17:179, 1967
23. Liliequist B: The roentgenologic appearance of spontaneous dissecting aneurysm of the cervical internal carotid artery. Vasc Surg 2:223, 1968
24. Lloyd J, Bannson HT: Bilateral dissecting aneurysms of the internal carotid arteries. Am J Surg 122:549, 1971
25. Ojemann RG, Fischer CM, Rich JC: Spontaneous dissecting aneurysm of the internal carotid artery. Stroke 3:434, 1972
26. Ehrenfeld WK, Wylie EJ: Spontaneous dissection of the internal carotid artery. Arch Surg 111:1294, 1976
27. Fischer CM, Ojemann RG, Roberson GH: Spontaneous dissection of cervicocerebral arteries. Can J Neurol Sci 5:9, 1978
28. Gee W, Kaupp HA, McDonald KM, et al: Spontaneous dissection of internal carotid arteries: Spontaneous resolution documented by serial ocular pneumoplethysmography and angiography. Arch Surg 115:944, 1980
29. Mehigan JT, Olcott C: The carotid "string sign." Differential diagnosis and management. Am J Surg 140:137, 1980.
30. Campbell FC, Robbs JV: Spontaneous dissecting aneurysms of the internal carotid artery. JR Coll Surg Edinb 26:286, 1981
31. Bradac GB, Kaernbach A, Bulk-Weischedel D, et al: Spontaneous dissecting aneurysms of cervical cerebral arteries. Report of six cases and review of the literature. Neuroradiology 21:149, 1981
32. Chapleau CE, Robertson JT: Spontaneous cervical carotid artery dissection: Outpatient treatment with continuous heparin infusion using a totally implantable infusion device. Neurosurgery 8:83, 1981
33. Friedman WA, Day AL, Quishing RG, et al: Cervical carotid dissecting aneurysms. Neurosurgery 7:207, 1980
34. O'Dwyer JA, Moscen W, Trevor, et al: Spontaneous dissection of the carotid artery Radiology 137:379, 1980

35. Epstein MA: Spontaneous carotid artery dissection in a 38-year-old man. Postgrad Med 68:103, 1980
36. Anderson CA, Collins CJ, Rich NM, et al: Spontaneous dissection of the internal carotid artery associated with fibromuscular dysplasia. Am Surg 46:263, 1980
37. McNeill DH, Dreisbach J, Marsden RJ: Spontaneous dissection of the internal carotid artery. Its conservative management with heparin sodium. Arch Neurol 37:54, 1980
38. Ehrenfeld WK, Stoney RJ, Wylie EJ: Relation of carotid stump pressure to safety of carotid ligation. Surgery (in press) 1982
39. Winslow N: Extracranial aneurysm of internal carotid artery: History and analysis of cases registered to August 1, 1925. Arch Surg 13:689, 1926
40. Marantz RA, Kirchner FR, Kishore P: Aneurysms of the petrous portion of the internal carotid artery. Surg Neurol 6:313, 1976
41. Weaver D: Retropharyngeal hemorrhage from the carotid artery. Trans Am Laryngol Assoc 85:222, 1964
42. Busby DR, Slemmon OH, Miller TF: Fatal epistaxis via carotid aneurysm and eustacian tube. Arch Otolaryngol 87:295, 1968
43. Weber RC, Barker WF: Aneurysms of the extracranial internal carotid artery. Arch Surg 99:501, 1969
44. Margolis MT, Stein RL, Newton TH: Extracranial aneurysms of the internal carotid artery. Neuroradiology 4:78, 1972
45. Rhodes EL: Aneurysms of extracranial carotid arteries. Arch Surg 111:339, 1976
46. Mokri B, Piepgras DG: Cervical internal carotid artery aneurysm with calcific-embolism to the retina. Neurology 31:211, 1981
47. Busuttil RW, Davidson RK, Foley KT, et al: Selective management of extracranial carotid arterial aneurysms. Am J Surg 140:85, 1980
48. Lane RJ, Weisman RA: Carotid artery aneurysms: An otolaryngologic perspective. Laryngoscope 90:897, 1980
49. Kirby CK, Johnson J, Donald JG: Aneurysm of the common carotid artery. Ann Surg 130:913, 1949
50. Young N: Bleeding from ear as sign of leaking aneurysm of extracranial portion of internal carotid artery. J Laryngol 56:35, 1941
51. Thapeid IM, Ashenhurst EM, Rozdilsky B: Spontaneous dissecting aneurysms of the internal carotid artery in the neck. Arch Neurol 23:549, 1970
52. Hardin CA: Successful resection of carotid and abdominal aneurysm in two related patients with Marfan syndrome. NEJM 267:141, 1962
53. Finney LA, David NJ: Aneurysm of the extracranial internal carotid artery: Report of a case and discussion. Neurology 14:376, 1964
54. Ledgerwood AM, Lucas CE: Mycotic aneurysm of the carotid artery. Arch Surg 109:496, 1974
55. Hammon JW, Silver D, Young WF: Congenital aneurysm of the extracranial carotid arteries. Ann Surg 176:777, 1972
56. Ehrenfeld WK, Hays RJ: False aneurysm after carotid endarterectomy. Arch Surg 104:288, 1972
57. McCollum CH, Wheeler WG, Noon GP, et al: Aneurysms of the extracranial carotid artery. Twenty-one years' experience. Am J Surg 137:196, 1979
58. Robinson NA, Flotto CF: Traumatic aneurysms of the carotid arteries. Am Surg 401:121, 1974
59. Elkin DC, Shumaker HB: Surgery in World War II (U.S. Army), *in* Vascular Surgery. Office of the Surgeon General, Deparment of the Army, Washington, D.C., 1955.
60. Salmon JH, Blatt EJ: Aneurysms of the internal carotid artery due to closed trauma. J Thorac Cardiovasc Surg 56:28, 1968

61. Crawford T: Pathological effects of cerebral arteriography. J Neurol, Neurosurg Psychiatry 19:217, 1956
62. Morris G: Relayed perforations of the internal carotid artery by an ingested foreign body. Br J Surg 56:711, 1969
63. Shipley AM, Winslow N, Walker WW: Aneurysm in the cervical portion of the internal carotid artery. An analytical study of the cases reported in the literature between August 1, 1925-July 31, 1936. Ann Surg 105:673, 1937
64. Fay T: Atypical facial neuralgia, a syndrome of vascular pain. Ann Otol Rhinol Laryngol 41:1030, 1932
65. Canaseal L, Mashiah A, Charlesworth D: Aneurysms of the extracranial carotid arteries. Br J Surg 65:590, 1978
66. Cooper A: Account of the first successful operation performed on the common carotid artery for aneurysm in the year 1808 with post-mortem examination in the year 1821. Guys Hosp Rep 1:53, 1836
67. Perdue GD: The significance of elongation and angulation of the carotid artery: A negative view. Surgery 77:45, 1977

E. Kieffer
J. Natali

25

Supraaortic Trunk Lesions in Takayasu's Arteritis

Takayasu's arteritis is a nonspecific panarteritis which may affect in various degrees the entire aorta and its branches as well as the pulmonary artery. Supraaortic trunk lesions appeared in the first description of the disease at the beginning of this century, when Takayasu, a Japanese ophtalmologist, described a retinal vascular disease of unknown etiology in a 21-year-old woman in 1908.[1] However, he failed to mention supraaortic trunk involvement in his case, and it was Onishi who established a correlation between vascular occlusive disease and the ocular complications in the discussion of Takayasu's presentation. During the next half century, only sporadic cases or small series were reported in the literature, and the disease was considered an exceptional one. During this period, progressive identification led to the use of a great number of descriptive terms. Pulseless disease, primary arteritis of the aortic arch, aortic arch syndrome, aortitis syndrome, nonspecific arteritis, young female arteritis, occlusive thromboaortopathy, and idiopathic medial aortopathy are some of the numerous synonyms used in the literature. Takayasu's arteritis remains the customarily used term in most countries. The possible involvement of the whole aorta and its collateral branches as well as its worldwide distribution have been recognized only recently. This has led to increasing recognition of the disease in the last 15 years. Its diagnosis must now be considered in a number of clinical situations including aortic arch syndrome, proximal occlusive disease of the upper limbs, atypical coarctation of the descending thoracic and/or abdominal aorta, and renovascular hypertension.

During the last 8 years, we have seen 87 cases, including cardiac, supraaortic, aortic, and renal localizations. Among them, 61 had supraaortic trunk involvement of various degrees and 33 of these latter were operated, mainly for cerebrovascular insufficiency. In a large number of patients, supraaortic trunk lesions were neglected and surgical management directed toward treatment of aortic and/or renal arterial lesions in order to control severe arterial hypertension.

The purpose of this review is to describe the diagnosis and management of supraaortic trunk lesions in Takayasu's arteritis based on a review of the literature and our own personal experience.

ETIOLOGY

Except in the Far East, Takayasu's arteritis has been considered a rare condition for a long time. Its frequency, however, seems definitely more important than believed initially. Numerous series reporting large numbers of patients have appeared recently in the literature.[2-14]

Clinical onset usually takes place in the second or third decade. Children are rarely affected but when they are, the disease may be particularly severe, with a rapidly unfavourable outcome.[10] In the rare cases when it occurs after the fourth decade, it may be difficult to differentiate from atherosclerosis. In early descriptions, only female patients were reported, and for a long time, some authors even considered this sex criterion as an absolute prerequisite for diagnosis. Females are, indeed, largely predominant, but male patients have also been encountered in as much as 10 to 15 percent of the recently reported large series.

The disease is more frequent in the Far East, particularly in Japan[4-6,14] and India,[12] but it has been reported in virtually all countries. The topography of the lesions and their course, however, have been shown to be slightly different from one continent to another. In France, a few cases are encountered in native people, but most of the patients come from North Africa or the French West Indies because of special medical relations with these countries.

The precise cause of the disease remains unknown. The congenital and infectious theories are now nearly completely abandoned. Yet, genetic predisposition is likely, as suggested by a few familial cases (as reported by Numano[15] and one personal case) and by HLA antigen determinations which show a significant increase as compared to control patients.[16] An immunological mechanism is probably involved, as suggested by the general symptoms of the preocclusive period; by the diffuse arterial involvement, including the pulmonary artery; and by the possible association with known immunological diseases (polymyalgia rheumatica, ankylosing spondylitis, lupus erythematosus, and polymyositis). Unfortunately, biological signs of immunological disturbances (presence of antiaorta antibodies and circulating immune complexes, and elevation of immunoglobulins and serum complement) are inconstantly found[17] and are nonspecific. Takayasu's arteritis is now considered as a nonspecific reaction to varied aggressions and is thought to be a syndrome rather than a definite disease. Among these aggressions, tuberculosis has frequently been incriminated as ascertained by clinical, pathological, and experimental facts.[2,10,12] The frequency of tuberculosis in most reported series of Takayasu's arteritis, however, probably does not exceed mere coincidence, and tuberculosis is certainly absent in many cases.

PATHOLOGY

Takayasu's arteritis may involve the whole aorta, from the aortic valve to the distal aortic bifurcation, and all of its branches, from the coronary to the renal and intestinal arteries. Involvement of the supraaortic trunks is present in the majority of cases, either isolated or in association with other aortic and/or arterial localizations. A topographical classification has been proposed distinguishing four types.[10,14] In type I, only aortic arch lesions are present. Type II concerns isolated thoracoabdominal aortic lesions. In type III, arch and thoracoabdominal lesions are associated. Type IV indicates pulmonary involvement, whatever the aortic lesion. Types I and III account for the vast majority of cases, reflecting the frequency of supraaortic trunk lesions, which may be present in as many as 90 percent of the cases. Although certainly valuable for diagnostic and prognostic purposes, however, this classification has important drawbacks. It does not take into account proximal aortic involvement (ascending aorta, coronary arteries, aortic valve), which is not infrequent and is of real prognostic significance.[6,18,19] Furthermore, it does not distinguish between proximal and distal lesions in the same aortic branch nor between occlusive and aneurysmal lesions.

Branch involvement often begins proximally at the origin of the artery, as part of the aortic disease. But the proximal part of the artery is sometimes spared from disease and involvement confined only to its distal part. Innominate and common carotid arteries are often involved through extensive lesions beginning at the aortic arch and extending up to the carotid bifurcation, which is usually normal (Figs. 25-1, 25-2, 25-3). Although proximal lesions may be encountered, subclavian artery involvement typically begins in the distal part of the artery, extending to the axillary or even brachial artery (Fig. 25-4). Vertebral arteries are usually normal, although their origin may be involved in an extensively diseased subclavian artery (Figs. 25-1, 25-2, 25-5). When both common carotid arteries are occluded or severely stenotic, the vertebral arteries may enlarge considerably and constitute the main collateral pathway to the brain (Figs. 25-1, 25-2, 25-5). Multiple lesions are common in advanced cases (Figs. 25-1, 25-2, 25-3, 25-5).

Lesions are usually occlusive in nature. Brain and/or upper limb ischemia are secondary to the hemodynamic consequences of the occlusive process. A few cases may be completely asymptomatic even in the presence of

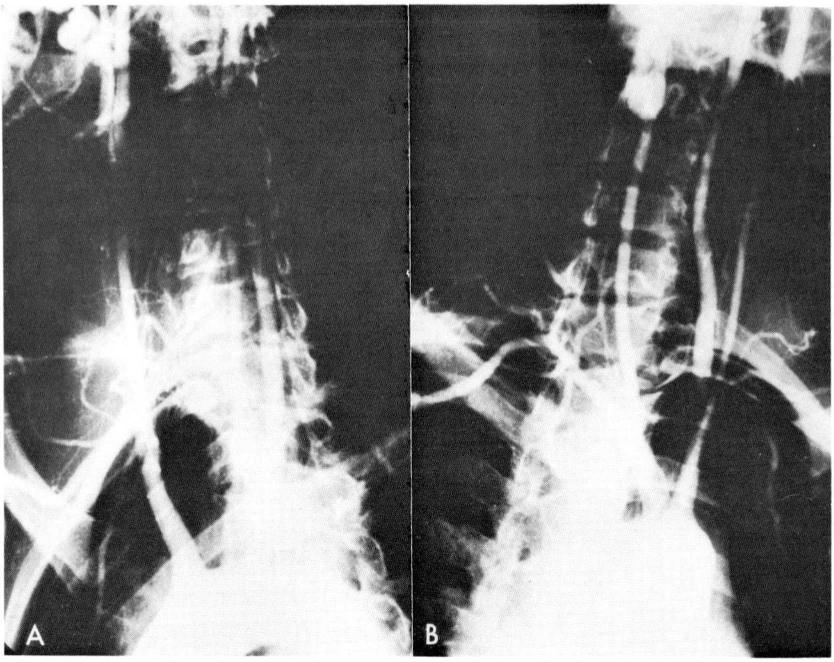

Figure 25-1A and 25-1B. Aortic arch syndrome. Tight stenosis of both common carotid and distal subclavian arteries. The carotid bifurcations are normal. Although stenosed at its origin on the subclavian artery, the vertebral artery is markedly enlarged.

severe anatomic involvement due to the proximal localization of the lesions and the many possibilities for collateral circulation (Figs. 25-2, 25-5). Arterio-arterial embolism is exceedingly rare, in contrast to the more common atherosclerotic lesions. Extensive occlusion due to superimposed thrombosis, however, may complicate severe proximal arterial stenosis, particularly in the carotid arteries. Nonstenotic involvement limited to parietal thickening is frequent, either isolated or in association with stenotic lesions. Aneurysms are present in a few cases.

Histological lesions begin and predominate in the adventitia and the external part of the media, which are affected by dense sclerosis[20] (Fig. 25-6). In the media, elastic fibers are often fragmented, accounting for the possible aneurysm formation. According to the clinical course of the disease, arterial sclerosis is associated with inflammatory lesions, including lymphocyte infiltrates and sometimes giant cells in varied proportions. The internal part of the media and the internal elastic lamella are usually normal. There is usually a strong intimal fibrotic reaction often with important intimal thickening.

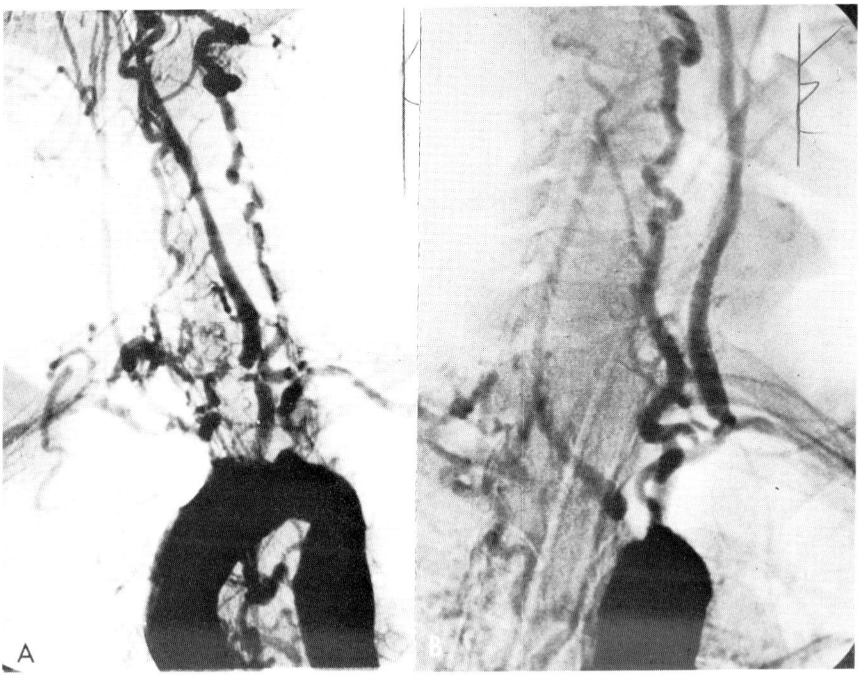

Figure 25-2A and 25-2B. Aortic arch syndrome. Multiple supraaortic trunk lesions with extensive collateral circulation through cervical arteries and left vertebral artery A descending thoracic aortic aneurysm is present.

This may be complicated by secondary atherosclerotic lesions and/or mural thrombosis.

CLINICAL MANIFESTATIONS

In typical cases, two distinct clinical periods are described in Takayasu's arteritis: preocclusive and occlusive phases.[10,21] The preocclusive phase is present only in one-third to one-half of the patients. At this early stage, Takayasu's arteritis appears as a general disease, whose diagnosis may be initially very difficult. General manifestations (fever, malaise, loss of weight, and anorexia) are constant and often associated with rheumatismal and cutaneous symptoms (myalgia, arthritis, skin rash, and erythema nodosum). Cardiac, pulmonary, and ocular symptoms are less frequent (tachycardia, pericarditis, dyspnea, cough, and episcleritis). Vascular symptoms and signs

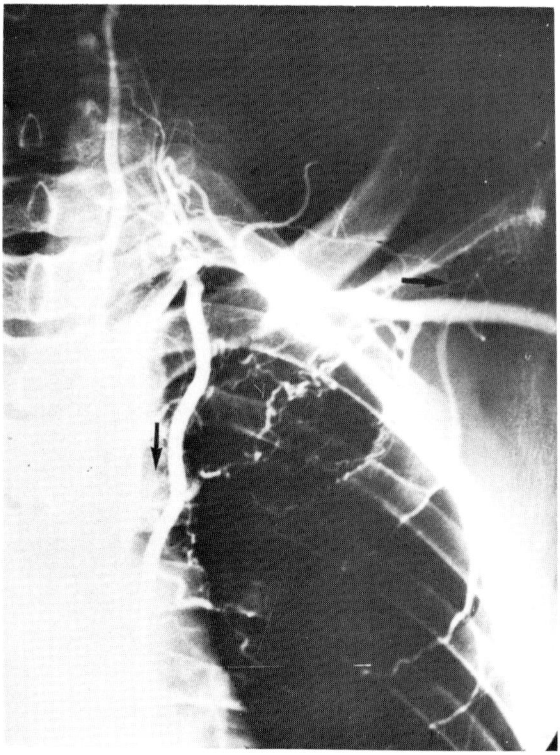

Figure 25-3. Distal subclavian lesion with revascularization through the internal mammary, upper intercostal and external mammary arteries.

are not yet present except in a few cases in which tenderness of the superficial arteries is present. The erythrocyte sedimentation rate is constantly elevated during this phase. Anemia, leukocytosis, and increase in α 2 and γ globulins may be present. Except in countries where the disease is common, it is frequently mistaken for more prevalent diseases such as rheumatic fever, typhoid fever, tuberculosis, or others. When symptoms are minimal and rapidly disappear spontaneously, no definite diagnosis is made. It is later that a retrospective diagnosis will be made, during the occlusive phase of the disease. Yet diagnosis at this early inflammatory stage is of utmost importance, since corticosteroids are probably capable of preventing the onset or limiting the extension of the arterial involvement.

The occlusive phase is characterized by the presence of arterial lesions which may vary in type and in topography. It is the apparent beginning of the disease when the preocclusive phase does not exist. Sometimes, it follows it

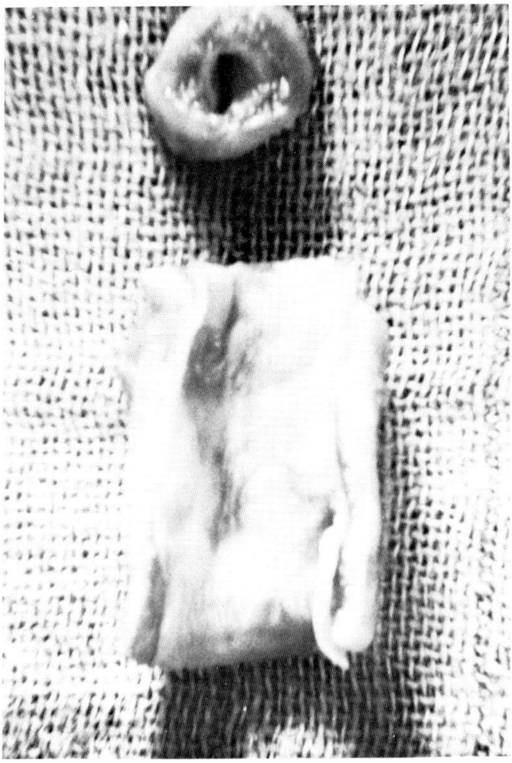

Figure 25-4. Gross appearance of a resected common carotid artery, showing adventitial and intimal thickening

without clinical discontinuity. More often, general symptoms of the preocclusive phase disappear spontaneously within a few weeks or months, and occlusive symptoms appear after an interval period of several months or even years. As already mentioned, although anatomic involvement of the supraaortic trunks is frequent, clinical symptoms are much less commonly present, due to the usual development of collateral circulation. In asymptomatic patients, physical signs include diminution of pulses and low blood pressure in the upper limbs as opposed to normal pulses and blood pressures in the lower limbs ("reversed coarctation"). Murmurs are usually heard at the base of the neck. The "aortic arch syndrome" includes three types of symptoms which may be associated in various ways. Cerebral symptoms are rare if one considers only focalized symptoms in the carotid or vertebrobasilar territories, whether transient or of a more durable type. Moreover, cerebrovascular accidents leading to permanent deficit or even death are possible but are more

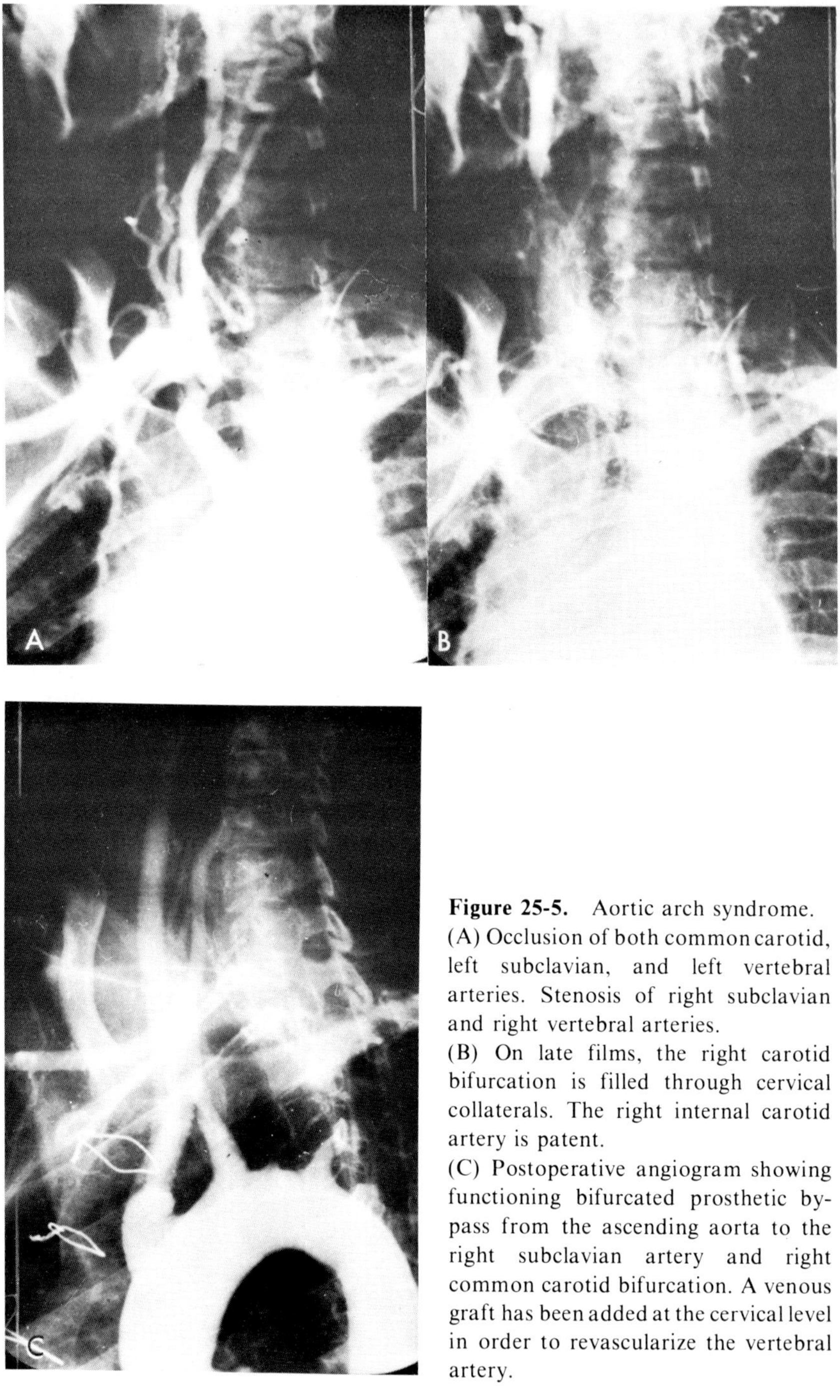

Figure 25-5. Aortic arch syndrome.
(A) Occlusion of both common carotid, left subclavian, and left vertebral arteries. Stenosis of right subclavian and right vertebral arteries.
(B) On late films, the right carotid bifurcation is filled through cervical collaterals. The right internal carotid artery is patent.
(C) Postoperative angiogram showing functioning bifurcated prosthetic bypass from the ascending aorta to the right subclavian artery and right common carotid bifurcation. A venous graft has been added at the cervical level in order to revascularize the vertebral artery.

often a result of severe uncontrolled arterial hypertension than a consequence of occlusive arterial disease. Nevertheless, a number of patients with multiple vessel involvement have a "low perfusion syndrome" which may constitute a considerable handicap in young patients' everyday lives. Upper limb ischemia is usually moderate, limited to forearm or hand claudication and/or Raynaud's phenomenon. Permanent ischemia with rest pain or necrosis is exceptionally, if ever, encountered. Facial ischemia is rare and only seen in advanced cases with multiple vessel occlusion involving at least the two common carotid arteries. They include jaw claudication; facial atrophy; ulceration of the palate, nose, or ear; and ocular complications such as bilateral ischemic cataract, possibly leading to total blindness.

Other localizations of the disease (aortic regurgitation, coronary insufficiency, and arterial hypertension secondary to atypical coarctation of the descending thoracic and/or upper abdominal aorta) must be carefully searched for and evaluated as they are important clues to the diagnosis and largely influence the prognosis of the disease.

Although noninvasive methods may be quite valuable, angiography is the definite method to investigate patients with Takayasu's arteritis. Due to the frequent extensive involvement, panaortography is necessary in order to locate all the possibly involved arteries.[9,22] It may be followed as necessary by selective angiograms according to the branch lesions found in one segment or another of the aorta on nonselective angiograms. Lesions are usually very typical in aspect, in topography, and by their associations (Figs. 25-1, 25-3, 25-5, 25-6). Supraaortic trunk lesions are typically different from those encountered in atherosclerotic occlusive disease. Aortic arch involvement is often major, and multiple lesions are frequent. Carotid lesions usually involve the entire common carotid artery, sparing its bifurcation and the internal carotid artery. Subclavian lesions usually involve and predominate at the distal part of the artery, often extending to the axillary and sometimes to the brachial artery. Associated stenosis of the descending thoracic aorta and/or upper abdominal aorta is highly characteristic and is a strong argument in favor of the diagnosis.[23,24] Angiographic diagnosis of isolated lesions of the distal subclavian artery may be difficult, but the clinical context helps differentiating them from fibromuscular dysplasia, radiation-induced lesions, or arterial complications of the thoracic outlet syndrome.

Young age, female sex, and ethnic origin also are important considerations in diagnosis. Pathologic examination and sometimes only the later evolution, however, may be the only definite clues to the disease. The presence of an inflammatory biological syndrome is neither constant nor specific, and its absence does not rule out diagnosis since the inflammatory phase may be completely absent and the patient may be seen for the first time during the occlusive phase.

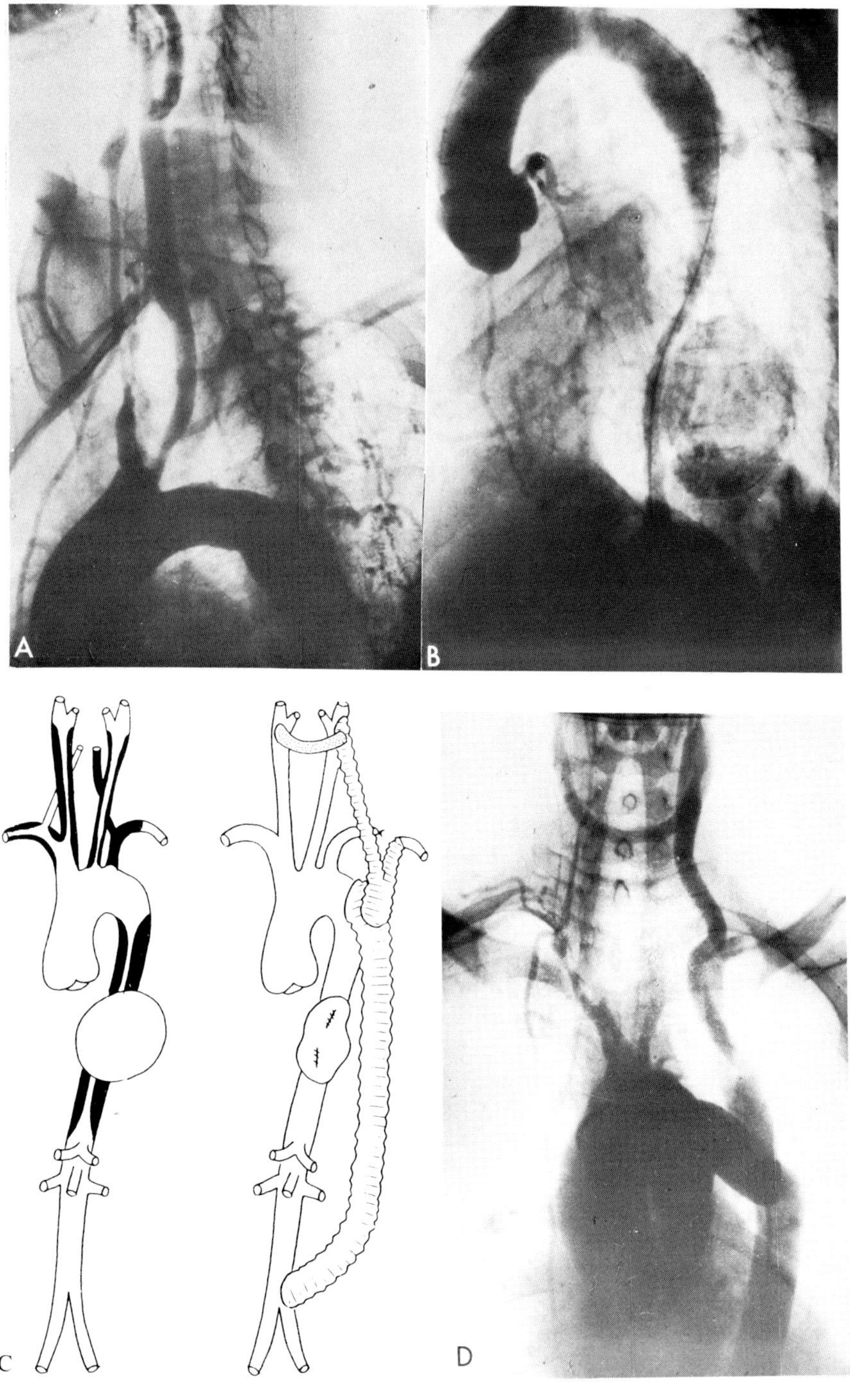
A
B
C
D

NATURAL HISTORY

The natural history of Takayasu's arteritis is not well known due to the lack of large, prospectively studied series of patients. A few cases proceed rapidly to death in a severe clinical condition associating multiple arterial occlusive manifestations and a persisting inflammatory syndrome. Death is generally of cardiac origin. These cases are very uncommon in Europe but have been reported from Japan,[6] India,[12] and Mexico.[10]

In the majority of cases the prognosis depends on ischemia secondary to occlusive aortic and/or arterial lesions. The major prognostic factor certainly is arterial hypertension secondary to atypical coarctation. Its presence reduces life expectancy to a few years[12] and represents the major cause of death in autopsy series.[10,25] Ischemic cerebrovascular accidents secondary to occlusive lesions of the supraaortic trunks are a less frequent cause of death or severe functional impairment. Multiple clinically significant lesions including retinopathy, arterial hypertension, cardiac localizations, and aneurysmal disease have also been shown to greatly diminish life expectancy.[6]

MEDICAL MANAGEMENT

In the absence of a known cause for the disease, there is no real treatment for Takayasu's arteritis, and one has to rely upon only symptomatic medical or surgical treatment.

Corticosteroids are the most useful symptomatic medication in the acute preocclusive phase of the disease, as they control the inflammatory process. Their use is sometimes contraindicated by severe uncontrolled arterial hypertension. If not, it is certainly important to use them in the inflammatory period. High doses, up to one milligram per kg weight, may be necessary during a few months, depending on clinical symptoms and repeated erythrocyte sedimentation rates. In our opinion, their long term prescription is not warranted since they are useless in chronic sclerotic lesions and may lead to

---

Figure 25-6. One-stage surgical management of multiple lesions.
(A) Aortic arch syndrome with proximal occlusion of the left subclavian artery, tight stenosis of innominate, right subclavian and both common carotid arteries.
(B) Atypical coarctation and saccular aneurysm of the descending thoracic aorta.
(C) and (D) Diagram and postoperative angiogram showing one-stage surgical management through combined left thoracotomy and cervical incisions: aortic bypass excluding the partially resected aneurysm; bifurcated prosthesis from the aortic bypass to the left subclavian and left common carotid arteries; venous crossover bypass between both common carotid bifurcations.

their own arterial and general complications. In a few cases, clinical or even purely biological inflammatory symptoms will reoccur during the follow-up period, necessitating further corticosteroid treatment. Antituberculous agents seem logical only in definitively proven active tuberculosis.

Other medical therapies such as antihypertensive medications, anticoagulants, antiplatelet aggregants, and vasodilators are intended to treat the ischemic consequences of the various arterial occlusions. They are used according to the clinical symptoms of the patients.

SELECTION FOR OPERATIVE THERAPY

Surgical management is logical only in chronic fixed lesions, whether stenotic or aneurysmal. A persistent inflammatory syndrome is a temporary contraindication to surgery due to the high morbidity and late recurrence rate which have been observed after operations performed under these conditions.[4,5,12,13,26,27]

Due to the important differences in symptomatology and their prognostic implications, a distinction must be made between lesions affecting only the upper limb vessels and those affecting the cerebral vessels.[7] Distal subclavian and/or axillary occlusive lesions are benign in nature, and in our opinion, only a few surgical indications are logical in these cases. Severely symptomatic cases should certainly be operated, especially on the dominant side. An arterial specimen may sometimes be needed as a clue to diagnosis and subclavian-axillary lesions are certainly the easiest to obtain. In still other cases with arterial hypertension secondary to atypical aortic coarctation, a reliable peripheral blood pressure cannot be measured due to bilateral upper limbs lesions. Although these lesions may be asymptomatic, we have performed a few unilateral revascularizations in these conditions.

Innomimate and/or common carotid artery lesions are more dangerous due to the frequent cerebrovascular symptoms in the cases of multiple lesions and to the unpredictable, infrequent, but real threat of an acute cerebrovascular accident. We think that these lesions must usually be operated on, except when truly asymptomatic in poor-risk patients or when an important neurological deficit is present. Good-risk patients, whether symptomatic or not, are best treated surgically in order to avoid cerebral complications and/or extensive carotid or vertebral occlusions which may be difficult or impossible to revascularize later on.[7] When the operation is performed through median sternotomy, a one stage treatment of all lesions is advisable, although it may sometimes be complicated by temporary cerebral edema.

Aneurysmal lesions deserve broad surgical indications, as in more common etiologies.

SURGICAL TECHNIQUES

General Considerations

Two types of reconstructive methods may be utilized.[25]

Direct techniques each have their own difficulties and limitations.

1. Endarterectomy is rather an intimectomy than the usual operation performed in atherosclerotic lesions. It is possible only when the artery has a normal diameter, when a cleavage plane is found through the parietal lesions, and if the remaining artery is of sufficiently good quality. It is simple only in relatively localized, well accessible lesions, which are rather rare. Its only theoretical advantage would be avoiding a prosthetic graft, but its durability is certainly low in Takayasu's arteritis.
2. Direct grafting applies principally to aneurysms, where the preferred method usually is intraaneurysmal grafting without resection of the aneurysmal sac.
3. Patch angioplasty is reasonably possible only in limited and moderately stenotic lesions. It is difficult to realize when dealing with tight or extensive stenoses.

These direct techniques also have two more inconveniences in common. Complete exposure of the diseased artery is necessary, and this may be difficult or even impossible due to periarterial fibrosis. In some situations, prolonged clamping may be needed, and this may be contraindicated when dealing with multiple lesions. For all these reasons, we have used the above mentioned methods only in a few selected cases.

The bypass principle certainly is the simplest method and is applicable to most, if not all, anatomical situations. The graft material used depends on the caliber of the operated artery. Dacron prostheses are suitable for large arteries, but we prefer autogenous venous or sometimes arterial grafts for the medium or small sized arteries.

Surgical management of supraaortic trunk lesions in Takayasu's arteritis differs according to the localization and the extension of the lesions.[7,13] Aneurysmal disease must be considered separately.

Isolated Lesions of the Subclavian and/or Axillary Arteries

These lesions may usually be operated on through a cervical approach. A venous bypass graft proceeding from the ipsilateral common carotid artery is the usual technique, but two conditions must be fulfilled: the common carotid artery must be healthy and a convenient venous graft obtained. The technique in itself is not difficult. The greater saphenous vein is first isolated in its upper part in order to make sure of its good quality and its sufficient caliber. The anticipated distal anastomotic site (usually the axillary, sometimes the brachial artery) is next isolated. The common carotid is then approached through a supraclavicular incision partially dividing the sternomastoid muscle. Its quality is appreciated by careful palpation. The proximal anastomosis is made side-to-end on the anterior aspect of the carotid artery. During this brief period of carotid clamping, we use no special measures of cerebral protection except for general heparinization (0.5 milligrams per kg weight) and keeping normal arterial blood pressure. The venous graft is tunneled behind the jugular vein, the clavicle, and the pectoralis muscles. The distal anastomosis is made end-to-side on the distal undiseased artery. A segment of diseased artery and sometimes a supraclavicular lymphatic node may be taken as pathologic specimens.

If a venous graft of insufficient length and/or quality is the only autogenous graft found, there are three remaining possibilities:

1. In cases of moderate or absent clinical symptoms, surgical abstention is logical. When the artery is completely occluded, an arterial biopsy may be the only procedure performed.
2. When the lesions are proximal and the clinical symptoms sufficiently important to warrant it, a prosthetic bypass using knitted Dacron or PTFE grafts may be done between the common carotid and the distal subclavian or proximal axillary arteries.
3. When the lesions are more distal and the clinical symptoms important, an upper thoracic sympathectomy is made through an axillary incision in the third intercostal space. A satisfactory clinical result may usually be obtained using this simple procedure, and late complications of small-sized arterial prostheses crossing a flexion crease are avoided.

In a few cases, either by preoperative angiogram or intraoperatively, the common carotid artery is found to be too heavily diseased in order to authorize the safe implantation of a bypass but not enough to warrant a proper revascularization procedure. In four such cases we have used bypasses from the thoracic aorta according to an unusual but interesting technique. Through an anterolateral thoracotomy incision in the third intercostal space, the venous or prothetic graft is implanted on the ascending or descending aorta using lateral clamping. It is tunneled through the pleural cavity and brought out through the second intercostal space to axillary region, where the distal anastomosis is completed. A concomitant upper thoracic sympathectomy may be realized easily. This technique has the distinct advantage of avoiding a median sternotomy incision which may be indicated some time later in order to perform more complicated surgery of the supraaortic trunks and/or thoracic aorta.

Other techniques of surgical management of occlusive subclavian arterial lesions used in atherosclerosis are rarely possible and have only exceptional indications in Takayasu's arteritis:

1. Direct common carotid-subclavian anastomosis is usually impossible due to distal extension of the lesions.
2. Endarterectomy is rarely if ever indicated, due to the extension of the lesions, the wide approach necessary for their complete exposure, and its rather poor early and late patency rates in medium-sized arteries.
3. Subclavio-carotid and crossover subclavio-subclavian or axillo-axillary bypasses, in our opinion, are contraindicated due to the frequent bilaterality of the lesions and the possibility of late involvement of the initially undiseased donor site.

Isolated Occlusive Lesions of the Innominate and/or Common Carotid Arteries

These lesions are best treated through median sternotomy. The usual proximal extension of the lesions makes limited local procedures (endarterectomy, resection and grafting, and patch angioplasty) rarely, if ever, possible, and their results have usually been poor.[5,7,13,27,28] The bypass principle is used in most cases.

Bypass proceeding from the ascending aorta is the technique of choice. The carotid bifurcation is first approached through a cervical incision, since it is usually the distal limit of the lesions. In most cases, the internal carotid artery is soft and patent. When it is occluded due to extensive thrombosis complicating proximal lesions, an isolated revascularization of the external carotid artery may be indicated. This is especially the case in the presence of ocular symptoms and/or if the intracranial internal carotid artery is revascularized through the ophtalmic artery and/or if an extracranial-intracranial anastomosis is anticipated. The ascending aorta is next approached through median sternotomy which is done separately or in continuity with the cervical incision according to the length of the neck region. When ascending aorta is soft and undiseased, a venous graft may be used if it is of sufficient caliber and good quality and if it is not necessary for another simultaneously or secondarily anticipated revascularization. If these conditions are not encountered or if the aorta is diseased and thick-walled, a 7, 8, or sometimes 10 mm knitted Dacron prosthesis has to be used. The aorta is partially clamped while maintaining the systolic arterial blood pressure between 100 and 120 mm Hg in order to allow easy placement of the clamps, to avoid its slipping, and to prevent aortic damage due to a sudden rise in blood pressure. A side-to-end anastomosis is made between the aorta and the venous or prosthetic graft using a continuous monofilament suture. When a prosthesis is used, especially if it is of small size, an interesting adjunct is to use a bifurcated prosthesis, keeping only one of its branches and the adjacent part of its body in order to allow for large bites in the aortic wall. If the ascending aorta is heavily diseased and/or calcified, it may also be necessary to excise a small piece of aorta in order to allow for correct expansion of the proximal anastomosis. The graft is brought to the cervical incision, the common carotid bifurcation is transsected, the origin of the internal carotid artery is longitudinally incised, and an end-to-side anastomosis is made using a continuous monofilament suture. If a prosthetic graft has been used, it must be isolated from the sternum by interposing the thymic remnants and subhyoid muscles which have been carefully preserved at the beginning of the operation.

Multiple Occlusive Lesions of the Supraaortic Trunks

Bypasses proceeding from the ascending aorta are best indicated in the management of this common condition. Many technical combinations may be imagined according to the numerous possible anatomical situations. In a few cases, multiple vein grafts may be used in a technique which is very similar to that used in aortocoronary bypass grafts. In most cases, a bifurcated knitted Dacron prosthesis is used to revascularize both carotid arteries, and secondary prosthetic or venous grafts are implanted on one or both limbs of the principal graft to revascularize axillary and/or vertebral arteries (Fig. 25-5). When the common and internal carotid arteries on one side are normal or completely occluded, the corresponding limb of the graft may be used to revascularize the subclavian artery or even the vertebral artery when it is particularly enlarged. In some cases, the subclavian and axillary arteries are diffusely diseased, but moderate or absent clinical symptoms do not warrant an associated upper limb revascularization. In these cases, an isolated vertebral artery revascularization is often indicated. It may be realized through a separate venous graft proceeding from the ascending aorta or from the body or one of the limbs of the aortocarotid prosthetic bypass graft. A direct anastomosis of the vertebral artery to the posterior aspect of the aortocarotid bypass may sometimes be performed. In our opinion, it is contraindicated to implant more than one bifurcated graft on the ascending aorta, even if the latter is long and lends itself easily to such a technique. A tracheal and/or venous compression is a likely complication of this technique, owing to the narrowness of the cervicothoracic inlet especially in young female patients two personal cases.[29] For this reason, it may even be preferable in a few cases to use only one large prosthetic tube graft to revascularize one carotid artery. The other revascularizations are then made separately at the cervical level from the aortocarotid graft.[29]

Aneurysms

Aneurysms of the supraaortic trunks do not add special technical difficulties. Distal revascularization is made through a bypass graft using a technique that is similar to that used for occlusive lesions. The aneurysm itself is treated either by exclusion if it is of small size and/or difficult to approach (i.e. subclavian-axillary aneurysms) or by resection if it is large, compressing the neighbouring structures, and/or easily approachable (i.e. innominate or common carotid artery aneurysms).

Alternative Techniques in the Unoperable Ascending Aorta

In a few cases, the ascending aorta cannot be used for proximal implantation of a bypass. This may be due to a previous or anticipated surgical procedure or, less infrequently, to a heavily diseased aorta, the lateral clamping of which introduces a potential risk of severe complications. Aortic disease of such importance may be anticipated preoperatively in the presence of major calcifications and absence of expansion of the ascending aorta but sometimes is appreciated only by intraoperative palpation. In such circumstances, a wise decision is either to abandon the anticipated revascularization or to choose another proximal anastomotic site.

1. Another supraaortic trunk may sometimes be used, usually the innominate artery, more exceptionally a distal subclavian artery which is rarely undiseased and may become occluded later on.
2. The descending thoracic aorta or a prosthetic graft replacing or bypassing it may sometimes be used (as reported by Veno et al.,[14] Kimoto,[30] and 2 personal cases). The left thoracic region, left upper limb, and neck are draped, and a posterolateral thoracotomy combined with a separate left cervical incision is made. The prosthetic graft is implanted proximally and then tunneled through the pleural dome and anastomosed to the left carotid and/or subclavian artery. When right supraaortic trunk lesions are to be treated, a crossover bypass may be done at the completion of the procedure or during a secondary procedure.
3. The supraceliac aorta, if undiseased, is easily approached through an upper median laparotomy and a vertical incision of the right diaphragmatic crus. The prosthetic graft is passed through the right pleural cavity and anastomosed to one or several supraaortic trunks. We have used this previously undescribed procedure in one of our cases.
4. The internal iliac and common femoral arteries might also be used, providing a thoracoabdominal aortic lesion is absent or has been previously treated. But the length and orientation of the graft will probably preclude long-term patency, thereby making indications for this procedure rather illogical in these young patients who are in good general condition.

Associated Procedures

Cardiac and/or coronary arterial lesions are best treated simultaneously if a median sternotomy is used for the management of supraaortic trunk lesions. In 2 cases of associated supraaortic and coronary lesions, we have first performed carotid revascularization using woven Dacron bypasses proceeding from the ascending aorta. Cardiopulmonary bypass was then instituted in order to anastomose saphenous vein grafts first on the distal coronary arteries and then on the aortocarotid prosthetic graft. This was intended to avoid a difficult proximal implantation on a heavily diseased ascending aorta, which could have compromised early or late patency of the vein graft, as mentioned in the few surgical cases reported in the literature.[18,19]

Atypical coarctations or, less frequently, aneurysms of the descending thoracic aorta, sometimes extending to the upper abdominal aorta, may often be associated. A one-stage procedure is sometimes possible, usually through a median sternotomy using an ascending aorta-abdominal aorta bypass,[33,34] more rarely though a left thoracic incision (Fig. 25-6). We have performed this extensive and time-consuming operation in four instances without complication. But we usually prefer a two-stage procedure, first revascularizing the supraaortic trunks through median sternotomy and then a few weeks later treating the aortic lesions through a left thoracic and/or thoracoabdominal incision.

PERSONAL EXPERIENCE AND RESULTS

During an 8 year period, we have seen 87 patients with Takayasu's arteritis. Clinical examination and panaortography showed supraaortic trunk involvement of various degrees in 61 of them, among whom 56 had occlusive lesions and 5 had aneurysms.

Thirty eight patients had isolated uni- or bilateral lesions of the subclavian and/or axillary arteries, and only 16 were operated on. In 10 patients, 11 carotido-axillary or carotido-brachial bypasses were performed through a cervical approach. Four patients had bypasses proceeding from the thoracic aorta. A venous graft was used in 14 instances; a prosthetic graft was used only once. Two more patients had an isolated upper thoracic sympathectomy. There was no mortality or major complication in this group. Postoperative occlusion occurred in 3 patients. Two of them underwent a second attempt at revascularization, which was successful in both cases.

Twenty-three patients had involvement of innominate and/or common carotid artery usually in association with subclavian and/or axillary lesions. Seventeen of them were operated through a thoracic approach. An isolated aorto-carotid bypass was used in only 2 cases. All other patients had multiple revascularisations proceeding from the thoracic aorta, using in most cases aorto-carotid tubular or bifurcated prosthesis bypass grafts from which venous grafts revascularizing the upper limbs or vertebral arteries were added at the cervical level. Eleven of these patients had associated surgery of aortic and/or renal lesions, 4 in the same session, 7 as a second procedure. There was one death in this group due to a hemorrhage from a suture line involving a heavily diseased ascending aorta. One patient presented cortical blindness, presumably due to embolism in the basilar artery, with major recovery. All surviving patients had a postoperative angiogram. Among the 49 arteries that were revascularized in these 16 patients, all except one were found to be patent.

In the whole series of 33 patients, 30 were completely asymptomatic in the postoperative period, while only 2 were only improved and one made worse.

Follow-up extended from 3 to 88 months (mean 39 months). There were no late deaths. Three patients had late arterial occlusions with recurrence of symptoms. One patient with mild chronic upper limb ischemia and an occluded carotido-axillary bypass was not reoperated. Two patients with neurological symptoms were successfully reoperated. The causes of the late failures were believed to be of a technical nature and not secondary to a recurrent inflammatory process, which was not encountered in our series and has been reported only infrequently in the literature.

CONCLUSIONS

Takayasu's arteritis is a rare but not exceptional disease. Its diagnosis is to be considered in several clinical circumstances, with aortic arch syndrome and atypical aortic coarctation being the most frequently encountered. There is no specific test for diagnosis that is based on a grouping of clinical, biological, pathological, and arteriographic facts. While corticosteroid therapy is the treatment of choice during the acute inflammatory phase, surgery is often indicated in the management of chronic noninflammatory occlusive or aneurysmal lesions. Results are good if the indications and the surgical techniques are satisfactory.

REFERENCES

1. Judge RD, Currier RD, Gracie WA, et al: Takayasu's arteritis and the aortic arch syndrome. Am J Med 32:379, 1962 (with a translation from Takayasu M. A case with peculiar changes of the central retinal vessels. Acta Soc Ophtalmol, Jpn 12:554, 1908)
2. Fiessinger JN, Tawfik-Taher S, Capron J, et al: Maladie de Takayasu: critères diagnostiques. Nouv Presse Med 11:583, 1982
3. Fraga A, Mintz G, Valle L, et al: Takayasu's arteritis: Frequency of systemic manifestations (study of 22 patients) and favorable response to maintenance steroid therapy with adrenocorticosteroids (12 patients). Arthr Rheum 15:617, 1972
4. Inada K, Katsumara T, Hirai J, et al: Surgical treatment in the aortitis syndrome. Arch Surg 100:220, 1970

5. Inoue T, Kawada K, Takeuchi S, et al: Surgical considerations of the aortic and arterial lesions due to nonspecific aorto-arteritis. J Thorac Cardiovas Surg 63:599, 1972
6. Ishikawa K: Survival and morbidity after diagnosis of occlusive thromboaortopathy. Am J Cardiol 47:1026, 1981
7. Kieffer E, Tricot JF, Maraval M, et al: Chirurgie des troncs supra-aortiques au cours de la maladie de Takayasu. J Mal Vasc 4:255, 1979
8. Kieffer E, Maladie de Takayasu. Rev Med 43:2311, 1980
9. Lande A, Rossi P: The value of total arteriography in the diagnosis of Takayasu's arteritis. Radiology 114:287, 1975
10. Lupi-Herrera E, Sanchez-Torres G, Marcushamer J, et al: Takayasu's arteritis. Clinical study of 107 cases. Am Heart J 93:94, 1977
11. Pokrovsky AV: Non-specific aorto-arteritis and its surgical treatment. J Cardiovasc Surg 19:623, 1978
12. Sen PK: Nonspecific Aortoarteritis. Bombay, New Delhi, Tata McGraw Hill Publishing Company, 1973
13. Thevenet A: Chirurgie des lesions multiples des troncs supra-aortiques à leur origine. Chirurgie 106:491, 1980
14. Veno A, Mishima Y: Surgical and nonsurgical late results of Takayasu's arteritis. Angeiologie 23:357, 1972
15. Numano F, Isohisa I, Kishi U, et al: Takayasu's disease in twin sisters: Possible genetic factors. Circulation 58:173, 1978
16. Numano F, Isohisa I, Maezawa H, et al: HL-A antigens in Takayasu's disease. Am Heart J 98:153, 1979
17. Bletry O, Balafrej M, Kieffer E, et al: Maladie de Takayasu. Conceptions étiologiques. Apport des examens biologiques. Artères et Veines 1:15, 1982
18. Thomas D, Dubourg O, Bletry O, et al: Les manifestations cardiaques de la maladie de Takayasu (cardiopathie hypertensive exclue). J Mal Vasc 7:7, 1982
19. Cipriano PR, Silverman JF, Pelroth MG, et al: Coronary arterial narrowing in Takayasu's aortitis. Am J Cardiol 39:744, 1977
20. Camilleri JP, Hofmann-Guillaume C: Maladie de Takayasu. Bases anatomopathologiques. Artères et Veines 1:9, 1982
21. Strachan WR: Prepulseless and pulseless Takayasu's arteritis. Post Grad Med 42:466, 1966
22. Chermet J, Kieffer E, Tubiana JM, et al: Maladie de Takayasu. Interêt d'une aorto-artériographie complete. Ann Radiol 24:464, 1981
23. Lande A: Takayasu's arteritis and congenital coarctation of the descending thoracic and abdominal aorta. A critical review. Am J Roentgenol 127:227, 1976
24. Lande A, Berkmen YM: Aortitis. Pathologic, clinical and arteriographic review. Radiol Clin North Am 14:219, 1976
25. Rose AG, Sinclair-Smith CC: Takayasu's arteritis. A study of 16 autopsy cases. Arch Path Lab Med 104:231, 1980
26. Austen WG, Shaw RS: Surgical treatment of pulseless (Takayasu's) disease. New Engl J Med 270:1228, 1964
27. Sunamori M, Hatano R, Yamada T, et al: Aortitis syndrome due to Takayasu's disease. A guideline for the surgical indication. J Cardiovasc Surg 17:443, 1976
28. Kieffer E: Chirurgie de la maladie de Takayasu. Problèmes tactiques et techniques, in Dubost C, Carpentier A (ed): Actualités de Chirurgie Cardio-Vasculaire de l'Hôpital Broussais. (troisième serie). Paris, Masson and Co., 1982
29. Crawford ES, DeBakey ME, Morris GC Jr, et al: Surgical treatment of occlusion of the innominate, common carotid, and subclavian arteries: A 10 year experience. Surgery 65:17, 1969
30. Kimoto S: The history and present status of aortic surgery in Japan particularly for aortitis syndrome. J Cardiovasc Surg 20:107, 1979

31. Lande A, Bard R, Bole P, et al: Aortic arch syndrome (Takayasu's arteritis). Arteriographic and surgical considerations. J Cardiovasc Surg 19:507, 1978
32. Cohen A, Manion WC, Spencer FC, et al: Occlusive lesions of the great vessels of the aortic arch. Surgical and pathological aspects. Arch Surg 84:628, 1962
33. Bloss RS, Duncan JM, Cooley DA, et al: Takayasu's arteritis: Surgical considerations. Ann Thor Surg 27:574, 1979
34. Kieffer E, Natali J: Ascending aorta-abdominal aorta by-pass. Technical considerations, indications and report of 15 cases, in Greenhalgh RM (ed): Extra-anatomic and Secondary Arterial Reconstruction. London, Pitman, (in press)

Norman R. Hertzer Edwin G. Beven
Floyd D. Loop Paul C. Taylor

26

Management of Simultaneous Carotid and Coronary Artery Disease

Myocardial infarction and stroke are the two leading causes of cardiovascular death in the United States. It is not surprising, therefore, that severe, simultaneous carotid and coronary artery disease may be documented in some patients initially under consideration for either myocardial revascularization or extracranial arterial reconstruction alone. Although multifocal atherosclerosis is common to all such patients, their referral for surgical management usually assumes one of two distinct courses.

First, a relatively small subset of those with known coronary artery disease (CAD) is found to have advanced carotid artery lesions preceding elective myocardial revascularization (Fig. 26-1). The incidence of postoperative stroke after aortocoronary bypass using contemporary methods for extracorporeal perfusion usually does not exceed 2 percent,[1-4] and many of these neurologic deficits are manifest as diffuse encephalopathy or intellectual impairment that does not specifically implicate extracranial occlusive disease as an etiologic factor. Because hemispheric neurologic complications might be expected to occur with greater frequency among patients with demonstrated carotid stenosis, however, several previous reports have recommended that carotid endarterectomy should be performed in selected patients as a staged or combined procedure at the time of myocardial revascularization.[5-9]

Secondly, coronary atherosclerosis is prevalent among patients found to have carotid disease that is sufficiently severe to warrant surgical correction, irrespective of whether the diagnosis of CAD has been recognized and established by coronary angiography (Fig. 26-2). Provided the operative stroke rate is not excessive, myocardial infarctions are principally responsible

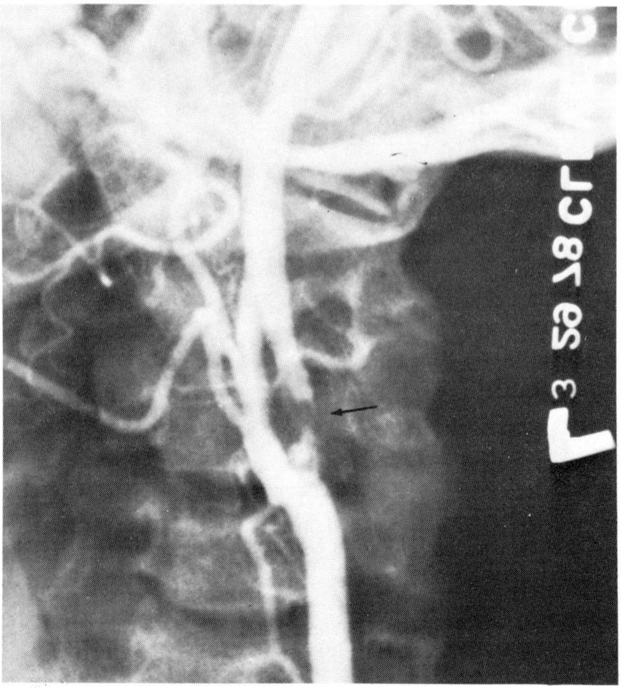

Figure 26-1. Carotid angiogram performed after asymptomatic carotid bruits were discovered in a patient scheduled for elective myocardial revascularization. Severe stenosis of the left internal carotid artery is present.

for the few postoperative deaths that occur after carotid endarterectomy.[10,11] Even more importantly, myocardial infarctions account for as many as 70 percent of all late deaths following successful extracranial arterial reconstruction and are especially common among patients suspected to have CAD on clinical grounds.[11-17] The incidence of fatal myocardial infarction during the late postoperative interval after carotid endarterectomy at the Cleveland Clinic has been shown to equal or surpass the total incidence of both fatal and non-fatal stroke in all age groups.[18] Accordingly, coronary angiography has been routinely employed before elective extracranial and other peripheral arterial operations at this institution since 1978.[19]

MANAGEMENT CONSIDERATIONS

Incidental Carotid Artery Disease

Although the topic has generated considerable controversy, the risk of postoperative stroke after cardiac or major peripheral vascular procedures among patients having severe, associated carotid artery disease *documented*

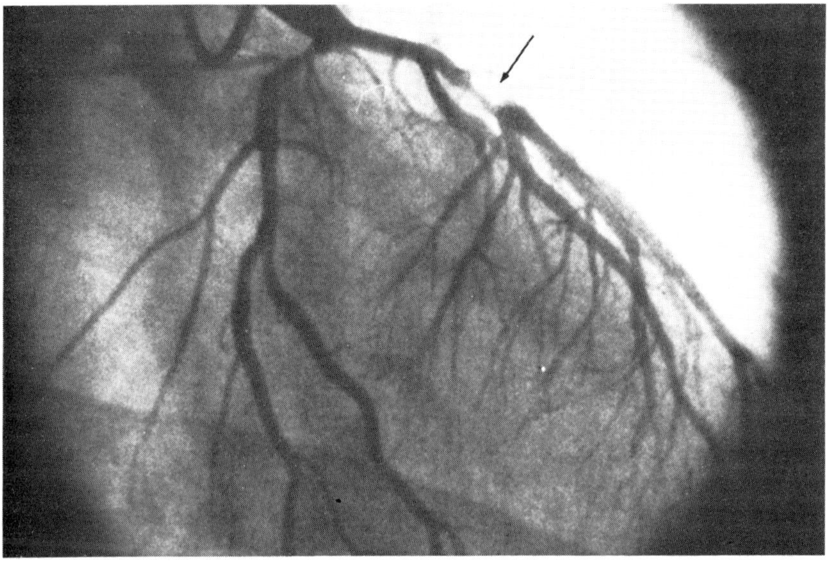

Figure 26-2. Cine coronary angiogram demonstrating severe stenosis of the left anterior descending coronary artery in a patient with symptomatic carotid occlusive disease.

by angiography has never been determined. Retrospective reports, such as those by Carney et al.[20] and Treiman et al.[21] have suggested that the incidence of perioperative stroke at the time of abdominal aortic reconstruction is no higher among patients with previous neurologic symptoms or asymptomatic cervical bruits than among those having no clinical indication of extracranial arterial disease. These and other similar retrospective studies have obvious limitations. Their conclusions are not based upon any objective assessment of the status of the carotid arteries and, even if appropriate for patients having elective aortoiliac revascularization, are not clearly applicable to those undergoing aortocoronary procedures in the setting of controlled hypotension required during cardiopulmonary bypass.

Other investigations have employed noninvasive cerebrovascular testing to quantitate the severity and risk of associated carotid disease in patients scheduled for other cardiovascular operations. Using such an approach, Barnes et al.[22] and Turnipseed et al.[23] reported that the incidence of postoperative stroke after myocardial revascularization was not significantly greater among those having positive noninvasive studies preoperatively. Although one of these reports[22] demonstrated a 15 percent incidence of neurologic symptoms within the first two years after abnormal noninvasive testing and the other[23] did not address the problem of late stroke, neither recommended that formal angiography or surgical management be considered even among patients with objective evidence of carotid disease. In comparison, Brewster et al.[24] obtained cerebral angiography on the basis of noninvasive test results in 31 of 100 consecutive patients with asymptomatic carotid bruits, and 19 of these 31 patients required endarterectomy. In this study, no late strokes occurred during follow-up periods of 6 to 21 months in patients who had normal noninvasive examinations or carotid reconstruction, including 34 who had other cardiovascular operations during this interval.

The ominous implications of symptomatic carotid atherosclerosis are universally accepted as indications for prompt angiographic investigation and appropriate arterial reconstruction to prevent eventual strokes. In addition, Thompson et al.[17] have demonstrated a statistically significant difference in the incidence of transient cerebral ischemic attacks (TIA) and late strokes in patients with asymptomatic carotid bifurcation bruits that were not evaluated by angiography. In this careful, long-term study of 270 patients, previously asymptomatic carotid bruits have been associated with eventual TIA in 27 percent of patients and with late strokes in 17 percent within a period of 20 to 32 months after their discovery, whereas only 4.5 percent of comparable patients have sustained either TIA or strokes during the same interval after prophylactic carotid endarterectomy. Cooperman et al.[25] have reported similar information in a series of 256 patients found to have asymptomatic carotid bruits at the time of lower extremity revascularization. Subsequent strokes occurred in 15 percent of patients having carotid bruits and in 4 percent of those without evidence of carotid disease, while TIA occurred in 20 percent and 12 percent of these two groups, respectively.

Clearly, obvious evidence of extracranial carotid disease, indicated on the basis of previous neurologic symptoms, physical examination, or noninvasive cerebrovascular testing, should not be disregarded in patients scheduled for other cardiovascular procedures simply on the grounds that the risk for perioperative stroke at the time of these other operations is low. Associated carotid disease should be evaluated and corrected on its own merit to avoid late neurologic complications, even if staged procedures before or after coronary artery bypass or other vascular operations are preferred.

Incidental Coronary Artery Disease

Although patients with severe carotid atherosclerosis comprise a relatively small subset of all those who require myocardial revascularization, the late mortality rate caused by myocardial infarction after carotid reconstruction suggests that CAD is far more prevalent in patients with recognized carotid disease. Improved patient selection and advances in the technology of intraoperative cerebral protection have enhanced the immediate safety of extracranial surgical procedures during the past 15 years, but the impact of fatal myocardial infarction on the late survival rate following successful operations has remained remarkably constant.

In a previous report from the Cleveland Clinic, postoperative survival rates at 5 years and at 10 years were 73 percent and 18 percent for all patients undergoing carotid endarterectomy, 78 percent and 24 percent for patients without clinical evidence of CAD, and 70 percent and 14 percent for those suspected to have CAD who did not undergo coronary angiography or myocardial revascularization.[11] Fatal myocardial infarctions caused 37 percent of the deaths that occurred within 5 years of operation and 38 percent of those occurring within ten years. In 1965, DeBakey et al.[14] reported 5-year survival rates of 68 percent for all patients following extracranial operations, 83 percent for patients without clinical evidence of CAD, and 64 percent for patients suspected to have CAD. DeWeese et al.[15] subsequently described a 5-year survival rate following carotid endarterectomy of 66 percent and found that myocardial infarctions caused 71 percent of all late deaths involving 24 percent of their entire series. Thompson et al.[16,17] observed that myocardial infarctions accounted for approximately three times the number of late deaths in patients with carotid atherosclerosis than did stroke, irrespective of whether the extracranial disease received surgical correction or no treatment at all.

In comparison, patients with documented CAD who undergo direct myocardial revascularization have been reported to sustain fewer cardiac complications after subsequent vascular and other major operations than otherwise would be expected. Ennix et al.[10] found that perioperative myocardial infarctions occurred at the time of carotid endarterectomy in 13 percent of patients who had angina pectoris and in only 0.8 percent of patients who had no clinical evidence of CAD. In this series of 1238 patients who underwent 1546 carotid procedures, the operative mortality rates were 1.5 percent for patients without CAD, 18 percent for those with angina pectoris who underwent carotid endarterectomy alone, and 3 percent for those with angina pectoris who had simultaneous carotid endarterectomy and myocardial revascularization. Crawford et al.[26] presented a series of 358 patients who required 484 subsequent operations at various intervals following direct myocardial revascularization, including 308 vascular procedures in 232 patients. Only four operative deaths (0.8 percent) occurred following these subsequent procedures, and only 12 patients (3 percent) died from cardiac causes within a 5-year follow-up period. The 5-year actuarial survival for 97 patients with carotid atherosclerosis and CAD was 73 percent following carotid endarterectomy alone and was 88 percent following carotid endarterectomy performed in conjunction with aortocoronary bypass. Such differences may become even more obvious in the future, as late survival after myocardial revascularization continues to improve because of technical advances and contemporary attempts to provide complete revascularization with multiple coronary bypass grafts.

Table 26-1 contains data concerning cumulative survival after combined carotid endarterectomy and myocardial revascularization for patients with

Table 26-1
Comparison of cumulative survival after combined carotid endarterectomy and coronary artery bypass with the results of previous reports for carotid endarterectomy alone.

Series	Patients	Cumulative Survival		
		1 Year	3 Years	5 Years
DeBakey et al.[14] (1965)	761	.913	.821	.723
DeWeese et al.[15] (1973)	102	.900	.770	.660
Bouchard et al.[13] (1975)	227	.911	.835	.777
Cleveland Clinic[11] (1981)	325	.941	.831	.726
Cleveland Clinic (combined)	289	.967	.925	.831

simultaneous carotid and coronary disease at the Cleveland Clinic,[27] together with comparable results that have been presented in previous reports after carotid endarterectomy alone.[11,13-15] Actuarial survival at 1, 3, and 5 years for patients whose CAD was documented and corrected by myocardial revascularization is consistently superior to that for patients whose preoperative evaluations generally were limited to their cerebrovascular circulation. From this perspective, it appears that recognition and management of severe, surgically correctable coronary atherosclerosis in patients with known carotid disease is as important as the diagnosis of carotid atherosclerosis among those already scheduled for myocardial revascularization.

SURGICAL APPROACH

Staged Carotid and Coronary Artery Procedures

A previous report from the Cleveland Clinic presented the early results of staged carotid endarterectomy preceding elective myocardial revascularization.[6] In a series of 59 patients who required a total of 65 carotid procedures, permanent postoperative strokes occurred after 1.5 percent of carotid operations but were entirely avoided at the time of subsequent aortocoronary bypass. Although the neurologic complication rate for staged operations is comparable to that for carotid endarterectomy under optimal circumstances, other studies have shown that serious cardiac complications may occur in some patients during the staging interval before myocardial revascularization. Bernhard et al.[5] and Morris et al.[8] encountered myocardial infarctions in 15 percent to 20 percent of patients during the period between prophylactic carotid endarterectomy and subsequent aortocoronary bypass, and recommended that simultaneous carotid and coronary operations should be seriously considered in order to reduce this risk.

Because of the possibility of interval complications between staged procedures, simultaneous carotid endarterectomy and myocardial revascularization presently are performed for most patients with severe or unstable CAD and associated carotid disease at the Cleveland Clinic. Nevertheless, staged operations are still preferred for (1) patients with chronic, stable angina pectoris without recent myocardial infarction or congestive heart failure, (2) stable patients who are candidates for coronary artery reoperation, (3) the rare asymptomatic patient with severe coronary atherosclerosis, and (4) patients with frequent TIA and severe carotid stenosis who are obviously in jeopardy of impending stroke unless immediate carotid endarterectomy is performed. In an attempt to eliminate the chance for cardiac complications between operations, myocardial revascularization usually is scheduled during the same hospital admission within 7 to 10 days after carotid endarterectomy.

Combined Carotid and Coronary Artery Procedures

Simultaneous carotid endarterectomy and myocardial revascularization are advisable for patients with associated carotid disease who have (1) severe lesions of the left main coronary artery, (2) diffuse CAD without satisfactory collateral circulation, and (3) severe CAD and any form of unstable angina pectoris. From 1973 through 1981, combined operations have been performed in 331 patients (mean age, 61 years) at the Cleveland Clinic, a subset representing 1.7 percent of the total of 22,100 patients (mean age, 54 years) who underwent myocardial revascularization at this institution during the same period of study.[27]

Technical Aspects

Early in this study period, median sternotomy customarily was performed as the initial procedure so that prompt cannulation for cardiopulmonary bypass could be done if myocardial function deteriorated during carotid endarterectomy. Because of advances in anesthetic techniques and the pharmacologic support of cardiac performance, carotid endarterectomy in recent years has been completed before sternotomy with substantial savings in operative blood loss. Since harvesting and preparation of the saphenous vein for aortocoronary grafting have usually been done at the same time as carotid endarterectomy, combined procedures have extended operating time only 45 minutes to 1 hour beyond that required for myocardial revascularization alone. Complete hemostasis and closure of the cervical incision were always delayed until intraoperative anticoagulation had been reversed and sternotomy closure had been completed.

Fifty-nine (18 percent) of the 331 patients had single aortocoronary grafts, 131 (40 percent) had double grafts, 113 (34 percent) had triple grafts, and 28 (8 percent) had four or more grafts. During carotid endarterectomy, an indwelling carotid shunt was inserted in 274 patients (83 percent), and only three of 185 operations since 1978 have been performed without shunts. Perfusion of the ipsilateral internal carotid artery was rarely interrupted for longer than 3 to 4 minutes during any operation done with the use of a shunt.

Patient Characteristics and Early Results

Of these 331 patients, 195 (58 percent) had functional Class III-IV angina pectoris, 308 (93 percent) had multiple-vessel CAD, 68 (21 percent) had over 50 percent stenosis of the left main coronary artery, and 185 (56 percent) had either segmental or diffuse impairment of left ventricular function. Severe, asymptomatic carotid stenosis that usually compromised lumen diameter by more than 70 percent was documented in 173 patients (52 percent), while the remaining 158 had experienced either TIA (38 percent) or completed strokes. Figure 26-3 contains graphic representation of the preoperative cardiac status and postoperative complications for the 331 patients who had combined operations, as well as for the group of 22,100 patients from whom they were selected. Differences in the prevalence of triple-vessel disease ($p < .01$), of left main coronary involvement ($p < .001$), and of ventricular impairment ($p < .01$) were statistically significant.

The hospital mortality rate for all 22,100 patients having myocardial revascularization from 1973 through 1981 was 1.9 percent. Postoperative strokes occurred in 1.8 percent, and 2.8 percent experienced perioperative myocardial infarctions. The mortality rate for the 331 patients who had combined operations was 5.7 percent. Postoperative neurologic deficits occurred in 9.0 percent, of which 4.5 percent were permanent, and 6.3 percent had perioperative myocardial infarctions. All of these differences were highly significant ($p < .001$). As indicated in Figure 1, however, associated extra-cranial disease was not the only risk factor identified in the study group. Mean age and the prevalence of left main coronary stenosis, multiple-vessel CAD, and impaired ventricular function in these patients were significantly higher than those found in the majority of patients without cerebrovascular disease undergoing myocardial revascularization. In addition, statistical data alone do not entirely reflect the desperate clinical situation of many of these patients who had incapacitating angina pectoris and diffuse CAD, compounded by impending stroke or severe carotid stenosis.

Table 26-2 contains comparable data concerning surgical management and the incidence of postoperative complications after combined procedures

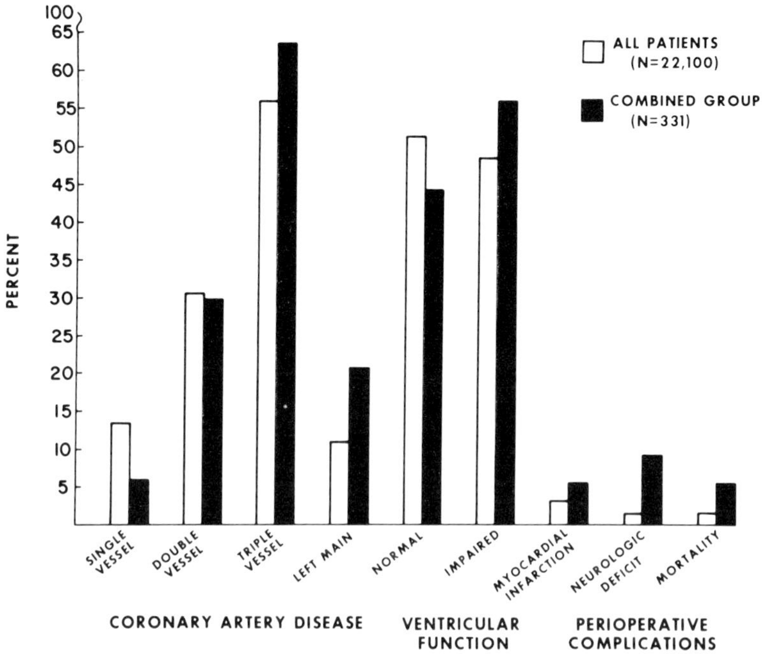

Figure 26-3. Graphic representation of the prevalence of preoperative risk factors and the incidence of postoperative complications for 331 patients who had combined operations at the Cleveland Clinic from 1973 to 1981, as well as for a total of 22,100 patients undergoing myocardial revascularization during this interval.

Table 26-2
Technical considerations and results during consecutive series of combined carotid and coronary operations at the Cleveland Clinic.[27]

Factors and Results	1973–1977 (N = 146) No.	%	1978–1981 (N = 185) No.	%
Coronary Artery				
Single bypass graft	35	24	24	13
Double grafts	67	46	64	35
Three or more grafts	44	30	97	52
Perioperative myocardial infarction	13	8.9	8	4.3
Operative mortality	8	5.5	11	5.9
Carotid Artery				
Intraoperative shunting	90	62	182	98
Perioperative neurologic deficit	18	12.3	12	6.6

during two consecutive periods of study, 1973 to 1977 (146 patients) and 1978 to 1981 (185 patients). During these intervals, there were obvious trends favoring multiple aortocoronary bypass grafting and the routine use of intraoperative carotid shunting. Together with advances in anesthetic methods, intraoperative myocardial protection, and the technology of postoperative care, these trends appear to be reflected in an improved incidence of perioperative myocardial infarction and neurologic deficit. This improvement has not yet achieved statistical significance, however, and the mortality rate for combined myocardial revascularization and carotid endarterectomy has remained relatively constant.

Late Survival

Three hundred thirteen of the 331 patients have survived combined procedures. For the purpose of this text, complete late information at a mean postoperative interval of 41 months has been obtained for all 289 patients whose operations were performed prior to July 1981. Thirty-seven (13 percent) of these 289 patients died at a mean interval of 34 months, and 24 (65 percent) of deaths were caused by cardiovascular diseases. Annual late mortality has ranged from 1.7 percent to 7.8 percent, and the 5-year cumulative survival presently is 83 percent ± 6 percent (S.D.). Figure 26-4 provides graphic representation of life table survival for these patients, for a normal

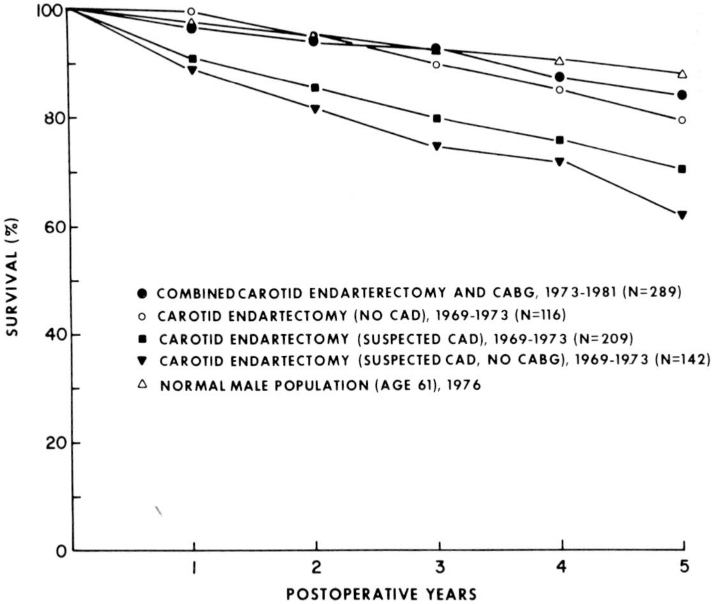

Figure 26-4. Life table survival curves for 289 patients after combined operations, for a normal male population of the same age,[28] and for 325 patients who survived carotid endarterectomy at the Cleveland Clinic from 1969 to 1973.[11]

male population of the same age (61 years),[28] and for 325 patients (mean age, 60 years) who survived carotid endarterectomy at the Cleveland Clinic from 1969 through 1973.[11] The 325 patients in this previous series include 116 who had no clinical evidence of CAD at the time of carotid endarterectomy and 209 who were suspected to have CAD on the basis of either the cardiac history or the preoperative electrocardiogram. Of the 209 patients suspected to have CAD, 67 eventually underwent coronary angiography and direct myocardial revascularization, while 142 had no further diagnostic studies with regard to cardiac disease.

Actuarial survival for the 289 patients who survived combined myocardial revascularization and carotid endarterectomy was not statistically different from that for the normal population or for patients without clinical indications of CAD who underwent carotid endarterectomy in the 1969-1973 series. Cumulative 5-year survival for patients with suspected but undocumented CAD from the earlier series was 62 percent ± 13 percent (S.D.). The difference in 5-year survival between patients in this subset and those who had combined operations exceeded two standard deviations and was statistically valid ($p < .005$).

Normal left ventricular function was present in 133 of the 289 patients surviving combined procedures, while 156 others had either segmental or diffuse ventricular impairment. Cumulative 5-year survival of 83 percent for each of these 2 subsets was identical (Fig. 26-5A). Fifty-seven patients had single coronary grafts, 118 had double grafts, and 114 had three or more grafts. Five-year actuarial survival for each of these subsets was 66 percent, 87 percent, and 92 percent, respectively (Fig. 26-5B). The difference in cumulative survival among patients receiving single grafts, the majority of whom had severe CAD but only limited targets for revascularization, did not achieve statistical significance. Crude late mortality, however, included 26 percent of those with single grafts, 8.5 percent of those with double grafts, and 5.3 percent of those with three or more grafts.

One hundred forty of the 289 patients had experienced neurologic symptoms preceding their combined operations, while the remaining 149 had asymptomatic carotid stenosis. Five-year cumulative survival rates for these two subsets were 81 percent and 84 percent, respectively (Fig. 26-6A). Unilateral carotid stenosis was present in 176 patients, and bilateral carotid disease exceeding 50 percent lumen stenosis had been documented in 113. Five-year actuarial survival was 86 percent for patients with unilateral carotid disease and was 78 percent for those having bilateral carotid stenosis (Fig. 26-6B). None of these differences was statistically significant.

Late Neurologic Complications

Eighteen (6.1 percent) of the 289 patients in the follow-up group have experienced late strokes at intervals of 4 to 85 months postoperatively (mean, 30 months). Limited clinical information was available for three of these

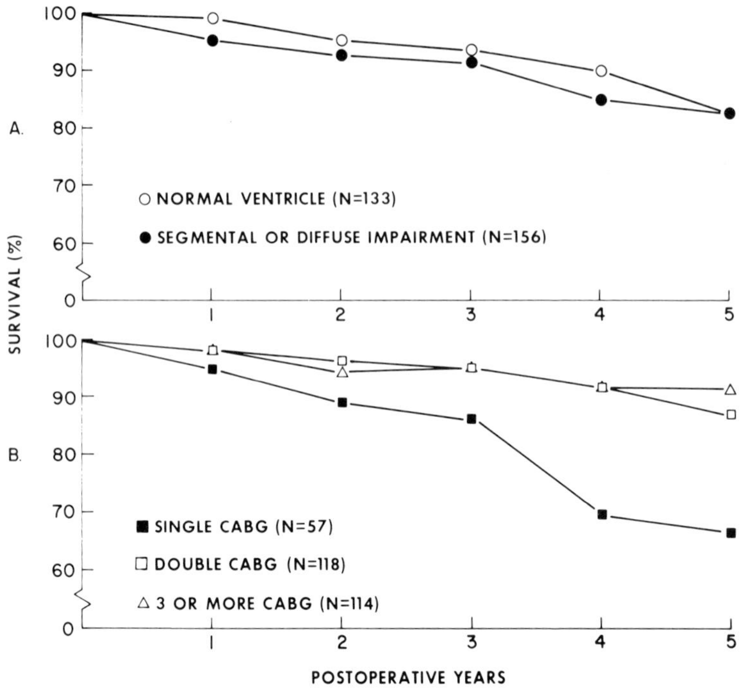

Figure 26-5. Life table survival curves after combined operations for (A) patients with normal ventricular function and those with segmental or diffuse ventricular impairment, and (B) patients having single, double, and three or more coronary artery bypass grafts (CABG).

patients. Of the remaining 15, late strokes appeared to involve the cerebral cortex on the same side as combined carotid endarterectomy in five (1.7 percent), the contralateral cerebral hemisphere in seven (2.4 percent), and the brainstem in three (1.0 percent). Four of these strokes were fatal.

Ten (5.3 percent) of 189 patients with less than 50 percent stenosis of the contralateral internal carotid artery at the time of combined carotid endarterectomy have developed late strokes. In comparison, late strokes have occurred in six (9.1 percent) of 66 patients who had over 50 percent stenosis of the contralateral internal carotid artery and in two (5.9 percent) of 34 patients with documented contralateral internal carotid occlusion. These differences were not statistically significant.

Additional Cardiovascular Operations

Fifty-seven patients (20 percent) have required a total of 67 elective peripheral vascular operations at some time after combined carotid endarterectomy and myocardial revascularization. Contralateral carotid reconstruction has been performed in 28 patients. Twelve of these patients

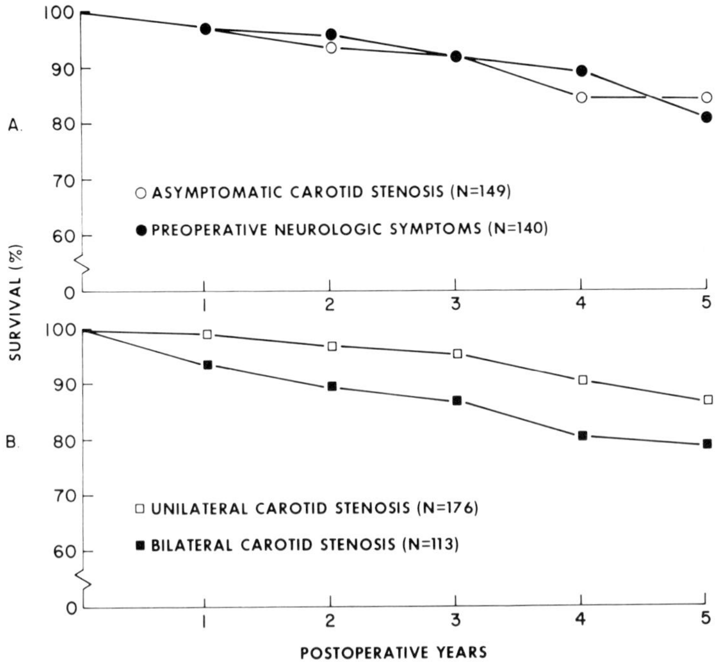

Figure 26-6. Life table survival curves after combined operations for (A) patients with asymptomatic carotid stenosis and those having preoperative neurologic symptoms, and (B) patients with unilateral carotid stenosis and those with bilateral carotid disease.

had planned, staged procedures to correct contralateral carotid disease that had been demonstrated at the time of their initial cerebral angiography, while 18 incidentally developed new neurologic symptoms or contralateral carotid stenosis during the late postoperative period. Three other patients have required reoperations because of recurrent carotid stenosis. The remaining 36 patients have undergone elective aortic aneurysm resection (11), aortoiliac (13) or femoropopliteal (7) reconstruction, renal revascularization (3), profundaplasty (1), or lumbar sympathectomy (1). Two postoperative deaths occurred, for a patient mortality of 3.5 percent and a procedure mortality of 3.0 percent.

SUMMARY

Experience with both staged and combined carotid endarterectomy and myocardial revascularization at the Cleveland Clinic indicates that either approach may be applied with a reasonable margin of safety in carefully selected patients with severe, simultaneous carotid and coronary artery disease. Routine surgical management of severe carotid disease demonstrated by angiography does not resolve the controversy concerning whether carotid reconstruction reduces the risk for stroke during myocardial revascularization, even though this risk is likely to be heavily concentrated among those who are proven to be candidates for either staged or combined procedures. The fundamental importance of late results in patients with severe, simultaneous carotid and coronary artery disease, however, too often is not addressed by studies that are limited to early postoperative complications. Since elective surgical correction of documented, simultaneous disease is associated with excellent late survival and a low incidence of subsequent stroke, it should be a serious consideration for a small but critical group of patients.

ACKNOWLEDGEMENTS

Mrs. Ramona Zurrer and Mr. Eric Christiansen, Research Associates, coordinated the retrieval of late postoperative data. Miss Geri Locher, Research Division, provided the statistical analysis. Miss Linda Maljovec assisted in preparation of the manuscript.

REFERENCES

1. Ashor GW, Meyer BW, Lindesmith GG, et al: Coronary artery disease. Surgery in 100 patients 65 years of age and older. Arch Surg 107:30, 1973
2. Brewer AC, Furlan AJ, Hanson MR, et al: Neurologic complications of open heart surgery. Computer-assisted analysis of 531 patients. Cleve Clin Quart 48:205, 1981
3. Loop FD, Cosgrove DM, Lytle BW, et al: An 11 year evolution of coronary arterial surgery (1967–1978). Ann Surg 190:444, 1979
4. Reul WJ, Morris GC Jr, Howell JF, et al: Current concepts in coronary artery surgery. A critical analysis of 1,287 patients. Ann Thorac Surg 14:243, 1972
5. Bernhard VM, Johnson WD, Peterson JJ: Carotid artery stenosis. Association with surgery for coronary artery disease. Arch Surg 105:837, 1972
6. Hertzer NR, Loop FD, Taylor PC, et al: Staged and combined surgical approach to simultaneous carotid and coronary vascular disease. Surgery 84:803, 1978
7. Mehigan JT, Buch WS, Pipkin RD, et al: A planned approach to coexistent cerebrovascular disease in coronary artery bypass candidates. Arch Surg 112:1403, 1977
8. Morris GC Jr, Ennix CL Jr, Lawrie GM, et al: Management of coexistent carotid and coronary artery occlusive atherosclerosis. Cleve Clin Quart 45:125, 1977
9. Rice PL, Pifarre R, Sullivan JH, et al: Experience with simultaneous myocardial revascularization and carotid endarterectomy. J Thorac Cardiovasc Surg 79:922, 1980
10. Ennix CL Jr, Lawrie GM, Morris GC Jr, et al: Improved results of carotid endarterectomy in patients with symptomatic coronary disease: An analysis of 1,548 consecutive carotid operations. Stroke 10:122, 1979

11. Hertzer NR, Lees CD: Fatal myocardial infarction following carotid endarterectomy. Three hundred thirty-five patients followed 6-11 years after operation. Ann Surg 194:212, 1981
12. Bauer RB, Meyer JS, Fields WS, et al: Joint study of extracranial arterial occlusion. III. Progress report of controlled study of long-term survival in patients with and without operation. JAMA 208:509, 1969
13. Bouchard JP, Fabia J, Simard D, et al: Carotid endarterectomy: Survival of 227 patients. CMA J 113:949, 1975
14. DeBakey ME, Crawford ES, Cooley DA, et al: Cerebral arterial insufficiency: One to 11-year results following arterial reconstructive operation. Ann Surg 161:921, 1965
15. DeWeese JA, Rob CG, Satran R, et al: Results of carotid endarterectomies for transient ischemic attacks—five years later. Ann Surg 178:258, 1973
16. Thompson JE, Austin DJ, Patman RD: Carotid endarterectomy for cerebrovascular insufficiency: Long-term results in 592 patients followed up to thirteen years. Ann Surg 172:663, 1970
17. Thompson JE, Patman RD, Talkington CM: Asymptomatic carotid bruit: Long-term outcome of patients having endarterectomy compared with unoperated controls. Ann Surg 188:308, 1978
18. Lees CD, Hertzer NR: Postoperative stroke and late neurologic complications after carotid endarterectomy. Arch Surg 116:1561, 1981
19. Hertzer NR, Young JR, Kramer JR, et al: Routine coronary angiography prior to elective aortic reconstruction. Arch Surg 114:1336, 1979
20. Carney WI Jr, Stewart WB, DePinto DJ, et al: Carotid bruit as a risk factor in aortoiliac reconstruction. Surgery 81:567, 1977
21. Treiman RL, Foran RF, Shore EH, et al: Carotid bruit. Significance in patients undergoing an abdominal aortic operation. Arch Surg 106:803, 1973
22. Barnes RW, Liebman PR, Marszalek PB: The natural history of asymptomatic carotid disease in patients undergoing cardiovascular surgery. Surgery 90:1075, 1981
23. Turnipseed WD, Berkoff HA, Belzer FO: Postoperative stroke in cardiac and peripheral vascular disease. Ann Surg 192:365, 1980
24. Brewster DC, Schlaen HH, Raines JK, et al: Rational management of the asymptomatic carotid bruit. Arch Surg 113:927, 1978
25. Cooperman M, Martin EW Jr, Evans WE: Significance of asymptomatic carotid bruits. Arch Surg 113:1339, 1978
26. Crawford ES, Morris GC Jr, Howell JF, et al: Operative risk in patients with previous coronary artery bypass. Ann Thorac Surg 26:215, 1978
27. Hertzer NR, Loop FD, Beven EG, et al: Combined myocardial revascularization and carotid endarterectomy. Operative and late results in 331 patients. J Thorac Cardiovasc Surg (in press)
28. National Center for Health Statistics: Vital Statistics of the United States (1976), Vol. II-Mortality, Part A, Table 5
29. Cutler SJ, Ederer F: Maximum utilization of the life table method in analyzing survival. J Chron Dis 8:699, 1958

Patricio Welsh
Roberto Pradier
Roberto Repetto

27

High Exposure of the Carotid Artery for Difficult Lesions

When fibromuscular dysplasia of the carotid artery was first described in the late 1960s,[1-4] it was thought to be a rare condition. Now, it is recognized as a cause of transient cerebrovascular symptoms, and surgical treatment has been proposed for patients who are symptomatic. Because the lesions of fibromuscular dysplasia are largely inaccessible, intraluminal dilation has been the surgical procedure of choice.

Blaisdell et al.[5] have suggested that the limits of accessibility of carotid lesions are defined by an imaginary line drawn on the arteriogram from the angle of the mandible to the tip of the mastoid process (Fig. 27-1). The purpose of this report is to describe the surgical technique which allows distal exposure and reconstruction of formerly inaccessible lesions. Much credit goes to Dr. Edwin Wylie[6] for the original idea. He not only published the first case report of this technique but was kind enough to explain it to the author personally.

PATIENT POPULATION

Cases coming to surgery on our unit consisted of 7 patients: 2 men and 5 women. Their ages ranged from 42 to 49 years, with the exception of 1 woman who was 66. All patients had transient ischemic attacks in the carotid artery territory appropriate to the surgical procedure. Hemiparesis was present in 5 patients, brachial paresis and aphasia in 1, and amaurosis fugax in 1. All patients experienced repetitive transient neurologic deficits. More than three episodes were recorded in 2 cases, and 1 exceptional patient had 90 episodes in

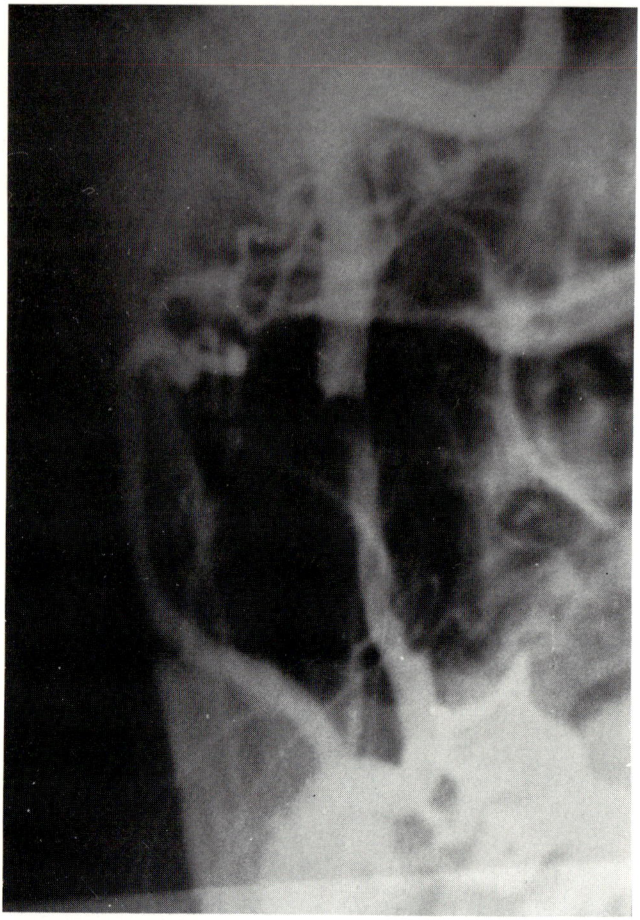

Figure 27-3. Close-up view of the arteriogram shown in Figure 26-2.

SURGICAL TECHNIQUE

The object of this technique of carotid surgery is to obtain safe exposure of the distal 6 to 8 cm of the internal carotid artery just below the entrance of the carotid into the calvarium. Access to this portion of the internal carotid artery is prevented by the vertical ramus of the mandible.

The angled cervical incision begins at the level of the tragus, proceeds 2 cm below the angle of the mandible, and then proceeds forward horizontally, parallel to the border of the mandible. The facial nerve is identified and exposed distally beyond its bifurcation. The mandibular insertion of the masseter muscle is sectioned and retracted upwards, exposing the bone to the

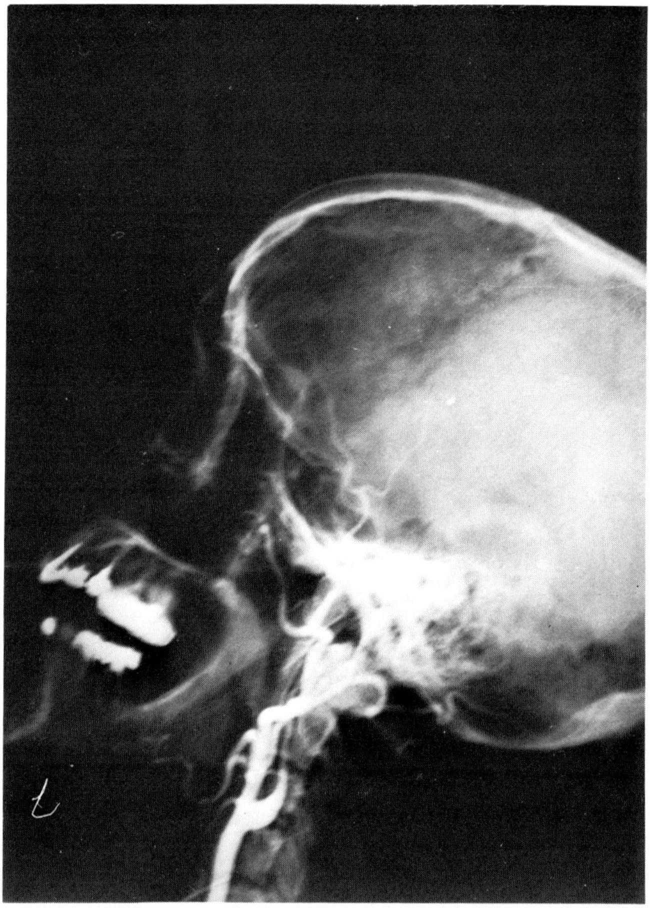

Figure 27-4. Arteriogram showing complete occlusion of the internal carotid artery.

mandibular notch. A subperiosteal osteotomy is done from the angle of the mandible to the notch. Two holes are drilled on either side of the proposed osteotomy before the bone is sectioned. Care should be taken to place the osteotomy as far posteriorly as possible in order to avoid injury to the inferior dental nerve. The anterior segment of the mandible is retracted forward, while the posterior segment with the parotid gland is rotated upward, over the temporomandibular joint.

Following division of the digastric muscle at its mastoid insertion, and the styloid process at its base, the hypoglossal and glossopharyngeal nerves are easily identified. They lie over the internal carotid artery, as shown in Figure 27-9.

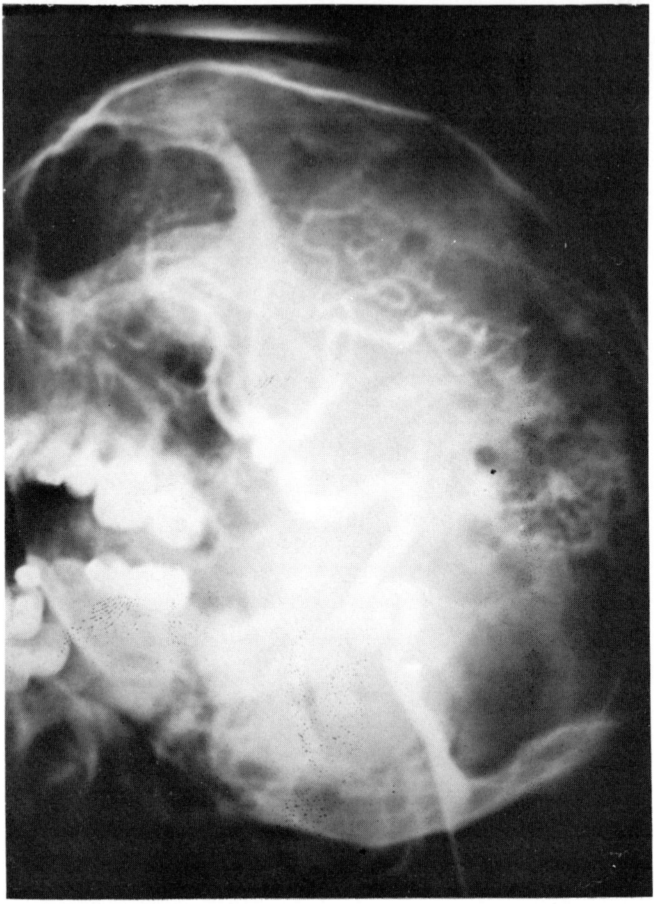

Figure 27-5. Arteriogram performed 2 months later shows a patent internal carotid artery with a saccular aneurysm due to fibromuscular hyperplasia.

The occipital artery, a branch of the external carotid, is divided in order to provide exposure of the entire carotid artery up to the base of the skull. Although the operative field is small, usually 1 to 2 cm of normal internal carotid artery can be identified below the base of the skull. It is in this area that an occluding clamp can be placed.

In 6 cases, resection of the diseased segment of the internal carotid artery was performed. This was replaced with autogenous saphenous vein in end-to-end fashion. The length of the resected segment varied from 3 to 7 cm. Thus, both the proximal and distal anastomoses were performed on the internal

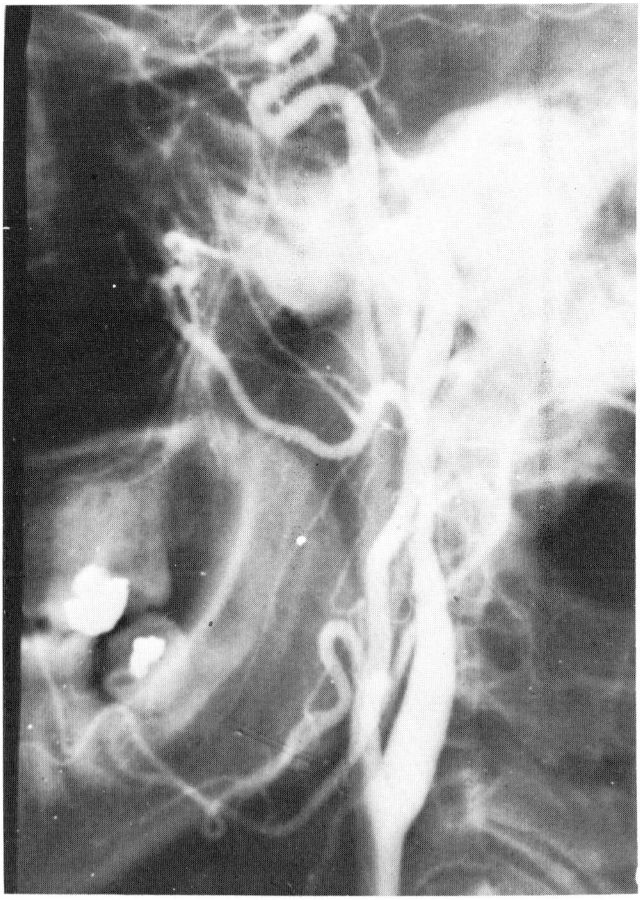

Figure 27-6. Carotid arteriogram showing stenosis of the internal carotid artery in a lateral position.

carotid artery. In all of these cases, the bifurcation of the carotid artery was normal.

As the vein graft was placed end-to-end to the proximal and distal internal carotid artery, the glossopharyngeal nerve was left in its place behind the vein graft. No intraluminal shunt was used in any of the 6 cases operated upon.

In one instance, the disease process was a dissection of the internal carotid artery extending through the foramen. In this instance, the lesion could not be corrected and the internal carotid artery was ligated.

No dental ligatures were used, but the mandible was reunited with wires passed through the previously placed holes on either side of the osteotomy.

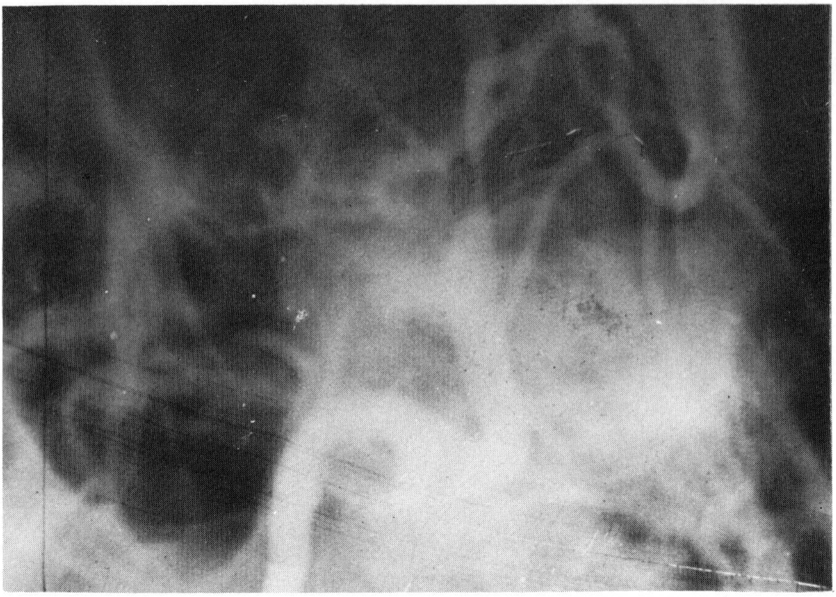

Figure 27-7. Frontal view of the lesion shown in Figure 26-6.

RESULTS OF SURGICAL THERAPY

Six patients had uneventful postoperative courses without neurologic symptoms. One patient had a postoperative hemiplegia, with partial recovery. The follow-up on these cases ranged from 18 months to 7 years. Postoperative arteriography was obtained in 3 cases (Figs. 27-10-27-12). Oculoplethysmography[7] was performed at yearly intervals, and, in all cases, normal OPG tracings have been obtained.

Four of the 7 patients had a peripheral facial palsy caused by traction on the facial nerve. In all instances, this remitted within 1 to 3 months. There have been no complications caused by the osteotomy of the mandible, and oral feedings were resumed on the second postoperative day in all instances. While there were no swallowing problems, actual chewing was restricted for a 3-week period postoperatively.

PATHOLOGY OF FIBROMUSCULAR DYSPLASIA

All segments of artery removed were subjected to pathologic study, and alterations were found in the intima, media, and adventitia in all cases. The

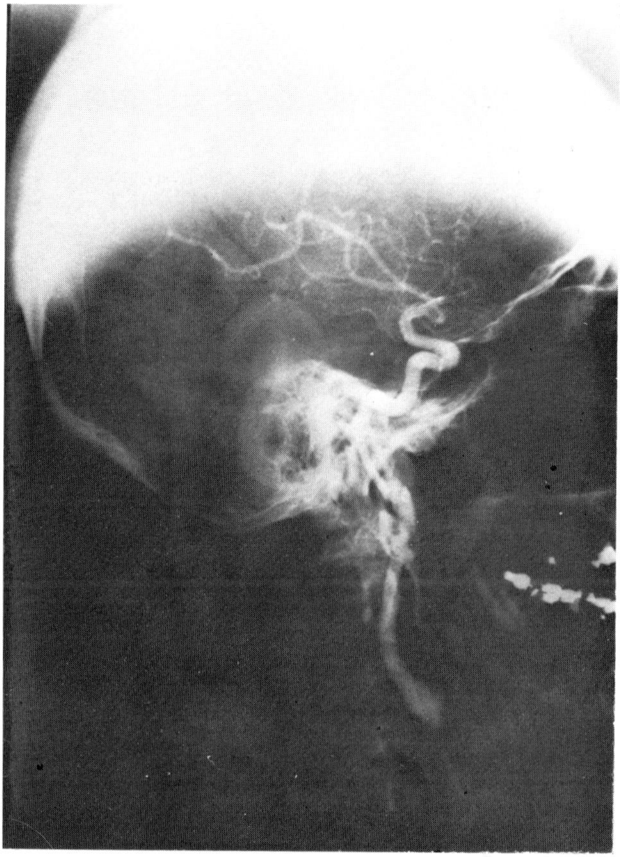

Figure 27-8. Dissecting aneurysm of the internal carotid artery.

most significant findings were in the media where smooth muscle was replaced by fibrous connective tissue. The medial and intimal fibrosis were apparently caused by the stenosis demonstrated on the arteriogram. The internal elastic lamina showed fragmentation and irregular thickening.

In 2 cases, a dissecting aneurysm with rupture of the intima was seen (Figs. 27-13 and 27-14). In both, it was a complication of a previously existing fibromuscular dysplasia. One of these was in the 44-year-old woman previously described, whose symptoms began after a motor vehicle accident.

In 1 case, a saccular aneurysm was the only finding and, in this instance, the arteriogram performed after a transient ischemic episode showed a complete occlusion while a later arteriogram showed patency of the artery.

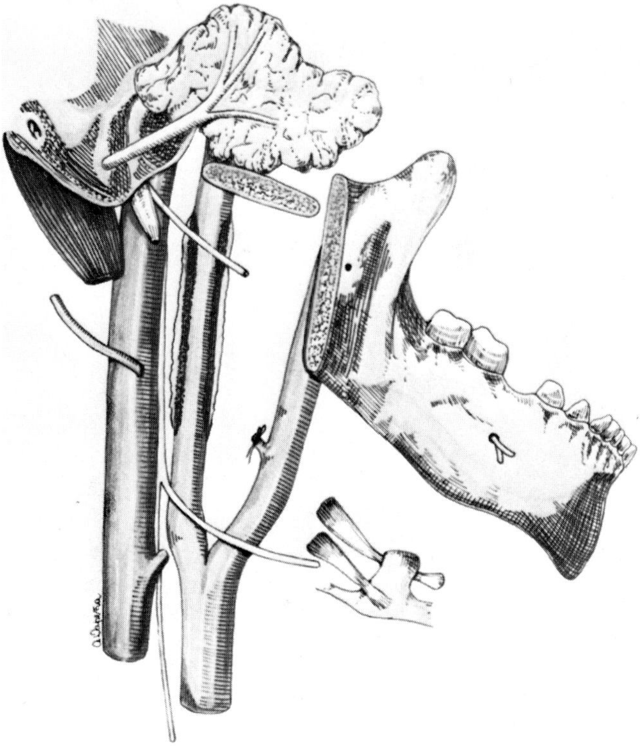

Figure 27-9. Artist's representation of the operative field.

DISCUSSION

While arteriosclerotic stenoses and occlusions of the internal carotid artery occur at the bifurcation, the lesions of fibromuscular dysplasia occur more distally. Fibromuscular dysplasia of the internal carotid artery is uncommon, and its natural history is not known. There is no doubt that it can produce severe neurologic deficit. Wylie and Ehrenfeld[6] reported a 22 percent incidence of stroke in such patients, and prolonged or transient neurologic deficits or amaurosis fugax occurred in two-thirds of their 86 patients. It is not surprising that the surgical patients described by Wylie and Ehrenfeld were strongly symptomatic as, at this time, surgery is not advocated in asymptomatic patients.

The pathogenetic mechanisms of symptom production in patients with fibromuscular dysplasia of the internal carotid artery are still poorly understood. It is probable that flow reduction occurs, and that this is caused by turbulence in the arterial stream resulting from alternating stenosis and

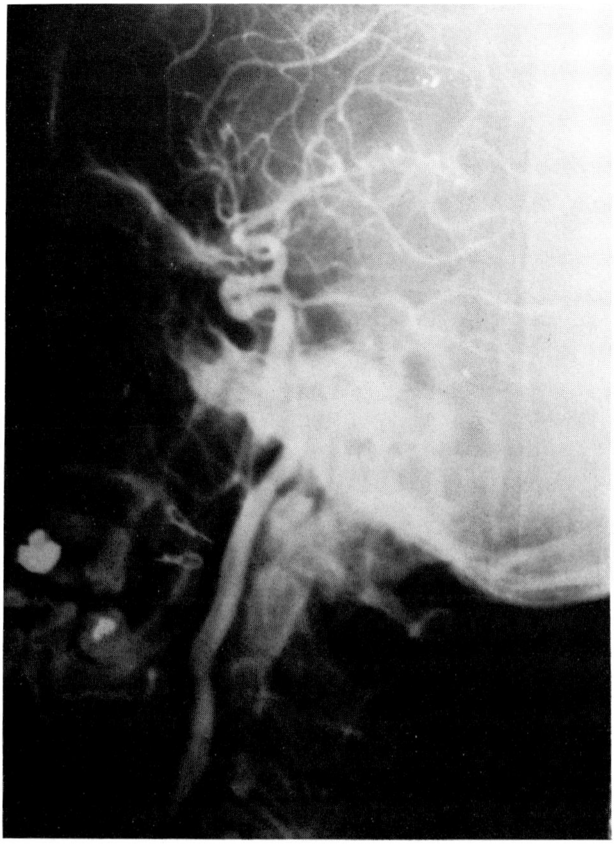

Figure 27-10. Postoperative carotid arteriogram following replacement of the internal carotid artery with vein graft. The mandible is sutured with wire.

dilation of the artery. Embolization of fibrino-platelet material developing on the irregular intimal surface and on fragmented intima is probable.

Fibromuscular dysplasia may also progress to a saccular aneurysm or dissecting hematoma of the arterial wall. This was demonstrated in one of the patients described above, who had a transient ischemic attack and an immediate arteriogram that demonstrated total occlusion of the internal carotid. A second arteriogram 2 months later demonstrated patency of the vessel. In another patient not described in this presentation, operated upon through a standard cervical incision, an identical process occurred.

When progressive stenosis of the fibromuscular dysplastic area occurs, or when a dissection of the wall of the vessel develops, fibromuscular dysplasia can cause cerebral infarction.[8]

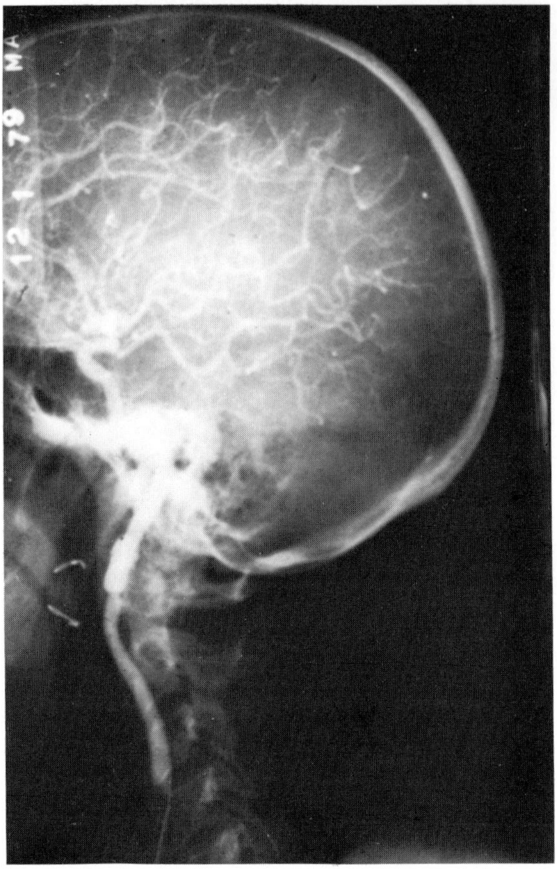

Figure 27-11. Postoperative carotid arteriogram. Replacement of the internal carotid artery with vein graft. Suture of the mandible with wires.

Isolated cases of rupture of the artery have been reported, and rupture of the intima shown on a postoperative arteriogram may be common.[9]

Fibromuscular disease of the internal carotid artery has been treated by the simpler surgical procedure of intraluminal dilation, as described by Morris, Lechter, and DeBakey,[10] Ehrenfeld and Wylie,[11] and Collins, et al.[12] Such dilation is not without risk, as shown by Effeney, Ehrenfeld, and Stoney,[13] who reported 11 neurologic complications in 130 operations.

Intraluminal dilation may be appropriate when the arteriogram shows a "string of beads" formation. That was the most common pattern in Wylie's series. Such dilation may not be as effective when there is a very tight stenosis due to severe medial and intimal hyperplasia. Intraluminal dilation is

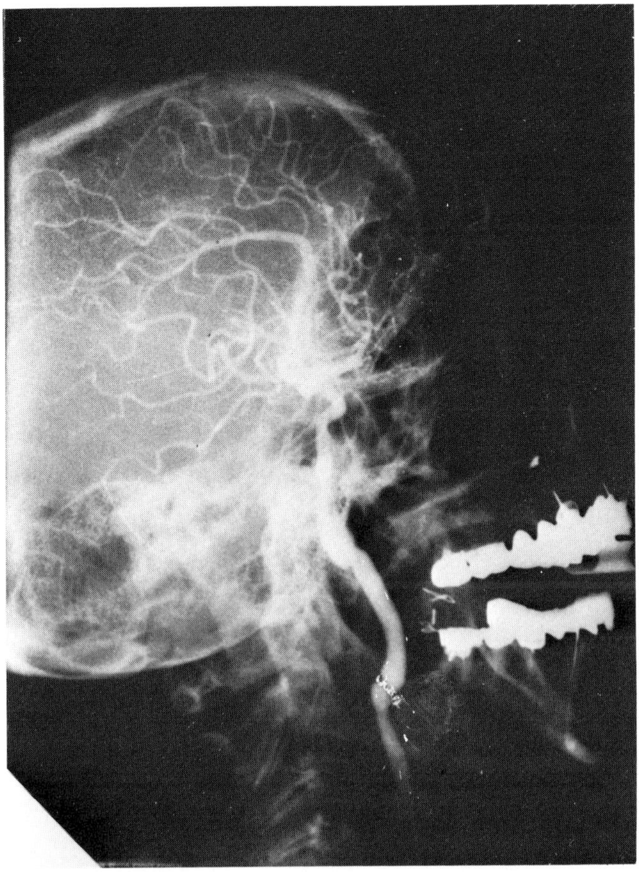

Figure 27-12. Postoperative carotid arteriogram. Replacement of the internal carotid artery with vein graft. Suture of the mandible with wires.

definitely dangerous when there is an intramural dissection present, as demonstrated by two of our cases. Certainly, the dilating instrument can be introduced into the false lumen in such cases. Intraluminal dilation cannot be used, of course, when the disease process is a saccular aneurysm, as demonstrated above.

In situations in which dilation is not appropriate, the ideal treatment is resection of the diseased segment and replacement with autogenous saphenous vein. It has been the object of this presentation to describe our approach to fibromuscular disease in the internal carotid artery which is not accessible by a standard surgical incision. The mandibular osteotomy described allows exposure of the entire length of the internal carotid artery up to the base of the

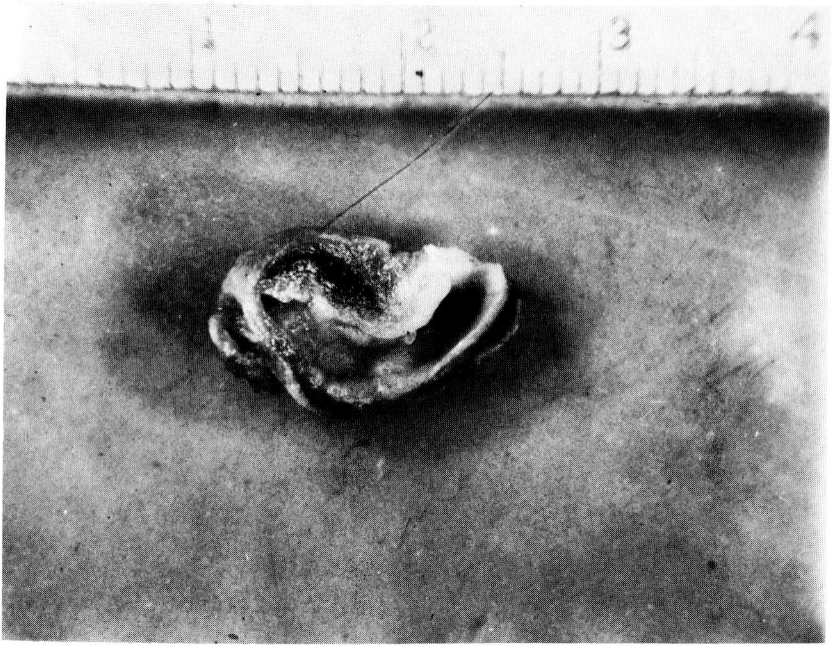

Figure 27-13. Specimen of internal carotid artery with a dissecting aneurysm.

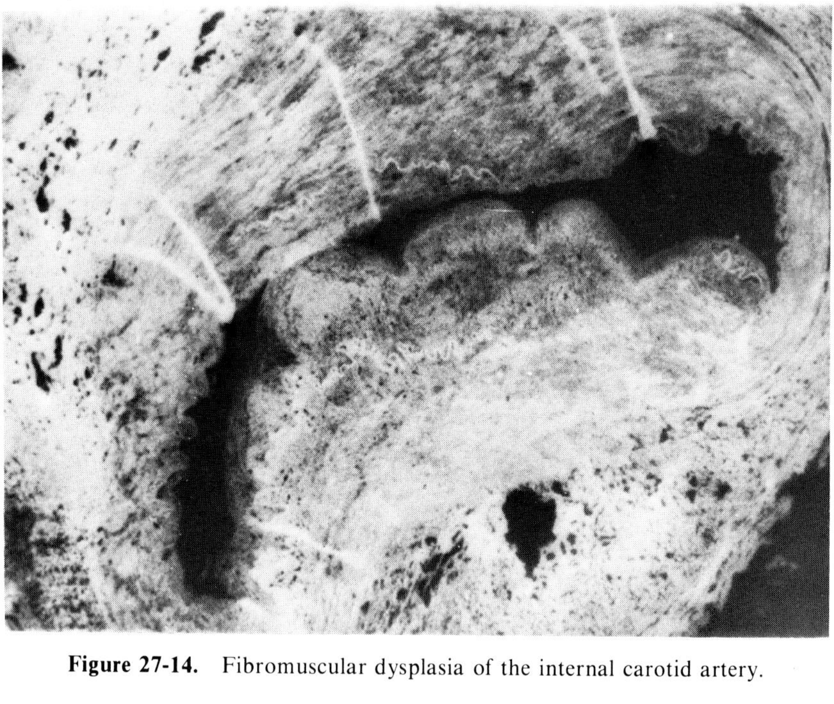

Figure 27-14. Fibromuscular dysplasia of the internal carotid artery.

skull. When this is done, it is possible to replace the most distal segment of the extracranial artery without complications of the mandibular osteotomy and create only temporary, mild discomfort in the patients selected for treatment.

REFERENCES

1. Palubinskas A, Ripley H: Fibromuscular hyperplasia in extrarenal arteries. Radiology 82:451, 1964
2. Wylie EJ, Binkley F, Palubinskas A: Extrarenal fibromuscular hyperplasia. Am J Surg 112:149, 1966
3. Houser O, Baker H: Fibromuscular dysplasia and other uncommon diseases of the cervical carotid artery: Angiographic aspects. Am J Roentgenol 104:201, 1968
4. Bergan JJ, MacDonald J: Recognition of cerebrovascular fibromuscular dysplasia. Arch Surg 98:332, 1969
5. Blaisdell W, Clauss R, Galbraith J, et al: Joint study of extracranial arterial occlusion. JAMA 209:1889, 1969
6. Wylie E, Ehrenfeld W: Extracranial Occlusive Cerebrovascular Disease. Philadelphia, WB Saunders Co, 1970, p 192
7. Kartchner M, McRae L, Morrison F: Noninvasive detection and evaluation of carotid occlusive disease. Arch Surg 106:528, 1973
8. Bostron K: Primary dissecting aneurysm of the extracranial part of the internal carotid and vertebral arteries. Neurology 17:179, 1976
9. Collins G, Rich N, Hobson R, et al: Fibromuscular dysplasia of the internal carotid arteries. Surgery 81:105, 1977
10. Morris G, Lechter A, DeBakey M: Surgical treatment of fibromuscular disease of the carotid arteries. Arch Surg 96:636, 1968
11. Ehrenfeld W, Wylie EJ: Fibromuscular dysplasia of the internal carotid artery. Surgical management. Arch Surg 109:676, 1974
12. Collins G, Rich N, Clagett P, et al: Fibromuscular dysplasia of the internal carotid arteries. Ann Surg 194:89, 1981
13. Effeney D, Ehrenfeld W, Stoney R: Why operate on carotid fibromuscular dysplasia? Arch Surg 115:1261, 1980

PART VIII

Carotid Surgery and Its Problems

John J. Bergan
William R. Flinn
James S.T. Yao

28

Cranial Nerve Injury in Carotid Surgery

Performance of carotid artery surgery has been influenced by historical developments in understanding cerebrovascular insufficiency. The concept of cerebral ischemia dominated thinking during the earliest periods of carotid reconstructive surgery. This led to development of intraoperative shunting techniques and the continuing attention to cerebral protection, which dominates discussion of carotid surgery today. Appreciation of the importance of embolic events in producing transient cerebral ischemia developed later. Now, it is understood that intraoperative embolic events are a major cause of neurologic deficit, and less attention is given to cerebral protection during carotid surgery. This and other technical advances have led to a lowering of the incidence of intraoperative neurologic deficit.

As the incidence of major operative neurologic sequelae has been reduced, it has become appropriate to turn some attention to the subject of cranial nerve injury. Although injuries to cranial nerves during carotid endarterectomy have little impact on the outcome of the procedure, they do produce physical discomfort and, occasionally, temporary disability. The frequency of cranial nerve injury during carotid surgery appears not to have decreased in parallel with the decrease in intraoperative stroke.

Prevention of cranial nerve injury in carotid surgery requires thorough knowledge of anatomy, precision in technique, and attention to detail during the operation. The nerves most commonly encountered during carotid endarterectomy include the great auricular nerve, the marginal mandibular branch of the facial nerve, the superior laryngeal nerve, the hypoglossal nerve, and the vagus and its branches.

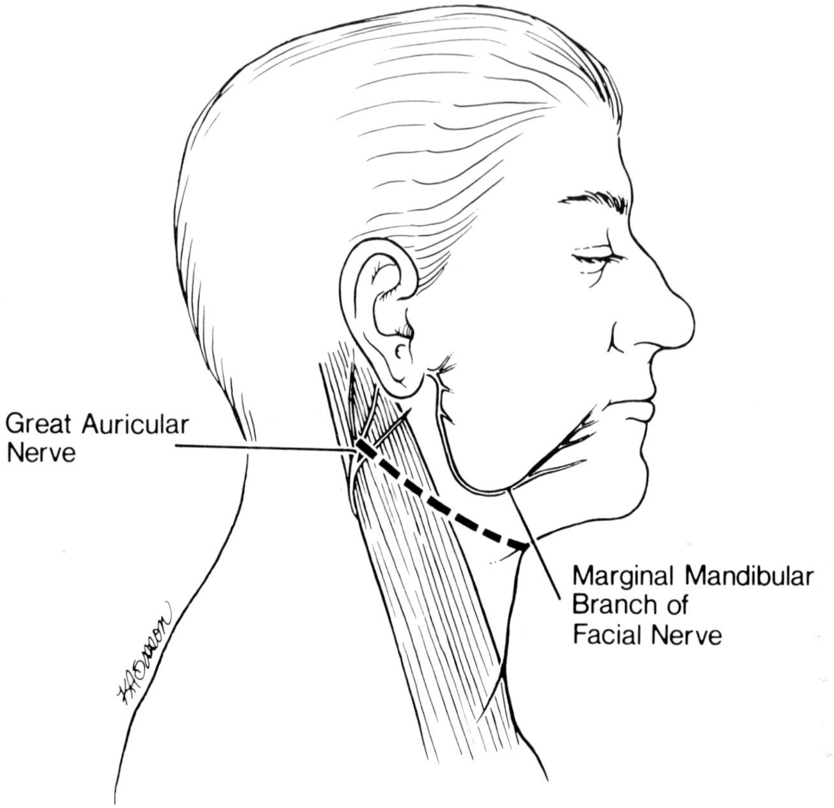

Figure 28-1. This artist's drawing shows the upper cervical skin crease placed in its usual location. The vulnerability of the great auricular nerve and the marginal branch of the facial nerve to trauma in the first stages of operative dissection is emphasized.

GREAT AURICULAR NERVE

As the operation of carotid endarterectomy proceeds layer by layer, each step exposes a different cranial nerve to injury (Fig. 28-1). In the upper cervical transverse incision, which is developed in the upper cervical skin crease, deepening the posterior portion of the incision exposes the great auricular nerve. Similarly, if the incision is made vertically along the anterior border of the sternocleidomastoid muscle, the upper portion of the incision may expose the greater auricular nerve. Fortunately, this nerve is a large structure and is easily seen. It arises from the second and third cervical nerves, and winds posteriorly around the sternocleidomastoideus muscle out of the operative field. After perforating the deep fascia, it ascends deep to the platysma and divides into anterior and posterior branches near the angle of the mandible. It is at this point that it is most subject to injury. The anterior branch, the portion of the nerve which is distributed over the face in the region of the parotid gland, is not subject to injury. However, the posterior branch, which supplies the skin over the mastoid process back of the auricula, the lobule, and lower part of the concha, is frequently damaged. Injury to the nerve may occur through direct trauma with the scalpel or indirect injury from electrocautery. The sensation of annoying numbness of the lobule of the ear may be permanent, but usually, it clears partially within 6 to 12 months.

MANDIBULAR BRANCH OF THE FACIAL NERVE

As the subplatysmal flaps are retracted for exposure of deeper structures, the marginal mandibular branch of the facial nerve may be injured. This nerve is not visualized during carotid endarterectomy, but as it descends below the angle of the mandible deep to the platysma muscle, it may be traumatized by self-retaining retractors placed for retraction of the superficial cervical fascia and platysma. The nerve may descend a variable distance below the mandible but usually is 1 cm below the mandible and parallel to it. As the patient's face is turned away from the surgeon during positioning and the chin is extended for exposure of the carotid bifurcation, the marginal mandibular branch of the facial nerve is drawn inferiorly, nearer to the operating field. Ultimately, the nerve turns cephalad, crosses the facial artery and vein, and supplies motor innervation to the muscles at the angle of the mouth and lower lip. This nerve is best avoided by careful placement of retractors deep to the platysma muscle in the superior musculo-cutaneous flap.

HYPOGLOSSAL NERVE

After the cervical fascia has been incised anterior to the sternocleidomastoid muscle and the avascular plane superior to the jugular vein developed, the common facial vein is divided to expose the carotid bifurcation (Fig. 28-2). Further exposure of the internal carotid artery distally may cause injury to the hypoglossal nerve. Usually, this nerve is 3 to 5 cm distal to the carotid bifurcation but may on occasion overlie the bifurcation of the carotid artery itself. As the hypoglossal nerve is exposed in the surgical field, it has already passed between the internal jugular vein and the internal carotid artery and has given off its descending branch, the ansa hypoglossi. In fact, the nerve can be identified by tracing back up the ansa to the main nerve trunk. The nerve disappears from the operative field by passing deep to the digastric muscle. The descending branch of the

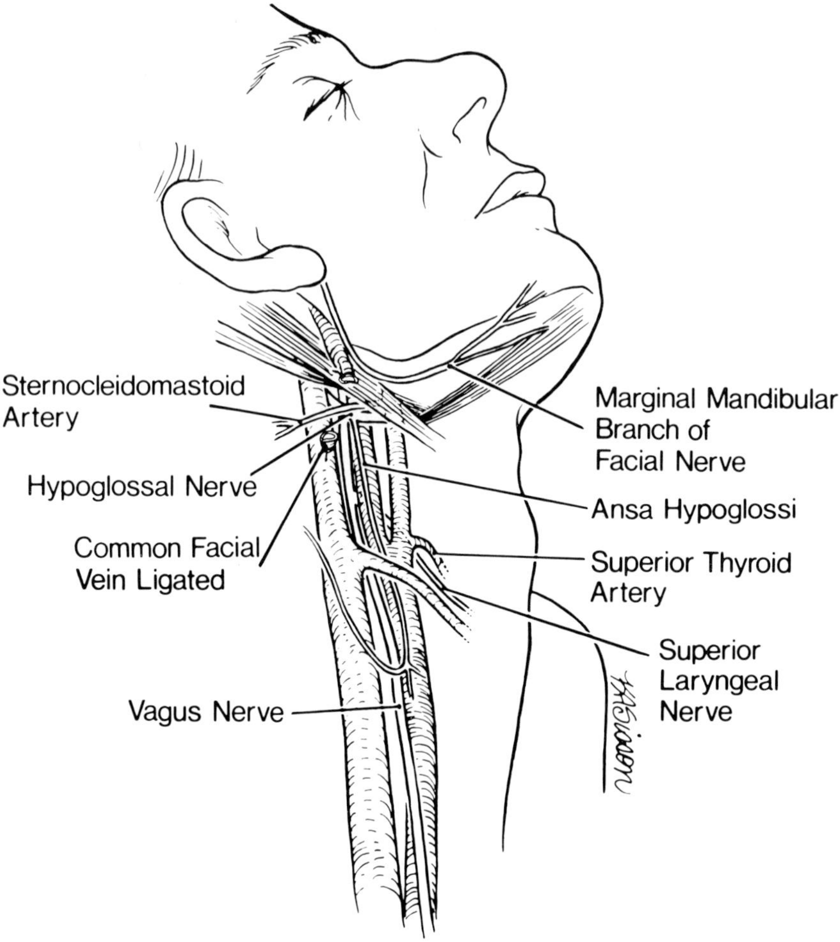

Figure 28-2. This artist's drawing shows the relationship of deeper structures in the region of the carotid bifurcation. The drawing exaggerates the sternocleidomastoid artery in order to show how division of this structure will allow the hypoglossal nerve to be moved superiorly and anteriorly for greater exposure of the internal carotid artery. The relationships of the superior laryngeal nerve to the superior thyroid artery and the vagus nerve to the carotid artery are indicated.

hypoglossal nerve limits the upward mobilization of the main nerve trunk. Therefore, it may be sacrificed, since it supplies only the omohyoid muscle.

Further mobilization of the hypoglossal nerve can be accomplished by dividing the sternocleidomastoid artery, a branch of the external carotid artery. When this is done, the nerve can be mobilized forward and retracted superiorly to expose the distal internal carotid artery. Identification of the sternocleidomastoid artery and its division is an important maneuver used to mobilize the hypoglossal nerve in situations where distal internal carotid artery exposure is mandatory. This occurs especially when the posterior plaque within the internal carotid artery ascends for an abnormally long distance within the lumen of the artery.

SUPERIOR LARYNGEAL NERVE

Of the various nerves which may be injured during carotid artery surgery, the superior laryngeal is the one that is least understood. It is subject to damage where it lies adjacent to the uppermost curve of the superior thyroid artery. At this point, the nerve passes posterior to the internal carotid and external carotid arteries, and is in the process of bifurcating into external and internal branches. Its proximity to the superior thyroid artery allows it to be damaged when the superior thyroid artery is mobilized extensively. It is the external branch of the superior laryngeal nerve which supplies the crico-thyroideus muscle. The internal branch supplies the mucosa of the larynx above the vocal folds. Therefore, the superior laryngeal nerve, and especially its external branch, is a most important nerve to avoid.

When the superior laryngeal nerve is transected, there is a lack of tenseness of the ispilateral vocal cord, and this produces an inherent inability to phonate high-pitched notes. It also produces easy fatiguability of the voice. The minor problems of swallowing which result from sensory loss (internal branch) are usually self-limited and resolve in 4 to 6 weeks. Injury to the superior laryngeal nerve can be avoided if the superior thyroid artery is ligated at its origin rather than mobilized extensively.

VAGUS NERVE AND ITS BRANCHES

Theoretically, the vagus nerve could not be injured in carotid artery surgery, but as one remembers that it is named for its wandering course, it is not surprising to encounter the rare situation in which the nerve lies anterior to the carotid artery. When it lies in an aberrant position, it is subject to direct surgical trauma. In its usual location, posterior to the carotid artery, it is not subject to direct trauma, but instead, may be injured by hematoma formation in the postoperative wound.

The recurrent laryngeal nerve is not subject to trauma within the operative field as it arises low in the neck. Blunt trauma to the vagus itself, however, may damage the recurrent laryngeal nerve fibers, or as indicated above, hematoma may impinge on the nerve and produce temporary damage.

DISCUSSION

A prospective study to determine the exact incidence of cranial nerve injury during carotid endarterectomy would be of interest. However, the results obtained would be pertinent only to the surgeon who performed the cases under study. Individual variations in technique produce cranial nerve injury during carotid endarterectomy, and conversely, it is nuances of technique that allow avoidance of cranial nerve injury.

In a prospective study of 123 patients who had preoperative otolaryngological examination, Hertzer et al.[1] found only seven who demonstrated cranial nerve injury. Interestingly, recurrent laryngeal nerve injury occurred in five, hypoglossal nerve injury in one, and superior laryngeal nerve injury in one. In a further study of 240 cases, Hertzer et al. identified 38 who sustained documented dysfunction of cranial nerves. Again, the recurrent laryngeal nerve was injured in 14, the hypoglossal nerve in 13, the marginal branch of the mandibular nerve in 6, and the superior laryngeal nerve in 5. In 25 of these 38 patients, postoperative dysfunction of a single cranial nerve was identified; however, 4 patients sustained injury to two cranial nerves, and 1 patient had injury to three nerves. Of greater interest was the fact that only 23 of the 38 patients had symptoms as a result of these cranial nerve injuries.

The use of tranverse neck incisions has probably served to increase the number of injuries to the hypoglossal nerve, and possibly, to the marginal branch of the mandibular nerve as well. The incision is close to and parallels the course of both nerves. Injury to either nerve is troublesome. Facial asymmetry is the price paid for injury to the marginal branch of the facial nerve. Tongue dysfunction can be a troublesome consequence of hypoglossal nerve trauma.

When bilateral carotid procedures are planned, hypoglossal nerve injury must be avoided studiously because bilateral hypoglossal palsy can cause upper airway obstruction, marked difficulty in deglutition, and destruction of speech.[2] Respiratory distress requiring tracheostomy may occur.[3,4] The incidence of hypoglossal nerve injury has been variously reported as 9.7 percent to 17.5 percent.[5,6] Certainly, hypoglossal nerve injury can be reduced to near-zero by careful attention to the anatomy of the nerve in the individual patient. Transection of the sternocleidomastoid artery under direct vision, as described, will further protect this nerve from injury.

Superior laryngeal nerve injury during carotid surgery occurs more frequently than has been suspected in the past.[1] Diagnosis depends upon laryngoscopic demonstration of cricothyroid muscle dysfunction but may be suspected in the patient who has a voice that tires easily. Difficulty with voice modulation in the upper registers is also a common symptom. This can be a considerable annoyance to the patient, even though it does not produce severe disability.

While it has been thought that injury to the recurrent laryngeal nerve is an unusual complication of carotid artery surgery,[7] careful attention to preoperative and postoperative study of patients undergoing carotid endarterectomy has indicated that injury to this nerve is common.[1] Mobilization of the common carotid artery should be done carefully, with strict adherence to the adventitial sheath, so that excessive manipulation of the carotid sheath containing the vagus nerve will not occur. Actual clamping of the carotid artery should be done under direct vision in an area where the artery is completely mobilized away from the vagus nerve.

Transection of the cranial nerves exposed to injury during carotid surgery rarely occurs. Nearly all patients with postoperative cranial nerve dysfunction exhibit little functional impairment. This is completely resolved within weeks to months in nearly every case. Therefore, it is retractor trauma, dissection injury, and electrocoagulation damage which produce the injury, not nerve transection.

When multiple or bilateral cranial nerve injuries occur, the manifestations of dysfunction may be of critical importance. The swallowing mechanism and laryngeal airway may be compromised.[2] Therefore, patients who require staged bilateral carotid endarterectomy are at the greatest risk for significant cranial nerve complications. In these patients, preoperative otolaryngologic examination should be considered following the initial carotid procedure.

REFERENCES

1. Hertzer NR, Feldman BJ, Beven EG, et al: A prospective study of the incidence of injury to the cranial nerves during carotid endarterectomy. Surg Gynecol Obstet 151:781, 1980
2. Verta MJ Jr, Applebaum EL, McClusky DA, et al: Cranial nerve injury during carotid endarterectomy. Ann Surg 185:192, 1977
3. Bageant TE, Tondini D, Lysons D: Bilateral hypoglossal nerve palsy following a second carotid endarterectomy. Anesthesiol 43:595, 1975
4. Imparato AM, Bracco A, Kim GE, et al: The hypoglossal nerve in carotid arterial reconstructions. Stroke 3:576, 1972
5. DeWeese JA, Rob CG, Satran R, et al: Surgical treatment of occlusive disease of the carotid artery. Ann Surg 168:85, 1968
6. DeWeese JA, Rob CG, Satran R, et al: Results of carotid endarterectomies for transient ischemic attacks—five years later. Ann Surg 178:258, 1973
7. Rainer WG, Feiler EM, Bloomquist CD, et al: Surgical approach to carotid artery insufficiency. Ann Thorac Surg 2:640, 1966

William E. Evans
James Hayes
Blair D. Vermilion

29

Speech and Mentation Impairments Associated with Carotid Artery Surgery

Injuries to nerves encountered in the surgical field during carotid endarterectomy appear to be more common than previously appreciated. DeWeese, in retrospectively reviewing a large series of surgical patients, noted a 9.7 percent incident of injury to cranial nerves or their branches.[1] Hertzer, in a prospective evaluation, found 15 percent with nerve dysfunction shortly after endarterectomy.[2] The preliminary report by Liapis in 1980 demonstrated a 27 percent incidence when prospective clinical evaluation was supplemented by specific detailed testing by a speech pathologist.[3]

In a more recent study, results of the prospective study by vascular surgeons and speech pathologists showed a very high incidence of cranial nerve dysfunction.[4] The surgical team evaluated patients by observation of tongue motion, ability to swallow, clear the throat and initiate the gag reflex, and by evaluation of gross speech. The patients were also evaluated with the use of direct laryngoscopy.

The speech pathologist supplemented studies with a more detailed evaluation of the specific nerve functions (especially as they relate to speech activities).

The hypoglossal nerve was studied by evaluation of tongue motility and by measuring tongue activity related to speech. Complete range of motion was measured in all planes. Articulation was subjectively evaluated and diadochokinesis assessed by measuring the patient's ability to repeat phrases such as "PUH-TUH-KUH." Assessment included the ability to accomplish these tasks by measuring the number of repetitions in 5 second intervals. Glossopharyngeal nerve functions were studied in a manner similar to that used by the surgeon. In addition, the reasonance chamber function of the pharynx was evaluated.

Branches of the vagus nerve function were assessed by evaluation of the superior and recurrent laryngeal nerves. The superior laryngeal nerve supplies the cricothyroid muscle, which tends to lengthen and thin the vocal cords, thereby producing pitches in the higher ranges. The recurrent nerve supplies the thyroarytenoid muscle, which tends to shorten and thicken vocal cords, producing low pitches. Normal vocal mechanics require an equilibrium between these muscle functions. To measure this equilibrium, patients were asked to glide from their lowest sound to their highest and then return. Additionally, the C, D, E, F and G pitches (pitch-pipe) were individually tested for the patient's ability to reach the pitch and to sustain the pitch for approximately 15 seconds. The latter test allows for an estimation of the patient's ability to maintain subglottic pressure, which requires integrated function of the vagal nerve branches.

Lastly, the speech pathologist gave an overall assessment of integrated speech activity by evaluating spontaneous speech activity.

Prospective evaluation was carried out in 116 patients undergoing 128 carotid endartectomies. There were 59 males and 57 females ranging in age from 34 to 87 years. Twenty-five additional patients having noncarotid vascular surgery requiring endotracheal intubation served as controls. The patients were evaluated preoperatively at 2 days, and at 6 weeks following operations. These results were compared to previous reports by Hertzer[2] from the Cleveland Clinic. Patients noted to have preoperative deficits were eliminated so that the determination of the risk of surgery in terms of the cranial nerve branches could be obtained.

RESULTS

Clinical evaluation by the surgeons was compared to that obtained by review of patients from the Cleveland Clinic and then to the findings of the more detailed assessment of the speech pathologist.

Clinical evaluation failed to demonstrate any postoperative glossopharyngeal nerve deficits at 2 days following surgery. Five percent had hypoglossal nerve function defects while superior-recurrent nerve deficits were identified in 14 percent. The incidence of hypoglossal nerve deficits was similar to that noted by Hertzer.[2] Superior-recurrent laryngeal nerve deficits were more frequently identified, but the number identified by laryngoscopy (8 percent) was the same.[4]

The more detailed evaluation by the speech pathologist identified a significantly greater number of defects. Integrated motor speech function was judged to be abnormal in 25 percent at 2 days postsurgery. Two glossopharyngeal deficits (1.5 percent) were found. Eleven percent of hypoglossal nerves functioned abnormally, and fully 35 percent showed dysfunction of the superior-recurrent laryngeal nerve ($p < .05$).

By 6 weeks, as expected, many abnormalities had resolved. The surgeons identified a 1.6 percent incidence of hypoglossal nerve dysfunction, and 4.5 percent still had laryngeal nerve changes, which is similar to the number of abnormalities noted by Hertzer.[2] The speech pathologist still could identify a significant number of changes. Integrated motor speech function was judged to be abnormal in 12 percent, 4 percent had hypoglossal nerve dysfunction, and 15 percent still had laryngeal defects.

The speech pathologist identified every abnormality found by the surgeon, even though half of these were grossly asymptomatic to the clinician by voice assessment and were identified by either laryngoscopy or evaluation of tongue motion.

No abnormalities of nerve function were identified postoperatively in the control group either by the clinician or the speech therapist.

DISCUSSION

The incidence of voice-related cranial nerve injuries is significant. The surgeon identified early postoperative abnormalities in 15 percent of patients undergoing carotid endarterectomy, which is similar to the reports of Hertzer[2] and Matsumoto.[5] Hypoglossal dysfunction at 6 weeks was noted in 1.6 percent, which is also similar to these reports. Our slightly higher incidence of superior-recurrent laryngeal nerve deficits probably reflects our interest in the problem.

The speech pathologist identified an injury incidence of 39 percent ($p < .05$). This increase reflects the more detailed evaluation carried out, particularly in identifying superior-recurrent laryngeal nerve dysfunction. Minor nerve changes result in speech abnormalities unidentified by gross evaluation. Most occur because of disequilibrium in the superior-recurrent nerve function and are identified only by the detailed studies employed by the speech pathologist.

Controls showed no evidence of motor nerve deficits. Hoarseness occasionally occurred, but detailed testing showed no evidence of nerve changes and in each instance, hoarseness cleared in several days. Since controls showed no evidence of nerve injury and since all preoperative abnormalities were eliminated, the findings of the study would appear to be indicative of the true incidence of nerve injury.

Results of the study indicate a significant incidence of postoperative nerve dysfunction. Careful surgical technique with clear separation of the nerves from the vessels to prevent direct nerve trauma should decrease the incidence of these injuries. Identification of nerve dysfunction is important, particularly in patients requiring staged bilateral carotid endarterectomy in terms of timing of the second side. Additionally, identification of nerve dysfunction allows early intervention by the speech pathologist.

CHANGES IN MENTATION FOLLOWING CAROTID SURGERY

Extensive data exist concerning the prevention of stroke by carotid endarterectomy. Quantitative proof of improvement of mental function following carotid surgery is more difficult to establish. Since the report in 1964 of Williams and McGhee,[6] numerous reports have appeared outlining possible mental changes following endarterectomy. Variability of the results of these studies raises serious questions concerning the suggested salutary effects of carotid surgery on intellectual ability. As pointed out by Hobson,[7] three pertinent questions must be answered concerning the effects of carotid surgery on intelligence. These are the following:

1. Are there consistent intellectual deficits in persons with carotid artery disease?
2. Does carotid endarterectomy improve intellectual function; does it prevent the progression of deterioration?
3. Do any physiologic events correlate with intellectual changes noted?

PRE-OPERATIVE INTELLECTUAL DEFICITS

Chason[8] reported a patient with bilateral carotid stenosis found to be impaired intellectually on the basis of the Weschler-Bellvue and Benton Visual Retention Tests. Grach,[8] however, was unable to confirm these findings. Sours[9] was also unable to show preoperative deficits. These authors conclude that bilateral carotid disease is not necessarily associated with intellectual deficits. Perry[10] found pre-endarterectomy patients to be significantly impaired on several subtests and on the impairment index of the Halstead-Reitan battery of neuropsychological tests when compared with the normal population.

In a study by Kelly,[11] controls were drawn from a group of surgical patients with no evidence of cerebrovascular insufficiency but with peripheral vascular disease. Control patients were matched by age and education with the carotid patients. By virtue of their peripheral vascular disease, controls had evidence of generalized arteriosclerosis. No difference could be established preoperatively between controls or test subjects on the neuropsychological or personality assessment.

Two studies by Haynes[12,13] failed to identify any differences between controls or test subjects preoperatively except in Part A of the Trails Making Test. Test subjects took significantly more time than controls to complete this part of the test. Controls in these studies were matched for age, education, race, and sex with the carotid group and drawn from a non-neurological surgical population.

Drake,[14] in evaluating patients in a large V. A. Hospital population, showed the greatest number of patients with "some" degree of intellectual loss in patients with bilateral carotid stenosis. Controls, who were elderly but without any evidence of cerebrovascular disease, had the least evidence of intellectual loss. Percentages of people with intellectual deficits in each group were 88 percent of bilateral carotid stenosis, 71 percent of unilateral carotid stenosis, 60 percent of surgically inaccessable cerebrovascular disease, and 33 percent of the controls.

POSTOPERATIVE ASSESSMENT

Postoperative comparisons are also variable. The two most recent studies by Kelly[11] and Haynes[13] showed the inherent problems with interpretation. Kelly,[11] as mentioned previously, could show no difference between controls and patients in the endarterectomy group preoperatively. Postoperatively, the endarterectomy group showed improvement on the Weschler Memory Scale and Controlled Word Association Test. This improvement was quantitatively different from the control group following operation. On the Hidden Figure Test and the Right-Left Discrimination Test, both control and endarterectomy groups showed improvement.

The State Anxiety Scale also showed improvement in both carotid and control groups. All other tests were essentially unchanged.

In Haynes'[13] evaluation, controls were not different from the carotid group preoperatively. Postoperative improvement on the WAIS verbal and performance scales was judged to be significant as was improvement on the Trails Making Test for the carotid group. It is of interest that although a mean change was noted for the carotid group, the postoperative mean was still not significantly different from the control group. Both controls and test subjects showed a decrease on the State Anxiety Level that did not differ. Endarterectomy patients did improve significantly on the Trait Anxiety Level (predisposition to respond with anxiety) postoperatively, whereas controls did not.

Another method of assessing any increase in intellectual function following carotid surgery is the use of a patient questionnaire. The questionnaire is designed to assess the patients' own subjective opinions of how they are functioning intellectually postoperatively, as well as the opinion of their families.

Two groups to use this type of assessment are Kelly's[11] and Wolfe's.[15]

Analysis of Kelly's[11] self-report indicated that carotid patients were no more likely to report that they were "better" in any category than were the controls.

Wolfe[15] did not employ a control group, but for comparison, questionnaires were sent to the patients and members of the patients' immediate families. In general, both the patients and their families felt that the patients' intellectual functioning had remained the same postoperatively. The patients responded to the questionaire items as follows: 75 percent felt that no change had occurred, 14 percent felt that they had become worse, while 11 percent had the impression of cognitive improvement. Family members responded as follows: 68 percent felt the patient remained the same, 10 percent felt the patient had become worse, and 22 percent felt the patient had improved following surgery.

Thus, the results of these questionnaires indicated no subjective improvement noted by the patient[11,15] or families.[15]

PHYSIOLOGIC CORRELATION

A major premise of any increase in intellectual functioning following carotid endarterectomy is that blood flow to the brain is increased. The only groups that have measured blood flow pre- and postendarterectomy are Perry[10] and Wolfe.[15] Perry[10] found a significant increase in blood flow from endarterectomy. However, no significant correlation between intellectual changes and blood flow changes could be made.

Wolfe[15] obtained similar results. There was a significant increase in blood flow pre- to postoperatively, but no correlation could be established between increased blood flow and increased intellectual abilities.

DISCUSSION

There are methodological shortcomings in the papers reviewed. These problems arise in the following areas:

1. Establishment of a neurological deficit prior to endarterectomy.
2. Control groups used (if any) and what constitutes a good control group.
3. Tests used to assess intellectual function pre- and postsurgically.
4. Types of patients studied.
5. Interpretation of statistical results.

It appears that great variability exists in the groups evaluated. Drake,[14] Perry,[10] and Sours[9] show evidence of a neuropsychological deficit in carotid patients when compared to controls preoperatively. Duke,[16] Grach,[8] Williams,[6] Kelly,[11] and Haynes[13] failed to find such deficits preoperatively when compared to controls.

This raises the question as to what constitutes a valid control group. Some have employed population normals as controls, but since age, generalized arteriosclerosis, education, and general level of health have a significant impact on neuropsychological testing, population normals are probably not the best control group. Several groups have used patients with generalized peripheral vascular disease, but without evidence of cerebrovascular disease as a control group. This type of control group approaches the ideal control group but still has some shortcomings.

The ideal control group would result from randomization of patients with cerebrovascular disease to surgical and nonsurgical groups. The problem with establishing a control group by randomization is obvious.

The control group that would best approximate the ideal is probably the one suggested by Matarazzo.[17] The control group was a subgroup of candidates for carotid endarterectomy who were initially tested and then retested in several weeks to show any retest variations not related to surgery. Surgery was then performed, and the group was retested in 6-8 weeks. This control group provided an approximation of a no-treatment group to compare with the effects resulting from operation.

The problem of appropriate tests of intellectual and neuropsychological function is also relevant. Which tests are most valid and which most closely allow approximation of the effect of intervention have not been clearly established. Additionally, all of the tests employed require patient cooperation necessitating concentration and motivation. How much these factors affect comparison of the results from pre- to postoperative is not well known. Anxiety also greatly affects performance and has only been marginally accounted for. Even the contribution of the tester becomes a factor. A prime example of this is in Reitan's Trails Making Test. Errors made by the patient are pointed out as they occur so that the testee completes the test with zero errors. The test is scored on basis of time of completion. This, therefore, requires not only the patient's concentration and activity, but also the reaction time of the tester to identify and point out errors and time for the patient to see and correct the errors. Interexaminer differences on this test are highly significant.[18] Finally, the practice effects must be accounted for. On the WAIS test, improvement of 1-9 points has been noted to occur simply on the basis of a second exposure to the test or testing methods. Goldstein[17] has attributed much of the change to the Halstead-Reitan test to this practice effect.[19]

Variability might also be predicted by the failure to accurately control the type of patients selected for the study. The samples have all been small so that the degree of stenosis or occlusion or the presence of bilateral disease might have an effect on the results. The extent of intracerebral arteriosclerosis may also contribute and has been poorly controlled. The degree of neurological involvement also has been a variable. Whether a difference exists between patients with asymptomatic carotid disease and those with TIA and/or stroke has not been clearly determined. In most studies, great variation in these factors exists in the same sample.

Of considerable importance is the selection and matching of patients and controls with respect to age and education. Age and level of education are both well known determinants of neuropsychological test results. Standardization of test scores is usually based on a cross-section of the general adult population. If a test subject has either more or less education than the standardization population, that subject will probably perform higher or lower than "normal."

Age can also be a significant variable when evaluating test scores of older patients. Some memory and learning functions that decline with age are also highly susceptible to the effects of organic brain disease. Age-graded scores are important to use for persons over 50-years-old and are essential to the evaluation of test performance on persons over 65.[18]

Kelly[11] reported significant differences in age and education for carotid patients classified as improved and not improved. Improved patients were younger and better educated.

Lastly, great variation from study to study exists in the interpretation of statistical results. Statistical significance does not imply practical significance. The assumption that if one measurement is larger than another, then a difference in the quantity of the measured variable exists is not necessarily valid. Mean scores mask individual variation. One or two outlayers may cause a shift of the entire group making it appear that greater changes are occurring than actually exist. Increases on any test may be a function of retesting or of the measurement error known to be characteristic of tests of intellectual and neuropsychological functioning. Also, as was pointed out by Williams and McGhee,[6] the placebo effect cannot be ruled out as accounting for change.

When one considers these multiple factors in light of the variability of results obtained, no clear-cut conclusions can be reached concerning the effect of carotid endarterectomy on mental functioning. Certainly anecdotal experience suggests that occasional patients are markedly improved by endarterectomy. There may, in fact, be a subgroup of carotid endarterectomy patients who do improve following surgery, but because of the lack of clarity on the studies to date, this group has not been clearly identified.

The final conclusion as to whether any increase in mentation occurs following carotid surgery awaits a larger, more detailed and better controlled study.

REFERENCES

1. DeWeese JA, Rob CG, Satran R, et al: Results of carotid endarterectomies for transient ischemic attacks—five years later. Ann Surg 3:258, 1973
2. Hertzer NR, Feldman BJ, Beven RG, et al: A prospective study of the incidence of injury to the cranial nerves during carotid endarterectomy. Surgery, Gynecology and Obstetrics, 151:781, 1980

3. Liapis CD, Satiani B, Florance CL, et al: Motor speed malfunction following carotid endarterectomy. Surgery 89:56, 1981
4. Evans WE, Mendelowitz DS, Liapis CD, et al: Motor speech deficit following carotid endarterectomy. Annual meeting Am Surg Assoc, Boston-April 23, 1982
5. Matsumoto GH, Cossman D, Callow AD: Hazards and safeguards during carotid endarterectomy. American Journal of Surgery 133:458, April 1977
6. Williams M, McGhee T: Psychological study of carotid artery occlusion and endarterectomy. Arch Neurol 10:243, 1964
7. Asken MJ, Hobson RW: Intellectual change and carotid endarterectomy: Subjective speculation or objective reality: A review. Journal of Surgical Research 23:367, 1977
8. Grach S, Hurwitz L, McDowell F: Bilateral carotid artery occlusive disease: A report of our patients. Arch Neurol 2:130, 1960
9. Sours J: Some neurological and psychiatric aspects of bilateral internal carotid occlusion. Journal of Mental Science 106:1063, 1960
10. Perry P, Drinkwater J, Taylor G: Neuropsychological tests and carotid artery disease. Brit J Surg 61:922, 1974
11. Kelly MP, Garron DC, Javid H: Carotid artery disease, carotid endarterectomy and behavior. Arch Neurol 37:743, 1980
12. Haynes D, King G, Dempsey R: Improvement of cognitive and personality changes after carotid endarterectomy. Surg Forum 26:288, 1975
13. Haynes CD, Gideon DA, King GD, et al: The improvement of cognition and personality after carotid endarterectomy. Surgery 80:699, 1976
14. Drake W, Baker M, Blumenkrantz J, et al: The quality and duration of survival in bilateral carotid occlusive disease: A preliminary survey of the effects of thromboendarterectomy, in Poole J, Siebert R, Whisnant J, (eds): Cerebral Vascular Disease. New York, Grune and Stratton, 1968
15. Wolfe V, Florance C, Mendelowitz D, et al: Cognitive changes in postcarotid endarterectomy. Unpublished data.
16. Duke R, Bloor B, Nugent G, et al: Changes in performance on WAIS, Trailmaking Test and Finger Tapping Test associated with carotid artery surgery. Percept Mot Skills 26:399, 1968
17. Matarazzo RG, Matarazzo JD, Gallo AE, et al: IQ and neuropsychological changes following carotid endarterectomy. J Clin Neuropsychology 1:97, 1979
18. Lezak MD: Neuropsychological Assessment. New York, Oxford University Press, 1976
19. Goldstein SG, Kleinknecht RA, Gallo AE: Neuropsychological changes associated with carotid endarterectomy. Cortex, September 308, 1970

Steven J. Eskind
Richard H. Dean

30

Blood Pressure Aberrations in Carotid Artery Surgery

Temporary instability in blood pressure is a well recognized and potentially catastrophic consequence of carotid endarterectomy. The incidence of temporary hypertension following carotid endarterectomy is reported to range from 20 to 56 percent,[1,2,3] while transient hypotension may occur in 28 to 50 percent of the patients postoperatively.[1,4,5] Whether it be hypertension or hypotension, the presence of side fluctuations in blood pressure following carotid endarterectomy can significantly and adversely affect the outcome of an otherwise technically successful operation. For this reason, understanding the etiology and methods of blood pressure stabilization is an important aspect of the surgical management of carotid artery disease.

CAROTID SINUS BARORECEPTORS

Although the exact etiology of postcarotid endarterectomy fluctuations in blood pressure remains unclear, "dysfunction" of the carotid sinus baroreceptor remains the most frequently cited cause.[1,2,3,4,5,6,7] The carotid sinus baroreceptors are bilateral stretch receptors located predominantly at the carotid bifurcation, which are important in maintaining a stable blood pressure during changes in cardiac output.[6,8,9] The reflex arc begins when afferent signals are generated from the stretch baroreceptors at the carotid sinus and travel along the carotid sinus nerve of Hering. Located within the areolar tissue between the internal and external carotid arteries, the carotid sinus nerve joins the glossopharyngeal nerve to continue centrally to the vasomotor center in the medulla. Following integration of these and other

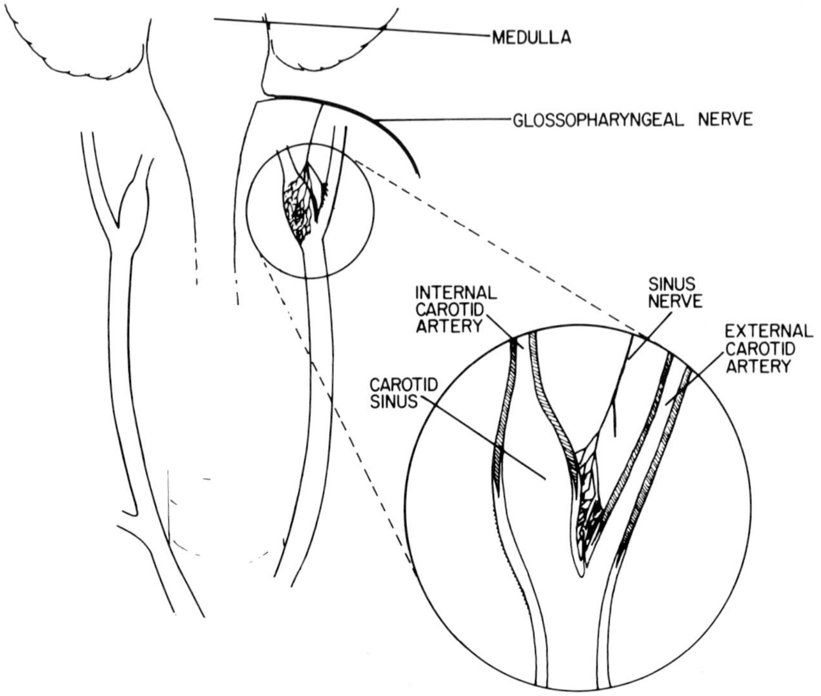

Figure 30-1. Drawing of the carotid sinus nerve baroreceptor reflex arc pathway. See text for further explanation.

stimuli within the medulla, cardiac and peripheral vascular tone are maintained through efferent signals transmitted down the vagus nerve and the sympathetic chain (Fig. 30-1).

The physiology of the carotid sinus baroreceptor reflex arc has been well-established in the normal population.[6,8,10] The stretch receptors in the walls of the carotid bifurcation are extremely sensitive to distension. In the presence of hypertension, the walls of the carotid vessels are stretched. This, in turn, stimulates the baroreceptors to generate an increased frequency of afferent signals being transmitted in the carotid sinus nerve. The compensatory response mediated within the medulla is a reduction in blood pressure and pulse rate. These changes are the result of inhibition in sympathetic mediated vasoconstrictor tone and increased vagal tone to the heart. In contrast, hypotension decreases stretch of the baroreceptors, which in turn causes decreased carotid sinus nerve activity. In a reciprocal fashion, the vasomotor medullary center responds with increased sympathetic vasomotor tone and decreased vagal stimuli to the heart, causing a rise in blood pressure and tachycardia (Fig. 30-2).

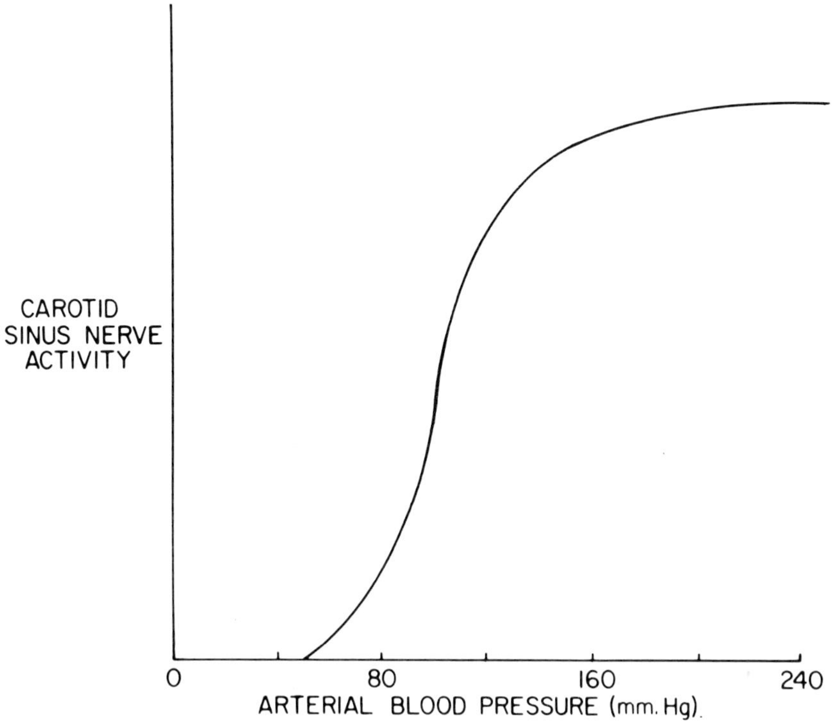

Figure 30-2. Graph of the relationship between the carotid sinus nerve activity and systemic blood pressure.

The integrity of the carotid artery reflex arc can be evaluated quite easily.[10] Normal baroreceptor function is evident with an increase in diastolic blood pressure above baseline occurring within 5 seconds after release of high intrathoracic pressure at the end of a Valsalva maneuver. An attenuated or absent functional reflex arc fails to produce this overshoot. Thus preoperative identification of a functional reflex arc might identify that patient prone to be hypertensive postoperatively if the carotid sinus nerve were denervated during carotid endarterectomy.

ASSOCIATED HYPERTENSION

Reviews evaluating the occurrence of perioperative hypertension associated with carotid endarterectomy provide disparate results and suggest an incidence of 20 to 56 percent.[1,2,3] This wide discrepancy may be explained by analyzing the definition of hypertension in each study. Whereas Lehv[2] defines postoperative hypertension as being a sustained blood pressure more than 15 mm Hg above mean preoperative blood pressure, Bove[1] defines hypertension as a rise in systolic pressure of more than 40 mm Hg above baseline. In contrast, Towne[3] defines postcarotid endarterectomy hypertension as a sustained elevation in systolic blood pressure exceeding 200 mm Hg. In any event, perioperative hypertension is common and requires appropriate therapy for its control.

Several causes of postoperative hypertension are possible and more than one origin may be present in any individual patient. The most frequently cited causes include reflex (baroreceptor) hypertension, neurogenic hypertension, hypercarbic anesthesia hypertension, and acceleration of pre-existent hypertension.

Carotid Baroreceptor Mediated Hypertension

Reflex postoperative hypertension due to dysfunction of the carotid sinus baroreceptor has received most attention of the respective possible causes of postcarotid endarterectomy hypertension.[1,2,3,6] The proposed mechanism whereby hypertension develops centers on denervation of the carotid sinus nerve. In the course of dissection during carotid endarterectomy, the carotid sinus nerve of Hering may be divided, thereby causing an absolute decrease in nervous impulses travelling to the medullary vasomotor center. This serves as a signal falsely indicating systemic hypotension. The reflex arc is completed with an inappropriate outpouring of sympathetic signals and decreased vagal tone to the heart. This, in turn, leads to hypertension and tachycardia. In this regard, Angell-James and Lumley and associates[6] reported a positive correlation between carotid nerve activity and blood pressure. Those patients who were hypertensive postoperatively had decreased carotid sinus nerve activity recorded at operation.

Not all patients respond to carotid sinus denervation in the same manner, however. In the series by Towne and Bernhard,[3] the incidence of postcarotid endarterectomy hypertension was 23.8 percent when the nerve was routinely divided as compared to 24.1 percent when the nerve was preserved. An explanation for this phenomenon has been reported by Appenzellar and Descarries.[10] They found that baroreceptor function tends to deteriorate with age as well as presence of cerebrovascular disease. In their series, carotid sinus receptor reflexes were absent in 33 percent of patients with chronic cerebrovascular disease. Bristow et al.[11] also showed a decrease in baroreceptor sensitivity and a resetting of the reflex arc toward a higher level of blood pressure in patients with essential hypertension. The preoperative functional integrity of the carotid sinus nerve can be determined by the valsalva maneuver. By identification of those patients not having an intact reflex arc preoperatively, a clearer definition of the incidence of carotid sinus nerve mediated hypertension might be ascertained.

Neurogenic Hypertension

Neurogenic hypertension can best be considered a complication of carotid artery endarterectomy because hypertension in this setting is secondary to deterioration in the neurologic status of the patient. Lehv[2] found that 69 percent of patients with a neurologic deficit developed postoperative hypertension compared to only 28 percent of neurologically intact patients. This increased incidence of hypertension occurred whether the neurologic deficit was an acute event or remote from the operation. Furthermore, 47 percent of hypertensive postcarotid endarterectomy patients showed deterioration of neurologic function. Caplan[12] described 2 patients who underwent carotid endarterectomy less than 5 weeks after an acute cerebrovascular accident. Both patients were asymptomatic, yet significant hypertension developed prior to onset of overt manifestations of an intracerebral hemorrhage. These case reviews emphasize that postcarotid endarterectomy hypertension can serve as the first sign of impending deterioration in neurologic function.

Two theories for the etiology of neurogenic hypertension have been popularized. The older concept suggests that in patients with a previous neurologic deficit, the increased pressure or flow through an abnormally permeable vascular bed within an ischemic area causes rupture of capillaries and hemorrhage into brain tissue.[3,12] The second theory suggests that the distal cerebral vascular bed is protected from systemic hypertension by the high grade carotid artery stenosis.[12] Following carotid endarterectomy, the fragile, distal vascular bed is exposed to a much higher perfusion pressure and is prone to rupture, which leads to intracerebral hemorrhage. Both theories agree that with intracerebral hemorrhage, intracranial pressure rises, which reflexively causes systemic hypertension.[13] Accordingly, postcarotid endarterectomy hypertension can be a manifestation of increased intracranial pressure due to revascularization of a previously ischemic area of the brain. Hypertension of neurogenic origin, therefore, tends to appear before overt manifestations of neurologic deterioration.

Hypercarbic Anesthesia Induced Hypertension

Hypercarbic anesthesia is a well-known cause of systemic hypertension. The physiologic effect of hypercarbic anesthesia results in activation of the sympathetic nervous system with increased release of catecholamines.[14,15] This response is mediated in the hypothalamus and medulla. The resulting hypertension is used as a method of providing cerebral protection during carotid endarterectomy. Subsequent studies have shown, however, that hypercarbia may result in an intracerebral steal syndrome and therefore it is not widely practiced.[16,17]

Acceleration of Pre-existent Hypertension

Postoperative acceleration of pre-existent hypertension is, by far, the most common etiology of postcarotid endarterectomy hypertension. Such acceleration is highly predictable, for these patients are volume and salt loaded perioperatively. Not surprisingly, on arrival to the recovery room, hypertension may be severe with diastolic blood pressures in excess of 120 mm Hg. Obviously, the more severe the preoperative hypertension, the higher the blood pressure will be postoperatively. In the review by Towne et al.[3] preoperative hypertension was the single most important determinant in the development of postoperative hypertension. In their studies, they show that 79.6 percent of patients hypertensive postoperatively were hypertensive preoperatively. Although other causes of postoperative acceleration of preexistent hypertension may be present, one can adequately explain their hypertension on the basis of injudicious volume and salt loading during the operative procedure.

Other Possibilities

Other theoretical and experimental considerations exist that also can explain postcarotid endarterectomy hypertension. Bunag et al.[18] described elevated renin levels soon after bilateral carotid occlusion in dogs. Hodge et al.[19] showed delayed hypertension with elevated angiotensin levels after bilateral carotid occlusion. Similarly, Bartter et al.[20] showed elevated aldosterone levels in dogs following carotid occlusion with preservation of the nerves of the thyrocarotid junction. Needless to say, such experimental findings are difficult to extrapolate to humans and require further investigation.

Clinical Considerations

The potentially devastating clinical significance of postcarotid endarterectomy hypertension is evident with even the most cursory review. In 2 studies, the incidence of neurologic deficits following carotid endarterectomy was less than 2 percent in the normotensive postoperative population as compared to 10 percent in the postcarotid endarterectomy hypertensive group.[1,3] In the extreme, 1 series[2] reported a 47 percent incidence of neurologic deficit in a group of postoperative hypertensive patients.

Preoperative identification of patients at risk of developing postcarotid endarterectomy hypertension might serve to reduce the incidence of this complication from the present average of 20 to 40 percent. Bove[1] showed that blood pressure instability did not correlate with age, indication for operation, or degree of ipsilateral or contralateral carotid artery disease. As previously mentioned, 2 groups of patients appear particularly prone to develop postoperative hypertension. The first group described by Lehv[2] are those patients who display a preoperative neurologic deficit due either to recent or remote cerebrovascular accidents. In such circumstances, intravenous steroid administration to decrease intracerebral edema is an important addition to antihypertensive therapy. The second group at increased risk for severe postoperative hypertension are the patients with preoperative hypertension, especially if they are inadequately controlled. Towne[3] reported that the hypertensive patient is not only at a greater risk of postoperative hypertension but also at increased risk for neurologic morbidity and mortality. In our experience, however, the presence of adequately treated postoperative hypertension has not been associated with an increased risk of postoperative neurologic deficits.

Careful monitoring of blood pressure both intraoperatively and postoperatively with intraarterial catheters is undoubtedly the most accurate method by which postoperative hypertension can be identified and appropriately treated. Since the appearance of hypertension may be delayed for up to 15 hours after operation,[1] a time during which the patient is typically neurologically stable and vital signs not as frequently recorded, postcarotid endarterectomy hypertension may go undetected if blood pressure monitoring is not continued. In our institution, all patients are monitored in this fashion in the intensive care unit for the first 24 hours postoperatively.

If the patient becomes hypertensive, aggressive pharmacologic measures are taken to reduce the systolic blood pressure to below 160 mm Hg and diastolic blood pressure below 100 mm Hg. Treatment begins with the infusion of nitroprusside, which is titrated to achieve the desired blood pressure. Then, the nitroprusside infusion is tapered as blood pressure comes under control with oral preparations. During this time, frequent neurologic evaluations are made to recognize the patient with hypertension of neurogenic origin. In this case, appropriate measures are taken to simultaneously reduce intracranial pressure.

Unfortunately, not all vascular surgeons agree with the need for postcarotid endarterectomy control of hypertension. Their contention is that, "the hypertensive response is due to a cerebral autoregulatory demand for increased perfusion pressure, possibly brought about by a declamping reactive hyperemia, cerebral edema and a consequent increase in cerebrovascular resistance."[21] Adherence to this opinion is particularly unwise since most studies demonstrate significantly increased neurologic morbidity and mortality in the setting of postcarotid endarterectomy hypertension.

PERIOPERATIVE HYPOTENSION

Hypotension in association with carotid artery surgery has been seen in 28 to 50 percent of patients.[1,4,5] The etiology of hypotension is easily explained in light of the carotid sinus reflex arc.[1,4,5,6,7] In patients with carotid artery disease, the rigid atheromatous plaque residing at the carotid bifurcation not only dampens the pressure waves reaching the carotid sinus baroreceptor but also reduces the distensibility of the carotid artery itself.[4,6] Both factors reduce the sensitivity of the carotid sinus baroreceptor. With restoration of flow following the completion of carotid endarterectomy, the vessel wall is thin and easily stretched at any given pressure. After endarterectomy, the undamaged baroreceptors become exposed to relatively higher pressures and are consequently stretched, producing increased baroreceptor discharge and increased activity in the sinus nerve of Hering.[6] This, in turn, results in increased vagal tone to the heart, decreased sympathetic vasomotor tone and, consequently, bradycardia and systemic hypotension. This centrally mediated reflex persists until the carotid sinus mechanism has been "reset."[1] According to Ransom,[14] hypotension is not related to preoperative neurological or general clinical status of the patient.

An example of postcarotid endarterectomy reflex hypotension is depicted in Figure 30-3. This patient was admitted with diffuse atherosclerosis and bilateral carotid artery bruits. Arteriography demonstrated bilateral high grade carotid artery stenoses. Following completion of carotid artery endarterectomy and within 3 minutes after carotid artery flow restoration, the patient developed severe hypotension (70/50 mm Hg) and bradycardia (55 beats/min). Prior to this, the patient's blood pressure had averaged 140/70 mm Hg with a pulse of 85 beats/min. A small bleeding site in the suture line required reclamping of the carotid vessels. Within 1 minute of reclamping, the pulse returned to 86 beats/min. and the blood pressure to 140/70 mm Hg. After release of the vascular clamps, blood pressure again fell to 70 mm Hg systolic and the pulse to 55 beats/min. The carotid sinus nerve was then locally infiltrated with approximately 2 ml of 1 percent xylocaine. This produced an immediate return of the blood pressure to 150/90 mm Hg and the pulse to 90 beats/min. These vital signs remained stable throughout the remainder of the operation. After the ensuing one and one half hours, the patient slowly began to drop his blood pressure to a low of 86/60 mm Hg and his pulse to 42 beats/min. At this point, an intravenous epinephrine infusion

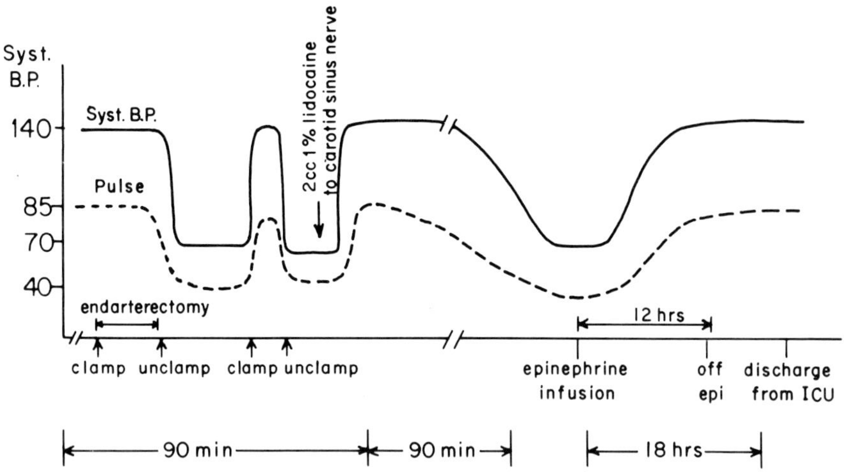

Figure 30-3. Graph of the blood pressure in a patient who exhibited a severe form of postcarotid endarterectomy hypotension that was mediated through the carotid sinus nerve reflex arc.

was begun with normalization of vital signs. Over the following 12 hours, the epinephrine was gradually stopped, and the patient experienced no further hypotensive spells. This patient dramatically illustrates the carotid sinus baroreceptor reflex arc mediation of postcarotid endarterectomy hypotension.

Obviously, there are several reasons why not all patients undergoing carotid endarterectomy experience hypotension postoperatively. Ransom et al.[14] and Tarlov et al.[4] showed that preoperative plasma volume expansion will decrease the frequency and severity of the hypotensive response to operation. Further, inadvertent operative trauma to the carotid sinus nerve may interrupt the reflex arc thereby masking any potential for hypotension. In addition, many of these patients will have lost their baroreceptor reflex due to the severity of the atherosclerosis at the carotid bifurcation. Interestingly, Tyden[5] reported that 80 percent of the patients who developed postcarotid endarterectomy hypotension had severe stenosing lesions, usually involving the entire circumference of the vessel wall. On the other hand, only 30 percent of patients with ulcerative lesions developed postcarotid endarterectomy hypotension.

The potential sequelae of transient hypotension in the untreated, diffusely atherosclerotic patient may dramatically affect the outcome of operation. Neurologic complications occurred in 7 percent of patients who were hypotensive after carotid endarterectomy in Bove's series.[1] Ransom et al.[14] reported that 40 percent of new postoperative neurological deficits appeared during or shortly after episodes of hypotension. It is unclear whether these cerebrovascular accidents were due to carotid artery thrombosis or due to intracranial arterial thrombosis during the period of poor perfusion. Nevertheless, either mechanism can produce catastrophic neurologic deficits in the face of hypotension. The potential for systemic complications is also increased in the setting of hypotension. Since these patients have generalized atherosclerosis and frequently have significant ischemic heart disease, periods of inadequate perfusion pressure can produce lethal consequences.

Postoperative hypotension due to increased baroreceptor activity can be avoided by routinely dividing the sinus nerve. This is not encouraged, however, since this removes an important autoregulatory mechanism. Rather than dividing the nerve, infiltration of the carotid sinus nerve with xylocaine is recommended in order to achieve local blockade. Although routine blockade is recommended by some surgeons, we prefer to employ this technique only if a dropping pulse rate or blood pressure is noted during operation. Such a selective use has been necessary in less than 5 percent of cases.

After excluding other causes of hypotension, postcarotid endarterectomy hypotension is treated in our center by pharmacologic support with epinephrine. Although neosynephrine may be equally useful, we begin an epinephrine infusion of 12 micrograms/ml at a rate of 15 ml/min and titrate the infusion to maintain a normal blood pressure. Other therapeutic modalities such as Tyden's[5] use of a small catheter left in the region of the carotid sinus nerve for postoperative xylocaine infusion appear to us to be less advantageous.

SUMMARY

Aberrations in blood pressure frequently affect patients undergoing carotid endarterectomy. Although there are several explanations for these hemodynamic changes, many are on the basis of carotid nerve dysfunction. Regardless of the etiology, however, postoperative instability of blood pressure may significantly contribute to increased morbidity and mortality of carotid artery surgery. Therefore, aggressive hemodynamic monitoring to identify aberrations in blood pressure and rapid institution of appropriate therapy to correct such changes should be a routine component of perioperative care of the carotid endarterectomy patient.

REFERENCES

1. Bove EL, Fry WJ, Gross WS, et al: Hypotension and hypertension as consequences of baroreceptor dysfunction following carotid endarterectomy. Surg 85(6):633, 1979
2. Lehv MS, Salzman EW, Silen W: Hypertension complicating carotid endarterectomy. Stroke 1(5):307, 1970

3. Towne JB, Bernhard VM: The relationship of post-operative hypertension to complications following carotid endarterectomy. Surg 88(4):575, 1980
4. Tarlov E, Schmidek H, Scott RM, et al: Reflex hypotension following carotid endarterectomy by carotid sinus nerve blockade. Acta Chir Scand Suppl 500:61, 1980
5. Tyden G, Samnegard H, Thulin L: Rational treatment of hypotension after carotid endarterectomy by carotid sinus nerve blockade. Acta Chir Scand suppl 500:61, 1980
6. Angell-James JE, Lumley JSP: The effects of carotid endarterectomy on the mechanical properties of the carotid sinus and carotid sinus nerve activity in atherosclerotic patients. Br J Surg 61:805, 1974
7. Crawford ES, DeBakey ME, Blaisdell FW, et al: Hemodynamic alterations in patients with cerebral arterial insufficiency before and after operation. Surg 48(1):76, 1960
8. Guyton AC: Short-term regulation of mean arterial pressure, in Textbook of Medical Physiology, 6th edition. Philadelphia, W. B. Saunders and Co., p 246, 1981
9. Matsumoto GH, Cossman D, Callow AD: Hazards and safeguards during carotid endarterectomy—technical considerations. Amer J Surg 133:458, 1977
10. Appenzeller O, Descarries L: Loss of baroreceptor reflexes in patients with cerebrovascular disease. Trans Am Neurol Ass 89:177, 1964
11. Bristow JD, Honour AJ, Pickering GW, et al: Diminished baroreceptor sensitivity in high blood pressure. Circ 39:48, 1969
12. Caplan LR, Skillman J, Ojemann R, et al: Intracerebral hemorrhage following carotid endarterectomy: A hypertensive complication. Stroke 9(5):457, 1978
13. Cushing H: Some experimental and clinical observations concerning status of increased intracranial tension. Amer J Med Sci 124:375, 1902
14. Ransom JHC, Imparato AM, Clauss RH, et al: Factors in the mortality and morbidity associated with surgical treatment of cerebrovascular insufficiency. Suppl I to Circ 39,40:269, 1969
15. Smith TC, Cooperman LH, Wollman H: The therapeutic gases, in Goodman Gilman (eds): The Pharmacological Basis of Therapeutics, 6th edition. New York, MacMillan Pub. Co., 1980, p 321
16. Fourcade HE, Larson CP, Ehrenfeld WK, et al: The effects of CO_2 and systemic hypertension on cerebral perfusion pressure during carotid endarterectomy. Anes 33:383, 1970
17. Thompson JE: Complications of carotid endarterectomy and their prevention. World J Surg 3:155, 1979
18. Bunag RD, Page IH, McCubbin JW: Neural stimulation of release of renin. Circ Res 19:851, 1966
19. Hodge RL, Lowe RD, Vane JR: Increased angiotensin formation in response to carotid occlusion in the dog. Nature 211:491, 1966
20. Bartter FC, Mills IH, Gann DS: Increase in aldosterone secretion by carotid artery constriction in the dog and its prevention by thyro-carotid arterial junction denervation. J Clin Invest 39:1330, 1960
21. Moore WS: Post-operative management and complications, in Rutherford RB (ed): Vascular Surgery. Philadelphia, W. B. Saunders and Co., 1979, p 1141

William H. Baker

31

Management of Stroke During and After Carotid Surgery

Stroke associated with carotid endarterectomy is a most dreaded complication. The aims of the operation are by and large to prevent stroke, not cause it. Although the incidence of this complication varies, in hospitals of excellence it ranges downward towards 1 percent. No one peripheral vascular service, therefore, has a vast experience in the management of these complications.

Loyola University Medical Center is not an exception to the above facts. Our experience with management of acute neurologic complications following carotid endarterectomy is anecdotal at best. Nonetheless, our material is being hereby reviewed in this chapter and a treatment plan formulated. The reader should examine the evidence, or lack of it, very carefully before adopting our theses.

ETIOLOGIES OF STROKE

Stroke during carotid endarterectomy may be caused by a variety of factors. In general, these factors may be divided from a surgical point of view into mechanical or "metabolic." This differentiation is more than of pure academic interest. A "metabolic" etiology stroke suggests that the physiology of the neurons has been upset in such a way as to prevent normal function. Regardless of the exact reason for the "metabolic" abnormality, the surgeon cannot reverse the neurologic status of the patient by going back to the operating room. Thus when the patient falls into this category of postoperative stroke, treatment will be nonoperative. Contrariwise, if the patient has a stroke on the basis of a mechanical etiology, i.e. an occluded endarterectomy site, perhaps a return to the operating room to restore normal cerebral blood flow will be beneficial. This latter view is not universally held.

During the past 6 years, 19 patients have had an acute neurologic event in the immediate perioperative period. These patients are detailed in Table 31-1. Discussion of these patients will form the basis for this chapter.

OCCLUDED CAROTID ENDARTERECTOMY

W.B., an 80-year-old man with hemispheric transient ischemic attacks, awoke neurologically intact in the recovery room. He became hypertensive and developed a neck hematoma. When returned to the operating room he was found to be hemorrhaging from numerous small arterial bleeders. The carotid was said to be pulsatile but was not meticulously examined. After his re-exploration for bleeding, the patient was slow to awaken and was maintained on a respirator. It was only after several hours that we realized that he had a dense hemiparesis. At autopsy, his carotid was found to be occluded.

V.D., a 72-year-old man, had left hemispheric transient ischemic attacks. Following a left carotid thromboendarterectomy, he had an uneventful time in the recovery room. That evening he was noted to have intermittent hand weakness by the nurses that was unreported. The next morning on rounds, it was found that he was neurologically intact, but 24 hours postendarterectomy he was unable to eat lunch because of hand paresis. In addition, he had mild aphasia but was able to converse fairly readily. Because we felt that his new symptoms were relatively acute, he was returned to the operating room where a thrombosed carotid was found. No distinct flap of distal intima was seen. The closure was not felt to be constricting. After a thrombectomy was performed, the arteriotomy was reclosed. The patient awoke with a dense hemiparesis and is currently a nursing home patient.

K.M., a 53-year-old male, had a left hemispheric stroke with good recovery. Angiographically, he had an occlusion on the left and a severe stenosis on the right. A right carotid endarterectomy was performed. After initially awakening, he developed a left hemiparesis and was unresponsive. At re-exploration, the origin of the carotid was pulsatile but an operative arteriogram (Fig. 31-1) revealed a total occlusion at the end of the endarterectomy site. The distal end point was tacked down and flow returned approximately 90 minutes post onset of symptoms. He recovered but is a severe neurologic cripple.

W.D., an 80-year-old man, had a right carotid endarterectomy for appropriate transient ischemic attacks. He was confused in the immediate postoperative period but awoke within hours neurologically intact. His postoperative noninvasive testing suggests that he has an occlusion of this artery.

B.G. and C.P. are discussed in the section on inappropriate timing of operation in patients with pre-existing neurologic symptoms, although their endarterectomy sites are presumed occluded.

These six postoperative occlusions do not give us a basis for recommending therapy. The first man's occlusion was unrecognized, and he

Table 31-1
Postendarterectomy Stroke

Patient	Age	Indication	Angiogram ICA L	Angiogram ICA R	Angiogram VERT L	Angiogram VERT R	Operation	Stump Pressure	Remarks
Occluded Carotid Endarterectomy									
K.M.	53	L H Stroke	100%	75%	0%	0%	R C TEA	13/11	Severe global deficit; thrombectomized, flow restored 90 min. (no shunt used); now has severe deficit.
W.B.	80	R H TIA	100%	50% Ulcer	0%	0%	R C TEA	36/30	Bleeding→re-exploration; awoke with global deficit→died. Occluded ICA at autopsy.
V.D.	72	L H TIA's	90%	25%	0%	0%	L C TEA	44/38	Intermittent weakness & aphasia reoperated at 30 hour for occlusion; awoke with severe deficit.
R.D.	80	R H TIA	Siphon 50%	90% plus Siphon 50%	0%	75%	R C TEA	17/16	Confused × 24 hour, noninvasive test→occlusion. Now intact.
B.G. C.P.	SEE INAPPROPRIATE TIMING OF OPERATION								
Hypoperfusion									
C.M.	49	V B TIA	100% CCA ICA	100% CCA	0%	50%	L SC → R ICA	N.D.	Hematoma→drainage; at 24 hour, aphasia and right hemiparesis; good recovery.
L.K.	76	V B TIA	90%	80%	0%	75%	L C TEA	80/70	EEG→slowing before and after clamping. Awoke confused. Mild right hemiparesis at 24 hour. Good recovery (see text).

Table 31-1 (continued)
Postendarterectomy Stroke

Patient	Age	Indication	Angiogram ICA L	Angiogram ICA R	Angiogram VERT L	Angiogram VERT R	Operation	Stump Pressure	Remarks
Occluded Carotid Endarterectomy									
M.B.	74	L H TIA	75%	25%	50%	100%	L C TEA	43/35	1/2 hour post-op→RUE paresis→ permanent mild deficit
O.G.	68	ASX	90%	80%	0%	0%	R C TEA	120/80	Had L C TEA one week prior. 10 hour after R C TEA had hypertension and seizures and right hemiparesis. 95% recovery.
J.S.	56	L H Stroke (old) R H TIA's	100%	60%	0%	0%	R C TEA	26/24	Abnormal EEG pre-op (L hem). Slowly progressive right hemiparesis. STA→MCA bypass pod #4 good recovery.
Embolus									
L.O.	65	Amaurosis Fugax	70%	0%	0%	0%	R C TEA	90/60	Post-op scotoma. Embolus seen in retina.
C.S.	65	L H TIA R H TIA	75%	75%	0%	100%	L C TEA Dacron patch angioplasty	75/60	R C TEA with recovery. One week later, L C TEA, Post-op ↑ BP. Pod #3→RUE paresis. Now, loss of fine motor control.
S.M.	71	ASX AAA	80%	100%	0%	0%	L C TEA	36/31	1 hour post-op→R H stroke; reoperated. Intraluminal thrombus removed. Permanent dense hemiparesis.
R.M.	61	L H RIND	50% Ulcer	50%	0%	0%	L C TEA	50/40	Amaurosis pod #1 coincident with loss of STA pulse. Rx ASA. ASX.

Inappropriate Timing of Endarterectomy									
B.G.	68	Mild dysphasia (2 weeks duration)	90%	25%	0%	0%	L C TEA	90/70	Pod #1 dysphasia, moderate. Pod #2 dysphasia, moderate; bruit gone; atrial fib.; Heparin rx. Pod #4 slight hemiparesis; acute MI. Pod #30 no weakness; mild dysphasia. Non-inv. test→occl. ICA.
C.P.	65	R H TIA's on Heparin. Mild deficit going to OR.	99%	50%	Not visualized		L C TEA	N.D.	Mild residual hemiparesis. Non-inv. test→ICA occl. Seizures developed late post-op.
O.S.	79	Mild RUE weakness. Mild aphasia. (10 days) on Coumadin.	50%	50%	50%	0%	R C TEA	63/50	Worsening of aphasia, new paresis. 95% recovery.
G.S.	70	Acute stroke on Heparin.	99%		Not visualized		L C TEA	50/40	Complicated heart disease (see text). Maintained on Heparin. Initial improvement. Pod #3→ hemorrhagic infarct.
A.C.	51	L H TIA's	75%	STA-MCA bypass	50%	100%	L C TEA	65/25	Slow waking. Hemiparesis at 24 hour. Wife reports he could not stand pre-op. Post-op A/G→ patent carotid. Occluded basilar artery. 50% recovery.

Table 31-1 (continued)
Postendarterectomy Stroke

Patient	Age	Indication	Angiogram				Operation	Stump Pressure	Remarks
			L ICA	R	L VERT	R			
Occluded Carotid Endarterectomy									
Occluded Second Lesion									
A.M.	63	L H TIA	50% see text (MCA 100%)	0%	0%	0%	L C TEA	56/46	Pod #6 aphasia. A/G→L MCA occl. STA-MCA bypass. 100% recovery.

L-left; R-right; ICA-internal carotid artery; CCA-common carotid artery; C TEA-carotid thromboendarterectomy; TIA-transient ischemic attack; H, hem-hemispheric; VB-vertebro-basilar; SC-subclavian; N.D.-not done; EEG-electroencephalography; RUE-right upper extremity; Asx-asymptomatic; STA-superficial temporal artery; p.o.d.-post-op day; AAA-abdominal aortic aneurysm; A/G-arteriogram; BP-blood pressure; MCA-middle cerebral artery; RIND-reversible ischemic neurologic deficit; non-inv.-non-invasive.

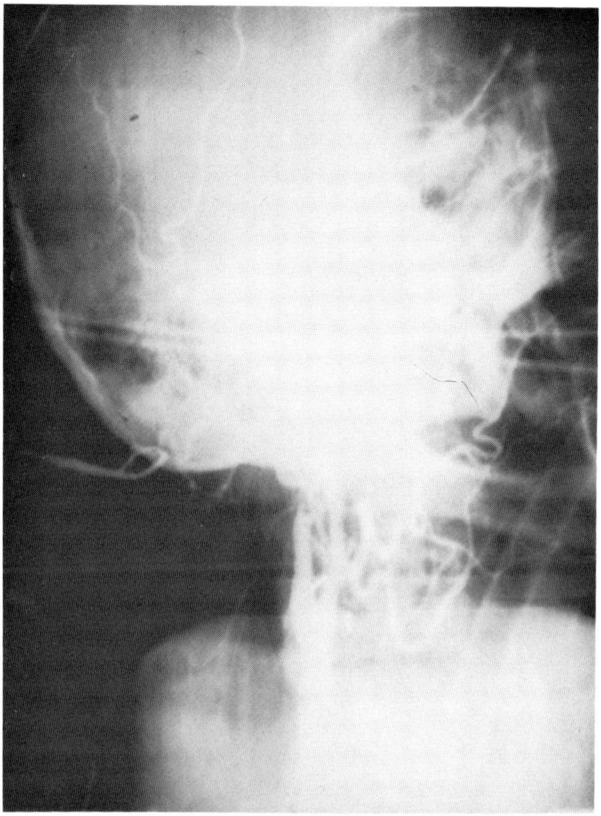

Figure 31-1. An operative arteriogram that shows a complete occlusion at the distal end of the endarterectomy site. A distal flap of intima was seen at reoperation.

subsequently went on to die. Had we reopened his thrombosed carotid artery, one can only speculate about his result. Reoperation in patient V.D. was in retrospect delayed several hours after the onset of neurologic symptoms and was detrimental. The third re-exploration restored flow after 90 minutes of ischemia and left a severe neurologic deficit.

The entire question of reoperation of patients with deficits is under review. For many years, operations on acute stroke of any kind were considered taboo. These operations were often ill conceived and done on patients with severe deficits after many hours of occlusion. The main objection to operation in the face of acute stroke is the conversion of a bland white infarct into a hemorrhagic infarct with worsening of the neurologic status of the patient.[1,2] In an area that is severely hypoxic and hypoperfused, there is damage not only of the neuronal tissue but also of the integrity of the blood vessels.[3] Restoration of a full head of pressure into these areas is said to lead to bleeding within the brain or a cerebral hematoma. This red infarct is associated with a severe worsening of the patient's clinical condition. This dogma continued to be espoused by most learned vascular surgeons until more recent reports suggested that operations for acute neurologic deficits under certain conditions may be justified.

In 1971, Najafi et al.[4] reported upon emergency carotid thromboendarterectomy, including 15 patients who occluded after angiography and 7 patients who occluded after carotid endarterectomy. These 7 patients awoke neurologically intact and later developed their deficit. As a group, 6 of these patients had a poor result (3 died), 5 were unchanged, and 11 were improved. Of interest, 4 patients with complete occlusions who were reoperated within one hour had total recovery from their hemiparesis.

More recently, Kwaan et al.[5] have reported on the successful management of early stroke after carotid endarterectomy. Three of their patients developed hemiplegia in the recovery room. The patients were immediately returned to the operating room, and under local anesthesia their wounds were reopened. A thrombosed carotid was found in each instance. The arteriotomy was opened, a thrombectomy hastily performed, and a shunt inserted to reestablish flow. Flow was restored within 20, 30, and 45 minutes. All recovered without deficit.

These good results with re-exploration can be contrasted with the poor results reported in this chapter. If anything is to be learned from these relatively few cases, it is that early exploration may be indicated, but late exploration is not. The time limit appears to be around one hour.

HYPOPERFUSION

Five of our patients had postoperative neurologic deficits because of hypoperfusion. This hypoperfusion is presumed to have occurred during the endarterectomy. It has been our policy not to use a temporary indwelling shunt during the performance of the carotid endarterectomy, relying instead on the adequacy of the collateral circulation. Whereas this policy is successful in almost all patients, there nonetheless remain others in whom collateral circulation is apparently inadequate.

L.K., a 76-year-old, had a left carotid endarterectomy for a 90-percent ICA stenosis. In addition, she had a proximal left common carotid stenosis that did not alter pressure and an 80 percent contralateral ICA stenosis. Intraoperative EEG showed 3-4 second periods of slowing both before and after clamping suggestive of ischemia, but no sustained changes were recorded. During the first postoperative day, she was confused. By the second postoperative day, she started to demonstrate a mild right hemiparesis. She continued to have a normal EEG. A CAT scan was likewise normal. Noninvasively, her operated carotid tested to be patent. She eventually had a full recovery. Although the etiology of this deficit is difficult to ascertain, we felt that she most likely had hypoperfusion. The brief episodes of slowing on the EEG before and during clamping suggestive of hypoperfusion support this point of view. The fact that she recovered indicates that the neurologic deficit was due to a reversible hypoxia.

C.M., a 49-year-old lady with multiple lesions, had a left-to-right subclavian-to-right internal carotid artery bypass. Her left internal carotid artery was occluded. Postoperatively, she required drainage of a neck hematoma and 24 hours later developed an aphasia with a right hemiparesis. It is hypothesized that during the performance of operation, her left or unoperated cerebral hemisphere became ischemic, developed edema, and thus led to her neurologic picture. Again, fortunately she recovered.

The third patient, J.S., a 56-year-old mover, had a total occlusion of a left internal carotid artery and a 60 percent stenosis of the right internal carotid artery. Eight years prior, he had had a left hemispheric stroke with full recovery. Currently, he was having right hemispheric transient ischemic attacks. A right carotid endarterectomy was performed. Back pressure was 25 mm Hg with a common carotid pressure of 150/80. Postoperatively, he awoke intact but soon thereafter began to develop right upper extremity paresis. This slowly progressed over the next 2 days and on postoperative day 3, he had a superficial temporal-middle cerebral artery bypass. His neurologic recovery was complete.

A fourth patient, M.B., a 74-year-old man, had a left carotid endarterectomy for left hemispheric transient ischemic attacks. The operated carotid was 75 percent stenotic and ulcerated. Although the contralateral carotid looked relatively normal radiographically, he had bilateral vertebral artery disease. In the recovery room he awoke neurologically intact but one-half hour later developed right upper extremity paresis. Noninvasively, his artery was patent. He has since recovered with but minimal paresis of a hand. Although he may have had an embolus, hypoperfusion cannot be ruled out.

O.G., a 68-year-old female, had an uneventful right carotid endarterectomy for transient ischemic attacks. One week later, a left carotid endarterectomy was performed. Ten hours after the second operation, she began to have seizure activity involving her left arm and leg. Her blood pressure at this time was 270/130. She was treated with diazepam and dilantin. A residual hemiparesis slowly cleared almost completely. It is presumed that intraoperative hypoperfusion led to contralateral hemispheric edema. This edema then produced the patient's symptoms. If the second operation had been delayed or if a temporary indwelling shunt had been used, perhaps this neurologic event could have been avoided.

In none of these patients can it be absolutely proven that they had intraoperative hypoperfusion. The evidence is particularly strong in those patients who had contralateral neurologic symptoms develop relative to a contralateral occlusion. The late development of these symptoms suggests that indeed it is not the immediate effect of hypoperfusion, but rather a late effect, i.e. the development of cerebral edema, that causes the neurologic picture.

Sundt et al.,[6] have correlated postoperative hyperperfusion using Xenon flow studies. In patients with a high grade carotid stenosis in whom there had been a very major increase in cerebral blood flow after the completion of endarterectomy, a pronounced increase in the retinal artery pressure was found. Sundt suggests that there was a paralysis of cerebral autoregulatory mechanisms in these patients. In their series, seizure activity or migraine variants were seen. In 2 patients receiving anticoagulant therapy, intercerebral hemorrhage occurred. Interestingly, they did not report the late development of symptoms such as in our patient population. This may be related to their liberal use of temporary intraarterial shunting. It is to be noted that of our 4 patients, 2 recovered completely, 1 recovered after the performance of a superficial temporal-middle cerebral artery bypass, and 1 recovered with a minor hand paresis.

EMBOLIZATION

Four patients in our series had symptoms presumably due to embolization.

One patient, L.O., a 65-year-old man, had a right carotid thromboendarterectomy for amaurosis fugax of the right eye. Postoperatively, he awoke with a scotoma, and an embolus could be seen in his retinal artery. Although this may have occurred before the performance of the operation, it must be presumed that this embolus was dislodged during the performance of the endarterectomy.

C.S., a 65-year-old female, had transient cerebral ischemia related to each cerebral hemisphere. A right carotid endarterectomy was performed, followed 1 week later by a left carotid endarterectomy. Following her second operation, she was slow in recovering. Hypertension was noted. On the third postoperative day, she had the sudden onset of a right upper extremity paresis. Noninvasive tests revealed the carotid to be patent, although she was not arteriogrammed. She had been maintained on aspirin and persantine.

This particular patient had a Dacron patch angioplasty closure of a very small carotid artery. It is presumed she embolized from the endarterectomized site or this Dacron patch. Her recovery has been complete in terms of strength, although she states she has lost the ability to control her fine motor function and no longer teaches a course in crocheting.

R.M., a 61-year-old male, had a left carotid endarterectomy for transient cerebral ischemia. On the first day postoperatively, he complained of an episode of amaurosis fugax in the left eye. At that time, the external carotid artery occluded with a disappearance of the superficial temporal artery pulse. It was presumed that the external carotid artery occluded and that some clot dislodged to his eye. He was placed on antiplatelet therapy and has been asymptomatic since.

S.M., a 71-year-old female, had a prophylactic carotid endarterectomy for an 80 percent stenosis and a contralateral internal carotid artery occlusion. The internal carotid artery back pressure was 36 with a common carotid artery pressure of 160. In the recovery room, she awoke intact but then developed the sudden onset of a hemiparesis. She was returned immediately to the operating room, but the carotid was found to be open. An arteriogram (Fig. 31-2) disclosed an irregularity within the endarterectomized artery. The arteriotomy was opened, a temporary indwelling shunt inserted, and the clot cleaned from the artery. No intimal flaps were seen during this time. The artery was reclosed. She recovered with a dense hemiparesis. Although the absolute etiology of this patient's stroke cannot be determined, it is presumed because of the suddenness of the onset of her symptoms and the findings at operation that an embolus did indeed occur. Hypoperfusion may also have been a contributory factor.

If the surgeon can make a diagnosis of embolus, further surgical therapy is ordinarily not indicated. An exception to this rule would be an operation to remove the source of the embolus so that a second and more devastating embolic attack does not occur. Operation per se will obviously not improve the clinical picture that has resulted from the first embolus. In our experience, most but not all of these embolic episodes leave relatively little permanent neurologic damage. The one exception occurred in a lady who had a contralateral occlusion and low back pressure. One might surmise that inadequate collateral circulation was responsible for the severity of her defect.

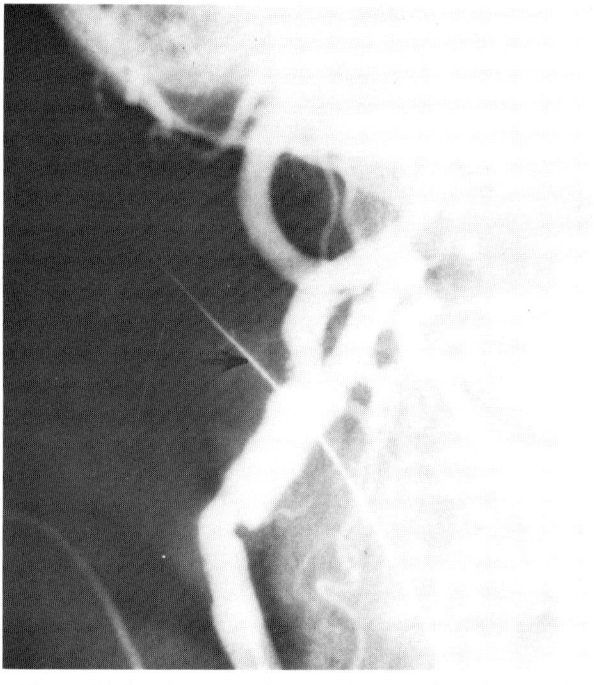

Figure 31-2. An operative arteriogram thrombus at the endarterectomy site.

INAPPROPRIATE TIMING OF ENDARTERECTOMY

Five patients in our series awoke with neurologic deficit as a direct result of poor patient selection. All of these patients had acute neurologic deficits preoperatively that were exacerbated by the performance of a carotid endarterectomy.

Two patients (O.S., B.G.) were recovering from relatively mild strokes. Both had had hemispheric transient ischemic attacks and on the last episode had had a residual neurologic deficit. Both had had relatively mild aphasias. One had a functioning hand that was obviously weak. Operation was indicated for continued TIAs despite adequate anticoagulation and a 90 percent ICA stenosis respectively. After the endarterectomy, both were minimally but perceptively worse after the operation. One man eventually had a 95 percent recovery of function and is enjoying retirement uneventfully. The second man had a myocardial infarction while in the hospital. He developed atrial fibrillation. A bruit which was initially present in his neck disappeared. Noninvasively, he had an occluded ICA. Whether or not the ICA was occluded because of technical reasons, embolus from his atrial fibrillation, or low flow past the endarterectomy site cannot be detemined. At late follow-up, he had no weakness but did indeed have an intermittent aphasia.

C.P., a 65-year-old lady had a 99 percent stenosis with waxing and waning neurologic deficit. An emergency operation was done during the midst of one of these attacks. She awoke with a residual mild hemiparesis. She later on developed seizure activity related to this cerebral hemisphere. She currently is functioning well. Noninvasively, the endarterectomized site is occluded.

A fourth lady, G.S., with severe valvular heart disease and a history of a thrombosed prosthetic aortic valve, had a femoral posterior tibial artery bypass of Gortex for threatened limb loss. She was being maintained on heparin when she developed an acute stroke. A CAT scan showed no hemorrhage. Arteriographically, she had a 99 percent stenosis. Because of the relative mildness of her deficit (50 percent hemiparesis) and the severity of her stenosis, an endarterectomy was performed. Heparin was maintained. Although at first she was better, 3 days later she became worse. A CAT scan disclosed that she had had a hemorrhagic infarction. She spent the next 3 months in and out of the hospital before dying.

Operation in this patient was ill advised. Her physicians were adamant against stopping heparin because of her prior cardiac valvular thrombosis. If her carotid stenosis had been left intact, perhaps her cerebral hemisphere would have been protected from hemorrhagic infarction. Although operation restored blood flow leading to temporary improvement, in the face of continued anticoagulation, this new full head of pressure next produced a hemorrhagic infarction.

ASSOCIATED LESIONS

Patient #1, a 63-year-old banker, had a left carotid endarterectomy for left hemispheric transient ischemic attacks. He had a known right middle cerebral artery occlusion, but the left middle cerebral artery was thought to be normal. Six days postoperatively, he had a left hemispheric transient ischemic attack. A second left hemispheric episode left him mildly aphasic. A repeat arteriogram showed that he had an occlusion of the middle cerebral artery on the left, which in retrospect was stenotic on his first arteriogram (Fig. 31-3). A subsequent superficial temporal-middle cerebral artery bypass was performed. Despite a postoperative subdural hematoma that required drainage, the patient has made a full recovery and has returned to work.

This case details the need for excellent preoperative arteriography as well as a complete and accurate interpretation. All too often, we are loathe to return the patient to the arteriographic suite if the films are not of perfect quality. Statistically, most stenotic lesions occur at the carotid bifurcation rather than distally in the arterial tree. Furthermore, the surgeon who operates in the neck has a tendency to focus his interpretation upon this area rather than equally examine the intracerebral arterial tree.

Inadequate films and their interpretation directly led to this patient's neurologic complication. Ideally, both lesions would have been recognized preoperatively. If the severity of the middle cerebral artery stenosis had been appreciated either by repeat angiography or by regional blood flow studies,

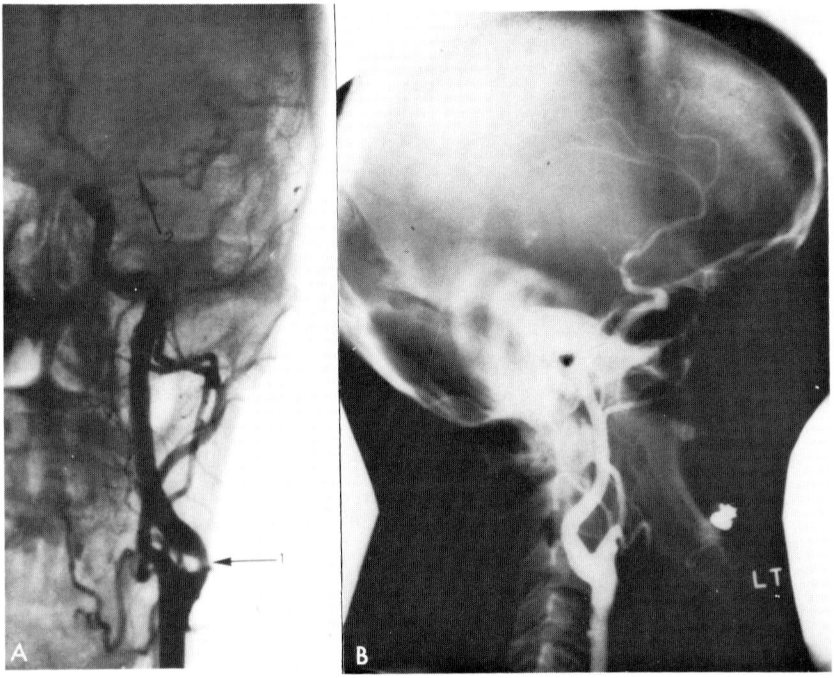

Figure 31-3. (A) Preoperative arteriogram (subtraction technique) showing a severe ICA origin stenosis and a poorly seen MCA stenosis.
(B) One week postendarterectomy. The MCA has occluded.

then he would probably have had a superficial temporal-middle cerebral artery anastomosis to bypass both lesions. A carotid endarterectomy in the neck could have been performed to prevent ocular and anterior cerebral ischemia. This plan would obviate his postoperative stroke. His eventual good result occurred despite our imperfect planning.

"METABOLIC" ETIOLOGIES OF STROKE

Nonoperative causes of the postoperative stroke include hypotension before, during, or after the operation. It is our policy to insert an indwelling radial artery catheter to monitor the patient's systemic pressure prior to the induction of anesthesia. Induction of anesthesia is a slow process designed to maintain hemodynamic stability. During the perfomance of the operation, the patient's blood pressure is always kept at a normal range for the patient. During the period of carotid clamping, the systemic pressure is, if needed, pharmacologically boosted into the high-normal range. In the postoperative period, the patient's lowest blood pressure minus 10 percent is established as a minimal requirement. No strokes secondary to hypotension are recorded in our series.

Hypertension is also well known to cause neurologic deficits. Although hypertension may in and of itself cause bleeding, in particular it may cause edema in an already ischemic brain. For those reasons, the patient's highest blood pressure plus 10 percent is kept as the upper limits of allowable blood pressure excursion. These limits are not strictly adhered to during the performance of the endarterectomy; in the postoperative period, blood pressure is watched extremely closely. Although hypertension was noted in some patients, we did not believe it to be directly responsible for the stroke. This association has been noted by others.[7]

The patients are also watched for development of hypoxemia. Although the hemodynamic parameters may be normal, inadequate ventilation for whatever reason leading to hypoxemia will sometimes tip the precariously balanced brain. In older patients in whom excessive doses of narcotics are given for pain, hypoventilation may be induced and hypoxemia will result. These patients must be supported with respiratory assist if need be until the medication is excreted or detoxified.

SUMMARY

Our current practice is as follows. The patient who develops a neurologic deficit is immediately re-examined; this procedure includes a supraorbital Doppler examination as well as direct Doppler audio analysis of the operated carotid artery. Immediate arteriography is not performed so as not to cause unnecessary delay. If there is any suggestion that the endarterectomy site is occluded, re-exploration is immediately performed using an indwelling shunt. All other patients are treated nonoperatively as outlined above. It is to be emphasized that this plan is based on anecdotal experience, and future modifications should be anticipated.

REFERENCES

1. Bruetman ME, Fields WS, Crawford ES, et al: Cerebral hemorrhage in carotid artery surgery. Arch Neurol 9:458, 1963
2. Wylie EJ, Hein MF, Adams JE: Intracranial hemorrhage following revascularization for treatment of acute stroke. J Neurosurg 21:212, 1964
3. Meyer JS: Importance of ischemic damage to small vessels in experimental cerebral infarction. J Neuro Pathol Exp Neurol 17:571, 1958
4. Najafi H, Javid H, Dye WS, et al: Emergency carotid thromboendarterectomy. Arch Surg 103:610, 1971
5. Kwaan JHM, Connolly JE, Sharefkin JB: Successful management of early stroke after carotid endarterectomy. Ann Surg 190:676, 1979
6. Sundt TM Jr, Sharbrough FW, Piepgras DG, et al: Correlation of cerebral blood flow and electroencephalographic changes during carotid endarterectomy. Mayo Clin Proc 56:533, 1981
7. Towne JB, Bernhard VM: The relationship of postoperative hypertension to complications following carotid endarterectomy. Surg 88:575, 1980

Wayne M. Swenson
William J. Gundlach

32

Carotid Endarterectomy in a Community Hospital

There has long been controversy over whether certain medical and surgical diseases such as acute leukemia, coronary artery disease, and carotid artery disease should be treated by physicians in community hospitals or only by physicians in large medical centers. The resolution of this controversy demands examination of results being achieved in smaller centers to determine if they match the excellent results being achieved in some large centers.

Carotid endarterectomy is widely held as effective therapy for the treatment of transient cerebral ischemic attacks and for the prevention of stroke. Perioperative mortality and morbidity have become acceptably low in some large centers because of better patient selection and because of improved operative technique and perioperative care. In an editorial in 1978, Hertzer[1] pointed out the disturbingly high incidence of complications following carotid endarterectomies reported from some community hospitals. He stated that carotid endarterectomy may be performed outside of major cardiovascular centers if "patients are properly selected and if the operation is frequently performed by a surgeon trained and experienced in extracranial cerebrovascular repair." This is a reasonable opinion; however, there was no information in the medical literature at that time indicating that acceptable results were being obtained in smaller centers. In 1979, we reported a low perioperative mortality and morbidity in a large number of patients who had carotid endarterectomies in a small community hospital.[2] Since that report, there have been several others with similar good results.[3-6] Our patients have also experienced a low incidence of stroke during long-term postoperative follow-up.

In this chapter, we review our experience with carotid endarterectomy in a small community hospital in Bismarck, North Dakota. We also review the experience of others in community hospitals who have reported their cases in the literature.[3–6]

MATERIALS AND METHODS

Description of Patients

This study includes 176 patients who underwent 210 consecutive carotid endarterectomies by the same surgeon during the period from June, 1969 through 1981. Most of the patients were referred by physicians in North Dakota from an area around Bismarck, extending approximately 200 miles.

There were 110 men and 66 women who ranged in age from 39 to 80 years. One-hundred-and-two patients had a history of hypertension or were found to have blood pressure readings greater than 150/90 millimeters of mercury. Eighteen patients had diabetes mellitus, and 21 had symptomatic peripheral arterial disease. The patients were examined by an internist either before or after referral.

Preoperative Assessment

All of the patients were evaluated by the vascular surgeon and a neurologist or neurosurgeon to determine the proper indications for operation. Direct carotid angiography or transfemoral angiography was performed on each patient. During the last 8 years of the study, transfemoral angiography was used exclusively to visualize all four extracranial vessels.

Neurologic symptoms of the patients were classified in a manner similar to that suggested by Thompson and Talkington.[7] Twenty-six patients had asymptomatic bruits, 67 had transient cerebral ischemic attacks, 22 had amaurosis fugax and 61 had symptoms of chronic cerebral ischemia. Chronic cerebral ischemia is defined as obvious cerebrovascular insufficiency with loss of memory, impaired mentation, or motor deterioration. Many of the patients in this latter category previously had had a completed stroke, and many of the significant carotid artery lesions were found incidentally while performing transfemoral angiography for evaluation of peripheral arterial insufficiency or coronary artery disease.

Indications for operation were based upon the 3 categories of clinical signs and symptoms and the finding of greater than 50 percent narrowing of the diameter of the carotid artery or an ulcerating plaque, or both. No patients with acute or progressing stroke were operated on.

Operative Technique

All of the endarterectomies were performed in an identical manner, as described by Julian and associates.[8] A Javid shunt was used in every instance. This shunt is beneficial because it allows an unhurried procedure, provides for protection of the cerebral circulation, and facilitates an accurate dissection of the plaque to its distal limits. It also forms a convenient stent for the arteriotomy repair and avoids creating unsuspected narrowed areas, should placement of sutures inadvertently be too far from the edge of the arteriotomy.

Heparin is not used systemically to obviate wound hematomas postoperatively. The Javid shunt, however, is immersed in a solution containing 1000 U.S.P. units of heparin in 250 milliliters of normal saline to help prevent the formation of thrombi in the tubing in the event that a slow run-off situation is encountered.

There are important steps that have been found to facilitate the procedure. The carotid artery is approached through an incision along the anterior border of the sternocleidomastoid muscle and carried down through the platysma. Bleeders are clamped and cauterized or tied with a 4–0 disposable suture. The omohyoid muscle belly is identified. The jugular vein is then identified because it is easier to locate than the carotid artery. Dissection is carried along the medial aspect of the jugular vein. A triangle is formed by the jugular vein, omohyoid muscle and the thyroid vein. Ligation of the thyroid vein exposes the common carotid artery. Sharp dissection rather than finger dissection is used to avoid dislodging plaque material from the carotid artery. Excessive manipulation of the artery is also avoided. The vagus nerve, which usually lies beneath the common carotid artery, is protected from injury. Dissection is carried around the common carotid artery, and an elevating vascular tape is placed around it. Dissection is then carried up to the superior thyroid artery which is surrounded with a tourniquet ligature or a temporary hemoclip. The external and internal carotid arteries are then dissected with care to avoid injury to the hypoglossal nerve. Sometimes the ansa hypoglossus is incised about 1 cm from the hypoglossal nerve to facilitate dissection of the internal carotid artery. The carotid body is not dissected. The distal extent of the plaque in the internal carotid artery is determined by palpation to determine if the Javid shunt can be inserted above it. A clamp is placed across the external carotid artery, and then one is placed across the common carotid artery. The internal carotid artery is then temporarily occluded by a vascular tissue forceps while an arteriotomy is made from the common carotid into the internal carotid artery beyond the plaque. The Javid shunt is then inserted into the internal carotid artery and seated well up into the siphon and held in place by a small Javid clamp. The shunt is allowed to fill by backflow and then it is inserted into the common carotid artery. Extreme care is taken to avoid air and plaque emboli while inserting the shunt into the common carotid artery. The shunt is gently pushed down into the common carotid artery and seated with a large Javid clamp. After the Javid shunt is in place, an unhurried dissection of the plaque ensues. After the plaque is removed, residual debris is removed and the arteriotomy is irrigated with copious amounts of solution containing 1,000 units of heparin in 250 milliliters of normal saline. After the arteriotomy site is clear of debris, it is closed with a running suture of 5–0 prolene. The proximal suture line is carried down to the carotid bifurcation. It is then tied in place with another suture. The common carotid artery is closed with 5–0 prolene until 1 cm of the arteriotomy remains. The cord tape previously placed across the internal carotid artery is simply elevated, as the Javid shunt is removed, to prevent backflow bleeding. This maneuver obviates the use of a vascular clamp on the internal carotid artery. The Javid shunt is now removed from the common carotid artery which is then temporarily occluded with a vascular clamp.

During final closure, backflow bleeding has been allowed by intermittently lowering the internal carotid artery vascular cord tape. After completing the arteriotomy, blood is initially allowed to flow into the external carotid artery to prevent any debris or air from traveling into the internal circulation. The average time from insertion of the Javid shunt until closure of the arteriotomy is 24 minutes. The platysma muscle is closed with a running suture of 4–0 Dexon, and the skin is closed with a subcuticular suture of Dexon or with skin staples. No drains are used.

RESULTS

The age range, sex distribution, and incidence of associated diseases in this series of 176 patients are similar to those reported by others. Radionuclide brain scans or computed tomography (CT) scans of the brain performed preoperatively in all of the patients showed only minor abnormalities, but no tumors or other unsuspected major abnormalities were detected. There was no correlation between findings on radionuclide brain scan or CT scan and the angiogram regarding the site of significance of the carotid artery lesion.

Perioperative morbidity and mortality were low (see Table 32-1). The morbidity from angiography was only 1.7 percent. An embolectomy at the needle puncture site was performed on 1 patient. No vascular injury resulted. In the 2 other patients, complete occlusion of an internal carotid artery developed, and an endarterectomy was required as an emergency measure. The patients recovered completely without neurologic deficit. One patient died within 3 weeks after operation of a myocardial infarction. The other patient, a 77-year-old man who had greater than 95 percent occlusion of both

Table 32-1
Complications of Carotid Endarterectomy in Community Hospitals

Series	Perioperative Deaths (%)	Perioperative Strokes (%)
Prioleau, Aiken, Hairston[15] (1977)	3.2	10.7
Easton and Sherman[16] (1977)	6.6	14.5
Gundlach and Swenson[2] (1979)	0.8	0.8
Haynes and Dempsey[3] (1979)	1.1	0.4
Carmichael[4] (1980)	0.2	2.1
Watson[5] (1981)	0.6	1.6
Kistner[6] (1981)	1.5	3.0
Present series updated	0.9	0.9

carotid arteries, died 1 day after carotid endarterectomy of a massive cerebral infarction. There were no other operative deaths. Postoperative neurologic morbidity occurred in 6 patients. Four had transient hemiparesis, and two had transient aphasia lasting for a few days. Only one other patient had a major stroke postoperatively which resulted in permanent hemiparesis.

Long-term follow-up was obtained 12½ years after the first patient had undergone carotid endarterectomy. This information was obtained by direct examination or by a questionnaire sent to the patient or the referring physician, or both. Death certificates obtained from the Bureau of Vital Statistics were also examined. Thirty-eight patients were dead. Twelve patients had had strokes, eight of whom died. One of the strokes occurred on the nonoperated side, and none of the other strokes were clearly related to the previous carotid operation.

Re-stenosis of the internal carotid artery developed in 3 patients. One was repaired 1 year after the initial endarterectomy and another 9 years after the initial endarterectomy. Neurologic symptoms did not develop during the period of re-stenosis. The third patient restenosed the same carotid artery on 2 occasions. The first repair was 18 months after initial endarterectomy, and the second was 6 months later. She experienced transient cerebral ischemic attacks during each period of re-stenosis. She has had no neurologic symptoms or other indications of re-stenosis during a 2-year follow-up period.

DISCUSSION

The purpose of this chapter is not to become embroiled in controversies over various technical aspects of carotid surgery, but to simply demonstrate that carotid surgery can be performed safely and effectively by a well-trained experienced vascular surgeon practicing in a small community hospital. The safety of the operation is measured by the mortality and serious morbidity associated with the operation. Its efficacy is measured by the prevention of strokes. Of the 176 patients in our series, 173 left the hospital with an excellent result. The incidence of perioperative mortality reported from some large centers approaches 1 percent. The incidence of permanent neurologic morbidity is 1 percent–4 percent.[1]

The efficacy of carotid endarterectomy in our hands is demonstrated by the occurrence of strokes in only 12 patients (7 percent) during the long-term follow-up period of 12½ years. Studies of the natural history of carotid artery disease in nonoperated patients have documented a stroke risk of 30–40 percent for patients with transient cerebral ischemic attacks related to the carotid circulation.[9–12] The low incidence of stroke in our patients compares favorably with that reported for patients treated with carotid endarterectomy in a large cooperative study.[13,14]

As we have previously mentioned, initial reports from community hospitals showed a discouragingly high incidence of perioperative death and strokes.[15,16] Hertzer[1] discussed these reports in his editorial in 1978 and concluded that "too many surgeons performed carotid endarterectomy on too few patients, for any surgeon to gain substantial experience with either patient selection or the operation."

It is gratifying that since our report in 1979, there have been at least 4 reports from community hospitals demonstrating similar good results from carotid endarterectomy with large numbers of patients (see Table 32-1).[3–6] Again, these data support Hertzer's view that "carotid endarterectomy may be expected to have optimal results if patients are properly selected and if the operation is frequently performed by a surgeon trained and experienced in extracranial cerebrovascular repair."[1]

CONCLUSION

One-hundred-and-seventy-six patients underwent 210 consecutive carotid endarterectomies in a small community hospital in Bismarck, North Dakota, during a period between June, 1969 through 1981. All operative procedures were performed by the same surgeon employing the Javid shunt. A less than 1 percent perioperative mortality and permanent neurologic morbidity resulted. The long-term postoperative stroke incidence was also low. Several other surgeons operating in community hospitals have reported similar good results.[3–6] These findings are comparable with those reported from large medical centers that have extensive experience in carotid endarterectomy.

Because carotid artery atheromatous disease is so common, patients should have easy access to safe and effective endarterectomy. Not all patients can be, nor need to be, referred to large medical centers for this operation because it can be safely and effectively performed within the community by well-trained, experienced vascular surgeons.

ACKNOWLEDGEMENTS

The authors thank Marie Albrecht for preparing the manuscript and Jane Hruby, R.N. for her assistance in collecting the data.

REFERENCES

1. Hertzer NR: Carotid endarterectomy and common sense (editorial). Surg Gynecol Obstet 147:235, 1978
2. Gundlach WJ, Swenson WM: Carotid endarterectomy in a community hospital. Surg Gynecol Obstet 148:720, 1979
3. Haynes CD, Dempsey RL: Carotid endarterectomy: Review of 276 cases in a community hospital. Ann Surg 189:758, 1979
4. Carmichael JD: Carotid surgery in the community hospital; 467 consecutive operations. Arch Surg 115:937, 1980
5. Watson MR: Carotid endarterectomy in a small community hospital. Am J Surg 141:543, 1981
6. Kistner RL: Carotid endarterectomy: 10-year experience at Straub. Straub Clinic Proc 46:17, 1981
7. Thompson JE, Talkington CM: Carotid endarterectomy. Ann Surg 184:1, 1976
8. Julian OC, Dye WS, Javid H, et al: A Handbook of Operative Surgery; Cardiovascular Surgery (ed 2). Chicago, Year Book Medical Publishers, 1970, p 114
9. Acheson J, Hutchinson EC: Observations on the natural history of transient cerebral ischemia. Lancet 2:871, 1964
10. Baker RN, Ramseyer JC, Schwartz WS: Prognosis in patients with transient ischemic attacks. Neurology 18:1157, 1968
11. Marshall J, Meadows S: The natural history of transient ischemic cerebrovascular attacks. Q J Med 33:309, 1964
12. Toole JT, Janeway P, Choi K, et al: Transient ischemic attacks due to atherosclerosis. A prospective study of 160 patients. Arch Neurol 32:5, 1975
13. Bauer RB, Meyer JS, Fields WS, et al: Joint study of extracranial arterial occlusion III: Progress report of controlled study of long-term survival in patients with and without operation. JAMA 208:509, 1969

14. Fields WS, Maslenikov V, Meyer JS, et al: Joint study of extracranial arterial occlusion. Progress report of prognosis following surgery or nonsurgical treatment for transient cerebral carotid artery lesions. JAMA 211:1993, 1970
15. Prioleau WH Jr, Aiken AF, Hairston P: Carotid endarterectomy: Neurologic complications as related to surgical techniques. Ann Surg 185:678, 1977
16. Easton JD, Sherman DG: Stroke and mortality rate in carotid endarterectomy: 228 consecutive operations. Stroke 8:565, 1977

PART IX

Long-Term Results of Carotid Surgery

James A. DeWeese

33

Long-Term Results of Surgery for Carotid Artery Stenosis

Carotid endarterectomies are currently being performed for patients with stenotic and/or ulcerated lesions at the carotid bifurcation who have demonstrated transient ischemic attacks (TIAs), reversible ischemic neurologic deficits (RINDs), completed strokes with little residual neurologic deficits, fluctuating strokes, and asymptomatic bruits in selected patients.

There has been a progressive improvement in the reported early results, and in general, the mortality rates are less than 1 percent and significant morbidity is less than 3 percent.

It is our purpose to discuss the late results of carotid endarterectomy beginning 1 month after operation. These will be discussed as they relate to (1) the endarterectomized carotid artery, (2) other extracranial cerebral vessels, and (3) mortality rates and causes of death.

IPSILATERAL ENDARTERECTOMIZED CAROTID ARTERY

The late results of carotid endarterectomy as they pertain to changes occurring in the operated artery are generally determined by an analysis of the following: (1) symptoms; (2) pathologic changes.

Symptomatic Results

There are many long-term follow-up studies that confirm the efficacy of carotid endarterectomy for relieving neurologic symptoms considered referable to lesions at the carotid bifurcation. These "classic" symptoms include amaurosis fugax or other symptoms of retinal ischemia, speech deficits, particularly if the lesion is on the side of the dominate hemisphere, and contralateral sensory and motor deficits. We have had the opportunity of following a group of 103 patients all of whom were operated on 5 and then 10 years previously for symptoms of transient ischemic attack.

There were 88 patients with "classic" TIAs. There were seven of the 88 patients who continued to have their preoperative symptoms or developed recurrent symptoms within 10 years. In addition, there were 4 patients who died of strokes considered referable to the operated carotid artery. In other words 11 percent of the 103 patients suffered late symptoms or death probably related to the operated carotid artery.[1,2] There were an additional 13 percent of the patients who continued to have nonclassic symptoms following their operation such as dizziness, syncope, headache, seizures, and confusion. Although it is possible that the failure to relieve these symptoms was due to persistent or new changes in the operated carotid artery, it is still strongly possible that the preoperative, and therefore the persistent postoperative, symptoms were related to vertebro-basilar or intracranial vascular lesions or other physical and emotional problems. It can be said with some certainty however, that at least 11 percent and not more than 24 percent of this group of patients had postoperative appropriate neurologic symptoms secondary to residual or new changes in their endarterectomized carotid artery. Thompson et al. reported a series of 293 endarterectomies for patients with transient ischemic attacks followed 6 months to 13 years.[3] There were 33 patients who were improved but continued to have postoperative symptoms, 4 who worsened, and 3 who improved and then worsened. There were therefore 40 of the 210 or 19 percent of the surviving patients who had symptoms possibly related to the endarterectomized vessel. The types of symptoms are not broken down into classic and nonclassic and the length of follow-up is not the same, but it can probably be stated that not more than 19 percent of the patients as compared to 24 percent of the patients in our series had late neurologic symptoms related to the endarterectomized carotid artery. Lees and Hertzer reported follow-up studies on 335 patients who underwent carotid endarterectomy for one of the several indications previously listed and were followed for a mean interval of 8.6 years.[4] There were 36 of 325 or 11.1 percent of the patients who developed transient ischemic attacks or strokes appropriate to the carotid artery operated upon, which again suggests that at least 11 percent of late neurologic problems are related to lesions of the operated artery. Fields et al. reported from the Joint Study of Extracranial Arterial Occlusion the long-term results of a group of patients randomized to carotid endarterectomy or nonsurgical treatment.[5] During an average 42 month follow-up, eight of 77 or 10 percent of patients who were operated upon for classic symptoms suffered transient ischemic attack in the carotid distribution. There were 73 patients operated upon who had nonclassic symptoms of which 49 percent had recurrent symptoms. There were 82 nonsurgical patients whose symptoms were classic and during the same follow-up period, 22 of them, or in other words 27 percent, exhibited recurrent classic symptoms. There were 63 patients with nonclassic symptoms, and 34 or 54 percent of them were symptomatic. Strokes occurred as a result of cerebral infarction in the same hemisphere as the original symptomatic carotid artery in two of 150 or 1.3 percent of operated patients as compared to 13 of 145 or 9 percent in nonoperated patients. Because of differences in reporting methods and length of follow-up, it is difficult to get an accurate estimate of the incidence of recurrent symptoms or strokes related to the operated carotid artery from all published long-term studies. It would be helpful if the life-table analysis method were used for reporting this type of information as suggested by Riles, Imparato, Mintzer, and Baumann.[6] A review of most of these reports, however, confirms our observations that approximately 10 percent of the patients followed for a significant period of time following carotid endarterectomy do develop recurrent symptoms or strokes possibly related to pathologic changes occurring in the operated artery.[7,8,9,10,11,12]

Pathologic Changes

The healing and pathologic changes occurring following endarterectomy have been evaluated in experimental studies, in late pathologic studies, by arteriography, and more recently by noninvasive testing.

Gryska, in 1959, removed intima and a portion of the media from the canine aorta and observed that the denuded area was covered by a thin thrombus which gradually organized and formed a firm collagenous layer, the surface of which resembled normal intima.[13] If the animals were placed on a high cholesterol diet and oral propylthiouracil, they developed, over a 5 month period, nonocclusive atheromatous changes in the wall of the aorta. Dirrenberger and Sundt studied the healing process of endarterectomized canine carotid arteries with light microscopy and scanning electron microscopy during the first 3 months after surgery. They observed the immediate formation of a fibrin-platelet carpet on the endarterectomized surface.[14] A thrombus layer then appeared causing occlusion in 52 percent of the vessels. By 48 hours, re-endothelialization was observed in the patent vessels, and by the end of a week, the mural thrombus had disappeared. At 3 months, re-endothelialization was complete. French and Rewcastle observed in humans that a new intimal layer completely covered the endarterectomized site within 30 days after operation and that further thickening and maturation occurred in time.[15]

There have been several reports on the pathologic changes observed when restenosis of the carotid artery has occurred. Acute thrombosis in the early postoperative period is usually attributed to the trauma of vascular clamps, the inadequate removal of the atheromatous plaque, or dissection underneath the intimal flap at the distal end of the endarterectomy. The lesions which cause recurrent stenosis and later occlusion demonstrate two distinctively different pathologic processes. Cossman, Callow, Stein and Matsumoto carefully examined seven pathologic specimens obtained at the time of operation for restenosis of endarterectomized carotid arteries.[16] They found that all seven specimens showed an exuberant myointimal hyperplasia which was characterized by stellate cells enmeshed in a fibromyxomatous stroma. There was a pronounced scarceness of lipid and no evidence of neovascularization or of deposition of hemosiderin or fibrin. These changes were not consistent with an atherosclerotic process or an organizing mural thrombus. All of these lesions occurred within the first 2 years after the original operation. At the time of the reoperation, no cleavage plane existed between the thickened myointima and the vessel wall, making a repeat endarterectomy very difficult. Cossman and other colleagues on another study operated on 16 carotid arteries for recurrent stenosis. They describe the microscopic pathologic findings on 1 patient to consist of myointimal proliferation and also indicate that no cleavage plane exists between this thickened myointima and the vessel wall.[17] They did not remove the other 15 lesions but describe them as having a smooth, white, glistening, fibrous thickening typical of myointimal hyperplasia. Operative management consisted of a patch angioplasty. Thirteen of their 16 lesions were also observed within 2 years of operation. Stoney and String examined 29 specimens of lesions causing restenosis.[18] Eleven of these lesions appeared within 15 months of the original operation, and the gross and microscopic description conformed to Cossman's description of "myointimal proliferation." They also described 20 lesions occurring 2 to 13 years following the original endarterectomy which showed the typical findings of atherosclerosis and at the time of reoperation, the endarterectomy dissection plane was developed easily in 16 of the 20 vessels. Hertzer et al. did describe atherosclerotic lesions in 7 of 9 patients who had restenosis within 2 years of operation and 6 of 16 whose lesions appeared 3 to 13 years following operation.[19] They, however, observed myointimal fibroplasia in only 2 of the 9 lesions appearing within 2 years and also observed myointimal hyperplasia in an artery which had restenosed 85 months following operation. In summary, it appears that myointimal fibroplasia is almost always responsible for restenosis occurring within 2 years and that recurrent atherosclerosis is almost always responsible for new lesions appearing greater than 2 years after the original operation. The myointimal fibroplasia lesion is best managed by patch angioplasty, whereas the recurrent atherosclerotic lesions may again be removed by endarterectomy. Imparato in a discussion of Stoney and String's paper, expresses the opinion that the neointimal fibroplasia is merely a different phase of true atherosclerosis.[18] He and others have expressed the opinion that routine vein patching might reduce the incidence of this phenomena. In summary, the incidence of restenosis was

3.4 percent and 3.6 percent in 2 years in Cossman's and his colleagues' experience, 1.5 percent in Stoney's and Strings' follow-up at 5 months to 13 years, and 1 percent in patients followed by Hertzer et al. for 0 to 20 years.[16,17,18,19] In general, these patients were all symptomatic, but in Hertzer's series it is indicated that 13 of 15 patients were recognized because of neurologic symptoms; but two of 15 were suspected of having recurrent problems because of a new bruit.[19] These 4 studies were reporting only recurrent stenosis which was operable and do not include those patients who may have had recurrent problems in the carotid arteries and remained asymptomatic or suffered completed strokes or death.

Stoney and String reported a very unusual cause of carotid narrowing secondary to external scarring.[18] Another unusual complication, which has been reported, is the development of false aneurysms particularly when patch grafts of either vein or prosthetic materials were used. These lesions may become symptomatic presumably because of the development of thrombus in the aneurysmal sac.[1,20,21] We have seen one true aneurysm develop in a patch graft in which a small piece of the anterior facial vein was used for the patch.

There have been a number of attempts to define the actual incidence of pathologic changes in endarterectomized carotid arteries. In one of our early series, information concerning the patency of the operated arteries was available in 98 of 227 operations.[22] The carotid artery was found to be patent by direct information provided by angiography, exploration, or autopsy in 36 instances. In an additional 56 cases, improvement in retinal artery pressures as measured by ophthalmodynamometry provided indirect information that the vessels were patent. Direct information revealed that in the remaining 6 cases, the carotid arteries were thrombosed. Ophthalmodynamometry was remarkably accurate in 19 patients in whom both direct information and retinal pressures were available. There were no false positive nor false negatives. Blaisdell,[23] Lim and Hall, in 1967, reported a prospective angiographic study. They obtained arteriograms before the incision was closed and in the early postoperative period on 95 vessels. In 9 patients the angiograms were again repeated 5 years later. In 26 instances, the arteriograms performed in the operating room revealed defects which compromised the lumen by 30 percent or more, and these were all corrected. Only one of 95 vessels was occluded in the early postoperative study, and this was in a patient in whom the lesion had not been completely corrected. Arteriograms or autopsies were obtained 5 years after operation in 15 patients, of which two demonstrated significant carotid arterial restenosis. Edwards and colleagues reported arteriograms on 30 patients (43 operated arteries) of 75 patients who underwent carotid endarterectomy 5 to 9 years previously.[24] Significant restenosis was found in 6 of 43 or 7 percent of the arteries. These were all producing symptoms. There was a less than 25 percent stenosis of 6 arteries, and 34 were 100 percent patent.

In summary, the restenosis rate was estimated to be 13 percent in 5 years in Blaisdell's series, 7 percent in 5 to 9 years in Edwards et al.'s study, and 6 percent at 1 month to 6 years by Schutz et al.[25]

During the past few years, noninvasive techniques have been used for the long-term follow-up after carotid endarterectomies. Kartchner and McRae followed over 700 patients. Significant recurrent stenosis was observed in 34 of 700 or 4.85 percent of the arteries.[26] Kremen and associates reported on the use of ocular pneumoplethysmography (OPG-GEE) on 173 postoperative carotid arteries 0 to 12 years after their procedure. There were 17 of 173 studies that were positive, and there was a presumed incidence of recurrent stenosis of 9.8 percent.[27] Only three of the patients were symptomatic, and it is interesting that six of the 17 arteries were totally occluded. Turnipseed et al. used Doppler imaging and spectral analysis of carotid flow to follow 70 patients at 1 week, 6 months, and yearly intervals.[28] The length of follow-up was not recorded. There were 29 patients with new or persistent bruits, but only seven of the bruits were thought to be caused by stenotic lesions of the internal carotid artery by noninvasive testing. Therefore, seven of 70 arteries, or 10 percent, did restenose following endarterectomy. Only 2 patients, or 2.9 percent, were symptomatic. Unfortunately, none of these studies were prospective studies of a significant number of consecutive patients followed by life-table analysis for a significant period of time. All of the available data, however, suggest that significant restenosis of an endarterectomized carotid artery may occur in approximately 10 percent of patients followed for 5 to 10 years after operation.

CONTRALATERAL CAROTID ARTERY

Atherosclerotic lesions may appear or progress in other extracranial cerebral vessels during the late follow-up of patients who have undergone carotid endarterectomy. The lesions most frequently associated with late neurologic symptoms are in the carotid artery contralateral to the endarterectomized vessel. We were able to make long-term observations on 77 patients who underwent carotid endarterectomy and demonstrated asymptomatic contralateral carotid stenosis at the time of their operation and compared this group of patients to 50 patients whose contralateral arteriograms appeared normal prior to their first operation.[29] All the patients were operated on at least 5 years prior to their last follow-up, and follow-up was terminated at the time of death, when the contralateral carotid artery became symptomatic, or at the end of 5 years. There were 14 of 67 or 21 percent of the patients who developed symptoms referable to the contralateral carotid artery. Classic TIAs were observed in 11 of 67 or 16.5 percent of the patients 10 to 48 months following their original operation. The other 3 patients (4.5

percent) suffered completed strokes at 6, 10, and 28 months and two of them died. Only 1 of the patients had TIAs prior to onset of their completed strokes. Of the 50 patients without demonstrable contralateral carotid stenosis, only 2 patients developed symptoms referable to the contralateral carotid artery within the follow-up period. One patient experienced a TIA, and 1 patient suffered a cerebrovascular accident without antecedent TIAs. Johnson et al. followed a group of patients following carotid endarterectomy from 6 to 42 months.[30] Of 77 patients with contralateral stenosis of greater than 10 percent and less than 100 percent, there were only 3 or 3.9 percent who developed symptoms appropriate to contralateral carotid artery lesions. Levin and Sondheimer in 1973 observed 60 patients from 2 to 12 years after carotid endarterectomy, who had greater than a 50 percent contralateral carotid stenosis.[31] Only 2 of their parents experienced TIAs. Levin et al., in 1980, presented a longer follow-up of 147 patients with ulceration or significant stenosis of the contralateral carotid artery.[32] They have been followed from 3 months to 20 years following their carotid endarterectomy. There were 9 of 137 or 6.6 percent of the patients who developed symptoms appropriate to disease of the contralateral carotid artery, and they underwent elective endarterectomy. Lees and Hertzer followed 48 patients who underwent carotid endarterectomy with significant contralateral carotid stenosis.[33] Over an 8.6 years mean follow-up period, 8 of 48 or 16 percent suffered late completed strokes. The number of TIAs which occurred is not recorded. This 16 percent incidence of neurologic events in the contralateral stenotic carotid artery following endarterectomy is similar to the incidence of 21 percent observed by ourselves. Johnson's lower incidence may be related to a shorter period of follow-up. The unique experience of Levin et al. is inconsistent with our observation and the observations of others who have followed asymptomatic carotid artery stenoses. Javid et al. followed 140 asymptomatic carotid artery lesions for 1 to 9 years with an average period of 3 years.[34] Eighty-six of the patients were available for repeated arteriograms, and 59 percent of the patients demonstrated increased severity of the degree of stenosis during follow-up. The rate of atheromatous change was increased in patients with hypertension and those with more significant degrees of stenosis on the initial study. They indicate that 11 patients died with profound neurologic deficit. They also state that "50 percent of patients who died from stroke had no symptoms referable to cerebral circulation prior to sudden development of neurologic insult." Humphries et al. followed-up 168 asymptomatic patients with carotid artery stenosis of more than 50 percent for a period up to 12 years.[35] During the period of follow-up, 30 of the 168 or 17.9 percent of the patients developed neurologic deficits. There were 26 patients with TIAs and 4 patients with completed strokes. Three of the 4 patients with completed strokes had TIAs prior to the final event. There is other evidence that completed strokes or progressive strokes frequently occur without warning sign of a TIA. In a retrospective analysis of the occurrence of TIAs prior to strokes in 112 patients, 47 percent of the patients had no previous TIAs. There were 53 percent of the patients who did have TIAs but 36 percent of these 59 patients had the onset of their first warning TIA less than 3 months prior to their completed stroke.[36] Thompson, Patman, and Talkington followed 138 patients with asymptomatic bruits for 1 to 124 months following detection.[37] There were 37 patients or 26.8 percent who developed TIAs and 24 patients or 17.4 percent who suffered completed strokes, of which 3 died.

There is some dispute as to whether patients with contralateral asymptomatic stenosis or whether any patient with an asymptomatic stenosis should undergo a prophylactic endarterectomy. There are those who prefer to follow such patients until they develop transient ischemic attacks or significant increase in the degree of stenosis as determined by noninvasive techniques or change of bruit. Unfortunately, there are many patients who develop their completed stroke or even fatal stroke without previous TIAs. In addition, the vessels can become inoperably occluded before the lesion is recognized. These arguments for prophylactic endarterectomy are also supported by the fact that the reported late results of patients operated on for asymptomatic stenoses are better than those for symptomatic patients.[38] Moore et al. suggest that a controlled study in which a life-table analysis was used for documenting the occurrence of late neurologic complications would be helpful in documenting the advisability of performing prophylactic endarterectomies. Until such study is available, however, it would appear that endarterectomy for asymptomatic stenosis is reasonable therapy for preventing stroke and prolonging survival in the hands of vascular surgeons who can offer a low operative morbidity and mortality.

LATE MORTALITY

There are a number of reports documenting a significant late mortality rate following carotid endarterectomy. Death occurred 1 month to 7 years following operation in 100 of 313 or 32 percent of patients reported by DeWeese et al. in 1971.[36] The indication for operation included TIAs, progressive and completed strokes, and asymptomatic stenoses. Other studies with long-term follow-up report include the following: DeBakey et al. reported a 25 percent mortality rate in a 1 to 11 year follow-up;[8] Edwards, Wilson, and Bennett reported a 29 percent mortality rate in patients in a follow-up period of 5 to 9 years;[9] Thompson et al. observed a 30 percent mortality rate in a follow-up period of 1 to 13 years;[3] Riles et al. reported a 22 percent mortality rate within 5 years of operation;[6] and Hertzer and Lees, utilizing a life-table analysis, reported a 5 year mortality rate of 27 percent and an 11 year mortality rate of 48 percent.[39] There are a number of factors that obviously affect this late mortality rate. We observed a 34 percent mortality rate within 5 years of carotid endarterectomy performed on 103 patients for TIAs.[1] The mortality rate was directly related to the age of the patient at the time of their operation. The mortality rate for patients age 50 to 59 was 18 percent, for ages 60 to 69 was 38 percent, and for age 70 to 79 was 52 percent. The mortality rate for patients with a previous history or findings of arteriosclerotic heart disease by electrocardiogram was 56 percent as compared to 27 percent for those patients without a positive history. Hertzer and Lees made similar observations on the significance of a preoperative history of arteriosclerotic heart disease.[39] They observed a statistically significant increased fatal myocardial infarction rate in 209 patients suspected of having coronary artery disease preoperatively as compared to 116 patients with no clinical evidence of coronary artery disease. The indication for operation also appears to have an effect upon the mortality rate. For example, we observed the mortality rate during a 1 month to 7 year follow-up period to be 22 percent for patients operated on for asymptomatic lesions, 27 percent for patients operated on for TIAs and 35 percent for patients operated on with progressive or completed strokes. Similar observations have been reported which suggest that the late mortality rate for patients operated on for more benign cerebrovascular symptoms has improved. Utilizing a life-table analysis, there was only a 17 percent mortality rate at 42 months in 72 patients who underwent endarterectomy for asymptomatic lesions.[38]

The cause of death is most frequently related to arteriosclerotic disease elsewhere, particularly in the coronary arteries. In a group of 103 patients who underwent carotid endarterectomy for TIAs, 50 percent of the patients died within 10 years.[2] The causes of death were as follows: myocardial infarction 60 percent, cerebrovascular accident 14 percent, ruptured aneurysm 2 percent, nephrosclerosis 2 percent, cancer 8 percent, and miscellaneous 14 percent. Hertzer and Lees observed a 48 percent mortality among 325 patients within 11 years who underwent carotid endarterectomy for various indications.[39] The causes of death and the percent of which they were responsible for death were as follows: myocardial infarction 37 percent, stroke 17 percent, cancer 10 percent, heart failure 6 percent, pulmonary embolism 2 percent, aorto-enteric fistula 1 percent, ruptured aortic aneurysm .5 percent, intestinal ischemia .5 percent, and other or unknown 26 percent. The cause of death was remarkably similar in several long-term follow-up studies. Complications of arteriosclerosis were common causes of death, and myocardial infarction or its complications was the single most common cause. Thompson et al. reported that 52.3 percent of late deaths were due to cardiac disease;[3] Edwards reported that 64 percent of patients died of coronary occlusion.[9] It is interesting that both Thompson and Edwards also report deaths due to ruptured aortic aneurysm.

Hertzer and Lees, in their retrospective study, presented information on the effect on mortality rate of the performance of myocardial revascularization as a staged or combined procedure in conjunction with carotid endarterectomy or as an incidental operation during the late follow-up period.[39] There was a statistically significant improvement in actuarial survival and reduction in the late mortality for patients with suspected coronary artery disease who received myocardial revascularization. Crawford and colleagues found that the 5-year actuarial survival for 97 patients with carotid stenosis and coronary artery disease was 73 percent following carotid endarterectomy alone and 88 percent following carotid endarterectomy in conjunction with direct myocardial revascularization.[40]

In summary, the late mortality rate following carotid endarterectomy is most directly related to the ages of the patients, their preoperative symptoms, and the degree of coronary artery disease present. The causes of death are most frequently secondary to complications of arteriosclerosis. These observations present a strong argument for the careful follow-up of these patients in hopes of discovering treatable lesions such as restenoses, contralateral carotid lesions, coronary artery disease, or abdominal aneurysms before irreversible damage occurs.

REFERENCES

1. DeWeese JA, Rob CG, Satran R, et al: Results of carotid endarterectomies for transient ischemic attacks—Five years later. Ann Surg 178:258, 1973
2. Rob C: Occlusive disease of the extracranial cerebral arteries: A review of the past 25 years. J Cardiovas Surg 19:487, 1978
3. Thompson JE, Austin DJ, Patman RD: Carotid endarterectomy for cerebrovascular insufficiency: Long-term results in 592 patients followed up to thirteen years. Ann Surg 172:633, 1970
4. Lees CD, Hertzer NR: Postoperative stroke and late neurologic complications after carotid endarterectomy. Arch Surg 116:1561, 1981
5. Fields WS, Maslenikov V, Meyer JS, et al: Joint study of extracranial arterial occlusion. JAMA 211:1993, 1970
6. Riles TS, Imparato AM, Mintzer R, et al: Comparison of results of bilateral and unilateral carotid endarterectomy five years after surgery. Surgery 91:258, 1982
7. Callow AD: The Leriche Memorial Lecture. J Cardiovas Surg 21:641, 1980
8. DeBakey ME, Crawford ES, Cooley DA, et al: Cerebral arterial insufficiency: One to 11-year results following arterial reconstruction operation. Ann Surg 161:921, 1965
9. Edwards WS, Wilson TAS, Bennett A: The long-term effectiveness of carotid endarterectomy in prevention of strokes. Ann Surg 168:765, 1965
10. Heyman A, Young WG Jr, Brown IW Jr, et al: Long-term results of endarterectomy of the internal carotid artery for cerebral ischemia and infarction. Circulation 36:212, 1967
11. Owens ML, Atkinson JB, Wilson SE: Recurrent transient ischemic attacks after carotid endarterectomy. Arch Surg 115:482, 1980
12. Riles TS, Imparato AM, Kopelman I: Carotid artery stenosis with contralateral internal carotid occlusion: Long-term results in fifty-four patients. Surgery 87:363, 1980
13. Gryska PF: The development of atheroma in arteries subjected to experimental thromboendarterectomy. Surgery 45:655, 1959

14. Dirrenberger RA, Sundt TM Jr: Carotid endarterectomy temporal profile of the healing process and effects of anticoagulation therapy. J Neurosurg 48:201, 1978
15. French BN, Rewcastle NB: Sequential morphological changes at the site of carotid endarterectomy. J Neurosurg 41:745, 1974
16. Cossman D, Callow AD, Stein A, et al: Early restenosis after carotid endarterectomy. Arch Surg 113:275, 1978
17. Cossman DV, Treiman RL, Foran RF, et al: Surgical approach to recurrent carotid stenosis. Amer J Surg 140:209, 1980
18. Stoney RJ, String ST: Recurrent carotid stenosis. Surgery 80:705, 1976
19. Hertzer NR, Martinez BD, Benjamin SP, et al: Recurrent stenosis after carotid endarterectomy. Surg Gynec Obstet 149:360, 1979
20. Gurdjian ES: Surgical considerations of 258 patients with carotid artery occlusion. Surg Gynec Obstet 110:327, 1960
21. Rainer WG, Guillen J, Bloomquist CD, et al: Carotid artery surgery: Morbidity and mortality in 257 operations. Amer J Surg 116:678, 1968
22. DeWeese JA, Rob CG, Satran R, et al: Surgical treatment for occlusive disease of the carotid artery. Ann Surg 168:85, 1968
23. Blaisdell FW, Lim R Jr, Hall AD: Technical result of carotid endarterectomy: Arteriographic assessment. Amer J Surg 114:239, 1967
24. Edwards WS, Wilson TAS, Bennett A: The long-term effectiveness of carotid endarterectomy in prevention of strokes. Ann Surg 168:765, 1965
25. Schutz H, Fleming JFR, Awerbuck B: Arteriographic assessment of carotid endarterectomy. Ann Surg 171:509, 1970
26. Kartchner MM, McRae LR: Noninvasive assessment of the progression of extracranial carotid disease, in Diethrich EB (ed): Noninvasive Cardiovascular Diagnosis, Current Concepts, chap. 2. Baltimore, Univ Park Press, 1978, p 13
27. Kremen JE, Gee W, Kaupp HA, et al: Restenosis or occlusion after carotid endarterectomy. Arch Surg 114:608, 1979
28. Turnipseed WD, Berkoff HA, Crummy A: Postoperative occlusion after carotid endarterectomy. Arch Surg 115:573, 1980
29. Podore PC, DeWeese JA, May AG, et al: Asymptomatic contralateral carotid artery stenosis: A five-year follow-up study following carotid endarterectomy. Surgery 88:748, 1980
30. Johnson N, Burnham SJ, Flanigan DP, et al: Carotid endarterectomy: A follow-up study of the contralateral non-operated carotid artery. Ann Surg 188:748, 1978
31. Levin SM, Sondheimer FK: Stenosis of the contralateral asymptomatic carotid artery—To operate or not?. Vasc Surg 7:3, 1973
32. Levin SM, Sondheimer FK, Levin JM: The contralateral diseases but asymptomatic carotid artery: To operate or not? Amer J Surg 140:203, 1980
33. Lees CD, Hertzer NR: Postoperative stroke and late neurologic complications after carotid endarterectomy. Arch Surg 116:1561, 1981
34. Javid H, Ostermiller WE, Hengesh JW, et al. Natural history of carotid bifurcation atheroma. Surgery 67:80, 1970
35. Humphries AW, Young JR, Santilli PH, et al: Unoperated, asymptomatic significant internal carotid artery stenosis: A review of 182 instances. Surgery 80:695, 1976
36. DeWeese JA, Rob CG, Satran R, et al: Endarterectomy for atherosclerotic lesions of the carotid artery. J Cardiovasc Surg 12:299, 1971
37. Thompson JE, Patman RD, Talkington CM: Asymptomatic carotid bruit: long-term outcome of patients having endarterectomy compared with unoperated controls. Ann Surg 188:308, 1978
38. Moore WS, Boren C, Malone JM, et al: Asymptomatic carotid stenosis: Immediate and long-term results after prophylactic endarterectomy. Amer J Surg 138:228, 1979

39. Hertzer NR, Lees CD: Fatal myocardial infarction following carotid endarterectomy: Three hundred thirty-five patients followed 6–11 years after operation. Ann Surg 194:212, 1981
40. Crawford ES, Morris GC Jr, Howell JF, et al: Operative risk in patients with previous coronary artery bypass. Ann Thorac Surg 26:215, 1978

PART X

Subclavian and Vertebral Artery Occlusion

Anthony M. Imparato
Thomas S. Riles

34

Surgery of Vertebral and Subclavian Artery Occlusions

Although the arrangement of arteries leading to the brain allows only one of the four extracranial arteries to supply the entire brain upon failure of the others,[1] nevertheless when only one of these vessels entering the circle of Willis becomes significantly narrowed or becomes the source of emboli, characteristic symptom complexes may occur. The severity depends upon 2 factors: the mechanism leading to ischemia, be it due to emboli or impairment of flow resulting from stenosis or occlusion, and the ability of the collateral circulation to compensate. It is generally agreed and is readily apparent from clinical observations, that carotid arterial insufficiency usually leads to ipsilateral cerebral hemispheric ischemia with contralateral motor and sensory deficits, ipsilateral visual disturbances, and if a dominant hemisphere is involved, to speech disorders. These are symptoms characteristic of disorders of the frontal parietal portions of the cerebral cortex, the distribution of the middle cerebral arteries.[2]

Visual symptoms may result from direct embolization to the retina as well. Vertebro-basilar insufficiency on the other hand, dependent upon the fact that the common midline basilar artery formed by the confluence of the vertebrals supplies arterial branches to the pons, thalamus, mid brain, and tempero-occipital portions of the cerebral hemispheres, results in symptoms characteristic of involvement of one or both pyramidal tracts, of the long sensory tracts, and of cranial nerves III-XI. Symptoms may be unilateral or bilateral, intermittent, progressive, or static. Specific symptoms of vertebral-basilar insufficiency include sensory and motor disturbances of one, two, three, or four limbs; diplopia; vertigo; headache; drop attacks with or without loss of consciousness; or combinations of these. When both carotid and vertebral arteries are involved in occlusive disease, symptoms characteristic of each system may occur together.[3,4] Occlusive lesions of the subclavian or innominate arteries ordinarily result in symptoms which result from basivertebral arterial insufficiency, or on occasion from carotid arterial insufficiency.[5] Rarely has it been possible to obtain a history of onset or worsening of symptoms with an exercise although this is said by some to occur in as many as 1/3 of patients (Table 34-1).

ANATOMY

The vertebral arteries originate as the first branches of the paired subclavian arteries at the base of the neck, course cephalad for a distance of one to two inches to enter the bony canal formed by the transverse processes of the cervical vertebrae, the foramina transversaria, through which they reach the base of the skull, there to exit from the canal and enter the cranium through the foramen magnum to join together to form the basilar artery. One intact vertebral artery may suffice to maintain adequate circulation to the brain stem, unless the contralateral one is a rudimentary structure whereupon compromise of the dominant vessel may be sufficient to produce ischemia.

Table 34–1
Symptoms of Cerebrovascular Insufficiency

A. Carotid Symptoms
   1. Hemiparesis
   2. Amaurosis Fugax
   3. Dysphasia
   4. Hemi-anesthesia
   5. Dementia

B. Vertebro-Basilar Symptoms
   1. Ataxia
   2. Vertigo
   3. Visual Blurring
   4. Diplopia
   5. Drop Attacks

C. Combined Carotid and Vertebro-Basilar Symptoms
   1. Dizziness
   2. Syncope
   3. Various Motor or Sensory Losses
   4. Dysarthria
   5. Combinations of A and B

D. Combinations of A, B and C
   1. Amnesia

Since approximately 80 percent of total cerebral blood flow comes from the carotid circulation, an adequate circle of Willis receiving inflow from patent carotid arteries may provide adequate perfusion of the posterior circulation even in the presence of extensive vertebral occlusive disease. The circle of Willis, however, is frequently incomplete, in an estimated 25 percent of humans having deficient posterior communicating arteries.[6] In the Joint Study of Extracranial Occlusive Disease, Hass et al. reported that 10 percent of patients with cerebrovascular ischemia have angiographic evidence of occlusive involvement of the posterior communicating arteries.[7] There is, therefore, great interdependence between carotid and vertebral circulations and therefore great variability in the ability of vertebral arterial lesions to produce ischemia.

The joining of the vertebral arteries into a common basilar artery predisposes to retrograde flow in one vertebral, usually the left, if its antegrade perfusion pressure is less than the contralateral vertebral by there being marked stenosis or occlusion of the origin of the ipsilateral subclavian, the so-called subclavian steal.[8]

Since the bony canal through which the vertebral arteries traverse the neck is formed by transverse processes of the cervical vertebrae, there are gaps in the canal through which the arteries may herniate leading to a rare condition of intermittent compression of the herniated loop of vertebral artery on head turning. This has resulted in characteristic symptoms when the contralateral vertebral artery has been either a rudimentary structure or the site of occlusive disease.[9]

The extraosseous portions of the vertebral arteries normally appear to be redundant from their subclavian origins to their entrances into the foramina transversaria, and from their exits from the foramina to their entrances into the skull via the foramen magnum. The redundancy results normally in relatively gentle curves without kinking, permitting head movements through a wide range without shutting off vertebro-basilar blood flow.

PATHOLOGY

Two aspects of pathology are of importance in determining the clinical syndromes resulting from arterial occlusive disease of the cerebral circulation, the one being the distribution of arterial lesions and the other the resulting patterns of cerebral ischemia or infarction. The distribution of arterial lesions has been studied in two ways, by postmortem examination of the extra and intracranial vessels of patients dying of cerebrovascular insufficiency syndromes and by exhaustive angiographic surveys of living patients presenting with symptoms. Both techniques yield similar results. Transiently symptomatic patients as well as those with frank cerebral infarcts have predominantly extracranial lesions at accessible sites in the neck, most commonly at the now familiar carotid bifurcations and at the origins of the vertebrals from the subclavian arteries.[7] In both areas, stenoses predominate over occlusion. The coincidence of atherosclerotic plaques involving both carotids and vertebrals is common. The coincidence is so frequent that Hutchinson and Yates proposed that the term caroticovertebral stenosis be applied to ischemic brain syndromes to give correct emphasis to the part played by atheromatous lesions involving arteries in the neck which supply the brain. They pointed out that the most commonly encountered brain infarcts, those of the cerebral hemispheres, were frequently associated with advanced lesions of the vertebro-basilar system as well as carotid lesions, further emphasizing the interdependence of the 2 systems in compensating for occlusive lesions.[10] The most commonly encountered arterial occlusive lesions are atherosclerotic and occur at stereotyped locations, sites apparently determined by local hemodynamic conditions.[11] This stereotyped pattern is observed in the basivertebral system. The lesions affecting the vertebral arteries most frequently encountered are atheromata of the first and second portions of the subclavian artery which encircle the origins of the vessels originating from them, namely the vertebrals, the thyrocervical trunks, the internal mammaries, and costocervical trunks. The most severe involvement, at least in patients subjected to angiographic study for cerebrovascular insufficiency syndromes, appears to be of the origins of the vertebral arteries. These atherosclerotic plaques rarely extend beyond the proximal 2-3 mm of the vertebral origins.[12] Beyond, the vessels may be singularly free of significant plaques along their entire course until the basilar artery is reached. Visible irregularities of the basilar artery, some of which are apparently produced by proliferative changes in the cervical vertebrae, are not infrequently seen on angiographic studies.[13] On occasion, however, there is total occlusion of a vertebral artery for variable distances beyond its origin, sometimes for only a short distance into the foramina transversaria, while at other times there may be total occlusion of only the most distal part of the vertebral artery, which may terminate in one of the intracranial branches, usually the posterior inferior cerebellar artery. Frequently associated with significant atheromatous disease of the vertebral artery origins are marked redundancy and kinking of the vessel before it enters the bony canal, sufficient to result in complete occlusion of the vessel on head turning.

The origin of the left subclavian artery from the aortic arch is a frequent site of severe occlusive atheromatous disease, and it is this critical stenosis proximal to the vertebral artery origin that results in subclavian steal. Less frequently, similar involvement of the innominate or even the right subclavian results in the steal phenomenon.

The frequently complex syndromes encountered in patients with extracranial arterial lesions and the patterns of cerebral infarcts found postmortem in patients dying of stroke attest to the interplay and interaction of carotid and vertebral systems in producing cerebral ischemia, emphasizing the need to study and evaluate both systems in symptomatic patients. Our own clinical experience further attests to the interdependence of the 2 systems both at the time of initial evaluation as well as in long term follow-up. Months or years following correction of symptomatic carotid lesions, significant stenoses may develop in the basivertebral system producing characteristic symptoms.

SELECTION OF PATIENTS

Lesions of the subclavian, vertebral, and innominate arteries are encountered relatively frequently in patients undergoing evaluation for ischemic brain syndromes. In the Joint Study of Extracranial Arterial Occlusion, 17 percent of all the patients had subclavian or innominate artery occlusion or stenosis of greater than 30 percent, but of these, only 168 or 15 percent with such lesions fulfilled the criteria of subclavian steal. Of these, 80 percent had associated lesions of other extracranial vessels. In an earlier phase of the same study reporting angiographic findings in 4748 patients, right vertebral arterial stenosis or occlusion occurred in 22 percent of all patients, and left involvement in 28 percent.[7] This high incidence of vertebral arterial lesions is attested to by our own experience but does not indicate the frequency of operative intervention required upon the vertebral system to alleviate symptoms. In a series of 1400 operative procedures performed in 1000 patients, operations upon the vertebral represented only 5.8 percent of the procedures while correction of subclavian steal or innominate artery lesions was performed in 2.5 percent, indicating the need for specific criteria in selecting patients for surgical correction of these lesions. Subclavian steal may be asymptomatic and appear only as a radiographic phenomenon. Unilateral vertebral arterial stenosis or occlusion in the presence of a patent contralateral vessel is usually well tolerated. Basivertebral symptoms in the presence of flow obstructing carotid lesions may be relieved upon correction of these carotid lesions.[14] In the early phases of the Joint Study, all accessible lesions of the carotid and vertebral arteries were deemed worthy of correction until it became apparent that symptoms could frequently be corrected by performing carotid procedures, indicating that basivertebral symptoms as seen by the vascular surgeon are probably due to impairment of flow rather than to embolization.[15] This is by no means a generally ascribed to point of view as indicated by the fact that Edwards and Mulherin found that 15 percent of 1700 patients with cerebral symptoms had significant stenoses of the proximal vertebrals, or subclavian arteries, or both for which surgical intervention was deemed necessary.[16] Our criteria[17] for operating upon the innominate subclavian vertebral system are more specific and rigid and are as follows:

1. Vertebral arterial operation—unilateral
   a. Bilateral flow obstructing vertebral stenoses or total occlusions with cerebral symptoms and no other accessible extracranial arterial lesions.
   b. Bilateral flow obstructing vertebral lesions and failure of symptoms to improve by correction of flow impeding carotid lesions.
   c. Bilateral flow obstructing vertebral lesions and bilateral internal carotid occlusions.
   d. Suspected embolization to the brain stem from subclavian vertebral lesions unilateral or bilateral.
2. Subclavian artery lesions
   a. Lesions proximal to the vertebral artery origin that could have been the source of emboli to the brain stem.
   b. Symptomatic subclavian steal as the only lesion.
   c. Symptomatic subclavian steal which fails to become asymptomatic after correction of flow impeding carotid lesions.
   d. Subclavian steal radiographically apparent, symptomatic or not, associated with unilateral carotid arterial occlusion and contralateral stenosis requiring operation upon the stenotic artery.
3. Innominate artery lesions[18]
   a. Flow impeding stenoses or total occlusions which are symptomatic.
   b. Embolization from nonstenotic innominate artery lesions recurring after correction of suspected ipsilateral carotid bifurcation lesions.

DIAGNOSIS

Diagnosis ordinarily is not difficult. Patients with basivertebral symptoms not infrequently will have neck bruits characteristic of extracranial arterial occlusive disease with or without specific localization of bruit over the subclavian arteries in the supraclavicular area. There are not infrequently pulse and blood pressure differences in the upper extremities, more frequently the pressure in the left arm being lower than that in the right. Although noninvasive studies by oculoplethysmography and various types of nonradiographic imaging have been useful for diagnosing carotid disease, these have not been found sufficient to delineate problems in the basivertebral system. Several angiographic studies are usually required for a full evaluation of the basivertebral circulation. The most satisfactory are those performed usually by catheter technique passed from the femorals to the aortic arch. The studies include arch angiography with visualization of the origins of the great vessels from the aorta, the cervical courses of both carotids, and vertebrals with special care taken to project clearly the true origins of the vertebrals from the subclavian. Frequently, there is overlap of subclavian and vertebral shadows and if such be the case, separate retrograde brachial injections are made to clarify the condition of the vertebral origins. In addition to the usual visualization of the carotids and the vertebrals in the neck, care is taken to ascertain that the vertebral arteries, one or both, join a patent basilar artery. One or both vertebrals may end either in mid or high neck or join only the lowermost portion of the basilar whose outflow may be only the postero-inferior cerebellar artery. A newly introduced digital intravenous technique has been useful for screening asymptomatic patients but frequently has not been sufficient to demonstrate clearly enough to plan surgical intervention the anatomy and pathology of the vertebral vascular system.

OPERATIVE TECHNIQUE

Vertebral Arterial Stenosis at Its Origin

Subclavian Vertebral Angioplasty[17] *(Fig. 34-1)*

Since most significant lesions of the proximal vertebral arteries have been combinations of vertebral ostial stenoses at their origins and marked tortuosity and kinking prior to their entrance into the bony canal, surgical intervention has been directed at correcting both abnormalities to result in unimpeded flow in all head positions and a configuration of the vertebral origin that might avoid the reoccurrence of ostial stenosis. To achieve this, a combination of plication of the redundant vertebral and subclavian vertebral roof patch angioplasty has resulted in overcoming the stenosis by creating a funnel shaped proximal vertebral artery without redundancy. Anaesthesia has been either cervical block or general inhalation anaesthesia with an endotracheal tube in place.

The incision is started parallel to the lower one-quarter of the anterior border of the sternocleidomastoid muscle and curved laterally to continue parallel to the upper border of the clavicle to approximately its midpoint. The platysma muscle is divided as is the origin of the clavicular head of the SCM muscle. The internal jugular vein is exposed to permit its medial retraction. The scalene fat pad is dissected free from all but its lateral attachment exposing anterior scalene muscle over which, deep to a thin fascial structure, courses the phrenic nerve from superior to inferior. The thin fascia over the phrenic nerve is incised, the nerve dissected free, and the scalene fat pad wrapped around the nerve posteriorly-to-medially-to-anteriorly providing a moist protected location for it. The anterior scalene muscle is divided and permitted to retract. The branches of the subclavian artery, namely the

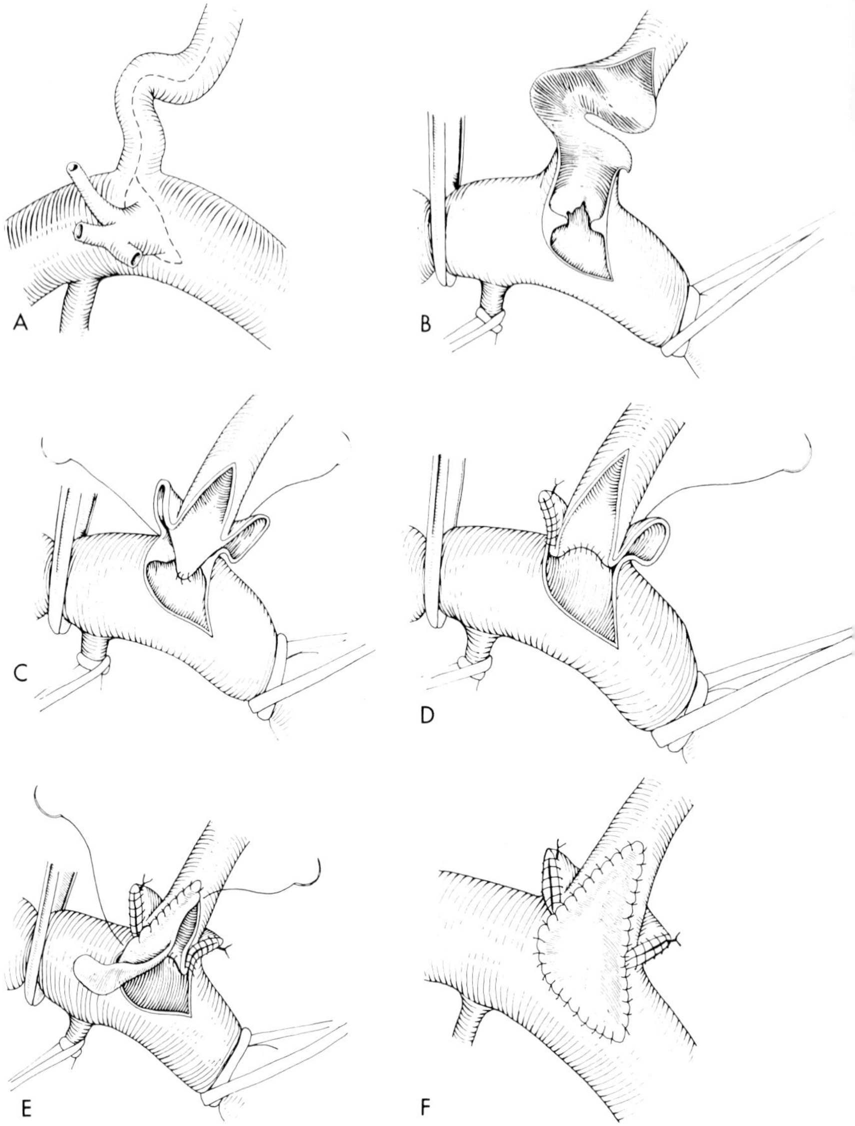

Figure 34-1. Vertebral-subclavian angioplasty performed by plication of the redundant vertebral artery and autologous roof patch of the subclavian vertebral junction.
(A) Line of excision of thyrocervical trunk, anterior wall of subclavian artery, and arteriotomy in proximal vertebral.
(B) Anterior wall of subclavian artery excised showing plaque at origin of vertebral and arteriotomy in the vertebral artery.
(C) Beginning plication of the vertebral artery—pulling the vertebral intimal surface down to cover the subclavian plaque.
(D) Plication completed, and "dog ears" oversewn on one side.
(E) Suture of vein roof patch over vertebral and subclavian arteries.
(F) Vein patch angioplasty completed.

vertebral, internal mammary, the thyrocervical trunk, and the costocervical trunk are exposed and controlled. The branches of the thyrocervical trunk require division to obtain access to the vertebral artery. On the right side, in securing control of the proximal subclavian artery, care is taken to protect the recurrent laryngeal nerve which winds around that artery. The vertebral artery is dissected free from its origin to its entrance into the foramena transversaria. Heparin is administered intravenously 3-5000 units. The vessels are clamped with suitable vascular clamps and the thyrocervical trunk origin resected extending the resultant subclavian arteriotomy upward towards the vertebral, across its origin along its course to beyond the most distal kink before its entrance into the bony canal. Plication sutures are used to shorten the vertebral and at the same time cover the plaque at the subclavian vertebral junction with normal vertebral artery intima. Autologous saphenous vein roof patch angioplasty is achieved to the subclavian and vertebral arterial opening over a small, usually 8 or 10, French catheter placed in the vertebral artery. Angiographic visualization of a completed angioplasty is performed either on the operating table or just prior to hospital discharge. The wound is closed without drainage.

Transposition of the Vertebral Artery to the Common Carotid Artery[16] (Fig. 34-2)

On occasion, division of the vertebral artery beyond the area of stenosis at its origin with its transplantation into the side of the common carotid artery has been performed. Surgical exposure is as for the subclavian vertebral angioplasty previously described except that division of the anterior scalene muscle is not required. The artery is exposed medial to the anterior scalene muscle and exposed to the entrance into the bony canal. The common carotid artery is dissected free for a variable distance below the crossing of the omohyoid muscle and clamped. Because the common carotid artery has usually had a thick wall at this level, patch angioplasty has been performed to provide a site for anastomoses of the vertebral by resecting 1 cm $\times$ ½ cm of the lateral wall of the carotid, closing the defect with a patch of autologous saphenous vein which is then incised to create an ostium to which the vertebral artery has been anastomosed.

Vertebral Arterial Lesions—Occlusive at the Origin

Autologous Venous Bypass from Either Carotid or Subclavian to the Vertebral Artery[19] (Fig. 34-3)

Vertebral arterial occlusions occurring at the origin extend a variable distance into the bony canal. Endarterectomy procedures have seemed

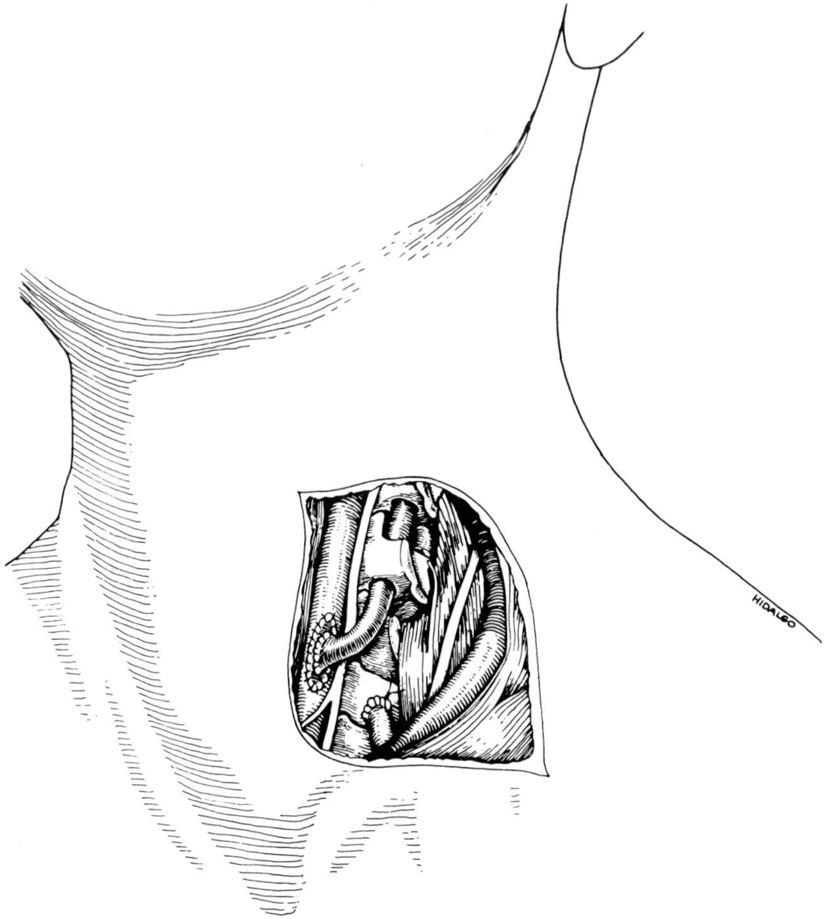

Figure 34-2. Reimplantation of the vertebral artery into the side of the common carotid artery as an alternative to vertebral subclavian angioplasty, using a vein roof patch on the common carotid artery if that artery is unusually thick walled.

hazardous in view of the friability of the subclavian and the small caliber of the vertebral so that in instances where the occlusion did not extend either intracranially or above C2-3, autologous venous bypass procedures have been performed. The foramen transversarium has been opened by removing the overlying bone, care being taken to control bleeding from the numerous small venules which surround the vertebral artery in the bony canal, and autologous reversed saphenous vein grafts have been sutured end-to-side to the subclavian artery or to the common carotid artery and end-to-end to the distal part of the vertebral artery.

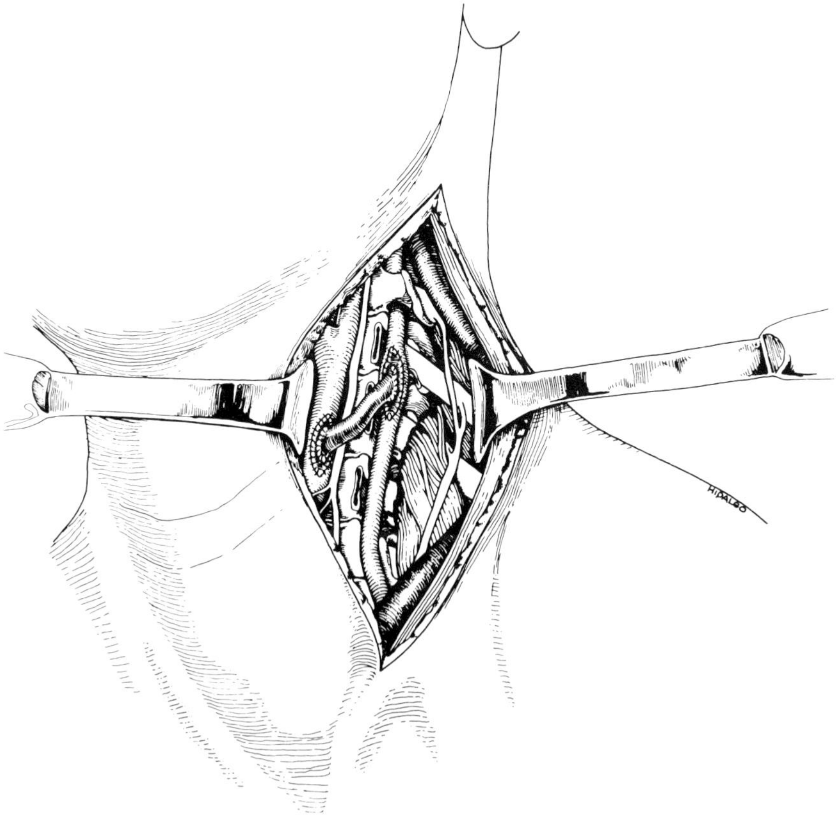

Figure 34-3. Vertebral occlusion. Carotid vertebral bypass with reversed autologous saphenous vein for vertebral artery occlusions extending into the foramina transversaria. Vein roof patches if necessary. The bony canal has been unroofed 3 segments.

Entrapment of the Mid Portion of the Vertebral Artery between 2 Segments of the Foramina Transversaria (Fig. 34-4)

On two occasions, one large vertebral has protruded between two segments of the foramina transversaria while the contralateral vessel was either occluded or atretic. These predominant vessels then become intermittently occluded on head turning causing drop attacks. On each occasion, the condition was corrected and symptoms were relieved by exposing the bony segments overlying the involved vertebral artery above and below the sites of entrapment and opening the anterior portion of the canal by removal of bone

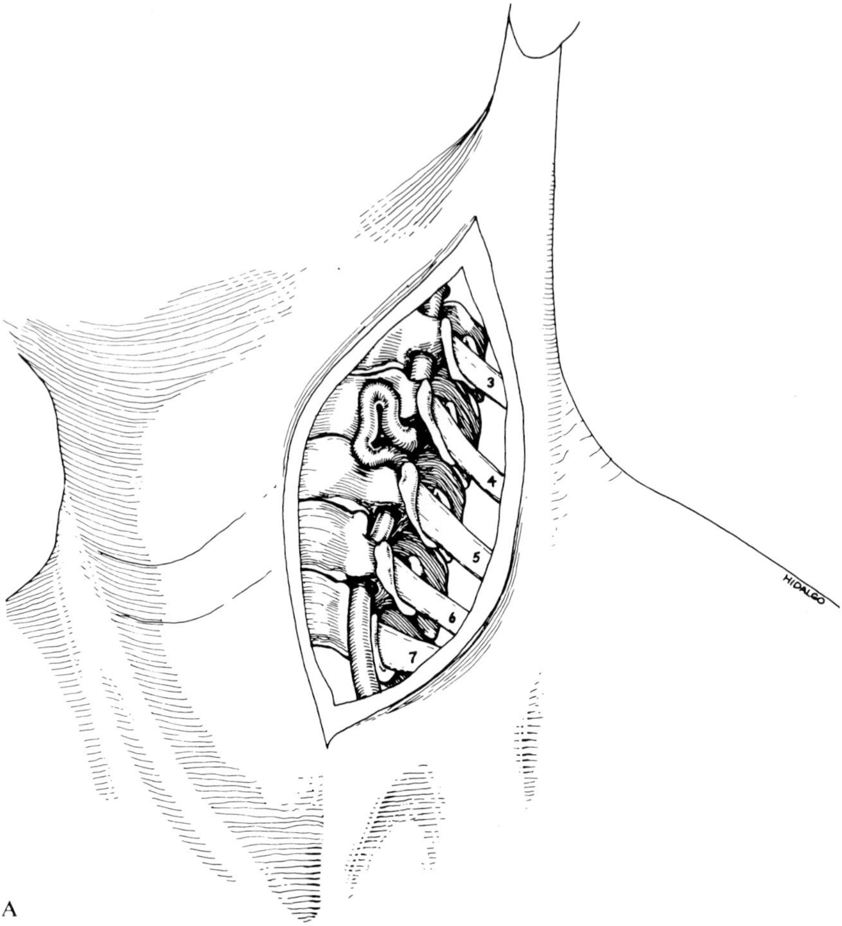

A

Figure 34-4. Relief of herniation of the vertebral artery.
(A) Herniation of vertebral artery between segments of the foramina transversaria.
(B) Herniation of vertebral artery between segments of the foramina transversaria, released by resection of segments of the anterior wall of the bony canal.

overlying the arteries, completely freeing them of constricting bands without resorting to resection of the redundant vessels.

Subclavian Steal Syndrome

Carotid Subclavian Bypass Graft[20,21,22] *(Fig. 34-5)*

Until the description of axillo-axillary bypass graft, the preferred treatment of symptomatic subclavian steal was by reversed autologous saphe-

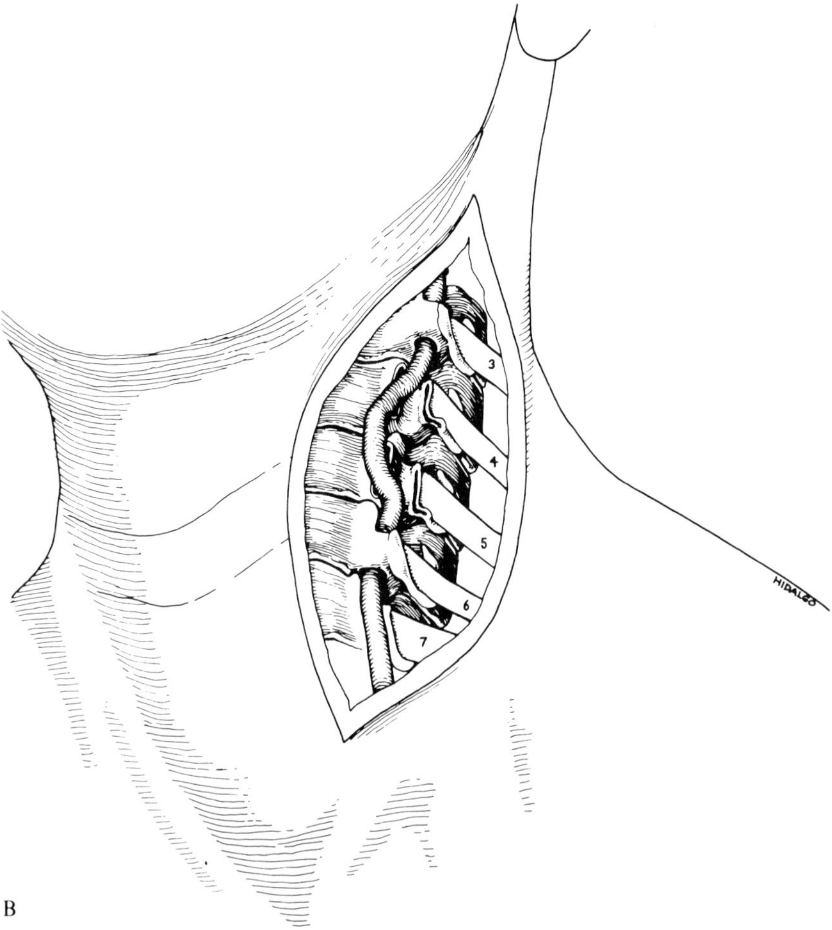

B

nous vein bypass graft performed through supraclavicular incisions without clavicular resection. This usually required division of the anterior scalene muscle for access to the subclavian. On occasion, extensive atherosclerotic changes in the 2nd and 3rd portions of the subclavian made the operation difficult. Nevertheless, flow dynamics in the vertebral were restored to normal correcting the steal without producing ipsilateral carotid steal.

Axillo-axillary Bypass Graft[23] *(Fig. 34-6)*

With the advent of the axillo-axillary bypass graft employing plastic prostheses, this has been the preferred operation for symptomatic subclavian steal. The operation is performed by making infraclavicular incisions bilaterally just below the coracoid processes, separating the edges of the

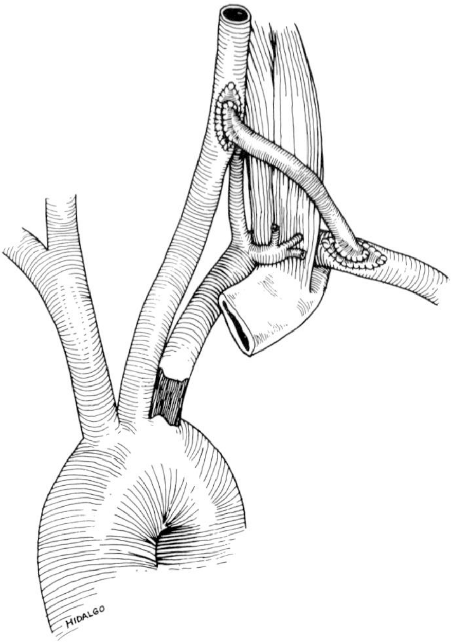

Figure 34-5. Subclavian steal. Carotid subclavian bypass using reversed autologous saphenous vein and roof patches on the carotid and subclavian arteries if necessitated by thick-walled carotid and subclavian arteries.

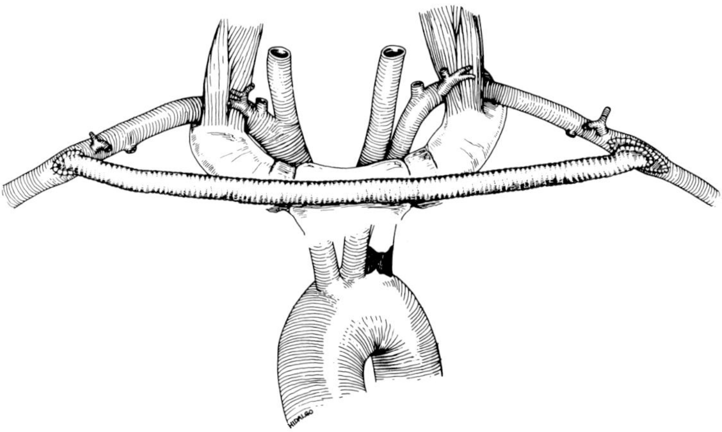

Figure 34-6. Subclavian steal. Axillo-axillary bypass using Dacron prosthesis with vein roof patches on the axillary arteries if those arteries are unusually small as they are apt to be on the occluded subclavian side.

pectoralis major muscles, dividing the origins of the pectoralis minor from the coracoid processes, dissecting the axillary arteries from amongst the cords of the brachial plexi, and connecting the two incisions through a subcutaneous tunnel, through which an 8 or 10 mm length of knitted Dacron is passed. The patients are heparinized. End-to-side anastomoses are performed between the ends of the preclotted prostheses and the axillary arteries. If those vessels are smaller than 5 mm in diameter, which may often be the case on the side of subclavian occlusion, autologous saphenous vein roof patch angioplasty is performed, and the vein patch then incised longitudinally to serve as a site for anastomosis of the plastic prosthesis.

Innominate Artery Lesions[24] (Fig. 34-7)

Innominate artery lesions can be managed satisfactorily in a number of ways, determined by the extent of the lesions and the mechanism producing symptoms, be it embolization or as more often seems to be the case, by interference with flow due to high grade stenosis. Since most lesions that

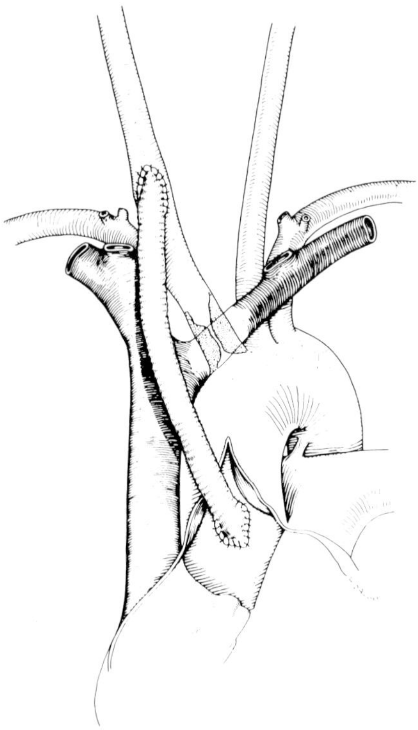

Figure 34-7. Innominate occlusion. Ascending aortic to common carotid bypass for innominate artery occlusion employing knitted Dacron prosthesis.

appear to be symptomatic involve the origins of the vessels with flow impeding stenoses, without encroachment upon either the common carotid or subclavian origins, extraanatomic bypass grafts either of the axillo-axillary or subclavian-subclavian bypass restore normal hemodynamics in the vertebral and carotid arterial circuits. Many innominate artery lesions, however, do not require surgical intervention. Direct surgical intervention has been employed only when the innominate artery was suspected of being the source of cerebral emboli. Direct aortic arch innominate artery endarterectomy via a sternum splitting incision with a lateral extension to the right hemithorax creating an operculum of the upper anterior chest wall has been performed with patch grafting of the innominate artery with Dacron and autologous vein. Partially occluding clamps have been placed on the aortic arch and endarterectomy performed in open fashion to the origin of the subclavian and right common carotid. This has been difficult to accomplish because of the difficulty in avoiding the left common carotid artery with aortic clamping and the added difficulty of controlling the plaque inevitably found in the aortic arch. More recently, endarterectomy for embolizing innominate lesions has been aban-

Table 34-2
Results of Vertebral Subclavian Angioplasty (N = 81) 1965–1980

		Died			Alive	
Years Follow-Up	Number	MI	CVA	Ca.	†V.B. Symptoms	Well
0–1 year	11	1				10
1–2 yrs.	17	1	1		2	13
2–3 yrs.	11					11
3–4 yrs.	9	1		1	1	7
4–5 yrs.	3	1	1			1
5–6 yrs.	3	1	1			1
6–7 yrs.	3					3
7–8 yrs.	2	1				1
8–10 yrs.	4					4
10–12 yrs.	4	1				3
12–15 yrs.	7					7
Total follow-up	74	7	3	1	3	61
Lost to follow-up	5					
Operative deaths	2*					
Total operations	81					

*Operative deaths: 1 stroke, 1 pulmonary embolus
†Recurrence vertebrobasilar symptoms: 1 proven basilar artery occlusion—patent vertebral angioplasty, 2 undiagnosed.

doned in favor of ascending aortic to right common carotid bypass with 8-10 mm knitted Dacron with closure of the innominate artery just proximal to the origin of the right subclavian, permitting retrograde flow into the subclavian and vertebral. The exposure for this approach has been through a full length sternum splitting incision without extension into the pleural cavity providing not only satisfactory exposure but a stable rib cage postoperatively avoiding the instability which sometimes results from the operculum incision.

RESULTS

The results of subclavian-vertebral angioplasties are tabulated in Table 34-2. Of 81 patients operated upon between 1965 and 1980, 61 are alive and well while 3 have recurrence of significant symptoms, one of whom has now proven basilar artery occlusion although the angioplasty remains widely patent.

The results of axillo-axillary bypass performed between 1973 and 1982 are tabulated in Table 34-3 and record that all are patent; that 18 are asymptomatic; that an additional 3 required carotid procedures, and of these, 1 had a cardiac pacemaker as well.

Table 34-4 summarizes the results of innominate artery operations and documents how infrequently the operation has been deemed necessary in our

Table 34-3
Results of Subclavian Steal: Axillo-Axillary Bypass—(N = 27) 1973–1982

Symptoms (N = 27)		
CNS	CNS + Upper Extremity	Upper Extremity
21	4	2
VB Symptoms 17 VB + Hemispheric 4		
Site of lesion: Left subclavian 18	Right subclavian 9	

Follow-up: 1–79 mos.		
Operative mortality	0	
Unrelated deaths	2	
Strokes	0	
Symptomatic relief	18	
Unrelieved	7*	
Uncertain	2	(early death)

*2 relieved by subsequent carotid endarterectomy
1 relieved by bilateral carotid endarterectomy and carotid pacemaker insertion.

Table 34-4
Innominate Artery (N = 4)

Results
Innominate endarterectomy 2
1–19 yrs.—alive and well
1–8 yrs.—alive and well
Aorto-common carotid bypass 2
1–6 yrs.—alive and well
1 —lost to follow-up

total series of 1400 extracranial operations for cerebrovascular insufficiency syndromes.

DISCUSSION

Lesions of the vertebral, subclavian, and innominate arteries are found relatively frequently in patients with cerebral vascular insufficiency symptoms but relatively infrequently require surgical correction for the relief of symptoms when compared to carotid artery lesions. It is not clear, however, that such lesions are innocuous even when clearly asymptomatic. In symptomatic patients, symptoms of basivertebral insufficiency appear to result from either failure of antegrade flow due to critical stenoses of vertebral or innominate arteries or from reversal of flow in vertebrals which originate distal to occlusive lesions of the subclavian or innominate arteries. Nevertheless coma-death occurs in patients who are followed for long terms after carotid operations from causes difficult to diagnose. Acute brain stem infarcts resulting in sudden death or in coma-death may be extremely difficult to diagnose even at postmortem examination, especially since examination of the brain stem is performed so seldom. Nevertheless, in the absence of evidence to suggest that nonstenosing lesions of the extracranial vessels supplying the posterior circulation result in ischemia as occurs in the carotid system by microembolization, and since basivertebral symptoms are so often ameliorated by correction of hemodynamically significant carotid lesions, we have continued to follow the rather strict indications for operation upon the vertebrals as previously outlined, at variance with some others who more aggressively correct vertebral lesions. In the selection of patients for operation, differential diagnosis of conditions unrelated to the cerebral circulation is essential. The most prevalent symptoms of basivertebral ischemia, light-headedness, dizziness, vertigo, transient ataxia, drop attacks, and frank syncope, may be caused in this age group in which arterial lesions are found, by transient cardiac arrhythmias including heart block, sick sinus syndromes, and hypersensitive carotid sinus reflexes; by convulsive disorders; and by aortic valvular stenoses. Indeed, more than one of these conditions may be found in the same patient demanding multiple procedures for the control of symptoms and perhaps the prevention of sudden death. Although there are those who have suggested that correction of vertebral arterial lesions is unnecessary, the finding in severely symptomatic patients of isolated bilateral vertebral arterial lesions, of bilateral vertebral lesions with bilateral carotid occlusions and the persistence of severe basivertebral symptoms including syncope, following carotid operations and subsequently relieved by unilateral vertebral angioplasty, attests to the need for operation in selected patients. Operation upon unilateral vertebral occlusion or stenosis in the presence of an adequate contralateral artery has never been necessary in our patient population and was performed only once in a patient with a proven surgically corrected contralateral vertebral stenosis. It is not unlikely that those patients who embolize from unilateral vertebral arterial lesions suffer such dire consequences from brain stem infarcts that they do not ever reach the vascular surgeon.

Subclavian steal and innominate arterial lesions seem to be well tolerated and most often appear to be asymptomatic. The correction of radiographically apparent subclavian steal without symptoms has not appeared to us to be an indication for prophylactic operation. Surgical techniques that have been employed for correction of various lesions encountered in the extracranial portion of this system are numerous. Angioplasty of the vertebral origin with or without plication at the subclavian vertebral junction appears to be the procedure most commonly employed for vertebral arterial stenoses at the origins. In our experience it provides a direct means of correcting the anatomical abnormalities, stenosis, and kink, which interfere with flow in the vertebral artery while changing the anatomical configuration which predisposed to the formation of the original lesion. Patch angioplasty with plication of the redundant vertebral results in a funnel shaped vertebral origin, quite different from its original right angle nontapered origin. Since intimal hyperplasia appears to be so intimately related to geometric configuration of arteries and to the resulting hemodynamic patterns, restructuring of the system seemed desirable and appears to have been justified by the durability of the results. Antiplatelet drugs, aspirin, and persantine are administered postoperatively to attempt to avoid suture line thrombus deposition which may also predispose to intimal hyperplasia. Vertebral-carotid bypass, which requires less dissection and is less traumatic to the phrenic nerve, has been avoided because of the need to clamp the common carotid artery, introducing the risk of cerebral embolization. The configuration of the resultant anastomosis may predispose to junctional hyperplasia. Transection of the vertebral and reimplantation either into the subclavian artery or into the transected stump of the thyrocervical suffers from the fact that those vessels are affected by the atherosclerotic process making anastomosis of an artery as small as the vertebral difficult and subject to either immediate reocclusion by thrombosis or to late reocclusion by progression of the atherosclerotic process in the subclavian. Operations for subclavian steal are even more numerous varying from ligation of the vertebral artery distal to the subclavian lesion to direct intrathoracic subclavian disobliteration or bypass procedures performed upon the subclavian artery including subclavian-subclavian bypass and carotid-vertebral bypass. The operation of axillo-axillary bypass employing plastic prostheses, however, is the most easily performed of all procedures avoiding deep dissection with possible bilateral phrenic nerve injuries which can occur during subclavian-subclavian bypass, and avoiding thoracotomy required for direct subclavian disobliteration or bypass, overcoming the need to clamp the common carotid artery required to perform carotid subclavian bypass. It has the added advantage of requiring a relatively short straight graft, unlike the long graft required for a femoral-axillary bypass. Axillo-axillary bypass has been durable with only one of 29 occluding over a period of ten years, satisfactorily correcting the steal and relieving the symptoms. The presence of the graft in the subcutaneous location even in women has not been disturbing to them. Indeed, it has been comforting to these patients to be able to feel the pulsations in the graft. Innominate artery procedures have been performed infrequently. The extraanatomical operation is preferable to all others if it can be used to effectively control subclavian or carotid steal syndromes, though alone it cannot be expected to eliminate embolization from innominate artery plaques. This latter phenomenon requires either the addition of interruption of that vessel, direct innominate endarterectomy, or aortosubclavian common carotid bypass grafting with innominate interruption, the last procedure being the preferred one in view of the difficulty of performing endarterectomy of the innominate artery at the level of the aortic arch. Operative mortality for all of these procedures is low as is the perioperative stroke rate. Various peripheral nerve palsies constitute the most common complication. Paralysis of a hemi-diaphragm from injury in mobilization of the phrenic nerve, Horner's syndrome from inferior cervical sympathetic chain injury and rarely, hoarseness from vagal or recurrent nerve injuries are the most common. Although usually transient, they are of sufficient concern to warrant warning patients preoperatively of their possible occurrence since such occurrences may be inevitable though justified to protect the brain stem from ischemic injury. There being no acceptable series of medically treated patients with basivertebral arterial insufficiency to which to compare surgical results, it is not possible to determine whether such operations either prolong life or prevent future strokes. It appears from life table analysis of results that the subsequent stroke rate in the vertebral artery operated group followed for as long as 14 years is unusually low in spite of the fact that as a group they seem to have the most extensive arterial involvement of the extracranial arteries.

CONCLUSIONS

Operations upon the carotid vertebral junction may be necessary in approximately 5 percent of patients who come for surgical treatment of cerebral vascular insufficiency syndrome. Operative procedures can be performed with a high degree of safety there being negligible mortality and a negligible stroke rate. The major complications are related to transient peripheral nerve palsies involving nerves in the area including the phrenic, cervical sympathetic, and rarely recurrent laryngeal or vagus. Operations upon the subclavian and innominate arteries are rarely required for cerebral symptoms. The most commonly required procedure is for subclavian steal syndromes; axillary-axillary bypass employing artificial prostheses has relieved symptoms and been performed with no mortality and no significant morbidity. Therefore, operations upon the innominate artery have been performed infrequently and then only for either embolization or for symptomatic flow impairment.

REFERENCES

1. Alpers BJ, Berry RG, Paddison RM: Anatomical studies of the circle of Willis in normal brain. Arch Neurol Psych 11:309, 1959
2. Myers KA: Reconstruction of vertebral artery stenosis. Aust NZ J Surg 47:41, 1977
3. Humphries AW, Young JR, Beven EG, et al: Relief of vertebrobasilar symptoms by carotid endarterectomy. Surgery 57:48, 1965
4. Ueda K, Toole JF, McHenry LC Jr: Carotid and vertebrobasilar transient ischemic attacks: Clinical and angiographic correlation. Neurology 29:1094, 1979
5. Herring M: The subclavian steal syndrome: A review. Am Surg 220, 1977
6. McHenry LC Jr: Cerebral Circulation and Stroke. Chapter II pp 42–44. Warren H. Green, Inc. St. Louis, Mo. 1978.
7. Hass WK, Fields WS, North RR, et al: Arteriography, techniques, sites and complications. JAMA 203:961, 968, 1968
8. Fields WS, Lemak NA: Joint study of extracranial occlusion VII Subclavian steal—A review of 168 cases. JAMA 222:1139, 1972
9. Imparato AM: Personal observation unreported cases
10. Hutchinson EC, Yates PO: Carotid-vertebral stenosis. Lancet 2:722, 1957
11. Gessner FB: Hemodynamic theories of atherogenesis. Circulation Research 33:259, 1973
12. Imparato AM, Lin JPT: Vertebral arterial reconstruction: Internal plication and vein patch angioplasty. Ann Surg 166:213, 1967
13. Powers SR, Drislane TM, Iandoli EW: The surgical treatment of vertebral artery insufficiency. Arch Surg 86:60, 1963
14. Ehrenfeld WK, Chapman RD, Wylie EJ: Management of occlusive lesions of the branches of the aortic arch. Am J Surg 118:236, 1969
15. Blaisdell WF, Clauss RD, Galbraith JG, et al: A review of surgical considerations. (Joint study of extracranial arterial occlusion as a cause of stroke) JAMA 209:1889, 1969
16. Edwards WH, Mulherin JLJ: The surgical approach to significant stenosis of vertebral and subclavian arteries. Surgery 87:20, 1980

17. Imparato AM, Riles TS, Kim GE: Cervical vertebral angioplasty for brain stem ischemia. Surgery 90:842, 1981
18. Mozersky DJ, Barnes RW, Sumner DS, et al: Hemodynamics of innominate artery occlusion. Ann Surg 178:123, 1973
19. Berguer R, Andaya LV, Bauer RB: Vertebral artery bypass. Arch Surg 111:976, 1976
20. Barner HB, Kaiser GC, William VL: Hemodynamics of carotid subclavian bypass. Arch Surg 103:248, 1971
21. Cook CH, Stemmer EA, Connolly JE: Effect of peripheral resistance on carotid blood flow after carotid subclavian bypass. Arch Surg 105:9, 1972
22. Diethrich EB, Garrett HE, Ameriso J, et al: Occlusive disease of the common carotid and subclavian arteries treated by carotid-subclavian bypass. Analysis of 125 cases. Am J Surg 114:800, 1967
23. Jacobson JH II, Mozersky DJ, Mitty HA, et al: Axillary bypass for the "subclavian steal" syndrome. Arch Surg 106:24, 1973
24. Julian OC, Javid H: Surgical Management of Cerebral Arterial Insufficiency. Current Problems in Surgery. Chicago, Yearbook Medical Publishers, Inc., March, 1971, pp. 6–18

Norman M. Rich G. Patrick Clagett
James M. Salander David W. Olson
Jerry R. Youkey John E. Hutton, Jr.

35

Extra-anatomical Bypass of Cerebrovascular Occlusions

The development of successful operative intervention in assisting patients who have had or have a potential compromise to their cerebral circulation associated with arteriosclerotic lesions of the aortic arch vessels and their branches occurred approximately 30 years ago. Carotid endarterectomy is well established as a procedure performed frequently and performed with excellent results. Nevertheless, this success appears to be associated with an increasingly older population with an increasing number of patients demonstrating progression of their generalized arteriosclerosis. In many major medical centers, there is an increasing demand for innovative approaches to provide extra-anatomical bypass procedures to assist patients who require complex cerebral revascularization.

Even with the most frequently performed operation currently utilized to help augment total cerebral perfusion and prevent distal intracranial embolization, we have altered our approach several times in performing carotid endarterectomy. Between 1967 and 1972, we performed 232 carotid endarterectomies under regional anesthesia.[1] There were 10 percent of the patients who required the use of general anesthesia and a temporary indwelling shunt because of the development of neurologic symptoms after temporary cross-clamping or the inability to tolerate regional anesthesia. The 30 day mortality was 2.6 percent. The incidence of fixed neurologic deficits was 2.2 percent, and the incidence of transient ischemic neurologic deficits was 3.0 percent. After several modifications, and prompted by multiple factors, we performed a prospective study between 1971 and 1976 performing 189 carotid endarterectomies under general anesthesia with the routine use of a temporary indwelling shunt.[2] The 30 day mortality was 0.5 percent. The incidence of fixed neurologic deficits was 2.6 percent, and the incidence of transient neurologic deficits was 2.6 percent. In our experience, the morbidity and mortality figures were not significantly different whether we used general anesthesia with a shunt or regional anesthesia without a shunt. In a prospective study that we reported in 1974, we also identified limitations in our experience in relying on carotid artery back pressure in attempting to determine whether or not patients would require a shunt during carotid endarterectomy.[3] In recognizing the systemic nature of generalized arteriosclerosis, it was noted that all patients in whom postoperative strokes occurred had multiple stenotic and/or occlusive lesion combinations.

The majority of patients with signs and symptoms of cerebrovascular ischemia will be managed successfully as outlined above. Also, the extensive experience with carotid endarterectomy has provided an opportunity to evaluate numerous modalities associated with protection of intracranial blood flow when more complex methods of cerebral revascularization are required. Five of our patients with the most complicated problems requiring complex cerebral revascularization in our experience had their cases reviewed in a report in 1978.[4] Prior to that report and subsequently, our experience has been similar to that reported from other large medical centers. It is well recognized that cerebrovascular symptoms associated with cerebral ischemia may be caused by a single lesion in the carotid arterial bifurcation or be associated with combined lesions of the innominate, carotid, subclavian, and vertebral arteries.

The concept for arterial bypass that does not follow the natural course of the artery has been popular for the past 20 years and is frequently termed "extra-anatomical bypass." Warren and Fomon described a series of procedures in 1966 which they described as "rerouting arterial flow to relieve ischemia."[5] These procedures were described as femoro-femoral, axillary-femoral, and carotid-carotid artery bypasses. Of particular interest is the use of the carotid-carotid bypass in anticipation of resection of a neoplasm and the involved carotid artery. Ehrenfeld, Levin, and Wylie, in 1968, described use of the autogenous greater saphenous vein for a subclavian-subclavian bypass with an extension to the right carotid artery in a patient with only one patent branch of the aortic arch.[6] Crawford and associates, in 1969, outlined the details of their extensive 10 year experience in managing occlusions of the innominate, common carotid, and subclavian arteries which established a trend toward extra-thoracic, extra-anatomical bypass procedures in the neck which have become popular in the past 10 years such as the subclavian-carotid bypass.[7] Moore, Malone, and Goldstone reviewed their experience in 1976 with extra-thoracic repair of branch occlusions of the aortic arch and provided valuable long term follow-up.[8] In 1977, Shumacker and associates reported an extensive review including their own personal experience in managing stenotic and occlusive lesions of the aortic arch branches.[9]

A variety of innovative arterial reconstructive procedures have been developed, particularly in the past 10 years, in highly-selected patients with multiple arteriosclerotic lesions, which are ulcerative, stenotic, and/or occlusive, to improve total cerebral perfusion and/or reduce the possibility of intracerebral arterial embolization. Some patients have had previous operative intervention, such as a carotid endarterectomy, and current symptoms may be related to subsequent failure of previous arterial reconstructions.

The importance of angiographic visualization of the aortic arch with selective four vessel visualization including cerebral circulation cannot be overemphasized (Fig. 35-1). Special subtraction techniques may be valuable in addition to obtaining use of several angles to allow optimal arterial visualization (Fig. 35-2). One of numerous combined occlusive lesions that might be associated with the consideration for complex cerebral revascularization is seen in Figure 35-3.

Among the great variety of arterial reconstructive procedures that may be considered, other than direct endarterectomy, for revascularization of the arch vessels are aorto-subclavian bypass, carotid-subclavian bypass, subclavian-carotid bypass, carotid-subclavian transposition, subclavian-subclavian bypass, axillo-axillary bypass and femoro-axillary bypass. DeBakey and associates outlined the first extensive experience in managing occlusive lesions of the innominate, carotid, subclavian, and vertebral arteries in their 1958 reports.[10,11] The subsequent 10 year experience of this group, reported in 1969 by Crawford and colleagues, outlined the transthoracic bypass graft principle with the bypass originating from the ascending aorta carrying flow beyond occlusions of the aortic arch vessels to a variety of locations including the subclavian, carotid, and axillary arteries[7] (Fig. 35-4). These authors emphasized that the increased morbidity associated with thoracotomy did not justify this approach in the elderly high-risk patient. They also emphasized that such extra-anatomical, extra-thoracic bypasses such as the subclavian-carotid bypass would avoid the additional morbidity of an intra-thoracic procedure. Figure 35-5 details 18 methods outlined by these authors of employing extra-thoracic bypass determined by the location and extent of the arteriosclerotic occlusive disease.

Emphasis will be placed on those extra-thoracic, extra-anatomical procedures that have been developed and utilized in the past 10 years.

AXILLO-AXILLARY BYPASS

Figure 35-6 is an artist's concept of the axillo-axillary bypass, which can be successfully employed with occlusive lesions in the left subclavian or innominate arteries. Myers, Lawton, and Sautter described the use of axillo-axillary arterial bypass for subclavian arterial revascularization in 1971.[12]

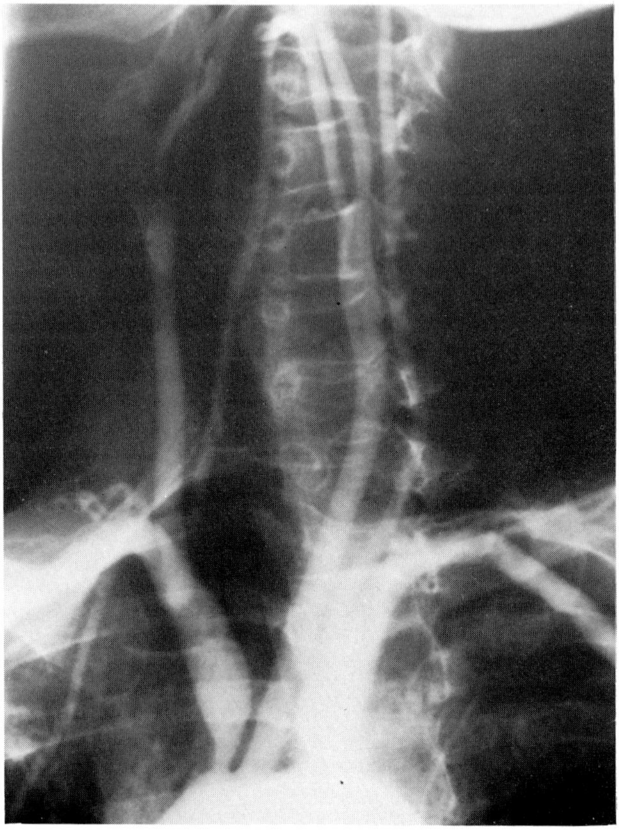

Figure 35-1. This aortic arch angiogram emphasizes the importance of visualizing the origin of the innominate artery, which is stenotic at its origin, the left common carotid artery, and the left subclavian artery arising from the aortic arch in addition to outlining the carotid bifurcations and origins of the vertebral arteries. To complete the evaluation, several views of these vessels, with appropriate selective four-vessel evaluation of the carotid and vertebral arteries to include intracranial arterial study, will be helpful in all patients and extremely important in some patients.

These authors utilized a 10 mm woven Dacron graft to perform an axillo-axillary bypass in a poor-risk patient under local anesthesia. The graft was still functioning at the time of the patient's death on the fifth postoperative day. Myers and co-workers in a subsequent 1979 report summarized their experience with 18 patients operated upon since 1972.[13] They revealed that they had 3 late graft failures, and they considered the axillo-axillary arterial

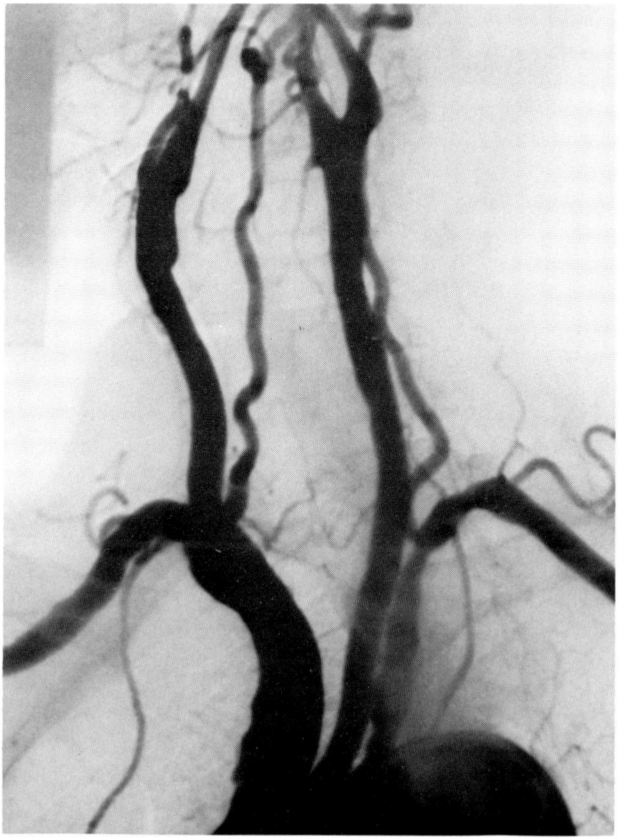

Figure 35-2. A subtraction study of the aortic arch vessels is often valuable in helping delineate the angiographic outline of the arterial anatomy. This is particularly true of the origins of the vertebral arteries. Moderate arteriosclerotic disease is obvious in the left subclavian artery and highlighted by this technique.

bypass to be the operation of choice for patients with subclavian steal syndrome.

Mozersky and co-workers in 1973 reported 3 cases of axillo-axillary bypass with 2 patients having innominate arterial lesions and the remaining patient having a subclavian arterial occlusion.[14] All three grafts functioned well. Another report in the same year, by Jacobson and colleagues, reported the use of axillo-axillary bypass for subclavian arterial revascularization and correction of the subclavian steal syndrome utilizing an autogenous greater saphenous vein graft as the bypass conduit.[15] Flow studies and arteriograms by Mozersky and co-workers and arteriograms by Jacobson and colleagues

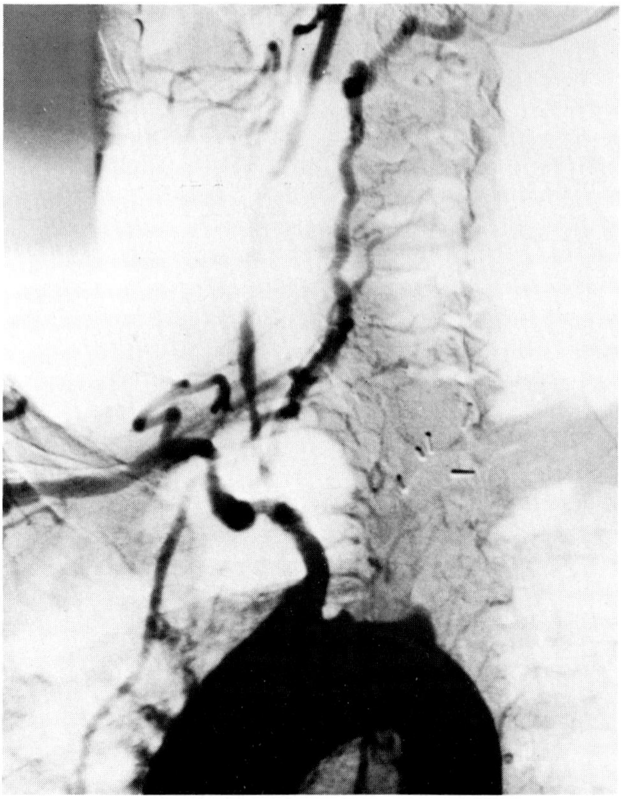

Figure 35-3. The marked contrast of this angiogram of the aortic arch by subtraction technique, compared to Figures 35-1 and 35-2, emphasizes the problems that can arise requiring consideration for complex cerebral revascularization. Both the left common carotid artery and the left subclavian artery are occluded at their origin, and significant arteriosclerotic disease is present throughout the right common carotid artery. Delayed films are important to outline the direction of collateral blood flow.

demonstrated that there was no steal from the donor arm and that this approach did reestablish flow in an antegrade direction in the involved vertebral artery.[14–16] Other investigators have duplicated the initial good results, and these include the reports by LeVeen and co-workers in 1974,[17] Dardik and Dardik in 1974,[18] Snider and associates in 1974,[19] and Lamis and colleagues in 1976.[20]

Bentley, Hollier, and Batson performed 10 axillo-axillary bypasses in New Orleans between 1975 and 1977.[21] Eight of their patients had lesions in

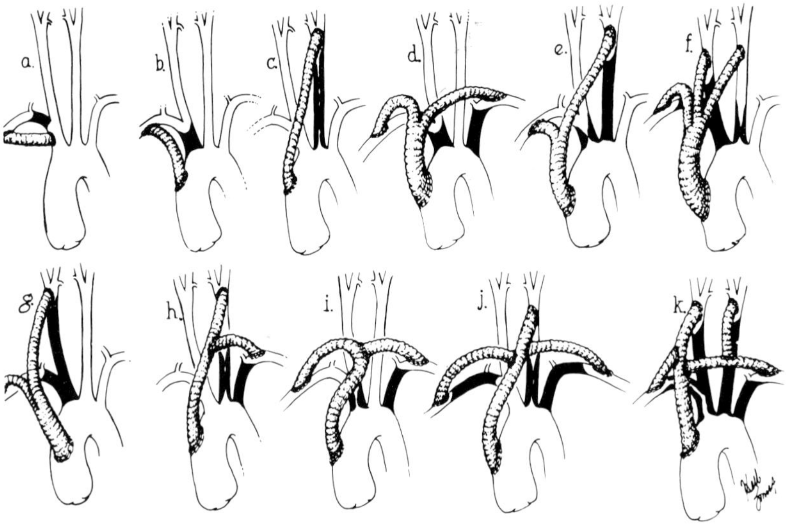

Figure 35-4. Diagrams show methods employing transthoracic bypass graft principle. Methods (a, c–g) are no longer employed either because they require grafts which are too large or because the occlusive process (a, e) is more suitably treated by extrathoracic operations (Crawford, ES, DeBakey, ME, Morris, GC, Jr and Howell, JF, Surgery 65:17, 1969).

the subclavian artery, and two had lesions in the innominate artery. They documented good results in that all of their patients were relieved of both central nervous system and upper extremity symptoms (Table 35-1). They experienced no operative complications, and the early graft patency was good. There were 2 patients who developed late graft thrombosis, which was alleviated by thrombectomy of the graft. These authors have recommended axillo-axillary arterial bypass for most innominate arterial lesions and they felt that this approach is useful in subclavian arterial revascularization in selected elderly, high-risk patients emphasizing that the procedure could be performed under local anesthesia.

The reported good results during the past 10 years with axillo-axillary arterial bypass include the disappearance of both previous central nervous system and upper extremity ischemic symptoms. A variety of conduits have been used ranging from Dacron to bovine to autogenous vein. The excellent patency rate of Dacron prostheses, however, emphasizes that it is probably unnecessary to sacrifice the autogenous greater saphenous vein or the cephalic vein, which would also add to the length of the procedure. There have been few complications reported. Hematoma formation can occur. Fortunately, the infrequent graft thrombosis has been easily remedied with thrombectomy.

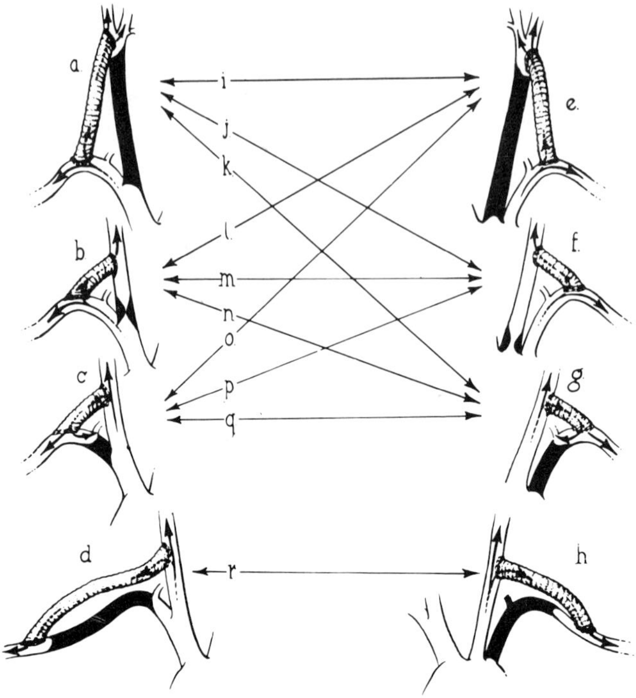

Figure 35-5. This diagram shows 18 methods of employing extra-thoracic bypass according to location and extent of obstruction in the Baylor University experience in Houston (Crawford, ES, DeBakey, ME, Morris, GC, Jr and Howell, JF, Surgery 65:17, 1969).

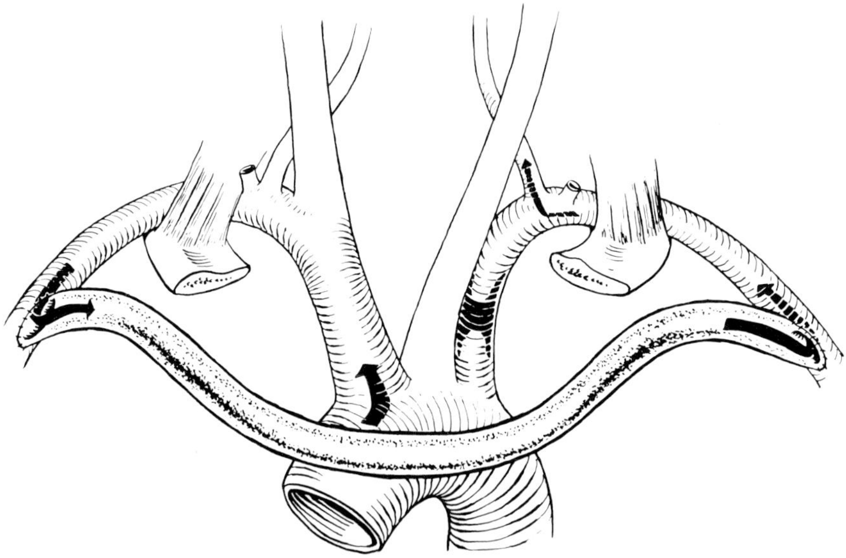

Figure 35-6. Axillo-axillary bypass, as depicted above, can be utilized to reverse flow in a subclavian steal syndrome with proximal left subclavian arterial occlusion.

Table 35-1
Clinical Features of 10 Patients Undergoing Axillo-Axillary Bypass

Case	Age/Sex	Follow-Up (Mos.)	Lesion	Symptoms	Complications
1	59/M	60	Left subclavian	Dizziness, claudication paresthesias	Graft thrombosis 8 months' postoperation*
2	54/M	59	Left subclavian	Dizziness, syncope, arm visual disturbance	
3	64/M	50	Left subclavian	Transient hemi-paresis, visual disturbance	
4	70/M	46	Left subclavian	Dizziness, arm claudication	
5	53/M	38	Innominate	Syncopal episode, arm weakness	
6	42/M	44	Right subclavian	Arm pain	Graft thrombosis 3 months' postoperation*
7	60/F	43	Innominate (left carotid)	Right amaurosis fugax, right upper extremity weakness	
8	45/F	42	Left subclavian	Claudication, paresthesias	
9	67/M	34	Innominate (left carotid)	Right amaurosis fugax, right upper extremity weakness	
10	58/M	32	Left subclavian	Dizziness	

*Both patients underwent successful graft thrombectomy.
From Bentley, FR, Hollier, LH and Batson, RC, Am Surg 48:70, 1982.

SUBCLAVIAN-SUBCLAVIAN BYPASS

The drawing in Figure 35-7 depicts the subclavian-subclavian bypass. Ehrenfeld, Levin, and Wylie, in 1968, described venous cross-over bypass grafts for arterial insufficiency including subclavian-subclavian bypass.[6] Finkelstein, Byer, and Rush, in 1972, described their management of 15 patients with subclavian steal syndrome treated by subclavian-subclavian

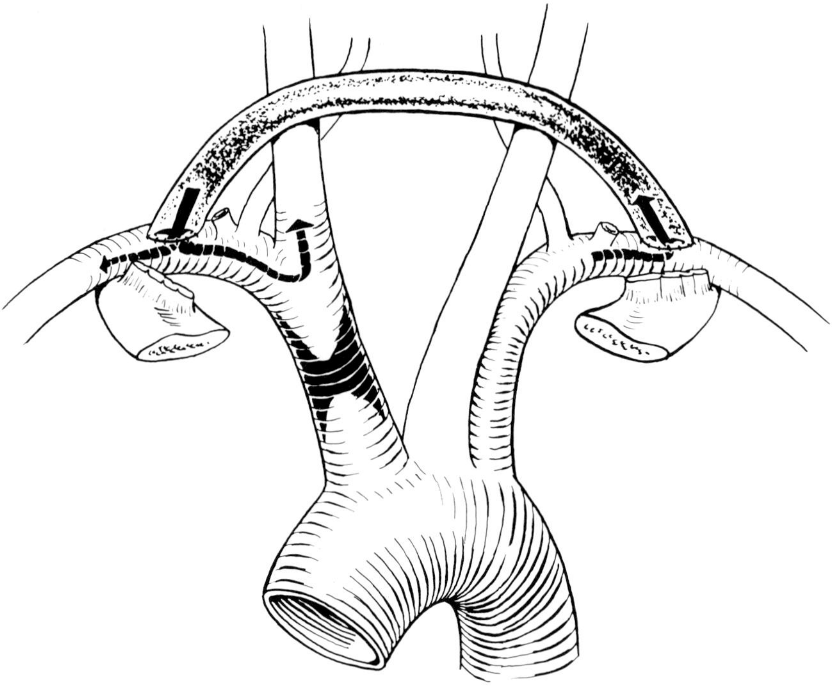

Figure 35-7. A subclavian-subclavian bypass, as noted in this artist's concept, can be utilized as an extra-thoracic, extra-anatomical bypass of an innominate arterial occlusion to reverse symptoms of cerebral ischemia and/or right upper extremity ischemia.

bypass.[22] Thirteen of these patients presented with central nervous system symptoms which were intermittent and similar to those symptoms found in patients with vertebrobasilar arterial lesions. These authors outlined using bilateral supraclavicular incisions with incision through the scalenus anticus muscle if required for optimum exposure, as the direct approach to the subclavian artery. Dacron prostheses were used in all reconstructions with no graft failures during their follow-up study which ranged from 6 months to 4 years. There was one patient who died in the immediate postoperative period of unrelated problems. There were no transient nor permanent neurological complications, and all patients remained free of symptoms throughout the follow-up period.

Forestner and co-workers evaluated the use of subclavian-subclavian bypass for correction of the subclavian steal syndrome.[23] They emphasized that alternate procedures were sought to avoid the potential problems associated with carotid artery-to-subclavian artery bypass, which might include possible compromise of the carotid circulation and/or production of cerebral embolization from the carotid graft suture line. These authors evaluated the hemodynamic changes associated with the subclavian steal syndrome and subsequent subclavian-subclavian bypass in the canine model in the experimental laboratory. They demonstrated that the subclavian-subclavian bypass achieved adequate restoration of cephalad vertebral arterial flow at the same time that it restored revascularization of the occluded subclavian artery.

SUBCLAVIAN-CAROTID BYPASS

Figure 35-8 is a line drawing of the subclavian-carotid bypass. Diethrich and co-workers, in 1967, analyzed their experience of 125 cases of carotid-subclavian and subclavian-carotid bypass in managing occlusive disease of the common carotid and subclavian arteries.[24] Included in this series was a

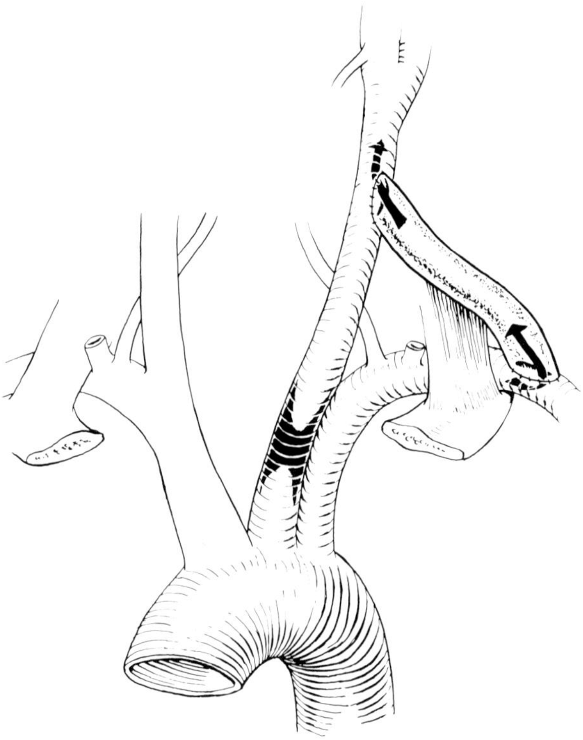

Figure 35-8. Subclavian-carotid bypass, as demonstrated in the above line drawing, can be utilized to restore proper arterial flow beyond occlusive lesions such as in the origin of the left common carotid artery.

group of 25 patients who presented with cerebrovascular insufficiency symptoms due to an obstructing lesion at the origin of the common carotid artery. The subsequent report by Crawford and co-workers in 1969, as previously described, provided additional emphasis for the value of this approach over the previously utilized intra-thoracic approach with aorto-carotid bypass.[7]

An extension of the subclavian-carotid bypass is the axillo-carotid bypass as championed by Bergan, Dean, and Yao in 1975 when they presented 2 cases of complex common carotid and innominate arterial disease.[25] They utilized an axillo-carotid bypass of autogenous greater saphenous vein with good results in this approach to complex cerebral revascularization. They emphasized that this specific operative technique would expand the surgeon's armamentarium. These authors identified the ease and safety of exposure and anastomosis of the axillary artery to make it a preferable donor vessel for extra-anatomical cerebral revascularization in the poor-risk, elderly patient population. In one of the two reconstructions, the autogenous vein bypass carried flow from the ipsilateral axillary artery to the internal carotid artery. In the second patient, a cross-over axillary-carotid bypass was utilized for cerebral revascularization.

To emphasize the numerous modifications that are possible, Hagood, Mozersky, and Fite utilized a subclavian-carotid bypass successfully during the staged palliative resection of recurrent carcinoma of the neck which presented a therapeutic dilemma.[26] They performed the subclavian-carotid bypass in an effort to reduce the dangers of cerebral ischemia, secondary infection, and hemorrhage associated with direct operative intervention of excision of the recurrent carcinoma of the carotid bifurcation which might have been done without vascular reconstruction. These authors performed a staged, extra-anatomic, distal subclavian-internal carotid bypass in the left neck utilizing autogenous greater saphenous vein. This was followed in 3 weeks by an en bloc resection of the carcinoma and involved carotid bifurcation.

CAROTID-CAROTID BYPASS

Figure 35-9 is the artist's interpretation of the carotid-carotid bypass. Warren and Fomon described use of the carotid-carotid arterial bypass in 1966.[5] A specific individual report by Manart and Kempczinski, in 1980, described success in managing a 62 year-old patient with severe stenosis of the innominate artery and stenosis of the proximal left subclavian artery with a carotid-carotid bypass graft.[27]

To again emphasize the number of variations that are possible, Bole and associates, in 1977, described an external carotid-to-external carotid cross-over vein bypass in a suprahyoid subcutaneous location to avoid an area of infection which required common carotid arterial ligation on one side.[28]

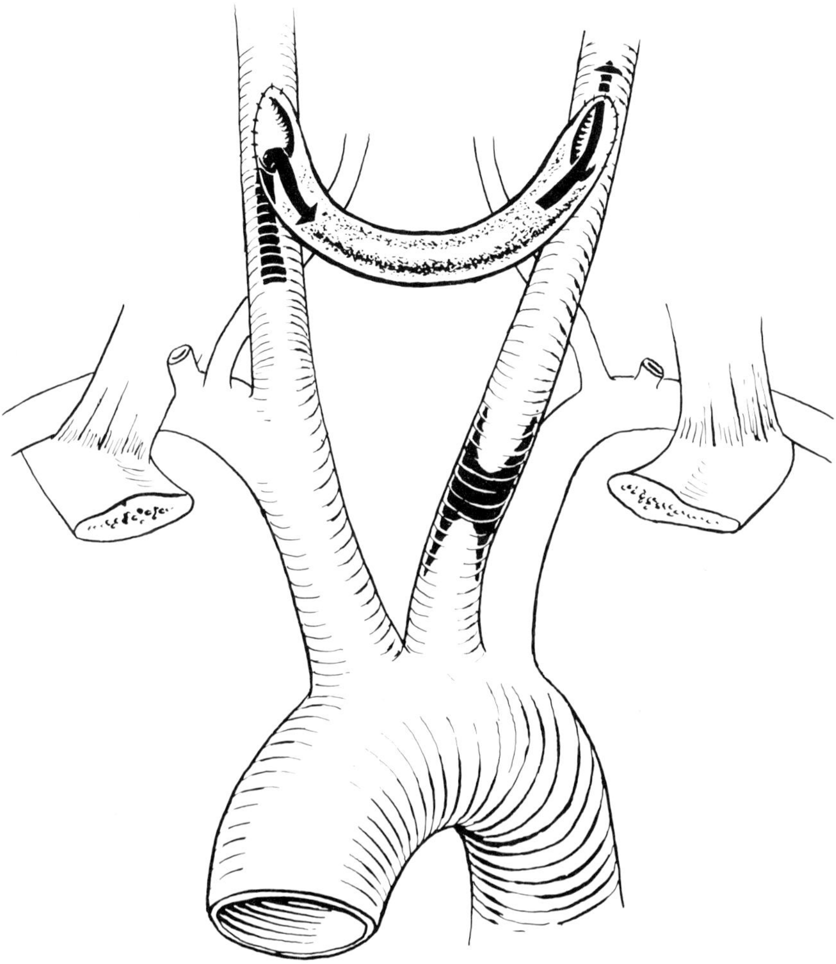

Figure 35-9. Carotid-carotid bypass has been successfully employed in proximal occlusive lesions such as that depicted in the drawing above in the patient with occlusion at the origin of the left common carotid artery.

OTHER EXTRA-ANATOMICAL BYPASSES

Sproul, in 1971, advocated the use of a femoro-axillary bypass graft as an alternative method of managing a patient with cerebrovascular insufficiency secondary to a complex problem including severe stenosis of the innominate artery, occlusion of the left common carotid artery, and occlusion of the left subclavian artery.[29]

Carotid-vertebral anastomosis was advocated by Clark and Perry who devised an alternate technique for correction of the subclavian steal syndrome. They were successful in anastomosing the external carotid artery in an end-to-end fashion to the vertebral artery after mobilization and transection of the vertebral artery in its second and third parts from the foramen transversarium followed by transposition under the sternocleidomastoid muscle.[30]

Mehigan and co-workers utilized subclavian-carotid transposition with an end-to-side replantation of the subclavian artery to the carotid artery for subclavian steal syndrome.[31]

COMMENT

Recognizing that the majority of patients with signs and symptoms of cerebrovascular ischemia will be helped by carotid endarterectomy, there are an increasing number of complex cerebral revascularizations, which challenge the surgeon's imagination. For the past 15 years, with procedures such as the subclavian-carotid bypass and more recently in the past 10 years, with increasing experience in utilizing the axillo-axillary bypass, there have also been patients who have required a combination of bypass procedures to provide adequate cerebral blood flow. Such procedures as the subclavian-carotid bypass avoid the additional morbidity of an intra-thoracic procedure. Nevertheless, it must be emphasized that additional hazards exist with arteriotomies in vessels that are otherwise normal. Questions arise such as the requirement for a temporary indwelling shunt when the carotid artery is approached as the donor vessel. In considering the numerous approaches, some operations are technically more difficult than others. As an example,

Table 35-2
Location and Extent of 412 Lesions in 299 Patients

Location	Extent of Obstruction		Totals
	Incomplete	Complete	
Innominate artery	40	26	66
Right common carotid artery	5	19	24
Right subclavian artery	30	29	59
Left common carotid artery	24	37	61
Left subclavian artery	69	133	202
Total	168	244	412

From Crawford, ES, DeBakey, ME, Morris, GC, Jr. and Howell, JF, Surgery 65:17, 1969

Table 35-3
Indications for and Results of Complex Cerebral Revascularizations

Case/Age, Yr/Sex	Principal Symptoms	Physical Findings	Risk Factors	Procedure	Complications	Results
1/69/M	Amaurosis fugax, dizziness	Bilateral cervical bruits, weak right radial pulse	Advanced age, prior myocardial infarction (MI), thiamine deficiency	Left to right subclavian-subclavian bypass, right carotid endarterectomy, extensions to both carotids	Bilateral supraclavicular seromas	Asymptomatic
2/41/F	Dizziness, vertigo, left arm weakness, progressive blindness in left eye	Right cervical bruit, absent left radial and temporal pulses	Hypertension, angina pectoris	Right to left subclavian-subclavian bypass, right vertebral endarterectomy, right carotid endarterectomy, extension to right carotid bifurcation	None	Dizziness abated, died of probable MI 8 months postoperative

Table 35-3 (continued)
Indications for and Results of Complex Cerebral Revascularizations

Case/ Age, Yr/Sex	Principal Symptoms	Physical Findings	Risk Factors	Procedure	Complications	Results
3/43/F	Dizziness, light-headedness, left upper extremity pain	Bilateral cervical and supraclavicular bruits, weak left radial pulse	MI-1969, angina pectoris, positive stress test	Right carotid endarterectomy, right to left axillo-axillary bypass, extension to left common carotid artery	None	Asymptomatic
4/45/M	Incapacitating dizziness	Bilateral cervical and infraclavicular bruits, weak right radial pulse	Hypertension, angina pectoris	Left to right axillo-axillary bypass	Transient hypotension	Occasional mild dizziness
5/49/F	Right amaurosis fugax	Bilateral cervical, supraclavicular, and infraclavicular bruits	Prior MI, angina pectoris, positive stress test	Left to right axillo-axillary bypass, extension to right common carotid artery	None	Asymptomatic

From Collins, GJ, Jr., Rich, NM, Andersen, CA and McDonald, PT, Arch Surg 113:706, 1978.

the subclavian-subclavian bypass may be more difficult than more direct exposure for a carotid-subclavian bypass in a patient with a proximal subclavian arterial occlusion and reversible flow in the vertebral artery distal to the occlusion. Many consider that the axillo-axillary bypass is easier to perform than the subclavian-subclavian bypass. The femoro-axillary bypass requires a longer graft in a superficial location where local pressure might result in thrombosis of the graft.

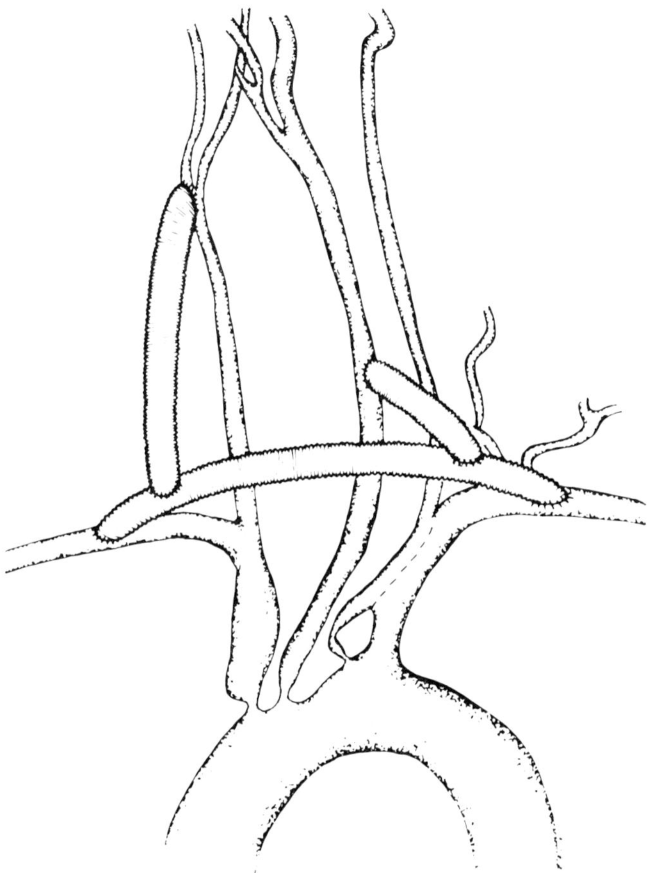

Figure 35-10. This schematic drawing shows sites of stenoses and operative procedures in a 69-year-old male who presented with symptoms of dizziness and amaurosis fugax. The complex cerebral revascularization procedures combined left to right subclavian-subclavian bypass, right carotid endarterectomy, and extension bypasses to both carotid arteries (Collins, GJ, Jr, Rich, NM, Anderson, CA, McDonald PT, Arch Surg 113:706, 1978).

Table 35-2 outlines the location and extent of arteriosclerotic involvement of the aortic arch vessels and major branches at the base of the neck. Obviously, combinations of involvement were frequent in this series. Identifiable progression of arteriosclerotic lesions in these locations emphasizes the importance for continued follow-up and periodic reevaluation of patients who require extra-anatomical bypasses for cerebral revascularization.

Moore and associates, in 1976, reviewed their experience between 1961 and 1975 in managing 26 patients with symptomatic occlusions of one or more branches of the aortic arch who underwent correction of 30 lesions by an extra-thoracic approach.[8] During that same interval, they had 465 operations on the extra-cranial cerebrovascular tree with this specific group of operations on the branches of the aortic arch constituting approximately 6.5 percent of the total operative experience for cerebrovascular disease. Our experience has been similar, which also emphasizes that these complex cerebral revascularization procedures are not required frequently.

Questions have existed regarding the hemodynamics of these extra-anatomical bypasses used in complex cerebral revascularization procedures. Both experimental and clinical investigation have demonstrated proper hemodynamic functioning.

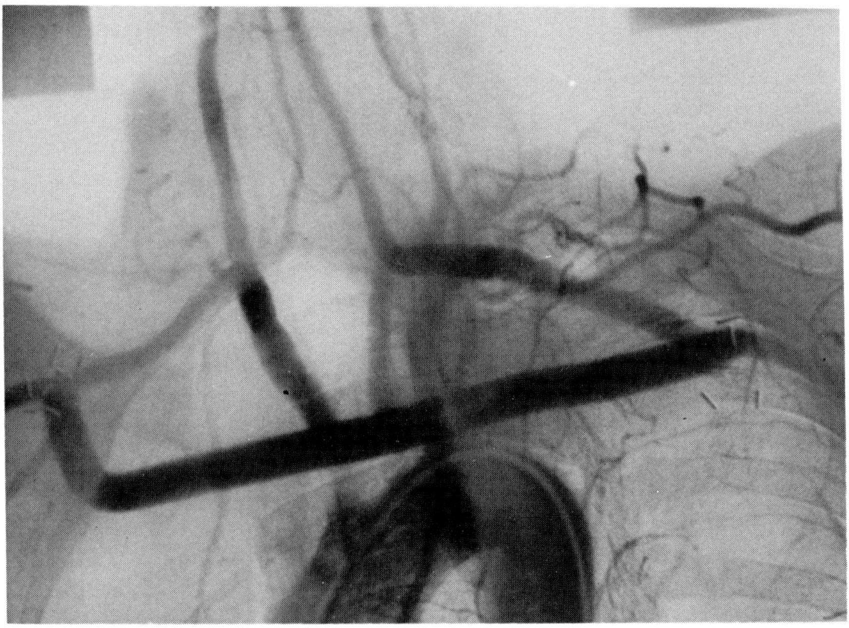

Figure 35-11. This subtraction study of an arch aortogram demonstrates filling of the axillo-axillary bypass utilized in a patient requiring complex cerebral revascularization.

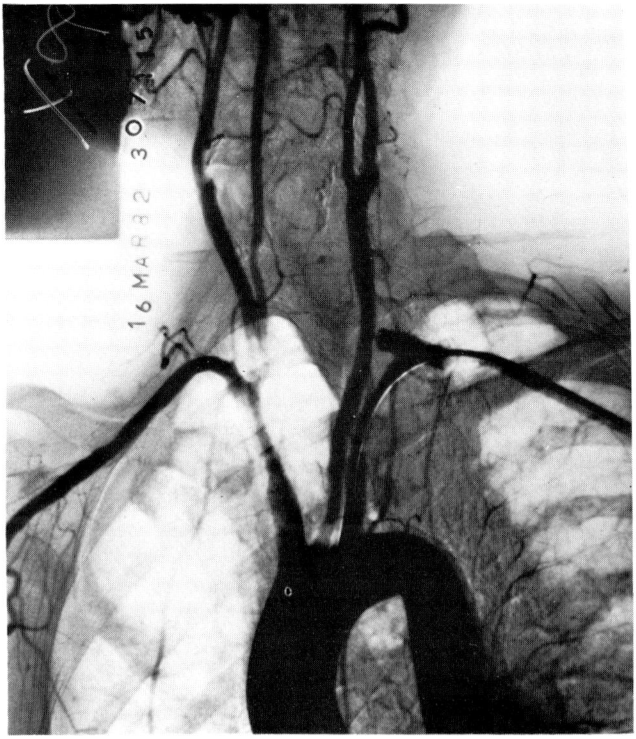

Figure 35-12. Severe stenosis is obvious at the suture line of a subclavian-common carotid arterial bypass on the left. This and other potential complications emphasize the importance for long-term followup in patients who require arterial reconstruction to reverse signs and symptoms of cerebral ischemia.

The importance of long term follow-up must be emphasized. Table 35-3 documents the indications and results of complex cerebral revascularization in our previously reported experience. Figure 35-10 provides the outline for one of these patient's problems identifying multiple arteriosclerotic lesions. Figure 35-11 outlines patency in an axillo-axillary bypass. In the long term follow-up, we have noted both the complications of suture line stenosis (Fig. 35-12) and progression of generalized arteriosclerosis (Fig. 35-13). While these extra-anatomical bypass procedures for complex cerebral revascularization are valuable adjuncts to the occasional management of patients with cerebrovascular ischemia, it is important to continue to document and analyze results and to provide the long term follow-up to document the degree of durability of these procedures.

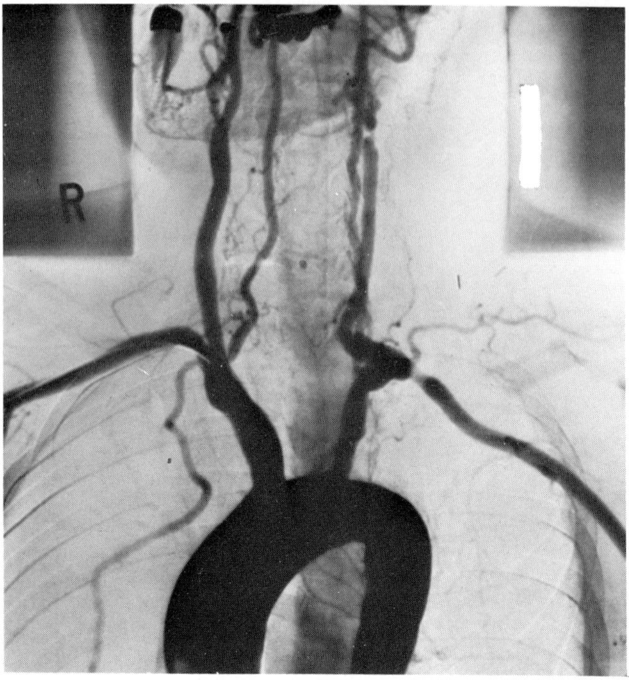

Figure 35-13. A long term follow-up of patients with generalized arteriosclerosis and previous operative intervention is emphasized by this patient who had a left subclavian-carotid bypass in 1976 in treatment of cerebral arterial insufficiency secondary to marked stenosis of the origin of the left common carotid artery. Six years later the patient returned with new symptoms and there is now marked stenosis in the bulb of the left carotid artery. The proximal left common carotid artery is now totally occluded.

ACKNOWLEDGEMENT

Gary G. Wind, MD, Assistant Professor of Surgery, Uniformed Services University of the Health Sciences, kindly provided the artwork in Figures 35-6–9.

REFERENCES

1. Rich NM, Hobson RW: Carotid endarterectomy under regional anesthesia. Am Surg 4:253, 1975
2. Andersen CA, Rich NM, Collins GJ Jr, et al: Carotid endarterectomy: Regional versus general anesthesia. Am Surg 46:323, 1980

3. Hobson RW, Wright CB, Sublett JW, et al: Carotid artery back pressure and endarterectomy under regional anesthesia. Arch Surg 109:682, 1974
4. Collins GJ Jr, Rich NM, Andersen CA, et al: Complex cerebral revascularization. Arch Surg 113:706, 1978
5. Warren WD, Fomon JJ: Rerouting arterial flow to relieve ischemia: Femoro-femoral, axillary-femoral and carotid-carotid artery bypass. Ann Surg 163:131, 1966
6. Ehrenfeld WK, Levin SM, Wylie EJ: Venous crossover bypass grafts for arterial insufficiency. Ann Surg 167:287, 1968
7. Crawford ES, DeBakey ME, Morris GC Jr, et al: Surgical treatment of occlusion of the innominate, common carotid, and subclavian arteries. A ten-year experience. Surgery 65:17, 1969
8. Moore WS, Malone JM, Goldstone J: Extrathoracic repair of branch occlusions of the aortic arch. Am J Surg 132:249, 1976
9. Schumacker HB Jr, Isch JH, Jolly, WW, et al: The management of stenotic and obstructive lesions of the aortic arch branches. Am J Surg 133:351, 1977
10. DeBakey ME, Morris GC Jr, Jordan GL, et al: Segmental thrombo-obliterative disease of branches of aortic arch. JAMA 166:988, 1958
11. DeBakey ME, Crawford ES, Cooley DA, et al: Surgical considerations of occlusive disease of innominate, carotid, subclavian, and vertebral arteries. Ann Surg 149:690, 1958
12. Myers WO, Lawton BR, Sautter RD: Axillo-axillary bypass graft. JAMA 217:826, 1971
13. Myers WO, Lawton BR, Ray JF III, et al: Axillo-axillary bypass for subclavian steal syndrome. Arch Surg 114:394, 1979
14. Jacobson JH II, Mozersky DJ, Mitty HA, et al: Axillary-axillary bypass for the "subclavian steal" syndrome. Arch Surg 106:24, 1973
15. Mozersky DJ, Sumner DS, Barnes RW, et al: Subclavian revascularization by means of a subcutaneous axillary-axillary graft. Arch Surg 106:20, 1973
16. Mozersky DJ, Sumner DS, Barnes RW, et al: The hemodynamics of the axillary-axillary bypass. Surg Gynecol Obstet 135:925, 1972
17. LeVeen HH, Piccone VA Jr, Diaz C, et al: A simplified correction of subclavian steal syndrome. Surgery 75:299, 1974
18. Dardik H, Dardik I: Axillo-axillary bypass with cephalic vein for correction of subclavian steal syndrome. Surgery 76:413, 1975
19. Snider RL, Porter JM, Eidemiller LR: Axillary-axillary artery bypass for the correction of subclavian artery occlusive disease. Ann Surg 180:888, 1974
20. Lamis PA, Stanton PE Jr, Hyland L: The axillo-axillary bypass graft. Further experience. Arch Surg 111:1353, 1976
21. Bentley FR, Hollier LH, Batson RC: Axilloaxillary bypass for subclavian and innominate artery revascularization. Am Surg 48:70, 1982
22. Finkelstein NM, Byer A, Rush BF Jr: Subclavian-subclavian bypass for the subclavian steal syndrome. Surgery 71:142, 1972
23. Forestner JE, Ghosh SK, Bergan JJ, et al: Subclavian-subclavian bypass for correction of the subclavian steal syndrome. Surgery 71:136, 1972
24. Diethrich EB, Garrett HE, Ameriso J, et al: Occlusive disease of the common carotid and subclavian arteries treated by carotid-subclavian bypass—analysis of 125 cases. Am J Surg 114:800, 1967
25. Bergan JJ, Dean RH, Yao JST: Use of the axillary artery in complex cerebral revascularization. Surgery 77:338, 1975
26. Hagood CO Jr, Mozersky DJ, Fulton WF: Staged palliative resection of recurrent carcinoma of the neck using an extra anatomic carotid bypass. Surgery 76:671, 1974
27. Manart FD, Kempczinski RF: The Carotid-carotid bypass graft. Arch Surg 115:669, 1980
28. Bole PV, Katz M, Cohen NH, et al: Carotid cross-over bypass: Cerebral revascularization after ligation of common carotid artery. J Cardiovasc Surg 18:533, 1977

29. Sproul G: Femoral-axillary bypass for cerebral vascular insufficiency. Arch Surg 103:746, 1971
30. Clark K, Perry MO: Carotid vertebral anastomosis: An alternate technic for repair of the subclavian steal syndrome. Ann Surg 163:414, 1966
31. Mehigan JJ, Buch WS, Pipkin RD, et al: Subclavian carotid transposition for the subclavian steal syndrome. Am J Surg 136:15, 1978

John J. Bergan
James S.T. Yao

36

Surgical Technique of Vertebro-carotid Reimplantation

Transient ischemia of the vertebro-basilar system presents symptoms that are much less stereotyped than those in the carotid territory. While vertigo is a common component of vertebro-basilar insufficiency, this alone is also a manifestation of labyrynthine disorders and therefore should not be considered a part of the vertebro-basilar insufficiency syndrome unless some other manifestations of brain stem ischemia are present.[1] These other manifestations may include transient hemiparesis, hemi-sensory deficits, and these, in turn, must be differentiated from cerebral hemispheric insufficiency. Similarly, homonymous hemianopsia can arise from ischemia of either the anterior or posterior circulation, but transient quadriparesis is most commonly of brain stem origin. Other symptoms which are commonly of brain stem origin include dysarthria, dysphagia, and transient impairment of function of the extra-ocular muscles. Finally, ataxia is a common manifestation of vertebro-basilar insufficiency.

Accurate arteriography is necessary for the identification of vertebral artery lesions and, in most instances, patients with vertebro-basilar symptomatology will also have internal carotid artery stenosis.

Since the mid-1960s, the traditional approach has been to attempt revascularization of the carotid system prior to considering vertebral artery revascularization.[2] Other approaches to correction of vertebro-basilar insufficiency have included trans-cervical ligation of the affected artery, a procedure which fortunately has not enjoyed widespread popularity,[3] bypass grafting[4] to the subclavian arteries by means of aorto-subclavian grafting, subclavian-subclavian, or axillary-axillary grafting, as well as direct bypass grafting to the vertebral artery itself.[5] Wylie's group[6] has favored trans-subclavian vertebral orifice endarterectomy, and this has proved to be an

PART XI

Extracranial/Intracranial Bypass

O. Howard Reichman

37

Extracranial/Intracranial Bypass: as Viewed by a Neurosurgeon

Anastomosis between the superficial temporal artery (STA) and a cortical branch of the middle cerebral artery (MCA) has become a firmly established operation for reliably providing new collateral circulation to the brain. The historical development of this procedure (performed at medical centers throughout the world since 1967), its rationale, and operative technique have been clearly described in the literature.[1]

Between August, 1970 and August, 1982 we have had occasion to perform 306 extra-intracranial bypass (EC-IC bypass) operations in 281 patients and have evaluated the resulting new collateral channel by at least one arteriographic study (usually performed several months after surgery) in 172 of these patients.

At this point, it seems appropriate to identify the major problems pertaining to EC-IC bypass and consider the need for continued investigation of these areas. A few important topics have, therefore, been selected for emphasis in this publication.

EXTENT OF PERFUSION AND LONG-TERM PATENCY

Skeptics of EC-IC bypass have emphasized the smallness in diameter of the STA and been concerned that it would be unable to provide a significant volume of flow. Actually, it has been repeatedly demonstrated, by using serial arteriograms, that the diameter of the STA gradually increases to an average measurement of 2.0 mm (range 1.3-2.8 mm).[2] This compares very favorably with the diameter of anterior or posterior communicating arteries, the major

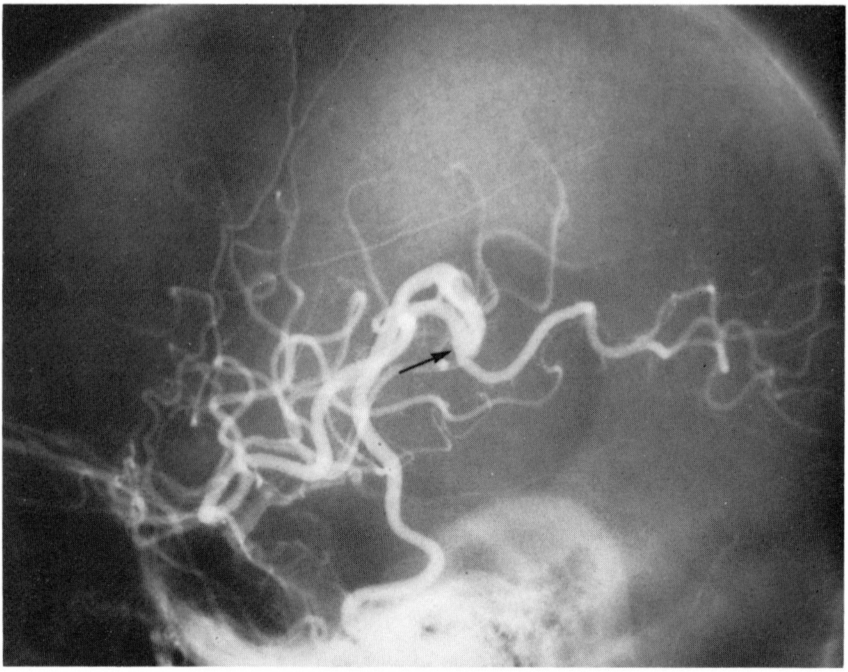

Figure 37-1. Sixty-one-year-old female with occlusion of right internal carotid artery and contralateral internal carotid artery stenosis. Arteriogram, performed 5 years after right EC-IC bypass, shows irrigation of entire middle cerebral territory through anastomosis (arrow).

sources of collateral circulation to the brain and recognized as major factors in the protection from, or development of, stroke relative to internal carotid artery (ICA) occlusive disease.

Review of 172 postoperative arteriograms evaluated the extent of perfusion into each of the four major MCA branches (ascending frontal complex, posterior parietal, angular, posterior temporal). Excellent perfusion (defined as filling three or four major MCA branches) was observed in 110 patients (Fig. 37-1) and fair perfusion (filling of one or two MCA branches) in 44 patients. Thus, 154 patients (90 percent) were considered a technical success. A technical failure was observed in 18 patients (10 percent) with poor perfusion in 11 and an EC-IC bypass occlusion in seven. Filling of three or four major MCA branches results in flow rates approximating 150 ml per minute, the normal range for MCA perfusion.[2]

Long-term patency has been observed regularly (Fig. 37-2) and the 9-year follow-up of a double branch EC-IC bypass graft is illustrated in Figure 37-3.

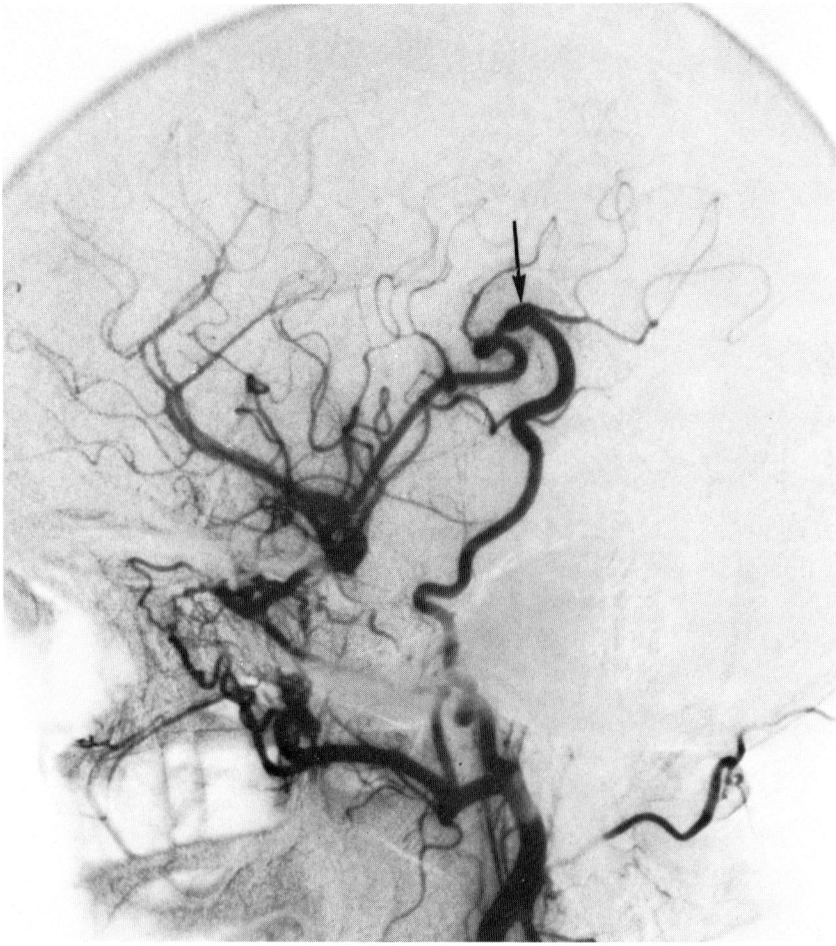

Figure 37-2. Forty-three-year-old female with bilateral internal carotid artery occlusion. Left carotid arteriogram, performed 5½ years after left EC-IC bypass, shows large superficial temporal artery irrigating entire left middle cerebral territory through anastomosis (arrow).

ACCURACY OF DIAGNOSIS

It should be indicated that episodic neurological dysfunction may frequently be difficult to specifically identify as arising from a minor focal seizure or represent cerebral ischemia. Furthermore, a detailed careful review of symptoms may not always provide an accurate diagnosis.

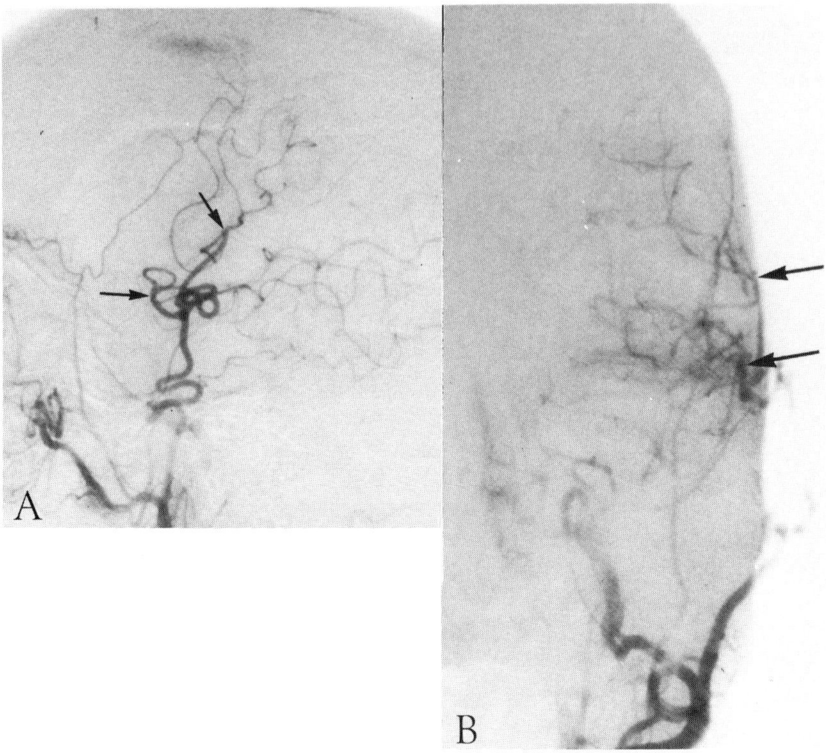

Figure 37-3. Twenty-five-year-old female with left middle cerebral artery stenosis. Selective left external carotid arteriogram performed 9 years after EC-IC bypass.
(A) Lateral projection shows separate anastomosis (arrows) for frontal and parietal branches of left middle cerebral artery with irrigation of entire middle cerebral territory.
(B) Frontal projection confirms separate anastomosis (arrows) for each branch of the superficial temporal artery and middle cerebral territory perfusion.

Similarly, abrupt or gradually progressive lasting neurological deficit may result from numerous neuropathological conditions other than cerebral vascular disease. With the initial benefit of excellent neurological consultation and a computed tomographic scan, the patient represented by Figures 37-4, 37-5, and 37-6 initially carried a diagnosis of stroke. Current arteriography did demonstrate stenosis at the origin of the internal carotid artery (Fig. 37-4), but head projections demonstrated evidence of tumor (Fig. 37-5) which was confirmed by tomographic scan (Fig. 37-6). Metastatic carcinoma was found at operation, but subsequent autopsy indicated no evidence of previous infarction.

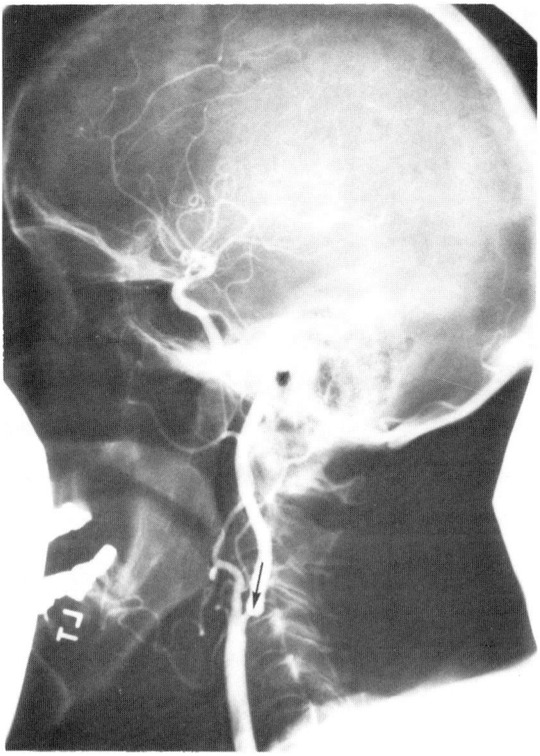

Figure 37-4. Sixty-five-year-old female with progressive thought disorder and dysphasia. An event 7 months prior to current problem had clinical manifestations and computed tomographic scan compatible with cerebral infraction. Current arteriogram demonstrates tight stenosis (arrow) of left internal carotid artery.

SELECTION OF PATIENTS

Selection of candidates has been made from the sub-group of patients having experienced temporary or relatively mild fixed ischemic neurological deficit associated with arteriographic findings of intracranial stenosis involving the internal carotid artery (ICA), ICA occlusion, MCA stenosis, MCA occlusion, or a combination of the above. It has now become clearly established that complete occlusion of a vessel does not preclude the possibility of subsequent ischemic attacks relative to the circulation beyond that occlusion.[3]

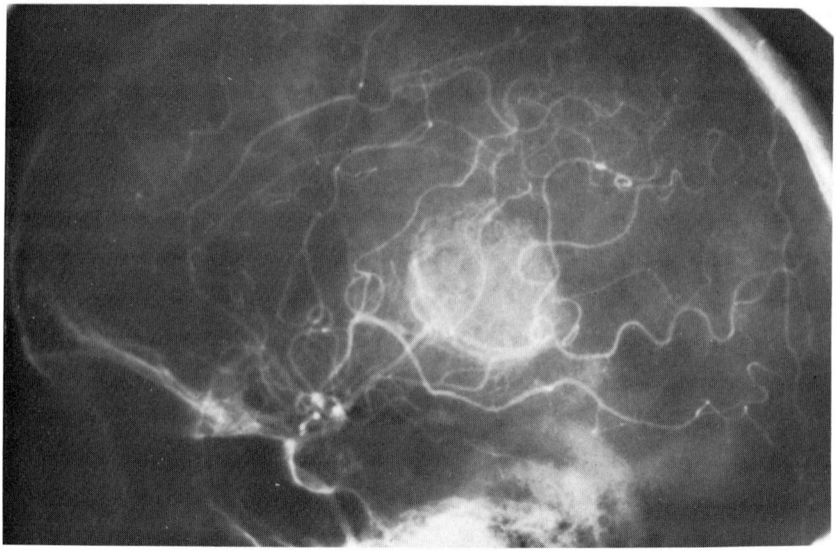

Figure 37-5. Later phase from head projection of same arteriographic study demonstrates "tumor blush" with localized downward displacement of posterior sylvian vessels conforming to anterio-inferior border of tumor.

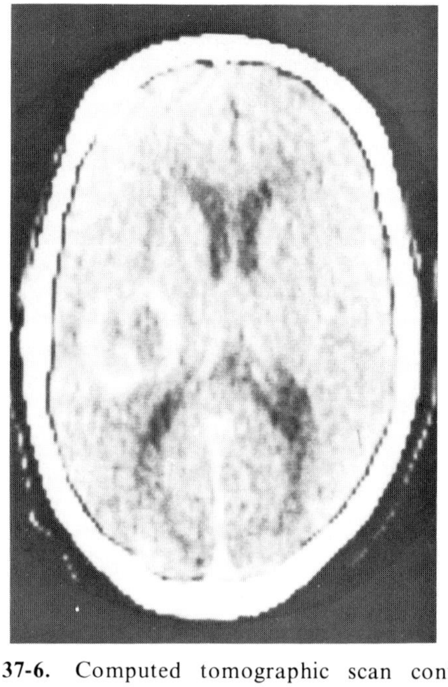

Figure 37-6. Computed tomographic scan confirms the presence of neoplasm deep in left cerebral hemisphere. Subsequent autopsy failed to demonstrate evidence of a previous infarction.

Selection of patients who will benefit from operation, however, is a very complex problem. Transient ischemic attacks may not always portend the subsequent development of stroke, and arteriographic lesions may resolve spontaneously. Conversely, arterial lesions frequently progress to complete occlusion associated with stroke. Furthermore, vessels having resolution of a threatening lesion may subsequently occlude resulting in sudden stroke.

CLINICAL BENEFIT

Absolute proof that EC-IC bypass has actual clinical value does not exist. Numerous experiences, however, strongly support such a conclusion in specific cases. Furthermore, the incidence of new stroke following EC-IC bypass is low,[4] particularly in comparison with other series of patients known to harbor intracranial occlusive vascular disease.

Figure 37-7 demonstrates the arteriographic findings of asymptomatic occlusion of anterior and middle cerebral arteries in a patient having a previous EC-IC bypass. In comparison, Figure 37-8 shows the arteriographic findings of a patient who had a fatal stroke resulting from middle cerebral artery occlusion. Such experiences are not uncommon to those neurological surgeons who have the opportunity of evaluating numerous patients in consideration of possible EC-IC bypass.

The ultimate evaluation of EC-IC bypass, as it relates to clinical benefit in a large population, awaits completion of the randomized, cooperative EC-IC bypass study currently in progress.[5]

INTRACRANIAL ICA STENOSIS

Atherosclerotic involvement of the intracranial internal carotid artery, because of its inaccessibility to surgery, has received relatively little attention even though it is a common lesion (either singly or in tandem with cervical ICA stenosis). As recently as 1980, Barnett reported, "No study can be found in the literature dealing with the natural history of intracranial or high cervical internal carotid stenosis."[5] A current published abstract summarizes a recent study attempting to clarify the history of this condition.[6] Fifty patients were followed for an average of 44 months. During the follow-up period, 18 percent developed a stroke and 46 percent died. It was concluded that this indeed represents a highly significant condition in terms of poor prognosis.

Medical treatment has consisted of anticoagulants or platelet-suppressive agents with unclear and, frequently, disappointing results. The development of EC-IC bypass has focused attention upon this lesion with some hesitancy.

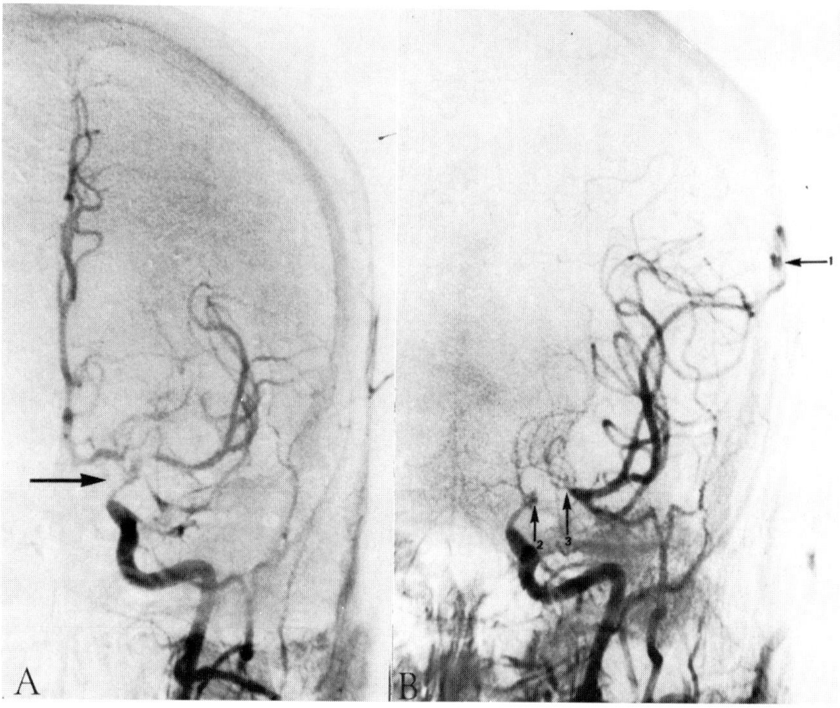

Figure 37-7. Forty-one-year-old male with numerous transient episodes of dysphasia and right hemiparesis.
(A) Left carotid arteriogram demonstrates tight stenosis (arrow) at intracranial bifurcation of internal carotid artery.
(B) Arteriogram, performed 6 months after EC-IC bypass, demonstrates excellent filling of middle cerebral territory through anastomosis (arrow 1). Occlusion of the left anterior cerebral artery, in addition to left middle cerebral artery occlusion (between arrows 2 and 3), has developed without any clinical manifestations.

Since the lesion is otherwise an inaccessible occlusive one, the EC-IC bypass offers an attractive surgical means of treatment. With significant flow continuing through the normal pathway, however, a stimulus for EC-IC bypass development is absent. Furthermore, the possibility of embolization poses a continuing threat, not clearly reduced by the bypass. It has been suggested that ligation of the internal carotid artery would remove the embolus-bearing portion of the artery from the ICA flow.[7] Internal carotid artery occlusion has been widely utilized for treatment of aneurysm but has a well-established risk.[8] The combination of EC-IC bypass and carotid artery ligation may provide a more suitable treatment for this condition.[9] Figure 37-9 illustrates a tight stenosis at the origin of the left internal carotid artery. In the same patient, Figure 37-10 illustrates an intracranial ICA stenosis in

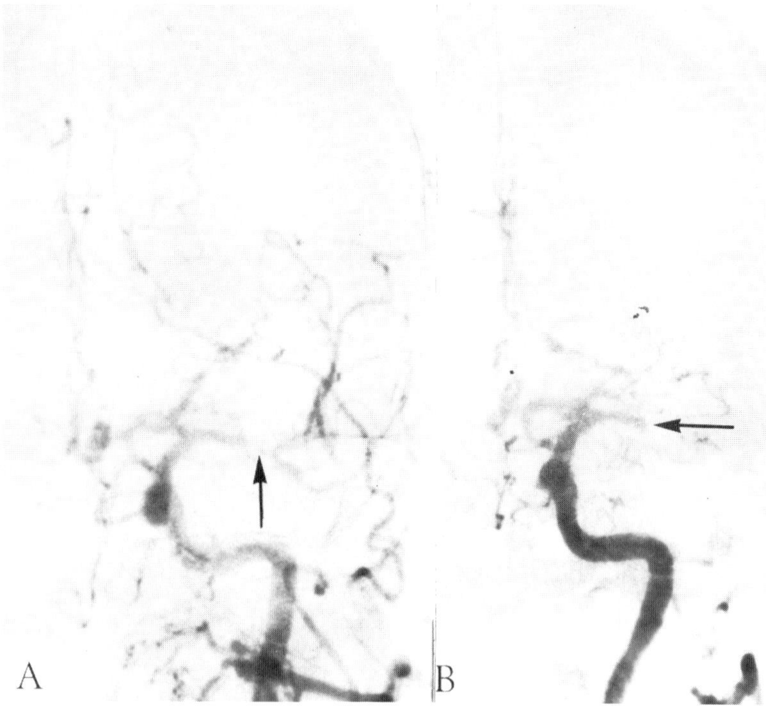

Figure 37-8. Seventy-five-year-old female with numerous transient episodes of dysphasia and right hemiparesis.
(A) Left carotid arteriogram demonstrates tight stenosis (arrow) of left middle cerebral artery.
(B) Occlusion (arrow) 5 months later, while undergoing preoperative preparation for EC-IC bypass, caused massive cerebral infarction, manifest by profound aphasia and hemiplegia and ultimately resulted in death.

tandem. This patient was treated with EC-IC bypass, illustrated by arteriography (Fig. 37-11) prior to ligation of the left internal carotid artery. Serial regional blood flow studies (Fig. 37-12) were helpful in understanding changes in perfusion associated with the several stages of treatment. Regional cerebral blood flow increased after EC-IC bypass but decreased after carotid ligation. Fortunately, the decrease in flow was not of a dangerous level. In the absence of EC-IC bypass, a more striking fall could have been associated with ischemic manifestations. However, carotid ligation continues to pose an unpredictable risk.

It is to be hoped that as surgical techniques improve, a more direct surgical approach to the intracranial internal carotid artery may be possible. The anatomical principles for operate exposure have been described.[10] With further development of surgical techniques, direct intracranial microsurgical

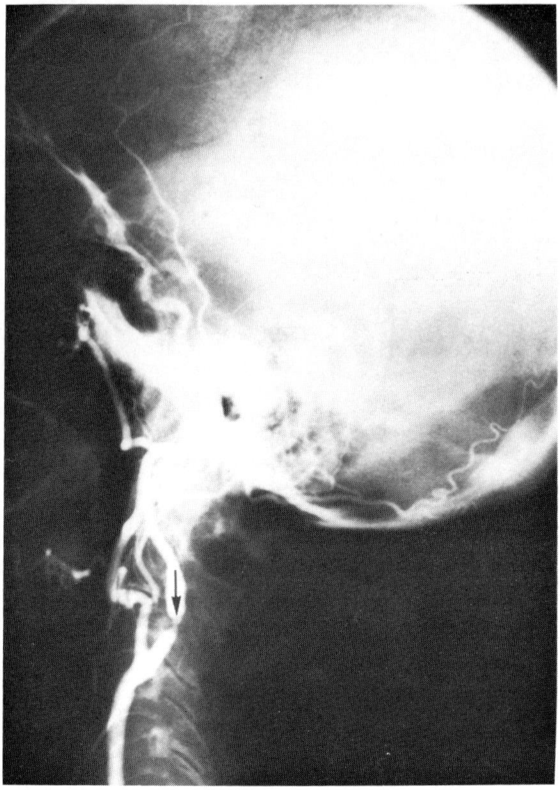

Figure 37-9. Sixty-five-year-old female who experienced three transient episodes of dysphasia and right hemiparesis. Left carotid arteriogram shows tight stenosis (arrow) of internal carotid artery at its origin.

ICA endarterectomy may become possible as Allen, Cohen, and Preziosi have described for the intracranial portion of the vertebral artery.[11]

VERTEBRO-BASILAR SYSTEM

Caplan has emphasized the need for more innovative methods in the treatment of patients experiencing serious difficulties attributable to occlusive disease involving the vertebral and basilar arteries or their branches.[12] Three innovative surgical methods are currently under investigation for improving perfusion in the vertebro-basilar system.

Sundt and Pepigras have summarized their experience in 16 patients with anastomosis between the occipital artery and the posterior inferior

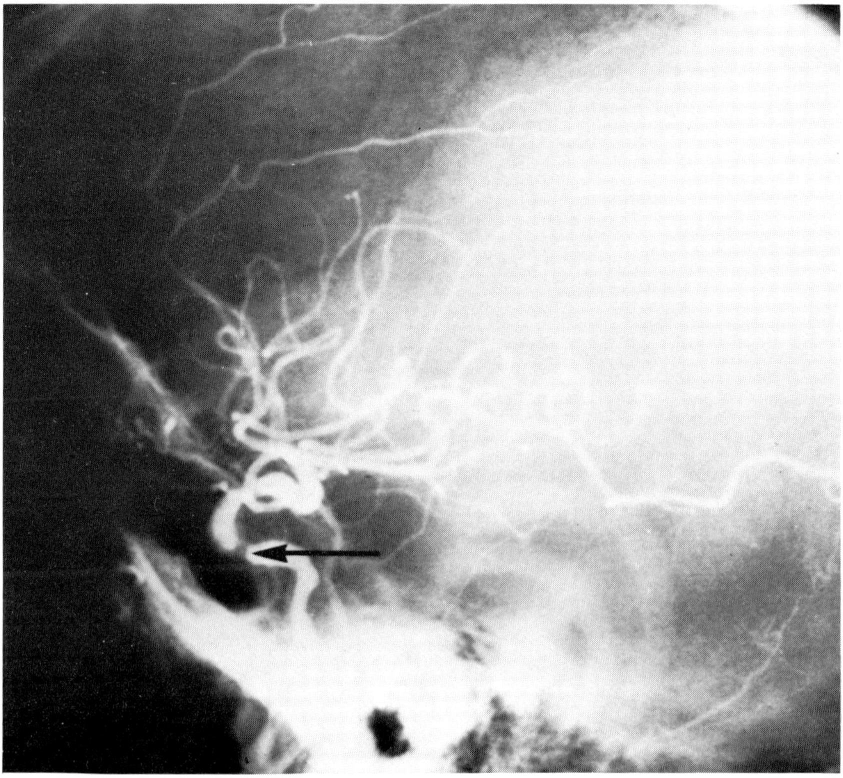

Figure 37-10. Intracranial stenosis (arrow) of left internal carotid artery in tandem.

cerebellar artery for vertebral artery hypoplasia or occlusive lesions located proximal to the posterior inferior cerebellar artery (PICA).[13] Preliminary results appear promising and have been confirmed in another group of 14 patients by Roski, Spetzler, and Hopkins.[14]

Allen, Cohen, and Preziosi have reported an innovative technique in 1 patient of microsurgical endarterectomy for a localized stenosis involving an intradural segment of the vertebral artery.[11] While we have not, as yet, actually performed this operation, it was considered, and probably would have been superior to occipital-PICA bypass in at least 1 patient of our series.

Ausman and co-workers have described their experience with STA to superior cerebellar artery anastomosis in 8 patients having basilar artery stenosis or occlusion.[15] While our clinical result in three such patients has not been gratifying, excellent collateral circulation to the upper brain stem was achieved. Figure 37-13 illustrates the arteriographic result following STA to posterior cerebral artery anastomosis and Figure 37-14 the arteriographic result following STA to superior cerebellar artery anastomosis. Choice of

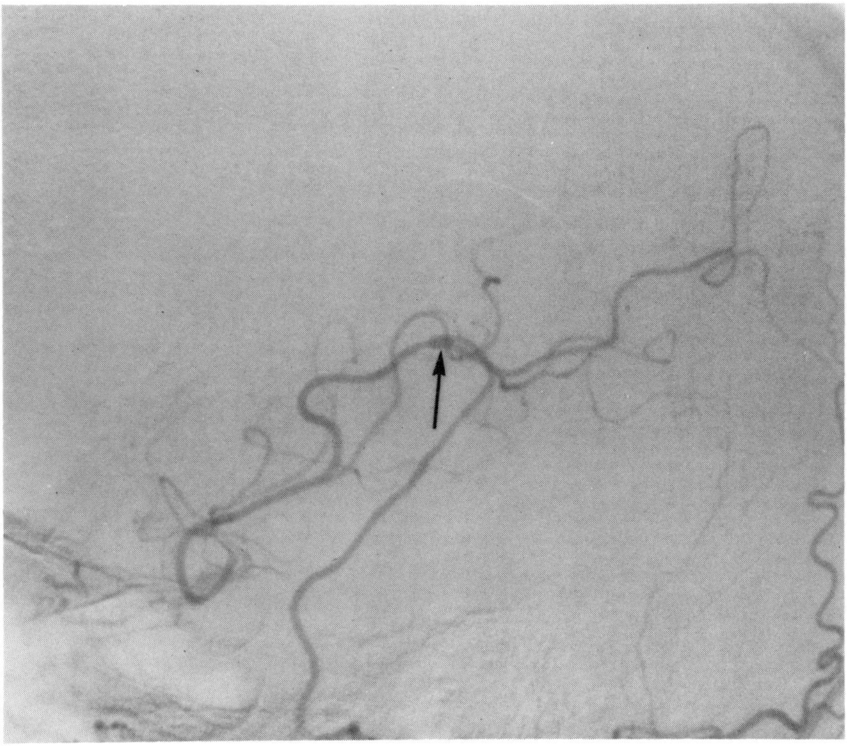

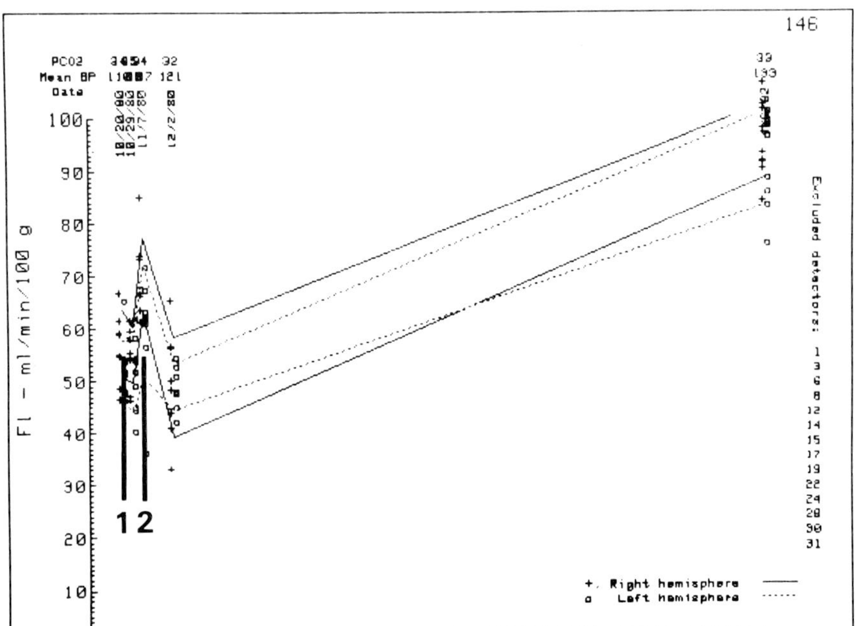

146
PCO2
Mean BP
Date
12/2/80
Fl - ml/min/100 g
1 2
Days
Excluded detectors:
+. Right hemisphere
o Left hemisphere

Figure 37-11. Subtraction version of selective left external carotid arteriogram shows patient EC-IC bypass with filling of a major division of left middle cerebral artery through anastomosis (arrow) even though a greater volume of middle cerebral flow is still derived from the internal carotid artery.

Figure 37-12. Serial comparison of five regional cerebral blood flow studies over a 510 day period using the inhalation ^{133}Xenon method with 32 detectors. Lower detectors have been excluded to eliminate air passage artifact. One standard deviation above and below the hemispheric mean value is plotted for each side. This study shows a bilateral increase in cerebral blood flow after EC-IC bypass (date 1), a bilateral decrease in cerebral blood flow after ligation of the left internal carotid artery (date 2), and ultimately, a bilateral increase in cerebral blood flow, presumed to reflect gradual enlargement of the EC-IC bypass developing during the 510 days of observation.

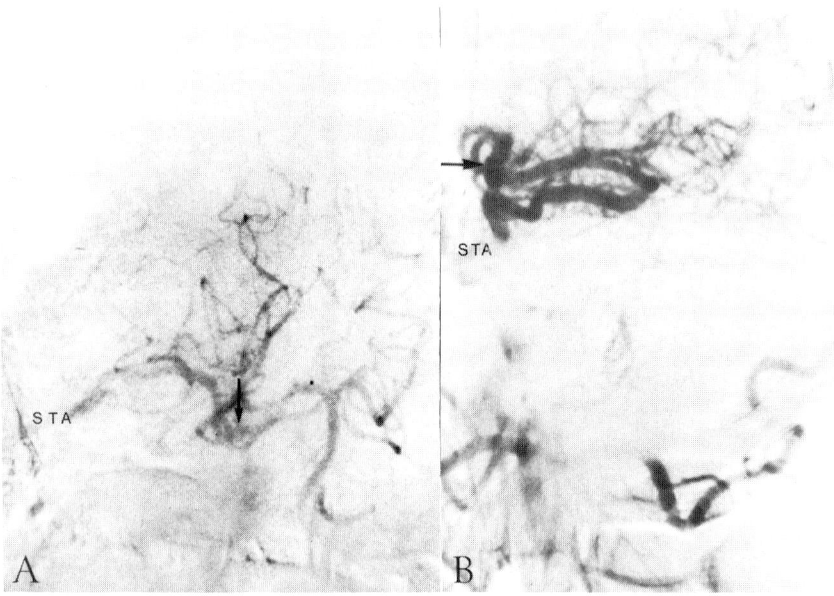

Figure 37-13. Sixty-two-year-old male with basilar artery stenosis. Selective right external carotid arteriogram performed 10 days after anastomosis between the superficial temporal artery (STA) and right posterior cerebral artery.
(A) Frontal projection shows STA coursing below right temporal lobe of brain to anastomosis (arrow) with posterior cerebral artery as it encircles brain stem. Perfusion includes both posterior cerebral arteries, both superior cerebellar arteries, the left anterior inferior cerebellar artery, and the basilar artery, retrograde to the level of stenosis.
(B) Lateral projection shows STA coursing, with a large backward loop, under the right temporal lobe toward anastomosis (arrow) to irrigate posterior cerebral arteries (above level of tentorium) and superior cerebellar arteries (beneath level of tentorium).

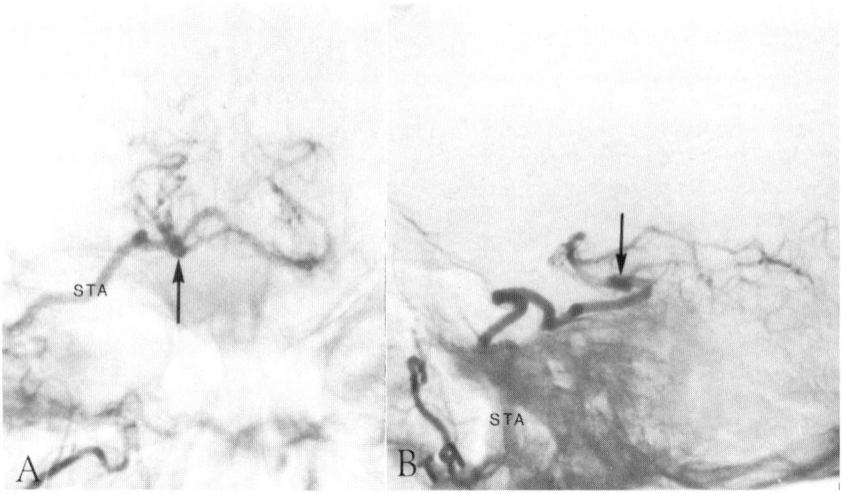

Figure 37-14. Sixty-one-year-old male with occlusion of right vertebral artery, intracranial stenosis of left vertebral artery, and stenosis at the origin of the right posterior cerebral artery. Selective right external carotid arteriogram performed 6 weeks after anastomosis between the superficial temporal artery (STA) and right superior cerebellar artery.
(A) Frontal projection shows STA coursing under right temporal lobe to anastomosis (arrow) with superior cerebellar artery as it encircles brain stem. Perfusion includes both posterior cerebral and both superior cerebellar territories.
(B) Lateral projection shows STA coursing, with a large backward loop, under the right temporal lobe toward anastomosis (arrow) to irrigate posterior cerebral and superior cerebellar arteries.

posterior cerebral or superior cerebellar artery depends upon the size or specific arterial pathology in each specific case, since either serves the upper brain stem equally well. With proper patient selection, this operation offers the prospect of substantially better treatment of patients with upper brain stem occlusive arterial disease.

ACKNOWLEDGEMENTS

The author wishes to express appreciation to Richard M. Raymond, Ph.D., David A. Wilson, Ph.D., Deanna Watson, R.N., and Louise A. Knasko, R.N. for assistance in providing regional cerebral blood flow material.

REFERENCES

1. Reichman OH: Extracranial to intracranial arterial anastomosis, in Youmans JR (ed): Neurological Surgery, ed. 2, chap 44. Philadelphia, W.B. Saunders, 1982, pp. 1584–1618
2. Reichman OH: Estimation of flow through STA by-pass graft, in Fein JM, Reichman OH (eds): Microneurosurgical Anastomoses for Cerebral Ischemia. New York, Springer-Verlag, 1978, pp. 220–240
3. Barnett HJM: Delayed cerebral ischemic episodes distal to occlusion of major cerebral arteries. Neurology 28:769, 1978
4. Tice LD, Chater NL: Microvascular bypass for stroke: Review of 203 patients. Angiology 31:6, 1980
5. Barnett HJM, Peerless SJ, McCormick CW: In answer to the question: "As compared to what?": A progress report on the EC/IC bypass study. Stroke 11:137, 1980
6. Marzewski DJ, Furlan AJ, St Louis P, et al: (Abstract) Intracranial carotid artery stenosis: Long-term prognosis. Stroke 13:113, 1982
7. Countee RW, Vijayanathan T, Hubschmann OR, et al: Carotid ligation for recurrent ischemia due to inaccessible carotid obstruction: Examination of the rationale of this treatment. J Neurosurg 53:491, 1980
8. Diaz FG, Ausman JI, Pearce JE: Ischemic complications after combined internal carotid artery occlusion and extracranial-intracranial anastomosis. Neurosurgery 10:563, 1982
9. Stephens HW Jr: Microvascular anastomosis and carotid artery ligation for fibromuscular hyperplasia and carotid artery aneurysm, in Fein JH, Reichman OH (eds): Microneurosurgical Anastomoses for Cerebral Ischemia. New York, Springer-Verlag, 1978, pp. 307–316
10. Paullus WS, Pait TG, Rhoton AL Jr: Microsurgical exposure of the petrous portion of the carotid artery. J Neurosurg 47:713, 1977
11. Allen GS, Cohen RJ, Preziosi TJ: Microsurgical endarterectomy of the intracranial vertebral artery for vertebrobasilar transient ischemic attacks. Neurosurgery 8:56, 1981
12. Caplan LR: Vertebrobasilar disease: Time for a new strategy. Stroke 12:111, 1981
13. Sundt TM Jr, Piepgras DG: Occipital to posterior inferior cerebellar artery bypass surgery. J Neurosurg 48:916, 1978
14. Roski RA, Spetzler RF, Hopkins LN: Occipital artery to posterior inferior cerebellar artery bypass for vertebrobasilar ischemia. Neurosurgery 10:44, 1982
15. Ausman JI, Diaz FG, Reyes RA, et al: Posterior circulation revascularization: Superficial temporal artery to superior cerebellar artery anastomosis. J Neurosurg 56:766, 1982

Roger M. Greenhalgh Peter Dawson
Richard Wise Terry Jones
Charles Mate-Kole

38

Extracranial/Intracranial Bypass as Viewed by a Vascular Surgeon

Unlike in the United States, in Britain, neurosurgeons have had relatively little interest in this operation. The vascular surgeons realize, however, that it is a procedure that they should have at their disposal. Fortunately, in our center, the vascular surgeon (Roger Greenhalgh) works in harmony with Mr. Robin Hillingworth, the neurosurgeon to the hospital. The arrangement is ideal. The neurosurgeon is aware of and takes great pains to avoid the slightest morbidity associated with a cooperative approach to the vessels on the surface of the brain, and the vascular surgeon is more conversant on a day-to-day basis with the need and indications for surgery on the arteries that supply the brain.

Viewed from the vascular standpoint, the operation is now well established, the technique is straightforward, and the only problem that remains to be solved is if and when this operation is indicated and what it can be expected to achieve. This chapter aims to set out very briefly what we are doing at present and some of our reservations.

During the time that we have performed the last 100 carotid endarterectomies, there has been a need in our center to perform extracranial/intracranial bypass on 24 occasions. This indicates that carotid endarterectomy is deemed to be required at least four times more commonly than extracranial/intracranial bypass in our practice. Our approach to the management of this problem is to treat transient ischemic attacks (TIAs), prolonged residual ischemic neurological deficits (PRINDs), and completed strokes in much the same way. If the patient's symptoms recover within 24 hours, we refer to this as a TIA, if the symptoms persist for more than 24 hours but less than 48 hours, we refer to this as a PRIND. If the signs persist for more than 3 days, we define this as a complete stroke. As soon as the patient comes under our care on day 1, we do not know into which category the patient fits. A consultant neurological opinion is requested at once to confirm the diagnosis of a carotid territory attack or a vertebral basillar territory attack. We next take steps to see if the patient has evidence of atrial fibrillation, polycythaemia or hypertension. For polycythaemia and hypertension, these are controlled and frequently attacks improve as a result. Such patients do not go on to angiography. In patients who have atrial fibrillation, it cannot be assumed that embolization is taking place from the heart, and the current practice is that these patients are sometimes considered for angiography.

At this stage, we perform an arch angiogram with selective carotid and intracranial views. Only this way can we determine the treatment profile for our patients. The patient receives this investigation either for TIA, PRIND, or for completed stroke from which there has been an excellent recovery. In summary, we are concerned about the risk of second more serious attacks and are unable to determine a satisfactory management profile without the arch angiogram. We concede that with the intravenous digital angiography and improving imaging possibilities, it might be possible to reduce the number of arch angiograms in the future.

Patients with a suitable extracranial lesion have this dealt with by surgery in the first instance. If there is minimal disease or if there is evidence of multiple site disease which is not amenable to surgery, then our patients are treated medically with antithrombotic drugs. It is important for the minimal and multiple site categories to be followed separately because a quite different prognosis from these 2 groups may be expected. Having performed any suitable extracranial corrective surgery, we are next concerned with the possibility of extracranial/intracranial bypass. This is performed by connecting the superficial temporal artery to a cortical branch of the middle meningeal artery. It is indicated for inaccesible disease of the intracranial internal carotid artery, for example near the syphon. It is also indicated for a symptomatic occlusion or stenosis of the main middle cerebral artery. The other indication of the bypass is for the occluded internal carotid artery above which there is a symptomatic carotid territory. We always perform CT scan, to see if there is any evidence of infarction of carotid territory, but the presence of an infarction does not rule out reconstructive surgery in our practice. CT scan does exclude neoplasms mimicking strokes and cerebral bleeds.

Of the 24 patients who had EC-IC bypass, 7 presented with TIAs, 2 of these patients having had a mild completed stroke in the past and residual transient ischemic attacks subsequently. Eight of our patients had a mild right-sided completed stroke, and 9 had a mild left-sided completed stroke. In these 17 patients, there was a definite but minimal neurological deficit, and the operation was performed within 1 and 12 months of the attack.

RESULTS OF EXTRACRANIAL/INTRACRANIAL BYPASS IN 24 PATIENTS

No patient died. There was no significant morbidity of the procedure. The patients' wounds all healed well and were hidden by the hair line. It was an excellent cosmetic result. The patients left the hospital approximately 7 days after the operation. All of the anastomoses were assessed at the time of surgery using a directional Doppler probe, and it was possible to show that blood was leaving the superficial temporal artery and passing in 2 directions along a cortical branch of the middle cerebral artery. In many cases, it was possible to see blood flowing through the thin cortical artery wall, and this was highly magnified by the operating microscope. In the postoperative period, the anastomosis was followed with a directional Doppler and in some cases with an arteriogram. All of the anastomoses stayed open and we confirm, as others have done, that the flow through the superficial temporal artery increases significantly during the follow-up period.

Two of our patients had slight but definite minor completed strokes in a follow-up period ranging from 2 months to 5 years. None of our patients have had transient ischemic attacks after this procedure.

Ten of the 17 patients had an apparently better gait, and the patients were more dextrous and according to our assessment by independent physiotherapists, 10 of the 17 were said to have improved. It is difficult to be certain whether this improvement would have occurred in any case as a result of dedicated rehabilitation. In 8 patients, an independent speech therapist claimed that improvement in speech had occurred.

Our impression has been that the operation is relatively easy to perform when a vascular surgeon is skilled in the use of microvascular techniques. The operation is reproducible, and the majority of patients claim that they feel better, but there is considerable doubt in our minds whether the patients really are better. We do not doubt that in many patients there is an increased blood flow to the brain. What we question is whether this increased blood flow to the brain is truly benefitting the patient in some objective way. We have, therefore, performed a psychological evaluation before and after our operations, and we have also performed some newer studies on cerebral blood flow to help answer these questions.

POSITRON EMISSION TOMOGRAPHY (PET)

The consequences of cerebral atherosclerosis on tissue perfusion can be studied objectively by techniques that measure regional cerebral blood flow (rCBF). Invasive methods to determine rCBF have been available since 1963.[1] The principle involves measuring the clearance of a freely diffusible, inert

vascular compartment on signal from tracer in the tissues leads to an overestimation of rOER, and hence $rCMRO_2$. This becomes increasingly significant when the volume of intravascular blood in a region is high (associated with vasodilatation) and the rOER low. Intravascular blood volume (rCBF) can be measured by emission-computed tomography after the patient has inhaled a tracer amount of carbon-11 monoxide (^{11}CO),[9] and this data used to correct values of rOER and $rCMRO_2$. The rCBV scan, by demonstrating areas of focal vasodilatation as areas of high rCBV, also provides important pathophysiological information in its own right.

It should be stressed that the $C^{15}O_2$ scan measures *tissue* perfusion. If there is shunting of blood away from the tissues by, say, an arteriovenous malformation, rCBF as measured by this technique reflects the low flow at capillary level and not the high flow through the larger vessels. This is a particular advantage when attempting to assess the effects of maneuvers designed to improve tissue perfusion, an advantage not shared by arterial flow meters, ultrasound techniques, etc.

Positron emission tomography (PET) and the ^{15}O steady state technique have been applied to several aspects of cerebrovascular disease and preliminary observations have been published, principally about pathophysiological changes after stroke.[10,11,12] Sequential studies early after the onset of stroke (Wise RJS, in preparation) have demonstrated that the change from high rOER to low rOER within the lesion occurs within hours, or at the most days, and is associated with a fall in $rCMRO_2$ (as infarction becomes established), with or without a variable degree of reflow. Over 50 patients with stroke have been studied, and no case of regional chronic ischemia or diminished perfusion reserve, either in the center or at the edge of the lesion, has been observed.

Figure 38-1 demonstrates the marked uncoupling between flow and metabolism that can occur after an acute stroke. Two days after the ictus, there was very low flow throughout the middle cerebral artery (MCA) territory of the right hemisphere. This was associated with a relatively greater depression of $rCMRO_2$ and rOER was also low—the pathophysiological pattern suggestive of established infarction. The same patient was studied again 10 days after the onset of his symptoms. At this time, there had been

---

Figure 38-1. Right hemisphere infarct studied at 2 days (above) and 10 days (below) after the ictus. Both rCBF and $rCMRO_2$ were very low in right middle cerebral artery (MCA) territory at 2 days. rCBF was depressed less relative to $rCMRO_2$ as reflected in the low rOER. The pattern of low rCBF, low $rCMRO_2$ and low rOER are strongly suggestive of established infarction—see text. At 10 days, there had been marked natural reflow in the infarcted region. There was no change in $rCMRO_2$. The rCBV scan at 10 days shows the focal vasodilatation in the infarct associated with the high reflow.

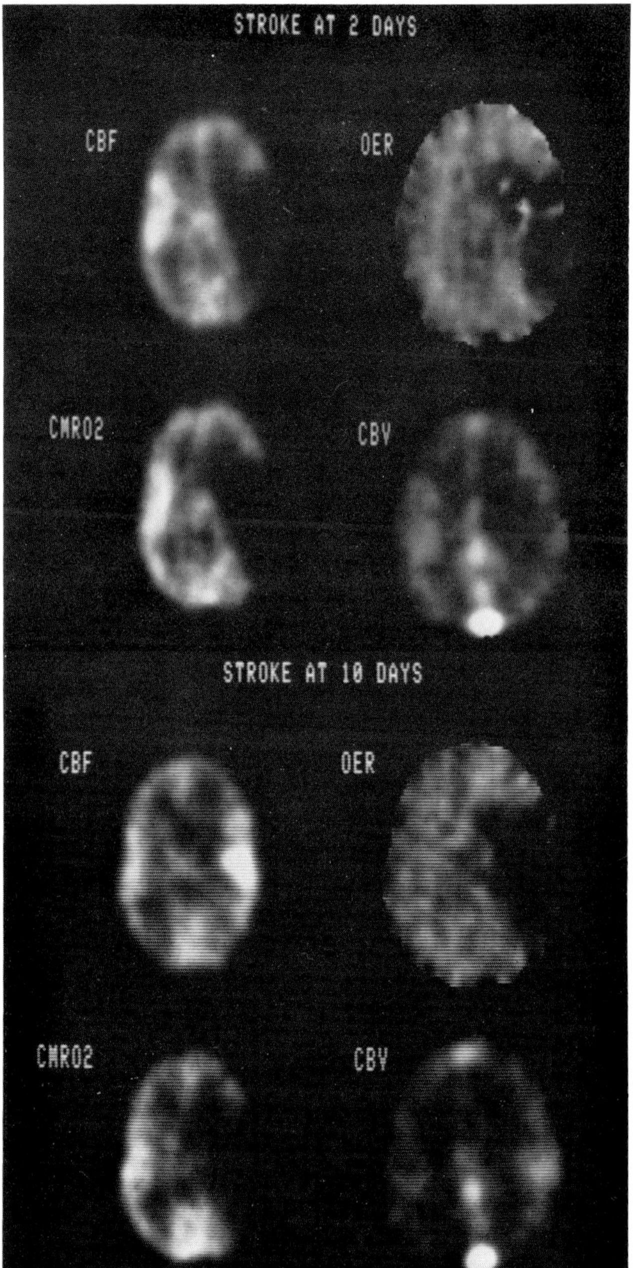
STROKE AT 2 DAYS
CBF
OER
CMRO2
CBV
STROKE AT 10 DAYS
CBF
OER
CMRO2
CBV

marked reflow in right MCA territory, and now rCBF in this region was 50 percent greater than that in left MCA territory. There was a corresponding area of high rCBV in the right hemisphere reflecting the focal vasodilatation. However, $rCMRO_2$ remained unchanged at a very low level. This case demonstrates how poorly rCBF reflects local cerebral function after a stroke.

Results from the studies (which include patients both with and without previous cerebral infarction) are being prepared for publication, but initial analysis has demonstrated that no instances of chronic ischemia were observed, and only rarely was a mild diminution in regional perfusion reserve seen. However, Baron JC et al.[13] have reported 4 patients who showed improvement in rCBF, with reduction of elevated rOER, after EC-IC bypass surgery. It is not reported what proportion these 4 cases made of the total referred for PET studies who were already being considered for vascular surgery on the basis of established criteria.

A demonstration, therefore, of persistent elevation of rOER in association with reduced rCBF would appear to be a good indication for vascular surgery. Present evidence, at least based on our experience, is that these cases are unusual, and only demonstrable by the use of PET scanning. Both transient cerebral ischemic attacks and the early stages of cerebral infarction are characterised by rapidly resolving ischemia, in the former by early return of rCBF and in the latter by tissue death.

Figure 38-2 illustrates typical studies, pre- and post- EC-IC bypass, in a patient with a large left cerebral hemisphere infarct. GB is a 39-year-old man who developed left cerebral hemisphere TIAs in October, 1981. At the end of October, he had a completed stroke with aphasia and right hemiplegia. Angiography demonstrated a total occlusion of the origin of the left internal carotid artery (ICA) and tight stenosis at the origin of the right ICA, with normal vertebral arteries. An x-ray CT scan confirmed the presence of a left posterior frontal nonhemorrhagic infarct. Two months after the stroke, a left EC-IC bypass was performed, followed by a right carotid endarterectomy 1 month later. Gradual improvement in the patient's aphasia and right hemiplegia was apparent preoperatively and appeared to be accelerated by the EC-IC bypass, but not by the right carotid endarterectomy. The images of CBF, OER, and $CMRO_2$ show no obvious change comparing the postoperative study (4 months after the EC-IC bypass) with the preoperative. The quantitative values for CBF, OER, and $CMRO_2$ in regions of the left hemisphere cortex, 4.5 cm above the cantho-meatal line, are shown in Table 38-2.

No recovery of $rCMRO_2$ was seen in the cortex at the edges or the center of the infarct after the EC-IC bypass. The fall in rCBF at the center of the infarct probably reflects partial recoupling of flow to an area of reduced metabolism in an old infarct.[11] The vascular surgery clearly did not increase tissue perfusion but if it had, this would have only resulted in the lowering of the already normal (edges of infarct) or low (center of infarct) rOER. Analysis

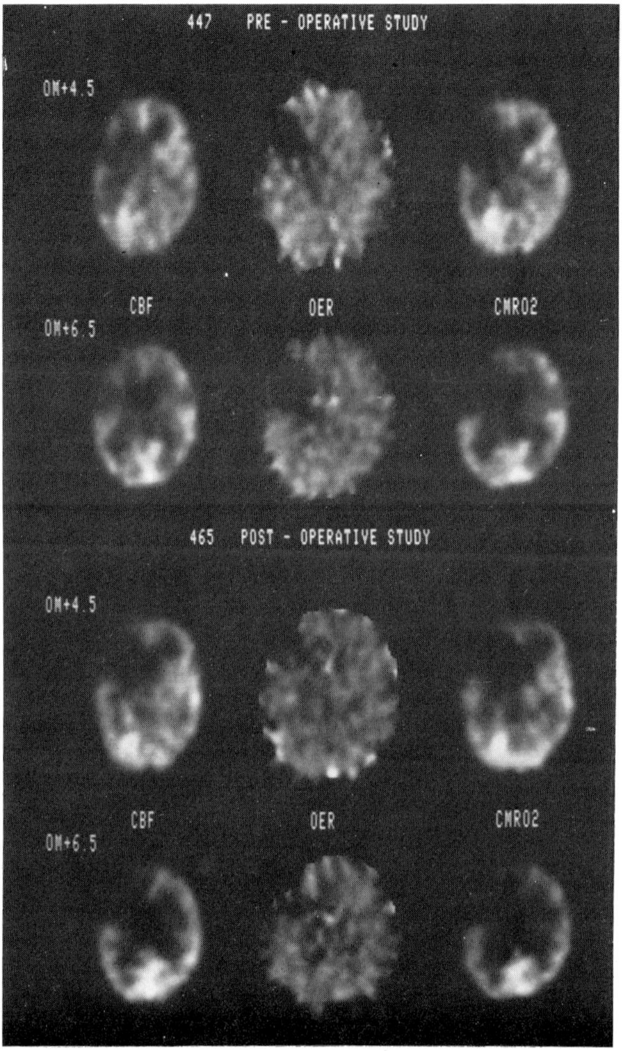

Figure 38-2. CBG, OER, and $CMRO_2$ images at 2 levels (4.5 cm and 6.5 cm above the OM line) in a patient with an established left hemisphere infarct before (above) and after (below) a left superficial temporal-middle cerebral artery anastomosis.

of cortex at 6.5 cm above the cantho-meatal line and subcortical grey and white matter similarly demonstrated no change in tissue perfusion or oxidative metabolism.

The resolution of the scanner does not allow complete separation of grey and white matter when defining the cortex. Therefore, the "cortical" values quoted in Table 38-2 include a proportion of white matter. This partial

Table 38-2

Region of Cortex	CBF (ml/100ml/min) Pre-op	Post-op	OER Pre-op	Post-op	$CMRO_2$ (ml/100ml/min) Pre-op	Post-op
Ant. Frontal	22.8	17.7	0.45	0.46	1.97	1.50
Post. Frontal	18.9	9.0	0.18	0.27	0.59	0.51
Ant. Temporal	29.0	33.5	0.48	0.46	2.70	2.90
Post. Temporal	30.5	35.6	0.51	0.48	2.98	3.25

volume effect is obviated by taking similar regions when comparing one study with another.

This illustrative case highlights the strengths and limitations of the technique. Objective comparison of oxidative metabolism pre- and postoperatively, coupled with the demonstration of absence of ischemia or diminished perfusion reserve preoperatively, are readily apparent from the quantitative data presented. There was some clinical improvement, however, in the patient's dysphasia and right hemiplegia between the two studies. This may reflect the plasticity of the brain, unaffected areas taking over functions normally occurring in infarcted regions, or the metabolic and functional recovery of regions of brain below the resolution of the PET scanner (this would be true, say, for the internal capsule).

Although PET studies on this patient demonstrated that vascular surgery perhaps was not helpful in relieving a critically low rCBF, associated with a high rOER, they could not provide evidence for or against the other indication for such surgery—to prevent further infarction if and when the right ICA stenosis progressed. The "prophylactic" rather than "curative" aspect of cerebral vascular surgery can only be investigated by controlled clinical trials.

It is becoming apparent, therefore, that PET has a useful role to play in studying at least some of the indications for, and the immediate impact of, the surgical treatment of cerebral atherosclerosis. Future studies done during induced, carefully monitored, mild hypotension, ethically justifiable only if capable of providing useful diagnostic information safely, may provide more insight, especially in patients considered to be suffering from TIAs induced by hypotensive episodes, or in those at risk who are about to experience hypotension during anesthesia and surgery.

PSYCHOLOGICAL EVALUATION

Psychological assessment should be part of a process of treatment and rehabilitation of any cerebrovascular disorder. It is not, in McFie's terms,[14] a single episode or "hit and run" with the patient. The need for psychological evaluation is to assess the existence of specific disabilities and dysfunction of corresponding areas of the brain. Neuropsychological tests attempt to measure at least aspects of language functioning, learning and memory, perceptual abilities, praxis, motor coordination and speed, and emotional behavior.

To many psychologists, microrevascularization is a new area and, therefore, only a handful of studies has been done. Evans and Austin[15] evaluated 11 males and 3 females undergoing the microrevascularization technique. Psychological measures used were to evaluate memory functioning, learning ability, perceptual and conceptual abilities, visual-motor coordination and speed. Their results suggested that 7 patients showed definite overall improvement.

Nine cases were reported earlier[16] in which the assessment was made of aspects of intelligence, verbal fluency, visual perception, and memory for verbal and visual material. It was found that left-sided surgery produced improvement on verbal tasks while right-sided surgery produced improvement on visuo-spatial tasks.

We have data for 15 patients who had EC-IC bypass. All 15 were assessed before surgery and 12 months after surgery. Tests used were of intelligence (Wechsler Adult Intelligence Scale), memory (Faces Recall Test and Words Recall Test), and object recognition test.

The results suggested that of the 15 patients, 5 showed definite improvement on these tests: (1) *Block Design,* which is a measure of visual constructive ability; (2) *Unusual Views,* which indicates an impairment of visual recognition; (3) *Arithmetic,* which measures calculation deficit; and (4) *Digit Span,* which provides a measure of the patient's immediate memory span (short-term memory). The results also suggested that certain factors might be crucial in predicting outcome of surgery. The two most important factors were side of surgery and the effects of having been a smoker. The results showed a trend that left-sided surgery produced more improvement than right-sided surgery. Nonsmokers performed better than smokers on most of the tests. Cigarette smoking may impair arterial blood supply to the brain and thus cause a functional deficiency that may show up on psychometric testing.[17]

Detailed results of our findings are not available because the study is still in progress and at this stage it is only possible to talk about trends.

CONCLUSION

Extracranial/intracranial bypass is now a well-established operative procedure. There is little doubt that it increases blood flow to the brain, and the patency figures are excellent. The morbidity of the procedure is minimal and subjectively, many patients appear to benefit. The psychological testing suggests that some patients are doing well, but the final results of this are awaited. The results of positron emission tomography give little comfort that EC-IC bypass or any form of cerebral revascularisation has much place in attempting to produce improvement in cerebral-functional deficit. As this does not in any way decry the procedure as a potential preventative measure, this potential value of the procedure will only be known as a result of further clinical trials.

REFERENCES

1. Lassen NA, Hoedt-Rasmussen K, Sorensen SC, et al: Regional cerebral blood flow in man determined by Krypton-85. Neurology 13:719, 1963
2. Stokely EM, Sveinsdottir E, Lassen NA, et al: A single photon dynamic computer assisted tomograph (DCAT) for imaging brain function in multiple cross sections. J Comput Assist Tomogr 4:230, 1980
3. Siesjö BK: Brain Energy Metabolism. New York, John Wiley & Sons, 1978
4. Siesjö BK: Cell damage in the brain: A speculative synthesis. J Cerebr Blood Flow Metabol 1:155, 1981
5. Phelps ME, Hoffman EJ, Huang SC, et al: ECAT: A new computerized tomographic imaging system for positron-emitting radiopharmaceuticals. J Nucl Med 19:635, 1978
6. Frackowiak RSJ, Lenzi GL, Jones T et al: Quantitative measurement of regional cerebral blood flow and oxygen metabolism in man using ^{15}O and positron emission tomography: Theory, procedure, and normal values. J Compt Assist Tomogr 4:727, 1980
7. Lammertsma AA, Jones T, Frackowiak RSJ, et al: A theoretical study of the steady-state model for measuring regional cerebral blood flow and oxygen utilisation using oxygen-15. J Comput Assist Tomogr 5:544, 1981
8. Lammertsma AA, Heather JD, Jones T, et al: A statistical study of the steady state technique for measuring regional cerebral blood flow and oxygen utilization using ^{15}O. J Comput Assist Tomogr In press, 1982
9. Phelps ME, Huang SC, Hoffman EJ, et al: Validation of tomographic measurement of cerebral blood volume with C-11 labelled carboxyhemoglobin. J Nucl Med 20:328, 1979
10. Ackerman RH, Correia JA, Alpert NM, et al: Positron imaging in ischemic stroke disease using compounds labelled with oxygen 15. Arch Neurol 38:537, 1981
11. Baron JC, Bousser MG, Comar D, et al: Noninvasive tomographic study of cerebral blood flow and oxygen metabolism in vivo: Potentials, limitations and clinical applications in cerebral ischemic disorders. Eur Neurol 20:273, 1981
12. Lenzi GL, Frackowiak RSJ, Jones T: Cerebral oxygen metabolism and blood flow in human cerebral ischemic infarction. J Cerebr Blood Flow Metabol In press
13. Baron JC, Rey A, Guillard S, et al: Non-invasive tomographic imaging of cerebral blood flow and oxygen extraction fraction in superficial temporal artery to middle cerebral artery anastomosis. Proc. 10th Salzburg Conf. Cerebral Vascular Diseases Amsterdam, Excerpta Medica, 1980
14. McFie J: Assessment of organic intellectual impairment. London, Academic Press, 1975
15. Evans RB, Austin G: Psychological evaluation of patients undergoing microneurosurgical anastomoses for cerebral ischaemia, in Austin GM (ed): Anastomoses for Cerebral Ischaemia. Springfield, Ill, C. Thomas, 1976
16. Greenhalgh R, Illingworth R, McFie J, et al: Extracranial to intracranial micro-revascularisation for the treatment of completed stroke. Br Med J 262:18, 1979
17. Weeks D: Do chronic cigarette smokers forget people's names? British Medical Journal 1627, 1979

INDEX

b
3 c
4 d
5 e
6 f
7 g
8 h
9 i
8 0 j